ALGINATES

Versatile Polymers in
Biomedical Applications and Therapeutics

Pharmaceutical Powder Compaction Technology

DRUGS AND THE PHARMACEUTICAL SCIENCES

A Series of Textbooks and Monographs

edited by

James Swarbrick

AAI, Inc.
Wilmington, North Carolina

ALGINATES

Versatile Polymers in
Biomedical Applications and Therapeutics

Edited by
Md Saquib Hasnain, PhD
Amit Kumar Nayak, PhD

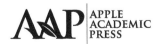

APPLE
ACADEMIC
PRESS

Apple Academic Press Inc.	Apple Academic Press Inc.
3333 Mistwell Crescent	1265 Goldenrod Circle NE
Oakville, ON L6L 0A2	Palm Bay, Florida 32905
Canada USA	USA

First issued in paperback 2021

Library and Archives Canada Cataloguing in Publication

Title: Alginates : versatile polymers in biomedical applications and therapeutics / edited by Md Saquib Hasnain, PhD, Amit Kumar Nayak, PhD.

Other titles: Alginates (Oakville, Ont.)

Names: Hasnain, Md Saquib, 1984- editor. | Nayak, Amit Kumar, 1979- editor.

Description: Includes bibliographical references and index.

Identifiers: Canadiana (print) 20190062118 | Canadiana (ebook) 20190062215 | ISBN 9781771887823 (hardcover) | ISBN 9780429023439 (PDF)

Subjects: LCSH: Polymers in medicine. | LCSH: Alginates. | LCSH: Biopolymers. | LCSH: Biomedical engineering

Classification: LCC R857.P6 A44 2019 | DDC 610.28/4—dc23

CIP data on file with US Library of Congress

Apple Academic Press also publishes its books in a variety of electronic formats. Some content that appears in print may not be available in electronic format. For information about Apple Academic Press products, visit our website at **www.appleacademicpress.com** and the CRC Press website at **www.crcpress.com**

ABOUT THE EDITORS

Md Saquib Hasnain, PhD

Md Saquib Hasnain, PhD, has over six years of research experience in the field of drug delivery and pharmaceutical formulation analyses, especially systematic development and characterization of diverse nanostructured drug delivery systems, controlled release drug delivery systems, bioenhanced drug delivery systems, nanomaterials and nanocomposites employing Quality by Design approaches as well as development and characterization of polymeric composites, and many more. To date, he has authored over 30 publications in various high impact peer-reviewed journals and 30 book chapters, and he has one Indian patent application to his credit. He is also serving as a reviewer of several prestigious journals. Overall, he has earned a highly impressive publishing and cited record in Google Scholar (H-Index: 12). He has also participated and presented his research work at over 10 conferences in India and abroad. He is also a member of scientific societies, including the Royal Society of Chemistry, Great Britain; International Association of Environmental and Analytical Chemistry, Switzerland; and Swiss Chemical Society, Switzerland.

Amit Kumar Nayak, PhD

Dr. Amit Kumar Nayak is currently working as Associate Professor at Seemanta Institute of Pharmaceutical Sciences, Odisha, India. He has earned his PhD in Pharmacy from IFTM University, Moradabad, India. He has over 10 years of research experience in the field of Pharmaceutics, Drug Delivery, Biomaterials especially in the development and characterization of polymeric composites, hydrogels, novel and nanostructured drug delivery systems. Till date, he has authored over 120 publications in various high impact peer-reviewed journals and 34 book chapters to his credit. Overall, he has earned highly impressive publishing and cited record in Google Scholar (H-Index: 31, i10-Index: 75). He has been the permanent reviewer of many international journals of high repute. He also has participated and presented his research work at several conferences in India and is a life member of Association of Pharmaceutical Teachers of India (APTI).

CONTENTS

CONTRIBUTORS

Mostafa M. Abd Al Aziz
Center for Materials Science, University of Science and Technology (UST), Giza, Egypt

Esraa A. Abdelsalam
Center for Materials Science, University of Science and Technology (UST), Giza, Egypt

Giovanni Amato
Department of Drug Science, University of Catania, Viale A. Doria, Catania, Italy

Younes Ahmadi
Department of Chemistry, Jamia Millia Islamia, New Delhi, India

Kholoud Arafa
Center for Aging and Associated Disease (CAAD), Giza, Egypt

Indranil Banerjee
Department of Biotechnology and Medical Engineering, National Institute of Technology, Rourkela, Odisha, India

Karina Bierbrauer
Centro de Excelencia en Productos y Procesos de Córdoba, Gobierno de la Provincia de Córdoba, Pabellón CEPROCOR, Córdoba, Argentina

Stefan Boskovic
Department of Chemical Engineering, University of Belgrade, Belgrade, Serbia

Branko Bugarski
Department of Chemical Engineering, University of Belgrade, Belgrade, Serbia

Claudia Carbone
Department of Pharmacy, University of Salerno, Fisciano, Italy

S. Viji Chandran
Department of Biotechnology, School of Bioengineering, SRM University, Kattankulathur, Tamil Nadu, India

Mario Contín
Universidad de Buenos Aires, Buenos Aires, Argentina

Isra Dmour
Faculty of Pharmacy, Al-Ahliyya Amman University, Amman, Jordan

Norma Beatriz D'Accorso
Universidad de Buenos Aires, Buenos Aires, Argentina

Sunil Kumar Dubey
Department of Pharmacy, Birla Institute of Technology & Science (BITS), Pilani, Rajasthan, India

Ibrahim M. El-Sherbiny
Center for Materials Science, University of Science and Technology (UST), Giza, Egypt

Nancy L. Garcia
Universidad de Buenos Aires, Buenos Aires, Argentina

Md Saquib Hasnain
Department of Pharmacy, Shri Venkateshwara University, Gajraula, Uttar Pradesh, India

Ankit Jain
Institute of Pharmaceutical Research, GLA University, Mathura, Uttar Pradesh, India

Sanjay K. Jain
Department of Pharmaceutical Sciences, Dr. Hari Singh Gour Vishwavidyalaya, Sagar,
Madhya Pradesh, India

Sougata Jana
Department of Pharmaceutics, Gupta College of Technological Sciences, Asansol, West Bengal, India

K. S. Joshy
International and Inter University Centre for Nanoscience and Nanotechnology,
Mahatma Gandhi University, Kottayam, Kerala, India

Doman Kim
Department of International Agricultural Technology, Institute of Green BioScience and Technology,
Seoul National University, Gwangwon-do, Republic of Korea

Kowthavarapu V. Krishna
Department of Pharmacy, Birla Institute of Technology & Science (BITS), Pilani, Rajasthan, India

Rapalli Vamshi Krishna
Department of Pharmacy, Birla Institute of Technology & Science (BITS), Pilani, Rajasthan, India

Deepak Kumar
Department of Applied Chemistry, Babasaheb Bhimrao Ambedkar University (Central University),
Lucknow, UP, India

Pramendra Kumar
Department of Applied Chemistry, M J P Rohilkhand University, Bareilly, Uttar Pradesh, India

Maria Rosaria Lauro
Department of Pharmacy, University of Salerno, Fisciano, Italy

Sabyasachi Maiti
Department of Pharmacy, Indira Gandhi National Tribal University, Amarkantak, Madhya Pradesh, India

Verónica Elena Manzano
Universidad de Buenos Aires, Buenos Aires, Argentina

Milan Milivojevic
Department of Chemical Engineering, University of Belgrade, Belgrade, Serbia

Sitansu Sekhar Nanda
Department of Chemistry, Myongji University, Yongin, South Korea

Amit Kumar Nayak
Department of Pharmaceutics, Seemanta Institute of Pharmaceutical Sciences, Ghiajodi, Odisha, India

Suraj Kumar Nayak
Department of Biotechnology and Medical Engineering, National Institute of Technology, Rourkela,
Odisha, India

María Natalia Pacho
Universidad de Buenos Aires, Buenos Aires, Argentina

Ivana Pajic-Lijakovic
Department of Chemical Engineering, University of Belgrade, Belgrade, Serbia

Kunal Pal
Department of Biotechnology and Medical Engineering, National Institute of Technology, Rourkela, Odisha, India

Pritish Panda
Department of Pharmaceutical Sciences, Dr. Hari Singh Gour Vishwavidyalaya, Sagar, Madhya Pradesh, India

Giovanni Puglisi
Department of Drug Science, University of Catania, Viale A. Doria, Catania, Italy

Dilshad Qureshi
Department of Biotechnology and Medical Engineering, National Institute of Technology, Rourkela, Odisha, India

Carlos A. Rodriguez Ramirez
Universidad de Buenos Aires, Buenos Aires, Argentina

V. Sanjay
Department of Biotechnology, School of Bioengineering, SRM University, Kattankulathur, Tamil Nadu, India

Francesca Sansone
Department of Pharmacy, University of Salerno, Fisciano, Italy

Preetam Sarkar
Department of Food Process Engineering, National Institute of Technology, Rourkela, Odisha, India

Snigdha S.
School of Chemical Sciences, Mahatma Gandhi University, Kottayam, Kerala, India

N. Selvamurugan
Department of Biotechnology, School of Bioengineering, SRM University, Kattankulathur, Tamil Nadu, India

Kalyan Kumar Sen
Department of Pharmaceutics, Gupta College of Technological Sciences, Asansol, West Bengal, India

Ravi Sheshala
Faculty of Pharmacy, Universiti Teknologi MARA Selangor, Puncak Alam Campus, Puncak Alam, Malaysia

Angela Singh
Department of Chemistry, University of Allahabad, Allahabad, Uttar Pradesh, India

Vandana Singh
Department of Chemistry, University of Allahabad, Allahabad, Uttar Pradesh, India

Gautam Singhvi
Department of Pharmacy, Birla Institute of Technology & Science (BITS), Pilani, Rajasthan, India

Miriam Strumia
Universidad Nacional de Córdoba, Departamento de Química Orgánica, Córdoba, Argentina

Seemadri Subhadarshini
Department of Biotechnology and Medical Engineering, National Institute of Technology, Rourkela, Odisha, India

Mutasem Taha
Department of Pharmaceutical Sciences, University of Jordan, Amman, Jordan

Joana Elisa Tasqué
Universidad de Buenos Aires, Buenos Aires, Argentina

Sabu Thomas
School of Chemical Sciences, Mahatma Gandhi University, Kottayam, Kerala, India

Ankita Tiwari
Department of Pharmaceutical Sciences, Dr. Hari Singh Gour Vishwavidyalaya, Sagar, Madhya Pradesh, India

Gabriela Valladares
Universidad Nacional de Tucumán, Departamento de Sanidad Vegetal, Tucumán, Argentina

Amit Verma
Department of Pharmaceutical Sciences, Dr. Hari Singh Gour Vishwavidyalaya, Sagar, Madhya Pradesh, India

Tin Wui Wong
Faculty of Pharmacy, Universiti Teknologi MARA Selangor, Puncak Alam Campus, Puncak Alam, Malaysia

Mithilesh Yadav
Department of Chemistry, Jamia Millia Islamia, New Delhi, India

Dong Kee Yi
Department of Chemistry, Myongji University, Yongin, South Korea

ABBREVIATIONS

βCD	beta-cyclodextrin
3D	three-dimensional
3D	tridimensional
5-ASA	5-aminosalycilic acid
5-FU	5-fluorouracil
AA	acrylic acid
AA	alginic acids
AAD	adipic acid dihydrazide
AAm	acrylamide
ABZ	albendazole
AC	aceclofenac
ACNs	anthocyanins
ADP	adenosine diphosphate
AgNPs	silver nanoparticles
ALG	alginate
ALG-PEGM	ALG–polyethylene glycol (PEG)–maleimide
ALP	alkaline phosphatase
APS	ammonium peroxydisulfate
ASP-ALG	styryl-pyridine-modified ALG
AZT	zidovudine
BG	bioactive glass/bioglass
BMP	bone morphogenetic protein
BMPs	biopolymeric microparticles
BMSCs	bone marrow stromal cells
BNPs	biopolymeric nanoparticles
BSA	bovine serum albumin
BTE	bone tissue engineering
BVZ	bevacizumab
CaP	calcium phosphate
CA	calcium alginate
CAN	ceric ammonium nitrate
CDDS	colon-specific drug delivery system
CDDS	controlled release drug delivery system
CF	cystic fibrosis

CMC	carboxymethyl cellulose
CN	cellulose nanocrystals
CNT	carbon nanotube
COL1A1	collagen 1 A
COL	collagen
CPC	calcium phosphate cement
CQD	carbon quantum dot
CS	chitosan
CS	chondroitin sulfate
CTG	carboxymethyl tamarind gum
CUR	curcumin
DCS	diclofenac sodium
DDS	drug delivery system
DLS	dynamic light scattering
DM	diabetes mellitus
DNA	deoxyribonucleic acid
DN	double network
DNR	daunorubicin
DOX	Doxorubicin
DP	degree of polymerization
DS	degree of substitution
DS	diclofenac sodium
ECM	extracellular matrix
ED	Entner Doudoroff
EDTA	ethylenediaminetetraacetic acid
EDX	energy dispersive X-ray
EE%	entrapment efficiency
EE%	encapsulation efficiency
EMF	external magnetic field
EPR	enhanced permeation and retention
EXE	exemestane
FA	folic acid
FDM	fused deposition modeling
FESEM	field emission scanning electron microscopy
FGF	fibroblast growth factors
FG	fibrinogen
FITC-BSA	Fluorescein isothiocyanate-labeled bovine serum albumin
FP-ALG	folate-phytosterol-ALG
FTIR	Fourier transform infrared
GA	gallic acid

GA	glutaraldehyde
GA	glycyrrhetinic acid
GAGs	glycosaminoglycans
GDL	glucono-delta-lactone
GDP	guanosine diphosphate
GE	ginger extract
GEL	gelatin
GFP	green fluorescent protein
GFs	growth factors
GG	guar gum
GGS-ALG	guar gum succinate–ALG
GI	gastrointestinal
GIT	gastrointestinal tract
GLSs	*Ganoderma lucidum* spores
GMA	glacidyl methacrylate
GMSCs	gingival mesenchymal stem cells
GO	graphene oxide
GR-HAP	glass-reinforced hydroxyapatite
HACC	hydroxypropyl trimethyl ammonium chloride chitosan
HA	hyaluronic acid
HA	hydroxyapatite
HAL	halloysite
HAP	hydroxyapatite
HCS	hydroxyl ethylacryl CS
HN	heparin
HNT	halloysite nanotube
HPMC	hydroxyl propyl methyl cellulose
IBSs	injectable bone substitutes
IBU	Ibuprofen
IDMC	indomethacin
INS	insulin
IPNs	interpenetrating polymer networks
LBG	locust bean gum
LbL	layer-by-layer
LCST	lower critical solution temperature
LG	Lakshadi Guggul
LPSA	lipopolysaccharide-amine
MDA	malondialdehyde
MFM	metformin HCl
MHC	metformin hydrochloride

MLV	multilamellar lipid vesicles
MMP	mitochondrial membrane potential
mMSC	mouse mesenchymal stem cells
MMT	montmorillonite
MNPs	magnetite particles
mPEG-g-CMCS	methoxypolyethylene glycol-grafted carboxymethyl CS
MPS	mononuclear phagocyte system
MSC	mesenchymal stem cell
MSN	mesoporous silica nanoparticles
MT	montmorillonite
MW	molecular weight
NaALG/PAVA	sodium alginate and poly(acrylamide-co-N-vinylcapro-lactam-co-acrylamidoglycolic acid)
NaALG-g-MMA	sodium alginate-g-methylmethacrylate
NCC	nanocrystalline cellulose
NFM	nanofiltration membranes
NGs	nanogels
NHS	N-hydroxysulfosuccinimide
NIC	nicotinamide
NiPAAM	N-isopropylacrylamide
NP	nanoparticle
NVCL	N-vinylcaprolactam
o/w	oil-in-water
OCN	osteocalcin
OCP	octa calcium phosphate
OLZ	olanzapine
OPN	osteopontin
OSA	sodium alginate oxidized
OSP	oyster shell powder
PC	pectin
PCL	poly(ε-caprolactone)
PCL	polycaprolacton
PDI	polydispersity index
PDLSCs	periodontal ligament stem cells
PEC	polyelectrolyte complex
PEG	polyethylene glycol
PEI	polyethyleneimine
PE	polyelectrolyte
PES	polyester
PGA	propylene glycol alginate

PGDF-BB	platelet-derived growth factor-BB
PG	polyglutamic acid
PLGA	poly(lactic-co-glycolic acid)
PL	polysaccharides
PLLA	poly-L-lactic acid
PLO	poly-L-ornithine
PNIPAM	poly(N-isopropylacrylamide)
PP	Peyer's patches
PPy-ALG	polypyrrole–ALG
PU	polyurethane
PVA	polyvinyl alcohol
pVEGF	plasmid encoding vascular endothelial growth factor DNA
RGD	arginine–glycine–aspartate
SA-PEG	stearic acid–polyethylene glycol
SA	sodium alginate
SBF	simulated body fluid
SCF	simulated colonic fluid
SD	spray-drying
SDDS	smart (stimuli-sensitive) drug delivery systems
SE-Cur	self-emulsifying curcumin
SEM	scanning electron microscopy
SFF	solid free-form fabrication
SF	silk fibroin
SGF	simulated gastric fluid
SIF	simulated intestinal fluid
SiRNA	small interfering
SIS	small intestinal submucosa
SLS	selective laser sintering
SME-Cur	self-micro-emulsifying curcumin
SMEDDS	self-microemulsifying drug delivery systems
SPI	soy protein isolated
SPP	solution plasma process
Sulfo-NHS	N-hydroxysulfosuccinimide
TCP	tricalcium phosphate
TEM	transmission electron microscope
TE	tissue engineering
TGF	transforming growth factor
TGF-β	transforming growth factor β
TIPS	thermally induced phase separation
TMX	tamoxifen

TNBS	trinitrobenzensulfonic acid
TNF	tumor necrosis factor
TNFR	tumor necrosis factor receptor
TPC	total polyphenol content
TPH	theophylline
TPP	tripolyphosphate
UV	ultraviolet
VEGF	vessel growth factor
VEGF	vascular endothelial growth factor
VF	venlafaxine
w/o	water-in-oil
w/w	water-in-water
WGA	wheat germ agglutinin
XRD	X-ray diffraction
ZnO	zinc oxide

PREFACE

Currently, the uses of biodegradable and biocompatible polymers extracted from natural origin are gradually increasing in various biomedical applications and in therapeutics. Among various natural biopolymers, alginates are the anionic polysaccharide group extracted in huge quantity from brown marine algae. These are biosynthesized from the bacterial strains. In nature, alginates exist as alginic acid salts of various metal cations found in the seawater, such as Na^+, Sr^{2+}, Mg^{2+}, and so forth. Sodium alginate, the sodium salt of alginic acid, is most extensively exploited to develop alginate-based systems for use in various biomedical, pharmaceutical, and cosmeceutical applications because of the nontoxicity, biodegradability, economic production expenses, and gel-forming ability in the aqueous milieu. Moreover, the abundance of hydroxyl groups and carboxyl groups in the molecular structure of alginates enable easy modifications. The improvements of the polymer characteristics of alginates through physical as well as chemical modifications may widen the scope of applications. Biomedical applications of alginates mainly include drug delivery and targeting, cell and enzyme encapsulations, growth factor delivery, protein and peptide delivery, delivery of herbal therapeutic agents and nutraceuticals, tissue regenerations, wound healing, and so forth.

This volume, *Alginates: Versatile Polymers in Biomedical Applications and Therapeutics,* contains 20 chapters that present current topics of interest and the latest research updates on the use of alginates as biopolymers in various medical applications and therapeutics. The topics of the chapters of this book include but are not limited to: Alginates: source, chemistry and properties; Recent advances of alginates as material for biomedical applications; Alginates: hydrogels, their chemistry, and applications; Alginate-based hydrogels: synthesis, characterization, and biomedical applications; Chemically modified alginates for advanced biomedical applications; Bionanocomposites of alginates, their chemistry and applications; Alginate and its applications in tissue engineering; Alginate-based scaffolds in bone tissue engineering applications; Alginate properties, pharmaceutical, and tissue engineering applications; Alginate: drug delivery and application; Chemical and physical modifications of alginate to improve its use as carriers in delivery systems; Updates on alginate-based interpenetrating polymer networks for sustained drug release; Alginate nanoparticles; Alginate-based nanocarriers in modern therapeutics; Alginate-based composites in drug delivery application; Hydroxyapatite–alginate composites in drug delivery; Alginate-based gastrointestinal tract drug delivery systems; Alginate hydrogels as colon-targeted drug delivery system; Alginate carriers for treatment of ocular diseases; Alginate carriers for bioactive substances: herbal natural compounds and nucleic acid materials.

This book particularly discusses the aforementioned topics along with emphasis on recent advances in the fields by experts across the world.

We would like to thank all the authors of the chapters for providing timely and excellent contributions. We also thank the publisher, Apple Academic Press, and Sandra Sickels for the invaluable help in the organization of the editing process. We gratefully acknowledge the permissions to reproduce copyright materials from a number of sources. Finally, we would like to thank our parents, other family members, all respected teachers, friends, colleagues, and dear students for their continuous encouragement, inspiration, and moral support during the preparation of the book. Together with our contributing authors and the publisher, we will be extremely pleased if our efforts fulfill the needs of academicians, researchers, polymer engineers, and pharmaceutical formulators.

—**Md Saquib Hasnain**
Shri Venkateshwara University, India

—**Amit Kumar Nayak**
Seemanta Institute of Pharmaceutical Sciences, India

CHAPTER 1

ALGINATES: SOURCE, CHEMISTRY, AND PROPERTIES

MITHILESH YADAV* and YOUNES AHMADI

Materials Research Laboratory, Department of Chemistry, Jamia Millia Islamia, New Delhi 110025, India

Corresponding author. E-mail: mithileshau99@yahoo.co.in

1.1 INTRODUCTION

Alginates (ALGs) are cell wall constituent of brown algae and have become very important biomaterial since its discovery in the late 19th century which is produced commercially from the coastal region by brown seaweeds harvesting. It is a naturally anionic biopolymer. The biocompatibility, low production cost, low toxicity, and gelation property in presence of divalent cations like Ca^{2+} enabled alginate to be suitable for numerous applications in the field of biotechnology, biomedical applications, medicine, beverage, and food industry (Gombotz and Wee, 1998). In addition to these properties, alginate has other unique properties, which enables it to be utilized as a matrix for delivery or entrapment of various biomolecules like cells and proteins (Williams, 2009). These properties are (i) encapsulation at room temperature without using organic solvent (Andersen et al. 2012); (ii) presence of an inert aqueous environment inside the matrix (Huebsch and Mooney, 2009; Ratner and Bryant, 2004); (iii) biodegradability in normal physiological condition (Suzuki et al. 1998); (iv) formation of highly porous gel which results in high diffusion of biomaterials and macromolecules (Peters et al, 2002); and (v) easy control of porosity by simple coating procedure (Liu et al, 2006). This chapter first describes the source of alginate, chemistry, and the properties of alginate are then discussed in details.

1.2   ALGINATE SOURCE

There are mainly two sources for the synthesis of alginate which are algal and bacterial sources based on the microorganisms used for the preparation of alginate (Smidsrod and Skjak-Bræk, 1990). The polysaccharide-based alginate was isolated from marine macroalgae for the first time in last century, but after 80 years a bacterial source (*Pseudomonas aeruginosa*) of the polysaccharide was identified from the mucoid strain of the *P. aeruginosa*, which is an alginate producer strain (Linker and Jones, 1966).

1.2.1   BACTERIAL SOURCE

There are mainly two kinds of bacteria which have been proven to secrete alginate, which are *Pseudomonas* and *Azotobacter*. Maximum research about the mechanisms of biosynthesis of bacterial alginate at the molecular level has been performed on the pathogenic bacteria, that is, *P. aeruginosa* or *Azotobacter vinelandii*, which is a soil-dwelling bacteria. Although these two types of bacteria make use of highly comparable molecular mechanisms for the biosynthesis of alginate, but they produce alginate which has different material properties and are used for different purposes. Some strains of *P. aeruginosa* which is called as mucoid strains produce high amounts of alginate to utilize it in the production of biofilms that is thick and highly structured (Nivens et al., 2001; Hay et al., 2009), while *Azotobacter* secrets a harder alginate that is because of the presence of higher concentrations of guluronate (G) residues in alginate structure which remains closely linked with the cell and permits the development of desiccation resistant cysts (Sabra and Zeng 2009). Mucoid *P. aeruginosa* which is alginate-producing strains was isolated from other cohorts of patients, for example, bronchiectasis and also from those patients who had middle ear or urinary tract and other cohorts of the infected patient but less frequently. ALG is also synthesized from a bacterial source named *A. vinelandii* in encystment process (encystment is a process that helps bacteria to survive under adverse environment). Another strain of *Azotobacter* called *Azotobacter chroococcum* also produce alginate. But the production of alginate needed a wider context so there was a need for the algal sources which are used for the isolation of alginate (Cote and Krull, 1988).

The first genes in alginate biosynthesis were discovered in *P. aeruginosa*, a bacterium, which was inspired by the medicinal importance of this bacterium as an opportunistic human pathogen that usually creates chronic infections in the lung of cystic fibrosis (CF) patients (May et al., 1991). The genes involved in biosynthesis of alginate at the molecular level for the tow bacteria (*Pseudomonas and Azotobacter)* are almost same even though they are little different in their regulation. All of the essential genes participating in the biosynthesis of alginate are limited within a single 12-gene operon which is initially described by Chitnis and Ohman (Chitnis and Ohman, 1993): algD, alg8, alg44, algK, algE (algJ), algG, algX, algL, algI, algJ (algV), algF, and algA. These genes are under the control of algD which is a promoter (Martin et al., 1993; Shankar et al., 1995), while evidence propose that another core promoter is present within the operon (Lloret et al., 1996; Paletta and Ohman, 2012). Even though the gene algC is not located within the operon but it is involved in lipopolysaccharide and rhamnolipid biosynthesis (Goldberg et al., 1993; Ye et al., 1994; Olvera et al., 1999). Apart from these 13 core genes, there are other genes which are involved in biosynthesis of alginate that is summarized in Table 1.1. The steps involved in biosynthesis of alginate can be divided into four: alginate precursor biosynthesis, polymerization, acetylation and epimerization/transfer, and spread (Iain et al., 2013):

TABLE 1.1 Genes Involved in the Biosynthesis of Alginate (ALG) in *Pseudomonas aeruginosa.*

Description gene	
GDP-mannose pyrophosphorylase/phosphomannose isomerase	AlgA
Phosphomannomutase	AlgC
GDP-mannose dehydrogenase	AlgD
Glycosyltransferase/polymerase-export function	Alg8
c-di-GMP binding-activation/membrane fusion protein	Alg44
Periplasmic protein/multiprotein comples assembly	AlgK
Outer-membrane porin/alginate export	AlgE
Mannuronan C-5-epimerase/biosynthesis	AlgG
Periplasmic protein with high sequence similarity to algJ/scaffold protein sequestering	AlgX
ALG lyase/biosynthesis	AlgL
ALG lyase (polyguluronate lyase)/biosynthesis	PA1167
O-acetylation	AlgI
O-acetylation	AlgJ
O-acetylation	AlgF
Member of *ntr*C subclass of two-component transcriptional regulatora (cognate sensor kinase is FimS)	AlgB

TABLE 1.1 *(Continued)*

Description gene	
Unknown function	AlgH
Regulatory component of two-component signal transduction system (cognate sensor kinase is FimS)	AlgR
Histone-like transcriptional regulator binds to *alg*D promoter	AlgQ
Histone-like transcriptional regulator binds to *alg*D promoter	AlgP
AlgR cognate sensor (alginate and motility regulator)	AlgZ
Homologous to *Escherichia coli*s Eglobal stress response factor	AlgU
Homologous to *E. coli*s serine protease DegS	AlgW
Homologous to *E. coli* RseP protease involved in activation of AlgU via regulated intramembrane proteolysis cascade	mucP
Periplasmic or outer-membrane protein involved in activation of AlgU through regulated intramembrane proteolysis cascade	mucE
ALG-specific c-di-GMP synthesizing enzyme	mucR
Homologous to *E. coli* serine protease DegP	mucD
Regulator	mucC
Anti s factor	mucB
Anti s factor	mucA
D-mannuronic acid	M

1.2.2   ALGINATE PRECURSOR BIOSYNTHESIS

The activated alginate precursor guanosine diphosphate (GDP)-mannuronic acid is formed in several enzymes induced cytosolic steps which facilitate the conversion of the central metabolite fructose 6-phosphate (Fig 1.1). At the initial stage, when the six carbon substrates enter the Entner Doudoroff (ED) pathway the synthesis starts and pyruvate forms which is directed to the tricarboxylic acid cycle. Later, by gluconeogenesis, oxaloacetate is converted to fructose-6-phosphate (Lynn and Sokatch, 1984; Narbad et al., 1988). There are three alginate-specific enzymes (AlgA, AlgC, and AlgD) which have been broadly characterized, catalyze these four alginate biosynthesis steps that convert fructose-6-phosphate synthesized in the initial step to mannuronic acid. The conversion of fructose-6-phosphate at first is catalyzed by bifunctional protein AlgA (phosphomannose isomerase active). Later, AlgC, which is phosphomannomutase enzyme converts mannose-6-phosphate to mannose-1-phosphate (Zielinski et al., 1992), followed by the conversion to GDP-mannose which is catalyzed by the GDP-mannose pyrophorylase activity of AlgA through the reversible hydrolysis of GDP (Shinabarger et al., 1991). At the final step, this is the rate determining step AlgD, also called GDP-mannose dehydrogenase catalysis the GDP-mannose irreversibly to GDP-mannuronic acid which acts as the substrate for the polymerization of alginate. The process of alginate biosynthesis is shown in Figure 1.1.

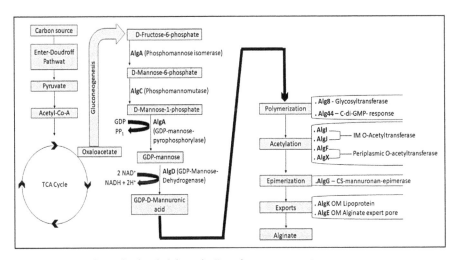

FIGURE 1.1 Biosynthesis of alginate in *Pseudomonas aeruginosa*.

Source: Adapted from Remminghorst and Rehm (2006).

1.3 POLYMERIZATION

There are at least two genes necessary for this step that are Alg8 (an inner membrane protein) and Alg44 protein (Remminghorst and Rehm, 2006b). Data collected from bioinformatics suggests that the inner membrane protein Alg8 is expected to be glycosyltransferase enzyme that catalyzes the transfer of sugar molecule from donor to an acceptor molecule. Other experimental data supports Alg8 has direct participation in the alginate polymerization which was observed that the over-production of alginate resulted by overexpression of Alg8 gene (Remminghorst and Rehm, 2006b), while another in vitro experiment revealed that a complete cell membrane is needed for the polymerization step to initiate which advocates that the Alg8 gene needs another gene for the expression (Hay et al., 2009; Oglesby et al., 2008; Remminghorst et al., 2009). The Alg44 gene plays an indirect role in polymerization step, which is not well understood, but polymerization of alginate did not occur upon deletion of this gene and also overexpression of this gene led to overproduction of alginate, which is similar to Alg8 gene (Oglesby et al., 2008; Remminghorst et al., 2009).

1.3.1 TRANSLOCATION AND ALTERATION

The translocation of new alginate which is resulted from polymerization step, across the concentrated gel-like matrix periplasm is done by a known multi-protein structure comprising of AlgG, AlgK, and AlgX which are periplasmic proteins (Jain and Ohman, 2005; Jain et al., 2003; Robles et al., 2004). These proteins help the alginate chain to translocate through the periplasm by protecting it against the degradative action of AlgL is periplasmic alginate lyase enzyme which interestingly takes part in the formation of periplasmic structure (Jain and Ohman, 2005).

1.3.1.1 ALGAL SOURCE

Currently, commercial alginates are produced from algal sources and are extracted from brown algae (*Phaeophyceae*), which are three species including *Ascophyllum nodosum, Laminaria hyperborea,* and *Macrocystis pyrifera,* and other sources are *Ecloniamaxima, Laminaria digitata, Sargassum, Lesonia nigrescens,* and *Laminaria japonica* species. In all of these species, alginate is present up to 40% by dry weight as a primary polysaccharide (Clementi, 1997; Pszczola, 1998; Sutherland, 1990; Konda et al., 2015). ALGs are present in intracellular matrix of brown algae as gels containing calcium, sodium, strontium, barium, and magnesium ions, which are found in seawater and by the ion-exchange equilibrium the counter ion composition can be determined (Yaphe and Morgan, 1959; Haug et al., 1974).

1.3.1.2 EXTRACTION

The extraction of alginate from algae sources comprised of different steps where at first step the algae are mechanically harvested and dried except *M. pyrifera*, which is processed in wet condition. After drying and milling of algal material, treatment with mineral acids is done to remove counterions by proton exchange. In the second step, sodium alginate is prepared by solubilizing insoluble alginic acid by neutralization process using sodium hydroxide (NaOH) or sodium carbonate (Na_2CO_3) as alkali. Centrifugation or other separation techniques like flotation and shifting followed by filtration is done to remove the precipitates. Sodium alginate is directly separated by treating the precipitate matter with mineral acid, alcohol, or calcium chloride which removes or degrades associated neutral homopolysaccharides like fucoidin and laminarin. At this stage, the alginate contains several cytotoxic impurities which make them unsuitable for biomedical applications. To remove these impurities further purification needs to be done. Thus, this method was not suitable for large-scale production as it is time-consuming and required expensive equipment for electrophoresis process. Therefore, another method of extraction was introduced by using Ba^{2+} ions because it has a higher affinity towards alginate than Ca^{2+} ions and the resultant product, that is, Ba-alginate gels are stable in neutral and acidic pH but disintegrate in alkaline pH. Impurities and nitrogen's could be eluted from Ba-alginate gel and pure alginate was obtained by treatment with different alkaline solutions followed by ethanol extraction (Zimmermann et al., 1992; Klöck et al., 1994). The schematic representation of alginate extraction is presented in Figure 1.2.

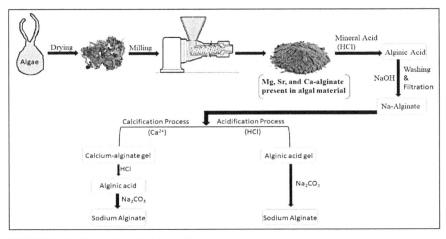

FIGURE 1.2 Extraction of alginate from algae.

1.4 CHEMISTRY

1.4.1 STRUCTURE

Before the identification of L-guluronate residue in 1955 (Fischer and Dörfel, 1955), D-mannuronate was considered as the major constituent of alginate. Later, the actual block copolymers of alginate were demonstrated by fractional percipitation using calcium and manganese salts and the mannuronate to guluronate ratio (M/G) dependence to its natural source were confirmed by Haug et al (Haug, 1959). Now, it is well understood that alginates are unbranched polysaccharides consisting of two linear binary copolymers having blocks of β (14)-linked D-mannuronic acid (M) and α-(14)-linked L-guluronic acid (G) residues. To determine the block composition of alginate, there are some standard chemical methods which involve the determination of M/G ratio (uronate composition) by complete acid hydrolysis, and partial acid hydrolysis of alginate (Carmeliet, 2005). On complete hydrolysis, high amount of degraded material was formed where the different copolymers of alginate structure were described in detail by partial hydrolysis followed by fractionation which resulted in formation of three fractions of different copolymer compositions, in which two insoluble or resistant fractions composed of homopolymeric regions of M (M-blocks) and G (G-blocks), and one soluble or hydrolysable fraction with almost equal proportions of M and G monomers having a high number of MG residues (Fischbach et al., 2009). Figure 1.3 shows the representative structure of alginate backbone.

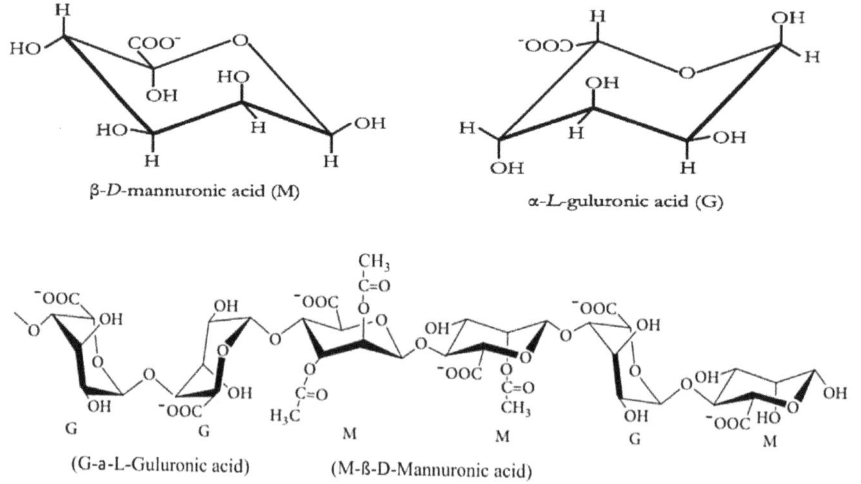

β-D-mannuronic acid (M)   α-L-guluronic acid (G)

(G-a-L-Guluronic acid)   (M-ß-D-Mannuronic acid)

FIGURE 1.3   Structure of alginate with the GM and MG residues.

Several mathematical models of alginate microstructure were derived but the most exact structural data are achieved by spectroscopy techniques like ¹H and ¹³C NMR among which ¹³C NMR is a powerful technique for sequence determination of alginates due to the presence of wide series of shifts, and sensitivity of the chemical shifts to the neighboring chemical unite. However, there are some disadvantages to ^{13}C NMR spectroscopy as all the carbon atoms may not have same nuclear overhauser enhancement even if they have same number of protons on them, and low sensitivity of ^{13}C NMR for quantitative work. Hence, ^{1}H NMR spectroscopy method is a useful technique for quantitative work where there are minor amounts of material available. From ^{1}H NMR spectrum, a clear method of determination of uronate composition (M/G ratio) using peak ratio and yield of GG, MM, GM, and MG fractions, was obtained (Penman and Sanderson, 1972). Later, ^{1}H NMR spectrum was used to study yield fractions of the four dimers GG, MM, GM, and MG (Grasdalen et al., 1977). The anomeric region in the ^{1}H NMR spectra of alginates by different M contents is shown in Figure 1.4. The following equation used in obtaining the monomer and dimer fractions, where Ia, Ib, and Ic are intensities of A, B, and C peaks, and F_G and F_M are the frequency of G and M residues, respectively (Grasdalen et al., 1979).

After normalization of $F_G + F_M = 1$, the mole fraction of M residue is derived.

Mole fractions and doublet frequencies are related by:

$$F_G = F_{GG} + F_{GM;} \text{ and } F_M = F_{MM} + F_{GM}$$

For long chains $F_{MG} = F_{GM,}$ so values for the doublet frequencies and M/G ratio can be calculated.

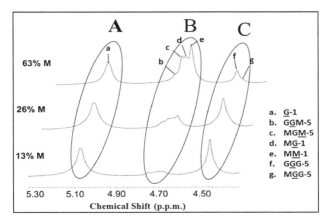

FIGURE 1.4   The anomeric region (in the 400 MHz) ^{1}H NMR spectra of alginate with different amount of M.

Source: Grasdalen et al. 1979.

1.5   PROPERTIES

The physical and chemical properties of alginates render them useful in many food and industrial applications. These characteristics include the ability to retain water and water-holding capacity; gelling, viscosifying and stabilizing properties; emulsifying properties; and temperature-independent sol/gel transition in the presence of divalent cations, such as calcium (Draget et al., 2005). ALGs bind easily with water and can produce high viscosity thickeners at low levels. The chemical composition and resulting physical properties of an alginate vary according to seaweed species, structure, and environmental conditions. "For example, some [species] may yield an alginate that gives a strong gel, another weaker gel; one may readily give a cream/white alginate, and another may give that only with difficulty and is best used for technical applications where color does not matter" (McHugh and Dennis, 2003). Growing environments are influential as well; the ion composition of alginates is determined by the ion-exchange equilibrium with the seawater in which the algae plant grew (Pawar et al., 2012). Another example, the amount of guluronate present in an alginate, is dependent on the seaweed sourced: the species, age at harvest, geographic location of harvest, and plant part extracted (Fett and Chandi, 1995).

1.5.1   PHYSICAL

ALG salts are odorless, white to yellowish-brown powders. ALGs have no discernable flavor. Forming a viscous, colloidal solution, the salts of alginic acid formed with monovalent cations are soluble in water (sodium alginate, potassium alginate, and ammonium alginate) (Kimica, 2014). As a 1% solution, the resulting pH is in between 5.0 and 7.5 (FMC biopolymer, 2006). Sodium alginate does not have a boiling or melting point. At temperatures, greater than 392°F (>200°C), sodium alginate will autoignite. ALGs are block copolymers comprised of two uronic acids, mannuronic acid (M-block) and guluronic acid (G-block), of varying composition and sequence (Yang et al., 2011). There is a correlation between the arrangement of the uronic acid blocks and the age of the plant and conditions of growth. The leaves of the same algae, *L. hyperborea*, have a very high content of guluronic acid when the plant grows unexposed coastal areas, compared to a lower G-content when the leaves float in placid waters.

1.5.2 CHEMICAL

The solubility of alginates is influenced by the total ionic strength of the solution, the free calcium concentration, and pH of the solvent (Van den Brink et al., 2009). Sodium, potassium, and ammonium alginates are soluble in hot and cold water (Saltmarsh, 2013). Table 1.2 outlines the solubility of different types of alginates in various solutions (Kimica, 2014). ALGs formed with divalent cations are insoluble; calcium and magnesium alginates do not dissolve in water but will swell when placed in water (Khotimchenko et al., 2001). Ammonium, potassium, and sodium alginates are insoluble in ethanol and ether (World Health Organization, 1997). Calcium alginate is slightly soluble in ethanol and will dissolve slowly in sodium polyphosphate and sodium carbonate. ALGs selectively bind with divalent cations, especially calcium, making them insoluble in high calcium solutions such as milk or hard water with high calcium content. All of the alginate types are listed in Table 1.2 and these are insoluble in fats, oils, and organic solvents.

TABLE 1.2 The Solubility of ALGs in Various Conditions.

Different kind of alginate	Acidic conditions Fruit juice, liquor, salad dressing, and so forth.	Alkaline conditions Kansui, and so forth.	In solution with divalent cations hard water, milk, and so forth.
Alginic acid	Insoluble	Soluble	Insoluble
Sodium alginate	Insoluble	Soluble	Insoluble
Potassium alginate	Insoluble	Soluble	Insoluble
Calcium alginate	Insoluble	Insoluble	Insoluble
Ammonium alginate	Insoluble	Soluble	Insoluble
Propylene glycol alginate (PGA)	Soluble	Soluble	Soluble

ALGs exhibit limited solubility at low pH. The soluble alginates will not hydrate in highly acidic systems (pH < 4–5). In more acidic conditions, alginic acid precipitates out of solution. The precipitation of alginic acid is caused by an abrupt decrease in pH below the pKa value of the alginate. ALGs with an alternating, heterogeneous structure (MG blocks) precipitate at lower pH compared with alginates containing a more homogeneous block structure (MM and GG). ALGs are stable in alkaline conditions up to a pH of 10, beyond which depolymerization occurs.

ALGs form chemically induced gels (Truong et al., 1995). The gel network is formed by inter-molecular association of divalent cations, such as calcium, with the polyguluronate sites of the alginate molecule. The cross-linking between carboxyl groups and divalent cations is the basis for gel formation. Therefore, the sol/gel transition of alginates is not temperature dependent. ALG gels can also be heated without melting.

1.5.3 DISSOLUTION

Algin dissolves readily in either hot or cold water. It is dissolved most easily when it is sifted into the water which is vigorously agitated. High-speed stirring and gradual addition of the algin increases the rate of dissolution and decreases the tendency toward lumping of the finer mesh products. When the formulation includes sucrose, dextrin, salts, or fillers, lumping can be prevented by dry-blending one of these materials with the fine-mesh algin before adding the mixture to water. Rapid solution rates can be obtained by first wetting the algin with ethanol, glycerol, or a similar water-miscible liquid before it is added to water or by preparing a slurry of the algin in the liquid and then rapidly adding the slurry to water with vigorous stirring. With good dispersion and agitation dissolution should be completed in a few minutes.

1.6 SOLUTION PROPERTIES

The properties of algin solutions can readily be changed to provide either long, short, or an intermediate type of flow. Algin solutions which contain no divalent or trivalent metal ions and those which contain polyphosphates to sequester the polyvalent metal ions have long flow properties. The measured viscosity is little affected by changes in the rate of shear. Increasing the amounts of polyvalent metal ions, among which calcium is particularly important, raises the viscosity and shortens the flow properties. This process is accompanied by an increase in thixotropy. Algin compounds which contain a small amount of calcium ions uniformly distributed along the chain molecules are particularly useful. These compounds have intermediate flow properties which can be readily adjusted to those of the long flow type by the addition of small amounts of polyphosphates, phosphates, or carbonates.

1.6.1 CONCENTRATION

Algin is available in a number of viscosity ranges under trade names with the viscosity of each product controlled within relatively narrow range. A high-viscosity algin has a viscosity of at least 2,000 cps at a concentration of 1% in water, while a very low viscosity product will have a viscosity of less than 10 cps at the same concentration.

1.6.2 TEMPERATURE

Algin solutions behave like other fluids in their independence of viscosity on temperature, for the change of viscosity with temperature. Over a limited range, the viscosity of algin solutions decreases approximately 2.5% for each degree of rise in temperature. This decrease is reversible the solutions regain their original viscosities upon cooling. However, if high solution temperatures are maintained for extended periods, there might be a progressive decrease in viscosity due to a partial depolymerization of the molecule. Algin solutions do not coagulate upon heating nor do they gel upon cooling, but they maintain their smooth flow properties over a wide temperature range.

1.6.3 pH

The viscosities of solutions of water-soluble algin salt change only slightly with changes in pH in the range of 4–10. There is a slightly higher viscosity near neutrality (pH 6–8) due to the repetitive effects of the negatively charged carboxyl groups which extend the chain and increase its water-binding capacity. Below a pH of 4.5, viscosity begins to increase because of the lesser solubility of the free acid. As the pH is lowered below four, the viscosity increases still more until a gel is formed at a pH of 3–3.5. In highly alkaline solutions, a gel forms at a pH of 11.5–12 if the gum concentration is above 1–2%, depending on the molecular weight of the algin. Algin solutions which contain calcium ions decrease in viscosity as the pH is raised above nine because of the ability of hydroxides and carbonates to tie up calcium ions. These solutions also gel at a pH of 11.5–12. Propylene glycol alginate is used in acidic solutions because the ester group hydrolyzes in alkaline media. This algin does not gel with acids.

1.6.4   GELS

Algin formulations gel at room temperature, and their setting time can be controlled. Water gels have excellent clarity. By altering the formulations, gels can be varied in texture from those which are soft and tender to those which are tough and elastic (Toft et al., 1986). As a result, algin gels are widely used for food, pharmaceutical, and industrial purposes. Algin gels are of three major types: calcium or other di- or trivalent metal salt gels, acid gels, combination of calcium salt, and acid gels (Fu et al., 2011; Draget et al., 1993). In general, gels are formed by the gradual and uniform release of either calcium or hydrogen ions or a combination of the two, throughout an algin salt solution. Setting time can be controlled by the addition of a limited amount of a compound, such as a phosphate or polyphosphate, which is capable of combining with a di- or trivalent metal ion. Formulations are available in which the whole ingredients are combined in a single powder. Since a large number of formulations are available for various purposes, the algin manufacturer should be contacted for specific recommendations.

To fully appreciate the potential of alginate's gel-forming properties, it helps to understand the chemistry behind gel formation. Regions of guluronate monomers, or G-blocks, in one alginate molecule can be linked to a similar region in another alginate molecule by means of calcium ions or other multivalent cations (Fig 1.5). The divalent calcium cation, Ca^{2+}, fits into the guluronate block structure like eggs in an egg box (Pawar and Edgar, 2012; Szekalska et al., 2016) (Fig 1.5). This binds the alginate polymers together by forming junction zones, resulting in gelation of the solution. There are three main components in a typical alginate gelling system— alginate, calcium salt, and sequestrant. ALG type and counterion, calcium source and the sequestering agent control the gelling system structure and the rate at which the gel forms. Hydration and uniform distribution of the alginate are essential to optimize a gel formation. The grade of alginate, calcium source and sequestering agents must be matched with the process and overall formulation to develop the final product (Fig 1.6).

1.6.5   FILMS

A wide range of water-insoluble and water-soluble films can be prepared from algin (Sirviö et al., 2014; Ionita et al., 2013). Films prepared from sodium alginate are water-soluble (Norajit et al., 2010), but calcium alginate

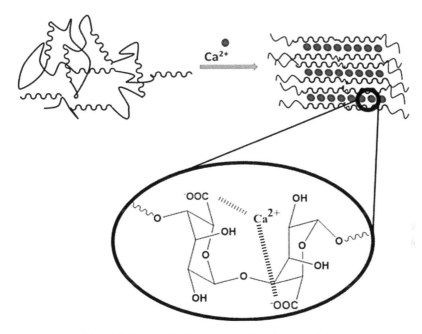

FIGURE 1.5   Calcium binding site in G-blocks and "egg box" model.

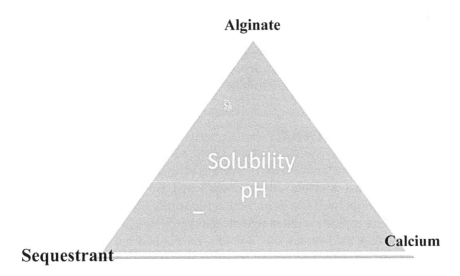

FIGURE 1.6   Factors influencing for alginate gel formation.

films are insoluble although they do swell in water. Many of these films are clear, tough, and flexible (Lacroix and Le Tien, 2005; Nieto, 2009). They resist penetration by greases, oils, fats, waxes, and organic solvents but transmit water vapor. Algin films are compatible with plasticizers such as glycerol and sorbitol (Jongjareonrak et al., 2006; Bergo et al., 2013; Aadil and Jha, 2016). Films are prepared by four basic methods such as evaporation of water from a cast film of a soluble alginate, extrusion of a solution of a soluble alginate into a precipitating bath which yields an insoluble alginate, treatment of a soluble film with a di- or trivalent metal salt solution or an acidic solution to form an insoluble film, and drying a cast film to drive off the ammonia from a solution of a di- or trivalent metal alginate that is soluble in excess ammonium hydroxide. Films can be made water-resistant by including in the formulation urea-formaldehyde resins which insolubilize the film when it is heated. They can also be made water-resistant by treatment with solutions of zinc chloride, zirconium oxychloride, or aluminum salts.

1.6.6   COMPATIBILITIES

Algin in solution is compatible with a large number of compounds (Esteban et al., 2011). Propylene glycol alginate is compatible with acids and, in many cases, with alkaline-earth metal salts. Acidic solutions which are strong enough to degrade the algin chain (below pH 2) lower the viscosities of propylene glycol alginate solutions considerably if kept for several days at room temperature; the rate is dependent on both pH and temperature. It concentrations below 0.5%, are soluble in acidic solutions above pH 1.5.

1.6.7   ALGIN IN FOODS

Algin has been eaten for hundreds of years as a constituent of kelp in specialty foods (Hadas and Srebnik, 2016; Cottrell and Kovacs, 1980; Littlecott, 1982), while algin itself has been used in foodstuffs for 30 years. Extensive animal feeding tests on sodium alginate and propylene glycol alginate have shown that they are wholesome, edible products and not allergens. Algin compounds have been specified as optional ingredients in Federal Standards of Identity for several foods. These include cream cheese, Neufchatel cheese, cheese spreads, French dressing, and salad dressing.

1.7   OTHER PROPERTIES

1.7.1   DISSOCIATION CONSTANT

The polysaccharide which has one-half of its carboxyl groups in the free acid form and the other half as the sodium salt has a pH of about 3.6 at a 1% concentration, which corresponds to a pH of 3.6 at this point. Because of the negative charge on the polymeric alginate ion, the apparent pK depends somewhat on the degree of neutralization. However, the addition of a salt represses the charge effect and gives a pK that is independent of neutralization if it is measured above the gel point. Thus, Saric and Schofield (1946) reported a pK of 2.95 for the dissociation of alginic acid in the presence of N potassium chloride.

1.7.2   EQUIVALENT WEIGHT

The equivalent weight of commercial alginic acid (as an acid) ranges 194–215. The theoretical equivalent weight for a hexuronoglycan is 176, however, the equivalent weight does not approach the theoretical value even if the solids have been determined by drying at 105° for 3 h. A major part of this difference might be due to water which is tenaciously held by the alginic acid. Attempts to remove this water with rigorous drying conditions degrade the alginic acid and in some cases, introduce additional acidic groups. Acidic groups in a degraded alginic acid might account for some of the reports of equivalent weights which approximate the theoretical value.

1.7.3   MOLECULAR WEIGHT

In kelp, algin has a very high molecular weight. By varying the processing conditions, algin can be produced which covers a wide range of viscosities and molecular weights. However, several different methods (Donnan and Rose, 1950; Vincent et al., 1955; Helmiyati and Aprilliza, 2017) indicate that commercial sodium alginates have molecular weights between 32,000 and 200,000 and a degree of polymerization of 180–930.

1.7.4   OPTICAL ROTATION

Reports of the $[\alpha]^{D}$ (Wang et al., 2002) of sodium alginate solutions vary from −113 to −148° (Black et al., 1952). Since specific optical rotation has little relation to quality and no relation to viscosity, it is seldom used.

1.7.5   ION-EXCHANGE PROPERTIES

Insoluble metal alginates behave as typical ion-exchange resins. When an insoluble metal alginate is allowed to equilibrate with a solution containing mixed cations, the composition of the metal ion mixture attached to the alginate is a function of both the concentration of the metal ion in solution and the dissociation constants of the metal alginates (Mongar and Wasserman, 1949).

1.8   CONCLUSION

This current chapter describes the source, properties, and chemical modification along with applications of alginate in different biological fields in brief. ALG is a colloidal hydrophilic polysaccharide obtained from bacteria (Pseudomonas and Azotobactor) and algae (*L. hyperborea, M. pyrifera, A. nodosum, Laminaria digitara, L. japonica,* and *Eclonia*). It is a linear copolymer containing -1, 4-linked D-mannuronic acid and α-1, 4-inked L-guluronic. Because of their special structural, enzymatic sequencing control and understanding of properties-sequence relationship alginates became an important polymer in different biological applications. The hydrophilicity, non-toxicity, biocompatibility, low cost, and water-solubility attracted researcher's attention in recent years. The water-soluble nature of alginates forms a gel in the presence of divalent cation like calcium ions. The reversible solubility of alginate enables the synthesis of alginate in different forms such as fibers, films, and microspheres, while the low mechanical strength of alginate has been improved by blending with other nontoxic biopolymers.

SUMMARY

ALG is a naturally occurring colloidal hydrophilic polysaccharide obtained from the various species of brown seaweed (phaeophyceae). Bacterial alginate is produced from Pseudomonas and Azotobactor. Commercial alginates are made from *L. hyperborea, M. pyrifera, A. nodosum, L. digitara, L. japonica,* and *Eclonia*. It is a linear copolymer consisting mainly residue of β-1, 4-linked D-mannuronic acid and α-1,4-inked L-guluronic. Because of their special structural sequencing of monosaccharide in one hand and our ability to act upon the alginate precursor by use of enzymatic controlled sequences, on the other hand, understanding of relationship between properties and sequence in natural alginates became a great opportunity to use this important polymer in different biological applications. On addition, production of alginate can be tailored by modification of bacteria during the regulation of biosynthesis of alginate which makes it more applicable for different applications. Other interesting properties of alginate such as nontoxicity, hydrophilicity, biocompatibility, a relatively low cost, and water-solubility, attracted researcher's attention in recent years. The water-soluble nature of it alginates forms a gel in the presence of divalent cation as the calcium ion. The reversible solubility of alginate enables us to synthesize alginate in different forms such as films, microspheres, and fibers. The undesirable properties of alginate such as low mechanical strength have been improved by blending with another nontoxic biopolymer.

KEYWORDS

- **alginate**
- **polymerization**
- **gels**
- **films**
- **biocompatibility**

REFERENCES

Aadil, K. R.; Jha, H. Physico⁺'Chemical Properties of Lignin–Alginate Based Films in the Presence of Different Plasticizers. *Iran. Polym. J.* **2016,** *25*(8), 661–670.

Andersen, T.; Strand, B. L.; Formo, K.; Alsberg, E.; Christensen, B. E. Alginates as Biomaterials in Tissue Engineering. In *Carbohydrate Chemistry: Chemical and Biological Approaches;* Rauter, A. P., Ed.; The Royal Society of Chemistry: Cambridge, UK, 2012; Vol. 37, pp 227–258.

Bergo, P.; Moraes, I. C. F.; Sobral, P. J. A. Effects of Plasticizer on Physical Properties of Pigskin Gelatin Films. *Food Hydrocolloids* **2013,** *32,* 412–415.

Black, W. A. P.; Cornhi, J. I.; W. J; Dewar, E. T. The Properties of the Algal Chemicals I.-The Evaluation of the Common British Brown Marine Algae as a Source of Alginate. *J. Sci. Food Agr.* **1952,** *3,* 542.

Carmeliet, P. Angiogenesis in Life, Disease and Medicine Angiogenesis in Life, Disease and Medicine. *Nature* **2005,** *438,* 932–936.

Chitnis, C. E.; Ohman, D. E. Genetic Analysis of the Alginate Biosynthetic Gene Cluster of *Pseudomonas Aeruginosa* Shows Evidence of an Operonic Structure. *Mol. Microbiol.* **1993**, *8,* 583–593.

Clementi, F. Alginate Production by *Azotobacter Vinelandii. Crit. Rev. Biotechnol.* **1997**, *17*(4), 327–361.

Cote, G. L.; Krull, L. H. Characterization of the Exocellular Polysaccharides from *Azotobacter Chroococcum. Carbohydr. Res.* **1988**, *18,* 143–152.

Cottrell, I. W.; Kovacs, P. Alginates. In *Handbook of water soluble gums and resins:* Crawford, H. B., Williams, J. Eds.;. McGraw-Hill, Auckland, 1980; pp 21–43.

Donnan, F. G.; Rose, R. C. Osmotic Pressure, Molecular Weight, and Viscosity of Sodium Alginate. *Can. J. Res.* **1950**, *28b,* 105.

Draget, K. I.; Simensen, M. K.; Onsøyen, E.; Smidsrød, O. Gel Strength of Ca-Limited Alginate Gels Made *in Situ. Hydrobiologia* **1993**, 260–261, 563–565.

Draget, K. I.; Smidsrød, O.; Skjåk-Bræk. G. Alginates from Algae. In *Polysaccharides and Polyamides in the Food Industry. Properties, Production, and Patents;* Steinbüchel, A., Rhee, S. K., Eds.; Verlag: Wiley, 2005; pp 1–30.

Esteban, E.; Urena, B.; Kitchens, C. L. Wide-Angle X-Ray Diffraction of Cellulose Nanocrystal, Alginate Nanocomposite Fibers. *Macromolecules* **2011**, *44,* 3478–3484.

Fett, W. F.; Chandi, W. Yields of Alginates Produced by Fluorescent Pseudomonads in Batch Culture. *J. Indust. Microbiol.* **1995**, *14,* 412–415.

Fischbach, C.; Kong, H. J.; Hsiong, S. X.; Evangelista, M. B.; Yuen, W.; Mooney, D. J. Cancer Cell Angiogenic Capability is Regulated by 3D Culture and Integrin Engagement. *Proc. Natl. Acad. Sci. U. S. A.* **2009**, *106,* 399–404.

Fischer, F. G.; Dörfel, H. Die Polyuronsauren Der Braunalgen (Kohlenhydrate Der Algen-I). *Z. Physiol. Chem.* **1955**, *302,* 186–203.

FMC Bio Polymer. MSDS: Protanal® LF 120 LS Sodium Alginate. "Product Specification Bulletin: PRONOVA SLM20." Philadelphia, PA". "Sales Specification: Keltone LVCR – Sodium Alginate." 2250200, **2005**, *2006,* 2012, 1–8.

Fu, S.; Thacker, A.; Sperger, D. M. et al., Relevance of Rheological Properties of Sodium Alginate in Solution to Calcium Alginate Gel Properties. *AAPS PharmSciTech.* **2011**, *12*(2), 453–460.

Goldberg, J. B.; Hatano, K.; Pier, G. B. Synthesis of Lipopolysaccharide O Side Chains by *Pseudomonas Aeruginosa* PAO1 Requires the Enzyme Phosphomannomutase. *J. Bacteriol.* **1993**, *175,* 1605–1611.

Gombotz, W. R.; Wee, S. F. Protein Release from Alginate Matrices. *Adv. Drug Delivery Rev.* **1998**, *31,* 267–285.

Grasdalen H; Larsen, B.; Smidsrød, O.; ^{13}C NMR studies of Alginates. *Carbohydr. Res.* **1977**, *56,* C11–C15.

Grasdalen, H.; Larsen, B.; Smidsrød, O. A p.m.r. Study of the Composition and Sequence of Uronate Residues in Alginates. **1979**, *68,* 23–31.

Hadas, H. H.; Srebnik, S. Structural Characterization of Sodium Alginate and Calcium Alginate. *Biomacromolecules* **2016**, *17,* 2160–2167

Haug, A. Fractionation of Alginic Acid. *Acta Chem. Scand.* **1959**, *13,* 601–603.

Haug, A.; Larsen, B.; Smidserod, O. Uronic Acid Sequence in Alginate from Different Sources. *Carbohydrate. Res.* **1974**, *32,* 217–225.

Hay, I. D.; Gatland, K.; Campisano, A.; Jordens, J. Z.; Rehm, B. H. Impact of Alginate Overproduction on Attachment and Biofilm Architecture of a Super Mucoid *Pseudomonas Aeruginosa* Strain. *Appl. Environ. Microbiol.* **2009**, *75,* 6022–6025.

Helmiyati, A. M. Characterization and Properties of Sodium Alginate from Brown Algae Used as an Ecofriendly Superabsorbent. *IOP Conf. Ser.: Mater. Sci. Eng.* **2017**, *188*, 12–19.

Huebsch, N.; Mooney, D. J. Inspiration and Application in the Evolution of Biomaterials. *Nature* **2009**, *462*, 426–432.

Iain, D. H.; Rehman, Z. U.; Moradali, M. F.; Wang, Y.; Bernd H. A. R. Microbial Alginate Production, Modification and its Applications. *Micro. Biotech.* **2013**, *6*, 637–650.

Ionita, M.; Pandele, M. A.; Iovu, H. Sodium Alginate/Graphene Oxide Composite Films with Enhanced Thermal and Mechanical Properties. *Carbohydr. Polym.* **2013**, *94*, 339–344.

Jain, S.; Franklin, M. J.; Ertesvag, H.; Valla, S.; Ohman, D. E. The Dual Roles of AlgG in C-5-Epimerization and Secretion of Alginate Polymers in *Pseudomonas Aeruginosa*. *Mol. Microbiol.* **2003**, *47*, 1123–1133.

Jain, S.; Ohman, D. E. Role of an Alginate Lyase for Alginate Transport in Mucoid *Pseudomonas Aeruginosa*. *Infect. Immun.* **2005**, *73*, 6429–6436.

Jongjareonrak, A.; Benjakul, S.; Visessanguan, W.; Prodpran, T.; Tanaka, M. Characterization of Edible Films from Skin Gelatin of Brown Stripe Red Snapper and Big Eye Snapper. *Food Hydrocolloids* **2006**, *20*, 492–450.

Khotimchenko, Yu. S.; Kovalev, V. V.; Savchenko, O. V.; Ziganshina, O. A. Physical–Chemical Properties, Physiological Activity, and Usage of Alginates, the Polysaccharides of Brown Algae. *Russ J. Mar. Biol.* **2001**, 53–64.

Kimica, Alginate: How to Use. 2009. http://www.kimica-alginate.com/alginate/how_to_use.html (accessed 2014, January 1).

Klöck, G.; Frank, H.; Houben, R.; Zekorn, T.; Horcher, A.; Siebers, U.; et al. Production of Purified Alginates Suitable for Use in Immunoisolated Transplantation. *Appl. Microbiol. Biotechnol.* **1994**, *40*, 638–643.

Konda, N. V.; Singh, S.; Simmons, B. A.; Klein-Marcuschamer, K. D. An Investigation on the Economic Feasibility of Macroalgae as a Potential Feedstock for Biorefineries. *Bioenergy Res.* **2015**, *8*, 1046–1056.

Lacroix, M.; Le Tien, C. Edible Films and Coatings from Non-Starch Polysaccharides. In *Innovations in Food Packaging*; Han, J. H., Ed.; Elsevier Science and Technology Books: San Diego, 2005; p 338.

Linker, A.; Jones, R. S. A New Polysaccharide Resembling Alginic Acid Isolated from Pseudomonads. *J. Biol. Chem.* **1966**, *241*, 3845–3851.

Littlecott, G. W. Food Gels—the Role of Alginates. *Food Technol. Aust.* **1982**, *34*, 412–418.

Liu, K.; Ding, H. J.; Liu, J.; Chen, Y.; Zhao, X. Z. Shape-Controlled Production of Biodegradable Calcium Alginate Gel Microparticles Using a Novel Microfluidic Device. *Langmuir* **2006**, *22*, 9453–9457.

Lloret, L.; Barreto, R.; León, R.; Moreno, S.; Martínez-Salazar, J.; Espín, G.; Soberón-Chávez, G. Genetic Analysis of the Transcriptional Arrangement of *Azotobacter vinelandii* Alginate Biosynthetic Genes: Identification of Two Independent Promoters. *Mol. Microbiol.* **1996**, *21*, 449–457.

Lynn, A. R.; Sokatch, J. R. Incorporation of Isotope from Specifically Labeled Glucose into Alginates of *Pseudomonas aeruginosa* and *Azotobacter vinelandii*. *J. Bacteriol.* **1984**, *158*, 1161–1162.

Martin, D. W.; Schurr, M. J.; Mudd, M. H.; Deretic, V. Differentiation of *Pseudomonas Aeruginosa* into the Alginate-Producing Form: Inactivation of MucB Causes Conversion to Mucoidy. *Mol. Microbiol.* **1993**, *9*, 497–506.

May, T. B.; Shinabarger, D.; Maharaj, R.; Kato, J.; Chu, L.; Devault, J. D.; Roychoudhury, S.; Zielinsky, N. A.; Berry, A.; Rothmel, R. K.; Misra, T. K.; Chakrabarty, A. M. Alginate

Synthesis by *Pseudomonas aeruginosa*: a Key Pathogenic Factor in Chronic Pulmonary Infections of Cystic Fibrosis Patients. *Clin. Microbiol. Rev.* **1991**, *4,* 191–206.

McHugh, D. J. A Guide to the Seaweed Industry, FAO Fisheries Technical Paper, *Food and Agriculture Organization of the United Nations,* **2003,** 441.

Mongar, J. L.; Wasserman, A. *Discuss. Faraday Soc.* **1949,** *7,* 118.

Narbad, A.; Russell, N. J.; Gacesa, P. Radio Labelling Patterns in Alginate of *Pseudomonas Aeruginosa* Synthesized from Specifically-Labelled *C Monosaccharide Precursors. *Microbios* **1988,** *54,* 171–179.

Nieto, M. B. Structure and Function of Polysaccharide Gum Based Edible Films and Coatings. In *Edible Films and Coatings for Food Applications;* Embuscado, M. E., Huber, K. C., Eds.; Springer: New York, 2009; pp 57–112.

Nivens, D. E.; Ohman, D. E.; Williams, J.; Franklin, M. J. Role of Alginate and Its O Acetylation in Formation of *Pseudomonas Aeruginosa* Microcolonies and Biofilms. *J. Bacteriol.* **2001,** *183,* 1047–1057.

Norajit, K.; Kim, K. M.; Ryu, G. H. Comparative Studies on the Characterization and Antioxidant Properties of Biodegradable Alginate Films Containing Ginseng Extract. *J. Food Eng.* **2010,** *98,* 377–384.

Oglesby, L. L.; Jain, S.; Ohman, D. E. Membrane Topology and Roles of *Pseudomonas Aeruginosa* Alg8 and Alg44 in Alginate Polymerization. *Microbiology* **2008,** *154,* 1605–1615.

Olvera, C.; Goldberg, J. B.; Sanchez, R.; Soberón-Chávez G The *Pseudomonas Aeruginosa* algC Gene Product Participates in Rhamnolipid Biosynthesis. *FEMS Microbiol. Lett.* **1999,** *179,* 85–90.

Paletta, J. L.; Ohman, D. E. Evidence for Two Promoters Internal to the Alginate Biosynthesis Operon in *Pseudomonas Aeruginosa. Curr. Microbiol.* **2012,** *65,* 770–775.

Pawar, S. N.; Edgar, K. J. Alginate Derivatization: A Review of Chemistry, Properties and Applications. *Biomaterials* **2012,** *33,* 3729–3305.

Penman, A.; Sanderson, G. R. A Method for the Determination of Uronic Acid Sequence in Alginates. *Carbohydr. Res.* **1972,** *25,* 273–282.

Peters, M. C.; Polverini, P. J.; Mooney, D. J. Engineering Vascular Networks in Porous Polymer Matrices. *J. Biomed. Mater. Res.* **2002,** *60,* 668–678.

Pszczola, D. E. Discovering Treasures of the Deep. *Food Tech.* **1998,** *52,* 74–80.

Ratner, B. D.; Bryant, S. J. Biomaterials: Where We Have Been and Where We are Going *Annu. Rev. Biomed. Eng.* **2004,** *6,* 41–75.

Remminghorst, U.; Rehm, B. H. Alg44, a Unique Protein Required for Alginate Biosynthesis in *Pseudomonas Aeruginosa. Fed. Eur. Biochem. Soc. Lett.* **2006,** *580,* 3883–3888.

Remminghorst, U.; Rehm, B. H. In Vitro Alginate Polymerization and the Functional Role of Alg8 in Alginate Production by *Pseudomonas Aeruginosa.* **2006b,** *Appl. Environ. Microbiol. 72,* 298–305.

Remminghorst, U.; Hay, I. D.; Rehm, B. H. Molecular Characterization of Alg8, a Putative Glycosyltransferase, Involved in Alginate Polymerisation. *J. Biotechnol.* **2009,** *140,* 176–183.

Robles-Price, A.; Wong, T. Y.; Sletta, H.; Valla, S. Schiller, N. L. AlgX is a Periplasmic Protein Required for Alginate Biosynthesis in *Pseudomonas Aeruginosa. J. Bacteriol.* **2004,** *186,* 7369–7377.

Sabra, W.; Zeng, A.-P. Microbial Production of Alginates: Physiology and Process Aspects. In *Alginates: Biology and Applications;* Rehm, B. H. A., Ed.; Springer Verlag: Berlin, Heidelberg, Germany, 2009; pp 153–173.

Saltmarsh, M.; Barlow, S. *Essential Guide to Food Additives;* 4th; Saltmarsh, M., Ed.; The Royal Society of Chemistry: Cambridge; 2013.

Saric, S. P.; Schofield, R. K. The Dissociation Constants of the Carboxyl and Hydroxyl Groups in Some Insoluble and Sol-Forming Polysaccharides. *Proc. R. Soc. A* **1946**, 185–431.

Shankar, S.; Ye, R. W.; Schlictman, D.; Chakrabarty, A. M. Exopolysaccharide Alginate Synthesis in *Pseudomonas Aeruginosa*: Enzymology and Regulation of Gene Expression. *Adv. Enzymol. Relat. Areas Mol. Biol.* **1995**, *70*, 221–255.

Shinabarger, D.; Berry, A.; May, T. B.; Rothmel, R.; Fialho, A.; Chakrabarty, A. M. Purification and Characterization of Phosphomannose Isomerase-Guanosine Diphospho-D-Mannose Pyrophosphorylase – a Bifunctional Enzyme in the Alginate Biosynthetic-Pathway of *Pseudomonas Aeruginosa. J. Biol. Chem.* **1991**, *266*, 2080–2088.

Sirviö, J. A.; Kolehmainen, A.; Liimatainen, A.; Niinimäki, J.; Hormi, O. E. O. Biocomposite Cellulose-Alginate Films: Promising Packaging Materials. *Food Chem.* **2014**, *151*, 343–351.

Smidsrød, O.; Skjak-Bræk, G. Alginate as Immobilization Matrix for Cells. *Trends. Biotechnol.* **1990**, *8*, 71–78.

Sutherland, I. W. *Biotechnology of Microbial Exopolysaccharides;* Cambridge University Press: Cambridge, UK, 1990.

Suzuki, Y.; Nishimura, Y.; Tanihara, M.; Suzuki, K.; Nakamura, T.; Shimizu, Y.; Yamawaki, Y.; Kakimaru, Y. Evaluation of a Novel Alginate Gel Dressing: Cytotoxicity to Fibroblasts in Vitro and Foreign-Body Reaction in Pig Skin in Vivo. *J. Biomed. Mater. Res.* **1998**, *39*, 317–322.

Szekalska, M.; Puciłowska, A.; Szymańska, E.; Ciosek, P.; Winnicka, K. Alginate: Current Use and Future Perspectives in Pharmaceutical and Biomedical Applications. *Int. J. Polym. Sci.* **2016**, *2016*, 1–17.

Toft, K.; Grasdalen, H.; Smidsrød, O. Synergistic Gelation of Alginates and Pectins. *Chemistry and Function of Pectins*, ACS Symposium Series 310; 1986; pp 117–132.

Truong, V. D.; Walter, W. M.; Giesbrecht, F. G. Texturization of Sweet Potato Puree with Alginate: Effects of Tetrasodium Pyrophosphate and Calcium Sulfate. *J. Food Sci.* **1995**, *60*, 1054–1059.

Van den Brink, P.; Zwijnenburg, A.; Smith, G.; Temmink, H.; Loosdrecht, M. V. Effect of Free Calcium Concentration and Ionic Strength on Alginate Fouling in Cross-Flow Membrane Filtration. *J. Membr. Sci.* **2009**, *345*, 207–216.

Vincent, D. L.; Goring, D. A. I.; Young, E. G. A Comparison of the Properties of Various Preparations of Sodium Alginate. *J. Appl. Chem. (London)* **1955**, *5*, 374.

Wang, L. Q.; Tu, K.; Li, Y.; Zhang, J.; Jiang, L.; Zhang, Z. Synthesis and Characterization of Temperature Responsive Graft Copolymers of Dextran with Poly(N-Isopropylacrylamide). *React. Funct. Polym.* **2002**, *53*, 19.

Williams, D. F. On the Nature of Biomaterials. *Biomaterials* **2009**, *30*, 5897–5909.

World Health Organization. Compendium of Food Additive Specifications. Addendum. Compendium, Rome: FAO – Food and Agriculture Organization of the United Nations, **1997**, *5*, 52.

Yang, J.-S.; Xie, Y.-J.; He, W. Research Progress on Chemical Modification of Alginate: A Review. *Carbohydr. Polym.* **2011**, *84*, 33–39.

Yaphe W; Morgan K Enzymic Hydrolysis of Fucoidin by Pseudomonas Atlantica and *Pseudomonas Carrageenovora*. Nature, London. **1959**, *183*, 761–762.

Ye, R. W.; Zielinski, N. A.; Chakrabarty, A. M. Purification and Characterization of Phosphomannomutase/Phosphoglucomutase from *Pseudomonas Aeruginosa* Involved in Biosynthesis of Both Alginate and Lipopolysaccharide. *J. Bacteriol,* **1994,** *176,* 4851–4857.

Zielinski, N. A.; Maharaj, R.; Roychoudhury, S.; Danganan, C. E.; Hendrickson, W.; Chakrabarty, A. M. Alginate Synthesis in *Pseudomonas Aeruginosa*: Environmental Regulation of the algC Promoter. *J. Bacteriol.* **1992,** *174,* 7680–7688.

Zimmermann, U.; Klöck, G.; Federlin, K.; Hannig, K.; Kowalski, M.; Bretzel, R. G.; et al. Production of Mitogen-Contamination Free Alginates with Variable Ratios of Mannuronic Acid to Guluronic Acid by Free Flow Electrophoresis. *Electrophoresis,* **1992,** *13,* 269–274.

CHAPTER 2

RECENT ADVANCES IN ALGINATES AS MATERIAL FOR BIOMEDICAL APPLICATIONS

MILAN MILIVOJEVIC*, IVANA PAJIC-LIJAKOVIC, and
BRANKO BUGARSKI

*Department of Chemical Engineering, Faculty of Technology and
Metallurgy, University of Belgrade, Karnegijeva 4,
Belgrade 11000, Serbia*

Corresponding author. E-mail: mmilan@tmf.bg.ac.rs

2.1 INTRODUCTION

Natural materials are among most desirable ones for biomedical applications due to their favorable properties although some synthetic polymers, alloys, and ceramic materials are widely used too, especially in cases where biomaterials lack some needed performances. However, natural materials are preferable in all cases where those lacks are not present. Among many desirable properties that one biomaterial should have are inherent biocompatibility, low toxicity, reproducible properties, low cost, mechanical stability, and easy manipulation. Numerous biomaterials indeed possess some of listed properties and are used for particular applications where these features are needed, but very little number of them have almost all of those attributes and are used in wide variety of applications. Alginates are one of those rare and there is a constant rise in a number of their investigations and applications. With increased research, some of their disadvantages have appeared but their favorable attributes have led to the broad investigations about ways to physically or chemically overcome those drawbacks.

Various aspects of alginates such as their properties, advantages, drawbacks, and ways of their chemical or physical modifications in order to tailor their properties to suit demanded applications, as well as, recent advances in the use of alginate and its derivatives for different pharmaceutical and biomedical applications, like drug delivery and controlled release of encapsulated drugs, wound healing, tissue engineering and regeneration, and some others, are discussed in the current chapter.

2.2 NATURAL SOURCES OF ALGINATES

Alginates are mostly available in the form of sodium salts products of alginic acid and they represent one of the most abundant families of the natural anionic polysaccharides. Having in mind that alginates may be produced not only by macroalgae but also by microalgae and some strains of soil bacteria, it may be said that their sources are almost unlimited. Alginates are unbranched (linearly structured), water-soluble biopolymers with high molecular weight (MW) (Milivojevic et al., 2015), and many favorable properties that have made them nowadays to be widely used and studied for many different applications, particularly biomedical and pharmaceutical (Giri et al., 2012; Lee and Mooney, 2012). Although nearly all alginic acid salts that are commercially available were derived from brown algae cell walls (Phaeophyceae such as *Ascophyllum nodosum, Durvillaea antarctica, Ecklonia maxima, Laminaria digitata, Laminaria hyperborea, Laminaria japonica, Lessonia nigrescens,* and *Macrocystis pyrifera*) (Rehm, 2009), they could be also produced as an exocellular polymer by some Gram-negative bacteria strains (*Azotobacter vinelandii* and many *Pseudomonas* sp.) (Hay et al., 2013), but, it is at the moment economically unfeasible. This ratio may be changed in future since alginates obtained by bacterial biosynthesis may give alginates with more defined physical and chemical properties than those derived from the seaweed (Lee and Mooney, 2012; Hay et al., 2013). In seaweeds, mixture of insoluble Ca^{2+}, Mg^{2+}, K^+, and Na^+ alginates salts constitute up to 40% of their dry weight, with percentage mostly dependent on algae species (i.e., 22–30% for *A. nodosum,* 22–44% for *L. digitata*, and 17–45% in *Sargassum* spp.) and their part (i.e., 25–44% in *L. digitata* fronds, 35–47% in *L. digitata* stipes, 17–33% in *L. hyperborea* fronds, and 25–38% in *L. hyperborea* stipes), growth season, and conditions (O'Sullivan et al., 2010). Those salts are mainly present in the intercellular spaces and cell walls of algae and give them not only the mechanical strength and flexibility but also serve as a water reservoir that prevents their dehydration if they are exposed to the air. The flexibility of alginates is connected to their composition, since they are, unlike cellulose, composed of two different sugar molecules, uronates (guluronic and mannuronic acid salts)

(Stojkovska et al., 2010). Those two building units may be linked together (usually 1000–3000 units in one molecule) in endless number of different combinations, making alginate chains partly flexible and partly stiff, and having MWs in the range between 32,000 and 400,000 g/mol (George and Abraham, 2006).

2.3 CHEMICAL STRUCTURE OF ALGINIC ACID

Alginates are natural polysaccharides present in algae, where they have a similar role as cellulose or starch in terrestrial plants. However, unlike cellulose, which is the polymer composed of only one type of molecule—glucose, alginates are unbranched copolymers composed of two types of molecules, both uronates. This composition gives them specific characteristics that differ from other natural polymers. They are made up of irregular ratios of β-D-mannuronate (M) and its C-5 epimer α-L-guluronate (G) linked by 1→4 glycosidic bonds (Sun and Tan, 2013). The β-D-mannuronic acid (M) and α-L-guluronic acid (G) are monosaccharides that have carboxylic acid at C_6 that was created by oxidization (O'Sullivan et al., 2010). The chain is constituted by these two acids joined together to form a blockwise pattern. The uronic acids have different conformations—4C1 for the β-D-mannuronic acid and 1C4 for the α-L-guluronic acid. When those acids are within the polymer chain acid monomers have tendencies to form energetically most favorable structure. This is 1C4 chair form linked together with an α-(1→4) glycosidic bond for GG-block, while for MM-block conformation is the 4C1 chair linked by β-(1→4) glycosidic bond. The types of acids being linked together have a great impact on the rigidity of chain. The GG-blocks have an axial/axial glycosidic bond and are thus buckled and stiff. The MM-block has a flat ribbonlike chain conformation because of its equatorial/equatorial glycosidic bond created by the already-mentioned large carboxylic group. The MG-blocks have an equatorial/axial glycosidic bond that causes their greater flexibility compared to the two previous types of blocks. Guluronic residues have a greater affinity for divalent ions (i.e., Ca^{2+}) than mannuronic ones and the give gels with higher strength. Considering this, the block rigidity should decrease this way: GG>MM>MG (Stokke et al., 1993a), but some recent findings have shown that the block components exhibit practically the same rigidity when analyzed separately (Vold et al., 2006).

After analyzing the structure of the alginates, it is obvious that they are a family of linear copolymers that have three types of blocks that have GG, MM, and MG residues—the homopolymeric G-blocks (GGGG) and

M-blocks (MMMM) and the heteropolymeric blocks (MGMG) whose percentages and distributions highly determine the physical and chemical properties of the molecule (Stojkovska et al., 2010), while the natural source dictates the mentioned ratio and the length of each building block. Because of those facts, there are at least 200 different alginates being manufactured today, primarily as a Na–alginate.

It is believed that only the G-blocks cross-link intermolecularly with divalent cations to form hydrogels, so to enhance the mechanical properties of the gel, typically the length of G-block and the MW should be increased (this can be done by using the alginate produced by the *Azotobacter*) (Hay et al., 2013). Any change in hydrogel composition, density, stiffness, viscoelasticity, or orientation affects the gel stability, drug release rate, and activity and phenotype of the encapsulated cells (Lee and Mooney, 2012).

2.4 PROPERTIES OF ALGINATES AND THEIR SOLUTIONS

There are many alginates properties that make them attractive polyelectrolytes and biopolymers for uses in many industries and the interest for the alginates is rising at this moment in many branches of biomedical and engineering sciences (Lee and Mooney, 2012; Milivojevic et al., 2015). In the presence of polyvalent cations (such as Ca^{2+}), they form gels very easily, while some other important and good properties that they possess are relatively high water solubility, natural abundance, relatively low cost, biocompatibility, bioadhesivity, biodegradability, nontoxicity, relatively nonimmunogenicity, sufficient transparency, relative stability, and ease of use (George and Abraham, 2006; Milivojevic et al., 2015). One not so good property of the alginic acid is its limited stability that forces the producers to transform it into different alginate salt forms that are stable (Onsøyen, 2001).

As it was mentioned before, gelling, stabilizing, and viscosifying properties can be changed by changing the composition and chemical structure of the alginates (Rehm, 2009). A challenging task for every researcher is to determine the exact composition and structure that is the best for wanted application, because they possess polydisperse MW which is affected by their natural (bacterial or enzymatic) sources. The main reasons for this heterogeneity are: production of the polysaccharides is under enzyme control, while genes do not affect it (Ertesvåg, 2015); alginate extraction process causes its depolymerization (Rehm, 2009); temperature, pH, contaminants, and free radicals also influence alginates stability (Milivojevic et al., 2015). This heterogeneity is one of the major drawbacks of alginates in their biomedical applications.

Several of the alginate gel's functional properties (porosity, swelling, stability, biodegradability, biocompatibility, strength, and immunogenicity) depend on the composition, structure, MW, and even on the gel-forming kinetics, and the gelling cation type (George and Abraham, 2006; Ertesvåg, 2015).

In order to eliminate this, many (bio)chemical techniques were combined to tailor alginate's properties as desired (by controlling their structure and the nature, location, and quantity of the substituents), which led to many derivatives being produced in the recent years (Pawar and Edgar, 2011).

2.4.1 BIOCOMPATIBILITY OF ALGINATES

Among alginate's properties, biocompatibility is a critical issue for their use in biomedical applications, especially for the long-term functioning on multiple therapeutic systems (Orive et al., 2005). They are considered as safe for in vitro and in vivo use (Lee and Mooney, 2012). The Food and Drug Administration regards alginates as generally safe (George and Abraham, 2006), and they are considered highly biocompatible, nontoxic, and nonimmunogenic (Rokstad et al., 2011), while when given orally, they are considered nontoxic and biodegradable (Cook et al., 2014), even though they are inherently nondegradable in mammals because of the lack of the needed enzyme—alginase—that is needed to split the polymer chains, and though many alginates available in the market cannot be removed by the body because their average MW is higher than the renal clearance of the kidneys (Al-Shamkhani and Duncan, 1995). To cope with their nondegradability by the human bodies, a partial oxidation of the alginate chains is an attractive approach (Lee and Mooney, 2012).

There is still an ongoing debate on the impact of the alginate's chemical structure on the biocompatibility of the alginates although many experiments took place. A clear difference was revealed between biocompatibility of the nonpurified and the purified alginates (Orive et al., 2005). It was observed that M-blocks triggered an immune response in some cases (Stokke et al., 1993b), as well as, in several animal in vivo models (Skjåk-Bræk et al., 2000). The G-blocks that have a polymerization degree of 10–20 were found to be nonimmunogenic (Otterlei et al., 1991). The alginates rich in M content are immunogenic and induce cytokine production 10 times more than high G alginates as shown in some studies (Otterlei et al., 1991), but in other experiments, little or no immune response was found around alginate implants (Zimmermann et al., 1992). This confusion is likely related to the purity of the alginates used in the reports because the immune response at the injection or implantation sites could be attributed to the impurities in the alginates or some other cause (Orive et al., 2005). The natural alginates could have various impurities such as heavy metals, proteins, endotoxins, and polyphenolic compounds and when the highly purified alginates (purified by a multistep extraction) were examined, it was observed that they did not trigger any significant foreign body reaction (Lee and Mooney, 2012).

2.4.2   GEL FORMATION AND METHODS OF GELLING

Gel formation may be the most useful of alginates, while the most preferable feature connected to the gelling is that three-dimensional (3D) gels are formed under very mild conditions. Those characteristics caused them to become one of the most used biopolymers in the industry and especially in the biomedical sciences. The biopolymers are able to absorb large amounts of the water owing to the abundant presence of hydrophilic groups ($-OH$, $-CONH-$, $-CONH_2-$ and $-SO_3H$). Thanks to this groups, polymers with the adequate composition in the right environment form complex hydrogel structures and become highly hydrated (up to and more than 95 wt.%) (Peppas, 1991; George and Abraham, 2006). The gel formation and its properties are dependent on the chemical structure, MW, and concentration of alginate and divalent ions (Ouwerx et al., 1998).

There are a few different methods that can be used to prepare those hydrogels: addition of polyionic cations, covalent or cell cross-linking, and thermal gelation (Lee and Mooney, 2012). The most important method among all mentioned is ionic cross-linking because the solgel transition in the presence of divalent cations (such as Ca^{2+}, Sr^{2+} or Ba^{2+}) is carried out under extremely mild temperature and pH, and may give nontoxic reactants (when Ca^{2+} cations are used), so this method is very suitable when the sensitive biomolecules are immobilized (such as nucleic acid, proteins, or living cells) (Mohan and Nair, 2005; George and Abraham, 2006; Rehm, 2009).

Mostly used chemical for the Na–alginate gelation is highly soluble calcium chloride ($CaCl_2$), so the gelation becomes fast and irreversible (Larsen et al., 2015), but also poorly controlled. The gelation rate is a critical factor that needs to be controlled since slower gelation gives the more uniform and mechanically strong structures (Kuo and Ma, 2001) and this rate can be done either by using the less soluble salts (such as $CaCO_3$ or

CaSO$_4$), or by lowering the temperature what lowers the ionic cross-linkers reactivity (Lee and Mooney, 2012).

The alginate polysaccharide affinity toward divalent cations increases in the following manner: $Mg^{2+} \ll Mn^{2+} < Ca^{2+} < Sr^{2+} < Ba^{2+} < Cu^{2+} < Pb^{2+}$ (Chan and Mooney, 2013). The affinity depends on the alginate's chemical structure (more G-blocks cause greater affinity), sequence, G-block length, and MW (Milivojevic et al., 2015). It is believed that only the G-blocks form so-called egg-box structure with divalent cations. According to the "egg-box" model of cross-linking, a chelate structure with divalent ions is formed when polyguluronate (GG)-blocks from one polymer molecule form a junction with the guluronate blocks of the adjacent polymer molecule, while the needed high degree of coordination of the ions is provided by the structure of the G-blocks (Pajic-Lijakovic et al., 2010). Thus, formed junctions are kinetically stable toward the dissociation. Polymannuronate (MM) units' divalent cation binding has normal polyelectrolyte properties.

The reported strength of the ion–block bond depends on the type of block, while the order of the ions is the same as for the affinity (Milivojevic et al., 2015):

GG-blocks: $Mg^{2+} \ll Ca^{2+} < Sr^{2+} < Ba^{2+}$;

MM-blocks: $Mg^{2+} \ll Ca^{2+} \ll Sr^{2+} < Ba^{2+}$;

MG-blocks: $Mg^{2+} \ll Ca^{2+} \ll Sr^{2+} \ll Ba^{2+}$

The rigidity of the alginate gels preserves the same ion order as affinity:

$Mn^{2+} < Co^{2+} < Zn^{2+} < Ni^{2+} < Ca^{2+} < Cd^{2+} < Sr^{2+} < Ba^{2+}$, $Cu^{2+} < Pb^{2+}$ (Rehm, 2009).

The mechanical properties of the formed hydrogels depend on the composition of the polysaccharides. It was found that the overall content of the G-blocks does not correlate with the gel strength, while this correlation was found with the length of these same blocks (Aarstad et al., 2013). The Young's modulus was very much influenced when 4~15 polyguluronate (GG) units were present (Rehm, 2009). Mechanical rigidity of the gel increases when the ionic binding is increased which was found in the alginates that are rich in G residues, that have long G-blocks and that have high MW (Kuo and Ma, 2001; Mohan and Nair, 2005). However, an increase in the MW is not desired because it leads to the increase in the viscosity which becomes a problem in processing (Kuo and Ma, 2008). This may be solved by using a combination of high- and low-MW molecules where the elastic modulus can be much increased while the viscosity is increased for a very small value (Kong et al., 2002).

Besides the ionic gels, the alginates are able to form the acids gels at pH below the pKa value of the mannuronic acid (pKa=3.38) and the gulu- ronic acid (pKa=3.65) (Milivojevic et al., 2015). The acid gels require the homopolymeric regions in the polymers and the most important stabilizing element is the G-block (Draget et al., 1994). The M-blocks also have a role in supporting the gels which are more of an equilibrium type (Draget et al., 1997), what differs from the ionic gels. To increase the stability, the alginic acid can be converted to propylene glycol alginate (PGA) when its free carboxylic group reacts with propylene oxide (Onsøyen, 2001). The acid's gels usage is very limited at the moment, except in some pharmaceutical uses (Mohan and Nair, 2005).

Alginate hydrogels can be covalently cross-linked, too. In this case, the nature of the cross-linking agent and the cross-linking density control the gel properties (Huang and Lin, 2017). As cross-linking agents, many different kinds of reagents (polycations) were used to form complexes which stabilize the gel network, improve its mechanical properties, or lower its permeability like poly-L-lysine (PLL) (Rajaonarivony et al., 1993; Quong and Neufeld, 1999; Ferreiro et al., 2002), poly(ethylene glycol)diamines (Lee and Mooney, 2012), aminopolyoxyethylene (Chen et al., 1998), DEAE-dextran (Huguet et al., 1996), chitosan (Coppi et al., 2001; Vandenberg et al., 2001), and proteins (Singh and Burgee, 1989; Lévy and Lévy, 1996). In these cases, the unreacted chemicals must be removed with special care because some covalent cross-linking reagents may be toxic (Reis et al., 2008).

A different approach that has been used is photo-cross-linking (by using laser light) that exploits covalent linking for in situ gel formation (Jeon et al., 2009). The alginate is first grafted with acrylate or allyl groups after which a covalent cross-linking by ultraviolet photopolymerization takes place to form strong and very deformable gels. The good side of this approach is that it can be carried out under mild conditions so it has a very good potential for stitchless surgeries, but some reagents can be harmful to the body because they could involve the use of a light sensitizer or an acid could be formed when reacting (Tanaka and Sato, 1972). The ability of these alginates for the cell adhesion could be further improved by incorporating Mg^{2+} ions in them since it affects their hydrophobicity (Yin et al., 2015). In addition, the elastic modulus, swelling behavior, or degradation rates of photo-cross-linked alginate hydro- gels could be controlled by varying the degree of alginate methacrylation, thus giving those materials a great potential to be used as therapeutic materials in regenerative medicine and bioactive factor delivery (Jeon et al., 2009).

Another interesting approach for preparing alginate gels is using freeze–thaw technique (Zhao et al., 2016a). Alginate polymers associate into certain structures during freeze solvent crystallization and after thawing those structures became the junction zones. It allows preparing alginate gels even at pH 4.0 and 3.5, two at which normally acid gels could not be formed. Thus, formed gels at pH 3.0 have increased gel storage modulus for almost two orders of the magnitude. The dynamic moduli and gel syneresis were influenced by a number of freeze–thaw cycles, alginate concentrations, pH values, and ionic strengths.

Thermosensitive hydrogels have a potential in biomedical applications, but alginate hydrogels were investigated only in few cases (Tan et al., 2012; Huang et al., 2016; Fang et al., 2017). The reason for this is that the alginate is not inherently thermosensitive and was overcome by preparing the structures that semiinterpenetrated polymer network through in situ copolymerizations. The most used gel of this type is poly(N-isopropylacrylamide), or PNIPAAM, because it undergoes a reversible phase transition around the temperature of the body in the aqueous media (Rzaev et al., 2007).

Although cell attachment on alginate gels is not possible, alginates modified with cell-adhesive ligands can cross-link with cells without the need for some other molecules (Ekerdt et al., 2013). This ligand–receptor links are weak, shear reversible, and can be formed many times, and when the gel structure is destroyed by shear forces, it needs only a few minutes to recover (Lee et al., 2003).

The most important technological properties of the alginate gels are their mechanical strength, porosity/diffusion, alginate distribution, shrink–swell capacity, and transparency (Milivojevic et al., 2015). They can become firm or soft, brittle or flexible, depending on the manufacturing process. Alginates that have high G-block content are strong, brittle, and have good thermal stability because of the greater affinity for divalent cations, while high M-block content causes weak, much tender, and elastic gels that are freeze–melt stable (Pawar and Edgar, 2011).

The gel's mechanical strength highly influence the gel's porosity/diffusion. High G-block content causes higher elastic moduli and higher diffusion rates (Pajic-Lijakovic et al., 2010) because their long G-blocks and short elastic parts are more stiff open when compared to the low G-block networks, which have long elastic blocks and are more dynamic and entangled (Milivojevic et al., 2015). The alginate gels are partly a solution and partly a solid (at the junction zones). Although they can have up to 99–99.5% water because of their good water-holding capacity, caused by the capillary forces, they retain their shape and resist stress as if they were a solid. These water molecules are entrapped in the gel by the alginate network but they are able to migrate (Imeson, 2009), so those gels can be used in many applications like cell immobilizations (Onsøyen, 2001). The levels of calcium in the gel determine whether the chains are temporarily or permanently associated: low levels cause temporary associations, high viscosity, and thixotropy, while high levels cause permanent associations (George and Abraham, 2006).

When the gel network is formed only by molecular entanglement or secondary forces (i.e., ionic, H-bonding, hydrophobic), or both, they are called physical or reversible gels (Milivojevic et al., 2015). These gels are not homogeneous because heterogeneity is created by the molecular entanglements or domains made by the secondary forces and because the free chain ends and loops are transient network defects (Hoffman, 2012).

The alginate hydrogel can be dissolved using the sodium citrate, phosphate or hexametaphosphate solution or when they are imposed to the intestinal fluid (Voo et al., 2016). Calcium cations can be detached from the network by soluble anions or just substituted by monovalent cations (Milivojevic et al., 2015).

Although there are different alginates that come from natural sources, today there is an existing need for making more alginates that possess desired physical and chemical characteristic (Milivojevic et al., 2015). If one wants to do this, the approach must be systematic and include everything from the genetics and biosynthesis to physical and chemical characteristics and processing. This path could lead to further research and increase the number of alginate's applications and make them usable in some potential new fields.

2.4.3   VISCOSITY OF ALGINATE SOLUTIONS AND GELS

Alginate solutions and gel viscosities are among their most important properties (Belalia and Djelali, 2014). There is a broad range of alginate applications that are mainly connected with their efficiency in controlling the rheology of aqueous solutions, since viscosity may be increased up to two orders in magnitude by addition of small amounts of alginate (up to 10 wt.%) (Mazur et al., 2014). A variable that has the strongest effect on the rheology of the alginate solution and gels is their MW (Fernandez and Norton, 2014). Alginate hydrogels are non-Newtonian, pseudoplastic fluids because of their shear-tinning characteristics (when shear rate increases, the viscosity drops) (Mitchell and Blanchard, 1974). The alginate's viscosity can be changed from low (free-flowing) to high (drip-free) values by changing the grade and the formulation. The shear sensitivity increases when the viscosity increases or when calcium or acid are introduced into the system or their levels are increased (Onsøyen, 2001).

The viscosity and the strength of the alginate gel determine the expansion and the flexibility of the gel and are influenced by the average MW (the length of the chains), the temperature, the solvent type, the ionic strength, the chemical structure (M/G ratio) (Draget et al., 1994; Ouwerx et al., 1998). As the MW increases, so does the viscosity (Rehm, 2009). The G-blocks increase the viscosity because the rotation around the glycosidic bonds is slightly obstructed so the polymer molecules in the solution are stiff; so, the solution of long stiff molecules is highly viscous. Temperature strongly influences the solution viscosity since an increase in the temperature of 1°C leads to a decrease of the viscosity of around 2.5% (Onsøyen, 2001).

2.4.4 SOLUBILITY OF ALGINIC ACID AND SALTS

Alginates are soluble in water but dissolve very slowly forming a viscous solution, while in ethanol and ether, they are insoluble. The alginate's solubility in the water is mostly determined by solvent's pH, medium's ionic strength, and the existence of the gelling ions in the solvent (Draget, 2009), while it can also be limited by the environmental conditions that do not change the ionic strength. The critical factor is the pH of the solution when it drops below the pKa of the uronic acids, phases separate, or hydrogel forms. The polysaccharide's precipitation with lowering the pH is also influenced by the MW and the composition (Milivojevic et al., 2015) because the MG-block-rich alginates have lower precipitation tendency than M- and G-rich alginates (probably because of their bond's higher conformational "disorders") (Hartmann et al., 2006).

2.4.5 STABILITY

Stability of solid alginates is related to their degree of polymerization (DP), while their depolymerization depends on alginate grades (low, medium, or high viscosity). High DP alginates are less stable compared to a low DP. Sodium alginates are the most stable form (particularly low viscosity), then comes propylene glycol and ammonium alginate, while alginic acid is the least stable among solid form of alginates. Hence, their storage should be in a cool and dry place. The stability of alginate solutions is higher than in solid forms and it is dependent on DP, presence of antimicrobial substances, and temperature and pH of the solution (Wasikiewicz et al., 2005).

The gel performance with the time is directly related to the hydrogel's stability (Leonard et al., 2004), which depends on the pH, the temperature, and the presence of contaminants. In both the acidic and the alkaline media, the sugar monomers' glycosidic linkages are susceptible to splitting (Smidsrød et al., 1966), which can happen even at the neutral pH in the presence of the reducing compounds, while all chain degradations are boosted by the temperature (Rehm, 2009). Alginate chains can be depolymerized by redox reaction by some free radicals like polyphenols and the enzyme lyase is able to degrade alginates to the unsaturated compounds (Milivojevic et al., 2015). Water solution of alginates can be degraded by bacterial activity (Polyzois and Andreopoulos, 1985). Alginates can be made to be photodegradable if this is needed (Narayanan et al., 2012). The safe handling conditions for alginates are a neutral pH and a limited heating (Milivojevic et al., 2015).

Alginate degradations may be consequence of some sterilization techniques such as autoclaving, heating, ethylene oxide treatment and gamma irradiation which could also cause polysaccharide damage (Draget et al., 1997). Since those sterilization techniques should be avoided, the recommended procedure is filtration over 0.22-mm filters (Rehm, 2009).

The calcium alginate gels' should not come in contact with sequestering agents of calcium ion such as citrate, phosphate, lactate, and EDTA because they will remove the cross-linking calcium from the network junctions (Zhu, 2007). High concentrations of competing ions will lower the network's stability, for example, Na^+ in a physiological saline solution (0.15 mol/L NaCl) (Rehm, 2009). Ionic alginate hydrogels have low stability in vivo because the ion exchange with monovalent ions in physiological media destabilizes the gel and causes its rupture (Thu et al., 1996b), but there are some strategies to overcome this problem (Nunamaker et al., 2007). The best strategy is to replace the Ca^{2+} ions with stronger binding ions—Ba^{2+} or Sr^{2+}—while using high G content alginates (Milivojevic et al., 2015). The biggest concern in this approach is the toxicity of these ions, but in one study there was no Ba^{2+} leakage detected from high G alginate hydrogels after extensive rinsing, while a significant stability increase was observed (Thu et al., 1996a). Another approach is in situ gelling (Nunamaker et al., 2007). An attractive strategy for overcoming this obstacle is by using stronger and more robust networks.

Gels with improved mechanical and swelling stability can be made by using the alginates with a high G content (>70%) and a long G-blocks (around 15 units). Strong complexes are made between alginates and polycations as well (Thu et al., 1996a). Another approach is to use alginate/ reduced graphene oxide double-network hydrogel (Zhuang and Yu, 2016). The covalent cross-links could be introduced in addition to the ion-induced ones. Alginate's covalent grafting with synthetic polymers, a combination of ionic and covalent cross-linking on the polysaccharide, the direct reticulation of poly(l-lysine) on alginate, and other techniques were attempted (Dusseault et al., 2008). The alginates with improved swelling stability in a saline solution were made by an enzymatic approach that led to the long alternating sequences in the polymer (Mørch et al., 2007).

2.5 CHEMICAL AND BIOCHEMICAL MODIFICATIONS

Various alginic acid derivatives that differ in the monosaccharide sequence and nature, or location and quantity of substituents can be created by a variety of strategies and combinations of different biochemical techniques (Hay et al., 2013). All this changes result in modulated alginate properties, among which the most important ones are mechanical strength, degradation, and addition of biofunctional moieties for better chemical or cell interactions, while others are solubility, hydrophobicity, certain protein affinity, and others (Pawar and Edgar, 2011; Szekalska et al., 2016).

Derivation by the chemical modifications is the most suitable approach to fulfill both: enhancement of existing and introduction of the new properties. For example, the ionic gel strength can be improved by additional covalent cross-linking, backbone hydrophobicity may be increased, and biodegradability can be improved. In addition, anticoagulant properties may be introduced or biochemical anchors for cell interactions can be provided in order to create the next generation of alginate biomaterials for new applications (Milivojevic et al., 2015).

The alginates have two types of functional groups (free hydroxyl and carboxyl groups) along the chain that can be modified to change the alginate's characteristics. The two secondary –OH (C-2 and C-3 positions) or the one –COOH (C-6 position) can be modified through their reactivity difference in order to selectively modify just one of them. However, it is a difficult task to selectively modify only C-2 or only C-3 hydroxyl group because of their minor reactivity differences (Szekalska et al., 2016). By functionalizing these two groups, aliginate's hydrophobicity, solubility, and/ or their physical, chemical, or biological properties can be changed, while another option for these changes is selective modification of just M or just G residues (Milivojevic et al., 2015).

Chemical modifications of the polysaccharides may enhance their degradability, cell surface interactions, hydroxyapatite (HAp) nucleation, and growth, heparin-like anticoagulation behavior or give desired hydrophobic–hydrophilic balance needed for better drug releasing. Most of the chemical modifications are achieved by means of oxidation, sulfation, esterification, amidation, or grafting methods (Milivojevic et al., 2015). The chemical modifications of the hydroxyl group can be done by oxidation, sulfation, reductive amination, covalent bonding to cyclodextrin, and copolymerization, while carboxyl group modifications can be done by esterification, amidation, and Ugi reaction (Milivojevic et al., 2015).

2.5.1 OXIDATION

The most commonly used method for alginate modification is periodate oxidation. However, the main drawback of this method is depolymerization that takes place when periodate oxidation is applied to polysaccharides (Vold et al., 2006). Sodium alginate can be oxidized by sodium metaperiodate that oxidizes C-2 and C-3 hydroxyl groups to aldehyde groups, thus converting the low reactivity groups to the high reactivity ones, which lead to big rotational freedom because of the C-2–C-3 bond break, while preserving carboxylate groups and thus retaining the ionic gel-forming ability. Partial oxidation may lead to accelerated alginate degradation in aqueous media which makes them suitable for controlled drug delivery use (Bouhadir et al., 2001a). Oxidized alginates are more susceptible to further modifications (Boontheekul et al., 2005) since they contain more reactive groups compared to native alginate (Reakasame and Boccaccini, 2017). However, oxidation leads to a big decrease of the viscosity due to the MW degradation and the extension of the polymer molecule by ring opening. The connection between MW drop in periodate containing solutions and the sequence and distribution of the M and G residues was recorded and alginates with long MG-blocks were seen to degrade faster than those with shorter MG-blocks (Scott et al., 1976). In addition, oxidation of alginate chains may reduce their stiffness (Gómez et al., 2007) and increase their degradation rate (Reakasame and Boccaccini, 2017).

2.5.2 REDUCTIVE AMINATION

Oxidized alginates that possess aldehyde groups are especially susceptible to reductive amination with alkylamine by using an appropriate reducing agent which provides conversion of carbonyl groups into amines. This fact was used in the preparation of some polymeric surfactants (Zhiyong et al., 2009). The amphiphilic properties (i.e., lower surface tension, solid azobenzene solubilization, or heavy metal adsorption) in practical applications were appended to them by adding the long alkyl chains (Milivojevic et al., 2015). After this modification, alginate microsphere beads had increased loading level of the hydrophobic drug of ibuprofen along with well-controlled release rate (Zhiyong et al., 2009). The monocarboxyl-terminated polyethylene glycol (PEG) and sodium alginate's derivative with added amine functionalities were obtained by using carbodiimide chemistry in aqueous solution to produce a new graft copolymer that retained the alginate's gelation characteristics. This was possible because PEG grafting leave carboxyl groups unchanged while giving increased pore dimensions, thus resulting in improved cell anchoring (Laurienzo et al., 2005). The alginate-g-PEG copolymers could be useful in applications where higher biocompatibility and bigger pores are required. The alginates with amphiphilic properties are preferable in making drug-loaded nanofibers where the mix of amphiphilic alginate derivative and a poly(vinyl alcohol) (PVA) showed greater electrospinnability compared to the sodium alginate and PVA mix (Giri et al., 2012). The amphiphilic alginate's drug release is found to be diffusion-limited; therefore; as the cross-linker density within the alginate hydrogel increases, the drug release rates decreases (Kashyap et al., 2005). Reductive amination can give gels that are softer (Gómez et al., 2006), with a better cross-linking features (Balakrishnan et al., 2005), increased thermal stability (Boanini, 2010), and higher drug loadings with better release rate control (Zhiyong et al., 2009). Reductive aminated oxidized alginate product was used for cell microencapsulation (Mahou et al., 2014).

2.5.3   SULFATION

Natural or synthesized polysaccharides that are sulfated, either enzymatically or chemically (with formamide and chlorosulfuric acid), have great blood-compatibility and even anticoagulant activity since the resulting molecule is very similar to the heparin (Alban et al., 2002). This alginate's derivative has been widely used as anticoagulant since alginate sulfates have a bigger influence on the intrinsic coagulation pathway compared to the anticoagulant behavior of heparin, but some undesired side effects may appear in the case of oversulfation (Shah et al., 1995). Sulfated alginate was used to dampen the inflammatory cytokine response (Arlov et al., 2016).

2.5.4   GRAFT COPOLYMERIZATION

The graft copolymerization is a very good technique for modifying the physical and chemical properties of natural alginates. By grafting two polymers, or a polymer and a monomer, chemical and physical properties of grafted molecules are superimposed onto the properties of alginates (Laurienzo et al., 2005). Grafting gives an abundance of the possibilities for further reactions. The sustained release of active molecules can be improved when synthetic polymers that introduce hydrophobicity and steric bulkiness are grafted to the alginates. Some, already existing grafting copolymers are composed of alginate and poly(acrylonitrile), poly(methyl acrylate), and poly(methyl methacrylate) induced by ceric ammonium nitrate (CAN), poly(N, N-dimethylacrylamide (PDMA) (Yadav et al., 2010), methyl ester of methacrylic acid (Yang et al., 2009), itaconic acid induced by CAN or benzoyl peroxide (Isiklan et al., 2011), PVA—to make ferromagnetic copolymers (Ma et al., 2008); amylose prepared chemoenzymatically—to make disintegrable beads (Omagari et al., 2010); poly (N-isopropylacrylamide) (PNIPAAm)—to make temperature/pH-responsive gels (Kim et al., 2002a); vinyl sulfonic acid—to improve metal ion uptake, swelling, flocculation, and biodegradability resistance (Sand et al., 2010). Various copolymers of acrylamide and sodium alginate were created by using microwave irradiation (Sen et al., 2010). Some biomedically and pharmaceutically valuable products were obtained by graft copolymerization of alginates (Tripathi and Mishra, 2012; Izawa et al., 2013).

2.5.5   COVALENT BONDING TO CYCLODEXTRIN

In some cases, covalent bonding to cyclodextrin may give materials with desired properties for different biomedical applications (Izawa et al., 2013; Ivancic et al., 2016).

2.5.6   ESTERIFICATION

The hydrophobic nature of the alginates can be increased by the addition of long alkyl chains (several alcohols) or aromatic group on alginate backbone. This can be easily done by esterification in the presence of the catalyst, which results in highly viscous solutions and strong hydrogels (Pelletier et al., 2001; Leonard et al., 2004). One of such commercially used derivatives is the PGA, made by esterification with propylene oxide, which may be used in tissue engineering applications (Rehm, 2009). Oleyl alginate ester prepared from alginate modified by esterification using hydrochloric acid reaction with oleoyl chloride demonstrates the potential for sustained release of vitamin D_3 (Li et al., 2011). Some authors prepared ester of alginate by the reaction between an alkyl halide and the carboxylic groups of alginate, previously transformed into their tetrabutylammonium salt (De Boisseson et al., 2004). Another approach is to graft aliphatic polyester poly(ε-caprolactone) on alginate in order to overcome some problems with intermolecular association that may be present when alkyl moieties are grafted onto polysaccharides (Colinet et al., 2009).

2.5.7 AMIDATION

Alginates can be modified by the amide bond when their carboxylic group reacts with different amines to enhance their properties (Yang et al., 2002; Galant et al., 2006; Gómez et al., 2006; Yang et al., 2011). The mucoadhesion may be enhanced when linear PEG chains are added to hydrogel (Bernkop-Schnurch, 2002), while alginate with poly(ethylene glycol acrylate) gives mucoadhesive material with enhanced sustained release ability (Davidovich-Pinhas and Bianco-Peled, 2011). Amidation of alginate was used for encapsulation of a peptide (Hurteaux et al., 2005).

2.5.8 UGI REACTION

The hydrophobically modified alginate can be created by the Ugi reaction—a condensation reaction that includes ketone or aldehyde, an amine, an isocyanide, and a carboxylic acid (Ugi, 1962; Bu et al., 2006).

2.5.9 POLYELECTROLYTE COMPLEXES

Another option for changing alginate properties are polyelectrolyte complexes (PECs) that can be made by mixing aqueous solutions of two oppositely charged polymers. They have the properties of both ingredients and may be useful for many biomedical applications (Rehm, 2009). A big number of polyanionic (alginate) and polycationic polymer complexes were investigated because of their potential employments in medicine and similar fields (Marón et al., 2004). Depending on the polycation's concentration, the exposure time and the gel dimensions, very stable beads can be formed since the strong electrostatic forces between the two molecules increase physical interactions and partially discharge the polymer. The problem of drug leaching during the preparation can be eliminated by mixing the alginate with polymers such as chitosan, pectin, ethyl cellulose, Eudragit, or Tanfloc (Gürsoy et al., 1998; Liu and Krishnan, 1999; Sezer and Akbuga, 1999; Jeon et al., 2009; Facchi et al., 2017). Among them, the chitosan is the most widely used because of the easy cross-linking enabled by the amino groups (Sezer and Akbuga, 1999; Marón et al., 2004; Rehm, 2009; Facchi et al., 2017). The hydrogels of chitosan–alginate complexes possess pH sensitivity and were used for oral delivery of peptide or protein drugs for obtaining microcapsules for cell encapsulations and as devices for controlled release of drugs and other chemicals (Polk et al., 1994; Hari et al., 1996). As a general rule, biomolecules that do not have ionic interactions with the negative charges present in the PECs are quickly released (within a few hours) and the release profiles have a more or less noticeable burst effect. The reduction of high protein diffusion rate in the alginate beads can be done by coating them with polycationic polymers soluble in water, such as chitosan, DEAE-dextran, PLL, poly-L-ornithine (PLO), poly-methylene-co-guanidine, amino-poly(oxyethylene), polyethyleneimine, or proteins (Lim and Sun, 1980; Tanaka et al., 1984b; Lévy and Lévy, 1996; Thu et al., 1996b; Wang et al., 1997; Quong and Neufeld, 1999; Coppi et al., 2001; Vandenberg et al., 2001; de Vos et al., 2006; Straccia et al., 2015). The coating changes gel porosity so the resulting complexes are better carriers for the protein drugs. The big problem with this approach is that it might trigger immunity reaction and a formation of a fibrotic capsule when implanted in the body due to the polycation presence on the hydrogel's surface. This problem can be reduced by adding a polyanion on top of the polycation, but whether a complete removal of inflammation is possible, still is unclear (Rehm, 2009).

2.5.10 IMPROVING CELL ADHESIVITY

The alginate structure inherently lacks signal sequence for the cell adhesivity and thus has low cell surface affinity (Sun and Tan, 2013). This can be overcome by adding the cell signaling moieties—cell-specific ligands or extracellular signaling molecules, usually by introducing collagen, oligosaccharides, fibronectin, or peptides as side chains (Rowley and Mooney, 2002; Yang et al., 2002; Donati et al., 2003). This functionalization makes alginates particularly good for scaffolds in cell culture and tissue engineering because their ligands are the key for promotion and regulation of cellular interactions and might help in controlling the growth, differentiation, and behavior of cells in culture (Lee and Mooney, 2012).

2.5.11   ALGINATE MODIFICATIONS LIMITATIONS

The two biggest limitations for alginate derivations are the alginic acid tendency for decomposition under acidic, alkaline, and reductive conditions and their absolute insolubility in organic solvents. Another big problem is the reduction of the gel's mechanical stability due to the nonselective chemical modifications and the side-chain groups that are mainly grafted on the alginate's G residues (Donati et al., 2003). This causes hampering of the gel formation, but it can be overcome either by chemoenzymatic synthesis that modifies only the non-gel-forming M residues (Donati et al., 2005), or by chemically grafting mannuronan (composed only by M residues) with methacrylate, and enzymatically converting M to G residues (Rokstad et al., 2006). This results in alginate with needed mechanical properties for tissue engineering usages.

Alginates with more precisely defined structure and properties (compared to seaweed alginate) can be made by bacterial biosynthesis that already provided alginates with up to 100% mannuronate (Valla et al., 1996; Hay et al., 2013). In addition, it can sequentially modify alginates through the enzymatic conversion of M residues in the chain to G residues. This is done by applying the mannuronan C-5 epimerases obtained from *A. vinelandii*, since the G residues in alginates are introduced by these enzymes (Ertesvåg et al., 1995). *A. vinelandii* encodes a family of seven exocellular isoenzymes that can epimerize alginates into many different derivatives that have short or very long G-blocks or MG-blocks, but bacterially biosynthesized alginates are partially O-acetylated (Franklin et al., 2004; Hay et al., 2013). This higher level of acetylation considerably amplify viscosity and pseudoplasticity (Donati and Paoletti, 2009), but degree of acetylation can be controlled by application of specific strains or mutants, as well as, by changing the growth media composition or cultivation conditions (pH, temperature, and aeration) (Díaz-Barrera et al., 2010).

The better control over bacterially biosynthesized alginates may be enabled by the further modifications of producing organism or by using recombinant enzymes in vitro as the recent development in the regulation of the bacteria genetics and the bacterial modifications have been shown

(Draget et al., 1997; Lee and Mooney, 2012). Understanding and harnessing all mentioned, as well as, the contrivance of new (bio)chemical mechanisms of alginate modification, could enable the production of alginates with improved properties for different biotechnological and medical applications (Hay et al., 2013).

2.6 APPLICATIONS

Alginic acid in the pharmaceutical industry is mainly used as thickener, stabilizer, viscosity and suspending increasing agent, tablet binder and disintegrant, as well as, for sustained release and release-modifying agent (Repka and Singh, 2009). Sodium alginate has similar applications as alginic acid but it could be also used as diluent in capsule formulation (Cable, 2009). Calcium alginate is mainly used as tablet disintegrant (Shah and Thassu, 2009), while other less used alginates, as ammonium and PGAs, are used as emulsifiers, humectants, color diluents, film formers, and suspending and viscosity-increasing agents (Nause et al., 2009).

Alginates have many pharmaceutical and biomedical applications, mainly in the form of beads, capsules, films, fibers, or as blends with certain polymers, in wound dressings (Lee and Mooney, 2012; Stojkovska et al., 2014), delivering of drugs (Lee and Mooney, 2012), proteins (Takka and Acarturk, 1999), cells (Park et al., 2002; Sanchez et al., 2003), and oligonucleotides (Lambert et al., 2001; Ferreiro et al., 2002), and in tissue engineering as protein or cell delivery scaffolds (Leonard et al., 2004; George and Abraham, 2006; Lee and Mooney, 2012). There are also some more specific usages of alginates as dental impression materials, in formulations for preventing gastric reflux (Milivojevic et al., 2015), and as chelators for removing radioactive toxins from the body (Rehm, 2009).

Alginates and its hydrogels are widely used for biomedical purposes when minimum inflammation is required since they are commonly considered as biologically inert (Chan and Mooney, 2013). Both, the alginates and the alginate hydrogels are mainly processed in the form of micro- and nanoparticles, capsules, films, fibers, sponges, mats or scaffolds, as blends, composites, or nanocomposites with natural or synthetic polymers (Rehm, 2009; Sun and Tan, 2013). A significant increase in alginate applications in recent years is mainly the consequence of the pharmaceutical industry's growing need for new materials (Rehm, 2009; Lee and Mooney, 2012). The most important factor that enabled this increase was the development of the methods for tailoring the structure and properties of alginates.

2.6.1 PHARMACEUTICAL APPLICATIONS

In this chapter, more emphasis will be given on alginate use in pharmaceutical applications such as tablet formulation and as scaffolds for drug and protein delivery systems, as well as some recent advances in that field.

Alginates are primarily used as thickeners, stabilizers, or gel-forming agent in the pharmaceutical industry, mostly in oral dosage forms, and also as depots for drugs localized in tissue and for controlled drug delivery. The rates of controlled release of the macromolecular proteins, even of small chemical drugs, can be adjusted in the desired direction by proper selection of the cross-linker type and methods of their bonding. The drugs encapsulated in alginate hydrogels can be taken orally or injected in a minimally invasive way which allows many applications in the pharmaceutical industry (Lee and Mooney, 2012; Szekalska et al., 2016).

2.6.1.1 ORAL TABLET FORMULATION

Although the application of alginate hydrogels in biomedical applications is growing, the most frequent use of alginate in pharmaceutical applications is still in oral dosage forms. Capsules and tablets with alginates are commonly designed either for the immediate release of the drug, when rapid absorption is needed, or for sustained release, when drug release is controlled. When used for immediate release, alginic acid is used in compressed tablets as a disintegrant, while sodium alginate is used as tablet-binding agent. If alginates are used for controlled release, they may be used either for coating of tablets and capsules or as binding agent in combination with other chemicals in order to give a kinetically predictable and reproducible drug release. One of the main reasons that have led to the alginate's wide usage in oral tablet formulation is their trait to preserve a gel (solid-like) attributes at gastric (acidic) conditions because of the mentioned acid gel formation. Thus, it protects the gentle compounds from gastric acid by preventing the convective flow of gastric juice and by being a buffering agent in the stomach when sodium or calcium alginate is used (Milivojevic et al., 2015).

2.6.1.2 DELIVERY OF SMALL CHEMICAL DRUGS

Alginates are highly suitable as immobilization matrix for drug delivery vehicles (Elnashar et al., 2010; Giri et al., 2012). Solid (dried) alginates are

preferably used for drugs with small molecular mass since they are more suitable for them (Sun and Tan, 2013). The oral drug delivery systems (DDSs)
must provide controlled drug release, which is one of its most important
functions, and this is done by usage of different dosage forms and preparation methods among which a controlled-release tablet is preferred for patient
compliance and pharmaceutical production (Zhao et al., 2014). Alginate
hydrogels were investigated as DDS for many low-MW drugs. Accurate
control over the delivery of single versus multiple drugs or sustained versus
sequential release as a response to outside conditions is very desirable in the
DDS. Dynamical control might improve the safety and the effectiveness of
drugs and make new therapies possible. The alginate hydrogel's on-demand
drug release as a response to outside conditions could be used for designing
active depots of many drugs (Lee and Mooney, 2012).

Mechanism of drug delivery for pure alginates is based on diffusion,
namely, alginate molecule after hydration creates a highly viscous hydrocol-
loidal layer which makes a diffusion barrier that decreases the rate of small
drug molecules migration. This alginate-based diffusion system can be either
in the form of the polymer membrane, where drug molecule is encapsulated
within a drug reservoir, or the polymer matrix, where the drug is homogeneously dispersed within a polymer matrix. Generally, alginate gels rich in
guluronic acid and with higher alginate concentrations are more effective
in drug retarding (Draget et al., 2001). The drug release mechanism is very
complex and determined by the drug diffusion, hydrogel matrix swelling and
dissolution, and reactivity of the drug/matrix (Hamidi et al., 2001). The pore
sizes, their volume fraction, and their interconnections, the drug molecule
size and drug molecule–polymer interactions control the drug diffusion.
Consequently, properly chosen hydrogel network must have desired properties (porosity, swelling, mechanical strength) in order to match the chemical
composition and cross-link density with the size and composition of the drug
(Hoffman, 2012). The drugs are released by two main mechanisms—diffusion through the network pores and polymer network degradation (Wee
and Gombotz, 1998), and it can be influenced by the right selection of the
alginate type and the formulation conditions since they affect the pore size
distribution, the network density, and the swelling (Eiselt et al., 2000; Thu
et al., 2000).

Drug diffusion is considerably linked to the average pore size, their
volume fraction, size distribution, and interconnection but the determination
of the specific influence of particular parameter is usually difficult so they are
commonly included together in a parameter called "tortuosity" (Hoffman,
2012). The alginate gel pore size is usually between 5 and 200 nm (George

and Abraham, 2006) and they are so big that diffusion of small molecules is close to the one observed in pure water so they rapidly diffuse even through nanoporous (pore size ~5 nm) hydrogels (Lee and Mooney, 2012). Even the large proteins (MW$>3 \times 10^5$ Da) can easily diffuse depending on their molecule size (Tanaka et al., 1984a). In the case of small drugs, significant drug losses may be present even during the preparation of delivery system so there is an obvious need to modify porosity which can be accomplished in many different ways (Kulkarni et al., 2001). One approach is the alginate cross-linking with polymers such as chitosan, pectin, natural gums, and Eudragit lead, while the second approach is to coat alginate beads with polycationic polymers soluble in water such as chitosan (Coppi et al., 2001; Vandenberg et al., 2001), PLL (Rajaonarivony et al., 1993; Quong and Neufeld, 1999; Ferreiro et al., 2002), proteins (Singh and Burgee, 1989; Lévy and Lévy, 1996), DEAE-dextran (Huguet et al., 1996), or amino-poly(oxyethylene) (Chen et al., 1998). The coated beads and microspheres have superior properties for oral delivery (George and Abraham, 2006), while the best approach for hydrophobic drugs is to use amphiphilic gel beads prepared by grafting alginate with other polymers (Lee and Mooney, 2012).

The gel swelling and dissolution kinetics need to be considered when applying alginic acid gels as a matrix in the DDS. The rate of swelling, swelling potential, and leakage of dissolved alginate increase as M residue content increases, while MW and bead particle size are the most important factor for acid gels with high G residue content and their influence becomes less pronounced as the M residue content increases. Based on this, it should be possible to make a DDS with a unique medical release profile (Milivojevic et al., 2015). In addition, the gel stability must be determined because it directly relates to the gel performance in time. Ionically cross-linked alginate gels notably lose their initial mechanical and swelling properties within a few hours in biological buffers that contain monovalent electrolytes or calcium chelators; thus, some approaches for increasing the gel stability and controlling gel permeability were developed and they commonly include frozen and freeze-drying cross-linking and polycation complex coacervation (De Boisseson et al., 2004).

The drug molecule–network chain interactions are determined by their compositions—alginates are mostly useful when a primary or a secondary bond between the alginate and the drug can be used for regulating the drug release kinetics. Consequently, the basic molecules can be retained in the network for longer time periods than acidic molecules. Their releasing can be started by introducing the non-gelling cations or Ca^{2+}-chelating compounds to the solution, which start degrading the network, while the introduction of an electrolyte, such as sodium chloride, causes deposition of the bounded Ca^{2+} ions and an increase in the capsule permeability. Neutral (bio)molecules that have low pI are dominantly released by diffusion mechanism where a ratio of their MW to the network mesh size determines the diffusion coefficient, and usually biomolecules that are ionically noninteracting with the alginate negative charges are released quickly (within a few hours) and their release profiles frequently show a more or less obvious burst effect (Leonard et al., 2004).

The composite spherical particles prepared from sodium alginate and amorphous lactose by spray-drying (SD) method showed good compatibility and excellent micrometric properties to be used as filler for direct tableting. These tablets have decreased drug release in an acidic solution and quick drug dissolution in a neutral solution when compared to the physically mixed sodium alginate and lactose particles with the same formulating percentage, while at the same time, the amorphous lactose thermal stability in SD composite was drastically increased due to the interactions with the sodium alginate (Takeuchi et al., 1998).

The chitosan–alginate PEC is particularly attractive for controlled drug delivery (Lee and Park, 1996) and its use for coating alginate beads to control the encapsulated molecule diffusion rate and for the bead structure's bulk modifications was investigated (Anal and Stevens, 2005). These systems can be used for immobilization of the polyphenolic extracts of some medicinal herbs, which have notable polyphenol content and antioxidant activity, in microbeads (Belščak-Cvitanović, 2011), or for preparing the capsules that contain eucalyptus essential oil that had strong in vitro anti-pathogen activity (Deladino et al., 2008).

Mucoadhesive DDS increases the drug residence time at the applied location and increased drug bioavailability and effectiveness (George and Abraham, 2006). Generally, polyanion polymers are better as bioadhesives than nonionic or polycation polymers and an increase in charge density results in better adhesion (Chickering and Mathiowitz, 1995); so, the alginate is a good choice for mucoadhesion (Kwok et al., 1989), and may be used as DDS for mucosal tissues, such as the gastrointestinal tract (Wee and Gombotz, 1998).

The number of researches that use different alginate-based DDS is growing, and there are numerous examples of their use for therapeutic agents. They have been used for drugs such as those for: high pressure and cardiovascular diseases such as pilocarpine (Cohen et al., 1997), carteolol (Séchoyo et al., 2000), dipiridamol (Jamstorp et al., 2010), nifedipine (Babu et al., 2007), diltiazem hydrochloride (Mandal et al., 2010), atenolol

(Rigo et al., 2006), prazosin hydrochloride (Kulkarni et al., 2010), trandolapril (Makai et al., 2008); antitubercular drugs (Ahmad et al., 2005; Ahmad et al., 2006; Ahmad et al., 2007); antibiotics such as ampicillin (Anal and Stevens, 2005), vancomycin (Lin et al., 1999), cefadroxil (Kulkarni et al., 2001), isoniazid (Choonara et al., 2011; Kajjari et al., 2012), rifampicin (Choonara et al., 2011), gentamicin (Iannuccelli et al., 2011), amoxicillin (Angadi et al., 2012), doxycycline (Giovagnoli et al., 2010); anti-inflammatory drugs such as diclofenac (Agnihotri et al., 2005; Wang et al., 2008), valdecoxib (Thakral et al., 2011), indomethacin (Xin et al., 2010), celecoxib–hydroxypropyl-β-cyclodextrin–PVP (Mennini et al., 2012), ketoprofen (Kulkarni and Sa, 2009); tumor therapy drugs such as cisplatin and rhenium-188 (Azhdarinia et al., 2005), mitomycin C (Eroglu et al., 2005), tamoxifen (Coppi and Iannuccelli, 2009), berberine hydrochloride (Zhu et al., 2011), daunomycin (Bouhadir et al., 2000), methotrexate (Bouhadir et al., 2001b); pulmonary drugs such as theophylline (Coilent et al., 2009), aminophylline (Gao et al., 2012); hepatoprotective drugs such as silymarin (El-Sherbiny et al., 2011); drugs for epilepsy and neuropathic pain like carbamazepine (Liu et al., 2010), drug for malaria like primaquine (Balakrishnan and Jayakrishnan, 2005); medication for the treatment of parasitic infestations like albendazole (Wang et al., 2011b), or for gene delivery (Douglas et al., 2006; Krebs et al., 2010).

2.6.1.3   PROTEIN DELIVERY

Many different types of carriers for protein delivery have attracted attention in the past decades since they can deliver large biomacromolecules such as proteins and genes, in a localized, as well as, in a targeted manner (Dang and Leong, 2006). Among them, alginates are the most widely used ones and many types of different alginate-based carriers (in the forms of hydrogels, porous scaffolds, or microspheres), as well as, alginate complexes with other materials, are explored, while some of them are even commercially applied (Leonard et al., 2004; George and Abraham, 2006).

The alginates have few preferable properties for protein drug delivery. Among them, the very mild conditions needed for protein incorporation minimizes their denaturation and enables retaining of their activity. The second one is alginate's ability to protect proteins from degradation until they are released (Lee and Mooney, 2012) because at low gastric pH, the alginate shrinks, thus preventing the release of the protein (Chen et al., 2004). Finally, the third is the mucoadhesive property of the alginates that results in an increase of the encapsulated protein bioavailability and decrease in therapeutic quantity since the protein transit time is postponed and the protein release can be localized to the desired area (George and Abraham, 2006).

There are some drawbacks, too, among which the biggest ones are the rapid release rates for many proteins, caused by the alginate's hydrophilic nature and gel's inherent porosity, and the low encapsulation efficiency (Lee and Mooney, 2012). An additional problem for protein encapsulation is the alginate matrices instability at higher pH which causes rapid dissolution. Namely, when they enter into regions of the gastrointestinal tract with higher pH, the alginic acid skin converts to a soluble viscous layer and hence creates conditions for burst release of protein and its denaturation (George and Abraham, 2006). Even though the alginate gel is relatively inert to proteins, sometimes a positively charged protein can compete with Ca^{2+} ions for carboxylic acid sites in alginate matrix and cause the protein inactivation (Espevik et al., 1993).

The encapsulated protein release is done by two mechanisms—by the diffusion through polymer network pores or by the polymer network degradation, the second one is in most cases undesired since it is commonly uncontrolled and lead to rapid release of proteins. Therefore, the preferable approach is the diffusion through the pores of the intact matrix where diffusion rate of proteins within the gel depends on their molecular mass and also could be further tuned by many different strategies for controlling this rate. Usually, the proteins are released by diffusion which rate is dependent on their MW (Tanaka et al., 1984a), while another considerably affecting parameter is the protein net charge. If the charge is negative, it increases the release rate and, if positive decreases, it because of the interactions with negative charge present in the alginate (Espevik et al., 1993).

Generally, the release rate can be notably reduced by reducing the gel matrix porosity by partial drying of the beads (Smidsrød et al., 1973). The protein entrapment is better, and the protein release rate is slower in alginates with high G content and with relatively high MW (George and Abraham, 2006). The protein release rate can also be changed by partial oxidation of the alginate by changing the gel degradation rate and making the protein release somewhat dependent on the degradation reaction (Silva and Mooney, 2010). The capability of alginate gel to reduce the diffusion rate is dependent on the amount of alginate present in the gel and increasing the concentration of alginate in the gels decreases the rate of protein diffusion through the pores (Holte et al., 2006). Gels made of G-rich alginate have the more open pore structure and allow higher protein diffusion rates (Milivojevic et al., 2015). Diffusion rates of protein immobilized in the alginate matrix could be significantly reduced by cross-linking the immobilized proteins to the alginate with 1-ethyl-3-(3-dimethylaminopropyl)carbodiimide (EDC) and N-hydroxysulfosuccinimide (Zhou et al., 2009). Another method to control the protein release rate from alginate matrix is the use of different ionic cross-linkers (i.e., Zn^{2+} vs. Ca^{2+}) in order to improve generally limited ability of alginate-based systems to control this rate (Jay and Saltzman, 2009). However, one of the mostly used approaches to reduce high protein diffusion rate is to coat or mix the alginate beads with polycationic water-soluble polymers such as chitosan (Coppi et al., 2001; Vandenberg et al., 2001; Chen et al., 2004; Silva et al., 2005; George and Abraham, 2006; Li et al., 2007; Kirzhanova et al., 2016), DEAE-dextran (Huguet et al., 1996), amino-poly(oxyethylene) (Chen et al., 1998; Sun and Tan, 2013), PLL (Rajaonar-ivony et al., 1993; Quong and Neufeld, 1999; Ferreiro et al., 2002; Lawuyi et al., 2007), poly-L-hystidine (Wang et al., 2005; Chen et al., 2012b), poly-L-arginine (Lan et al., 2008; Wu et al., 2008), PLO (McQuilling et al., 2011), poly (lactic-co-glycolic acid) (Zhai et al., 2015), or proteins (Singh and Burgee, 1989; Lévy and Lévy, 1996; Rahmani and Sheardown, 2017). This approach is based on the fact that when alginates are exposed to polycations (i.e. PLL) diffusivity of small molecules is reduced. The average diameter of pores on the gel surfaces is significantly decreased when MW of those polycations is decreased and/or exposure time extended (Gong et al., 2003). When alginates are mixed with proteins, they form complexes if proteins are below their isoelectric point (pI) since the proteins in this region have a net positive charge. Thus, obtained alginate–protein complex stability and formation mostly depend on pH, ionic strength, and alginate/protein ratio. The complexation may be easily reversed by changing pH or ionic strength. Therefore, those complexes have the potential for pH/ion-sensitive drug or protein delivery (Rahmani and Sheardown, 2017). The quick release rate and bad encapsulation efficiency can be further fixed by cross-linking, by appropriate encapsulation techniques, or by increasing the protein–gel interactions (George and Abraham, 2006). The efficient encapsulation of high pI proteins, such as lysozyme or chymotrypsin, was observed in ionically cross-linked alginate microspheres as these proteins and sodium alginate can be physically cross-linked (Wells and Sheardown, 2007). Hydrophobic modification of the alginates is good approach for certain proteins, including bovine serum albumin (BSA), Hb, and *Helicobacter pylori* urease because the encapsulation yield was very high (70–100%) and no protein release was detected after several days (Leonard et al., 2004). The gelation procedure for those proteins was based on the presence of network physically stabilized by the intermolecular hydrophobic interactions of the alkyl chains linked to the alginate backbone, and not on the commonly used Ca^{2+} cross-linking. The hydrophobic parts directly interact with the proteins and thus retain them, even beside a relatively large porosity. The addition of surfactants, which disrupt intermolecular hydrophobic junctions, or of lipases, which hydrolyze the alkyl chain–polysaccharide ester bond, can cause the dissociation of the physical network and give the desired controlled protein release (Leonard et al., 2004).

Alginates were widely used for entrapment of wide number of different proteins such as melatonin (Lee and Min, 1996b), heparin (Edelman et al., 2000), hemoglobin (Huguet et al., 1994; Chen et al., 2012), myoglobin (Matricardi et al., 2006), vaccines (Kim et al., 2002b; Romalde et al., 2004), fibrinogen (Chevalier et al., 1987), fibroblast growth factor (Tanihara et al., 2001; McQuilling et al., 2011), BSA (Vandenberg et al., 2001; Lin et al., 2005; Wu et al., 2008; Zhai et al., 2015), albumin (Polk et al., 1994), human serum albumin (Lévy and Lévy, 1996), doxorubicin (Rajaonarivony et al., 1993), IgG (Chevalier et al., 1987; Gray and Dowsett, 1988), lysozyme (Zorzin et al., 2006), vascular endothelial growth factor (Drury and Mooney, 2003), hydrocortisone (Yuk et al., 1992), α-interferon (Saez et al., 2012), proteases papain (Sankalia et al., 2005), subtilisin (Simi and Abraham, 2007), adenoviruses (Park et al., 2012), plasmid DNA (Quong and Neufeld, 1999; Nograles et al., 2012), bone morphogenetic protein (Priddy et al., 2014), and, most of all, insulin (Silva et al., 2006; Ye et al., 2006; Martins et al., 2007; Reis et al., 2007; Sarmento et al., 2007; Zhang et al., 2011).

2.6.2   BIOMEDICAL APPLICATIONS

In this chapter, more emphasis will be given to using alginates in biomedical applications such as wound treatment, bone, cartilage, cardiovascular, nerve and other tissue engineering applications, and dental materials uses, as well as, some recent advances in that field.

Alginates have many advantageous properties, such as biocompatibility, hydrophilicity, nonimmunogenicity, and ease of gelation so they meet the requirements for many biomedical applications (Lee and Mooney, 2012; Khan and Ahmad, 2013). The biomaterial should interact with the body in order to heal; augment; or replace tissue, organ, or a body function (Williams, 2009). It should accomplish as many functions of the extracellular tissue matrices as possible, and thus to control the host responses (Lee and Mooney, 2012). Recently, alginates regained attention because of their natural origin and structural similarity to glucosaminoglycans, the important constituent of the living tissue exocellular matrix (Bhattarai et al., 2006; Lee and Mooney, 2012). In some cases, bioactive molecules can be released from gels, either alone or in combination with growth factors or trace elements, for enhancing the tissue repair (Silva et al., 2007).

The use of alginates in advanced biomedical therapies inevitably demands an in-depth knowledge of their chemical characteristics, structure, and function dependencies in order to adequately prepare specific alginate that is able to meet needed characteristics. Generally, the alginate gel matrix for biomedical applications should have high mechanical and chemical stability; defined pore size with narrow distribution; controllable swelling and degradability; and low content of immunogenic, pyrogenic, and toxic compounds (Orive et al., 2004).

2.6.2.1   WOUND DRESSING

The applications of alginates as wound dressing materials is one of the most promising and most used ones. The alginates were used for wound dressing for acute and chronic wounds, especially for exudating wounds such as leg ulcers, pressure sores, and surgical wounds (Qin, 2008b; Rehm, 2009). Reasons for this are numerous, but there are few that are crucial. The first is that calcium alginate is a natural haemostat (Barnett and Varley, 1987), so the wound dressings based on alginate can be used even for bleeding wounds. The second reason is that alginate sponge dressing absorbs the exudates and provides a desirable moist environment for wound healing by preventing its drying (Balakrishnan et al., 2005). This moisturizing effect can also help in avoiding the secondary injury when dressing is peeled off (Sun and Tan, 2013). They also have very good flexibility (for high M-blocks) and strength (from high G-blocks), and are transparent so the healing can be easily monitored (Thomas et al., 2000). In addition, body tolerates them very well when they come in the contact (Milivojevic et al., 2015), since their structure is similar to the tissue extracellular matrices (Lee and Mooney, 2012), and their long-term biocompatibility and stability were verified (Becker et al., 2005). Finally, alginates may be combined with different materials (i.e., Ag nanoparticles, chitosan, etc.) to form an antibacterial wound dressing, which is of utmost importance since wounds often provide favorable environments for infections which can delay healing (Balakrishnan et al., 2005; Sun and Tan, 2013).

Commercially available alginate-based wound dressings are numerous, produced by many different companies and include AlgiSite™, Algosteril®,

Kaltocarb®, Kaltogel®, Kaltostat®, Melgisorb®, Restore®, Seasorb™, Sorb-
alon®, Sorbsan®, Tegagen™, (Gong et al., 2003; Paul et al., 2004). Based
on the nature of their action, the wound dressings are classified as passive,
interactive, or bioactive products (Paul et al., 2004). The first dressing type
is the oldest, such as gauze and tulle, and it mainly acts as a barrier that
prevents pathogen entry while allowing the wound exudates evaporation
(Boateng et al., 2008). The second one is mainly made of polymeric films
that are translucent and water vapor permeable, but bacteria impermeable,
and are recommended for low exuding wound, while in the third type are
materials that deliver active substances to wound either by delivering bioactive compounds or by being made of them. When used as third class, the
alginates are combined with chitosan, proteoglycans, collagen, and non-
collagenous proteins (Paul et al., 2004; Balakrishnan et al., 2005; Straccia
et al., 2015). Among the mentioned polymers, the usage of alginates for
(epi)dermal wounds started some decades ago. They were particularly used
in non-woven alginate fiber dressings because they offer many advantageous features when compared to the traditional dressings since they can
successfully maintain a moist environment which causes rapid granulation
and re-epithelization of damaged tissue's (Thomas, 2000). Some alginate
dressings (i.e., Kaltostat®) can enhance wound healing by stimulating
monocytes to produce high levels of cytokines, while some (Sorbsan® and
Kaltostat®) activate human macrophages, that are thought to regulate the
healing process, to secrete tumor necrosis factor alpha (Thomas, 2000).

Alginate-based dressings can be used for bleeding wounds, too, because
calcium alginates are naturally hemostatic (Barnett and Varley, 1987;
Thomas, 2000). As they are hydrophilic they can be easily removed without
much trauma and pain (Paul et al., 2004; Stojkovska et al., 2014), reducing
the possibility for bacterial infection (Lee and Mooney, 2012). The positive
effect on wound healing is obviously displayed by the alginate molecule,
but it is discussed whether the release of Ca^{2+} ions from calcium alginate
promote early stage of wound healing, since these ions act as a modulator in
keratinocyte proliferation and differentiation in the homeostasis of mammalian skin (Lansdown, 2002).

There are many different types of alginate-based wound dressing and
differences between the various types may influence not only their handling
characteristics but also influence wound healing (Thomas, 2000). Alginate
dressings are made by ionically cross-linking an alginate solution with Ca^{2+}
ions to form a gel and then processed to make freeze-dried porous sheets
(foam) or fibrous non-woven dressings, so the dry alginates dressings absorb
wound fluid when applied and re-gel, but they can also supply water to a dry

wound (Lee and Mooney, 2012). Calcium alginates hence appear to be a suitable topical treatment of diabetic foot lesions from the points of healing and of tolerance (Lalau et al., 2002). Nowadays one of the most used types of alginate gels, in the wound management industry, is in the form of fibers. They have become well established and many improvements have been made to enhance the absorption and gel-forming capabilities, anti-microbial properties, and develop alginate fibers with novel functional ingredients (Qin, 2008a).

Although alginate gels are already used clinically in wound healing, their role is generally passive so many more functional and bioactive alginate wound dressings are researched. In addition, although calcium alginate may improve some cellular aspects of wound healing, it has no effect or even may have adverse effects on others (Doyle et al., 1996). Bioactive agents for enhancing the tissue repair, such as drugs or growth factors, can be integrated into the alginate as they show a good maintenance of local concentrations of biological factors, such as proteins, over an extended period of time (Silva et al., 2007).

Many different bioactive molecules that suit specific needs were added in alginate wound dressings: dibutyryl cyclic adenosine monophosphate (Balakrishnan et al., 2006), serratiopeptidase and metronidazole (Rath et al., 2011), stromal cell-derived factor-1 (Rabbany et al., 2010), fucoidan (Murakami et al., 2010), curcumin (Li et al., 2012; Yuvarani et al., 2012), zinc (Agren, 2009), or silver nanoparticles (Wiegand et al., 2009; Hooper et al., 2012; Stojkovska et al., 2014). Later were revived for clinical use because of the constant increase of existing antibiotic-resistant microorganisms (Monteiro et al., 2009) since the silver nanoparticles have strong antimicrobial activity and trigger extensive inhibitory biocide spectra for many bacteria (Guzman et al., 2012; Radzig et al., 2013), fungi (Panácek et al., 2009), and viruses (Xiang et al., 2011).

Alginate can be also used in combination with other polymers for wound dressing and a combination with a chitosan was clinically tested for treatment of chronic ulcers (Paul et al., 2004). A similar application was for alginate/antacid anti-reflux preparations, composed and tested in vitro in order to provide symptom remedy by forming a physical barrier on top of the stomach contents. Formed rafts showed effectiveness for a range of liquid products and proven to be very cohesive, buoyant, voluminous, resistant to reflux, and durable under conditions of movement (resilient). In addition, the product showed a wide range of acid neutralizing capacities (Hampson et al., 2005).

Accurate control over the sustained versus sequential release or the single versus multiple drug delivery as a response to changes in the external environment is very desirable for the future in wound dressing materials (Lee and Mooney, 2012).

2.6.2.2 TISSUE ENGINEERING

When an injury, a disease or something else, causes a certain tissue or organ failure, either partly or completely, it may be regenerated, repaired, or replaced with the natural or synthetic (artificial) substitute. Tissue engineering is usually among the last options in managing organ loss. It is aimed toward replacing or repairing missing or damaged organ or tissues by means of distributing to the demanded area supporting scaffolds with or without different types of functional cells, or immobilized growth-promoting molecules, signal molecules, or DNA that encode those molecules. Repair and replacement can be used in situations where surgery and implants have success, but even though this is a fairly successful option, there exists a need for developing materials that can replace and regenerate human tissues (Kamitakahara et al., 2008). Tissue engineering can include the use of scaffolds, therapeutics that will promote tissue repair and healing (e.g., growth factors), as well as, use of stem cells (Guo and Dipietro, 2010). Among them, scaffolds are most extensively used issue in tissue engineering. The first option for organs that are unhealthy or injured is extracorporeal blood circulation through polymeric membrane exchange device, which is mainly passive, but, in last few years, can contain entrapped or encapsulated cells from the patient (autogenic) or from other human, or even from animal (bioartificial or biohybrid) (Hoffman, 2012). The goal of today's tissue engineering is to provide patients that had a loss or a failure of an organ or a tissue, with a man-made replacement. The tissue or the organ is regenerated by repairing it through the cell delivery (Hunt et al., 2010a; Giri et al., 2012) and hydrogels are a good choice for that because they ensure a space for tissue formation and control the structure and function of the tissue. The appropriate cross-linking approach for each cell type and the target tissue is desirable in order to deliver cells in a targeted fashion (Bidarra et al., 2014). However, this cannot be done without a profound understanding of tissue biology and extracellular matrix in order to realize appropriate tissue regeneration.

The biomaterial scaffold has a key role in most tissue engineering strategies since it directs the organization, growth, and differentiation of cells in the engineered tissue. Therefore, the scaffold should provide a physical support for the cells, as well as, the chemical and biological cues needed in forming functional tissues. The basic requirements for appropriate biomaterial are to have the appropriate physical strength, to be nontoxic (and its degradation products too), non-immunogenic, with the rate of degradation similar to the rate of new tissue formation. And most of all, the biomaterial should be able to "crosstalk" with the cells on the molecular level in a controlled and precise manner, similar to the natural interactions within the tissue, or in other words to be biomimetic (Leor et al., 2005).

Alginate gels, solely and in combination with many other polymers were tested as a biomaterial scaffold (delivering vehicle) for proteins or cell populations that can regenerate or engineer tissues or organs (Kuo and Ma, 2001; Lee and Mooney, 2012). Alginates are one of the most promising and one of the most investigated biomaterials for tissue engineering for many reasons. They are biodegradable, biocompatible, and easily reshaped under very mild conditions (Milivojevic et al., 2015), their high water content permits good nutrient and gas transport and provides an aqueous environment similar to those found in soft tissues (Lum and Elisseeff, 2003), and they induce minimal inflammatory response when implanted in vivo (Marijnissen et al., 2002). Alginates are stable against the action of mammalian enzymes although they can be dissolved and eliminated in vivo through the kidneys. All this made them be one of the most used gels in transplantation and cell therapy as a selective immune barrier for protecting the transplanted cells from the immune system of the host (Lim and Sun, 1980; Rokstad et al., 2002). Furthermore, alginate ability and ease of chemical modification are also very important since they inherently lack mammalian cell adhesivity and consequently have low cell surface affinity. Therefore, they need to be chemically modified by functionalizing them with cell signaling moieties (Milivojevic et al., 2015), so the ease of covalently incorporating cell membrane receptor peptide ligands (oligosaccharides, collagen, fibronectin, or peptides), needed for cell adhesion improvement, spreading, and growth within the gel matrix, is a big advantage when compared to a more hydrophobic alternatives such as PLGA (Hoffman, 2012). This functionalization is crucial in many tissue engineering applications and the adhesion ligand type and their spatial organization in hydrogel are main variables since they can regulate cell phenotype and the regenerated tissue resultant function. Presence of cell-binding peptides, especially the sequence arginine-glycine-aspartic (RGD) acid tripeptide, in the structure of the alginate scaffold could be advantageous because these peptides mimic the cell–matrix interaction typical of the ECM. Those peptides are widely used as model cell adhesion ligands and it was observed that the spacer arm length between RGD acid and the alginate chain is a crucial parameter in regulating cellular response. The number of adherent cells in the gel and the growth rate also depend on the bulk RGD density in the hydrogel, while the cell response is dependent on the cell adhesion peptides' affinity for them. The RGD acid incorporated in alginate hydrogels makes possible control of interacting myoblasts phenotype (Rowley and Mooney, 2002), chondrocytes (Degala et al., 2011), osteoblasts (Comisar et al., 2007), ovarian follicle (Kreeger et al., 2006), and bone marrow stromal cells (BMSCs) (Wang et al., 2003; Bidarra et al., 2010), but multiple ligands or combination of ligands and soluble factors might be needed for a proper tissue or organ replacement (Lee and Mooney, 2012).

The hydrogel degradability is an important property for tissue engineering biomaterials and sometimes they need to be non-degradable and sometimes degradable or dissolvable for releasing growth factors and creating pores for penetration and proliferation of living cells (Eiselt et al., 2000; Hoffman, 2012). Limited stability of ionic alginate gels in vivo is a property that quickly and frequently have unpredictable degradation profile (Hunt et al., 2010b), which is mainly caused by ion exchange with monovalent ions present in a physiological media (Thu et al., 1996a), but, on the other hand, covalently cross-linked alginates create matrices with enhanced mechanical properties (Milivojevic et al., 2015). The alginate gel degradation in a culture media can be delayed by adding orthosilicic acid (Birdi et al., 2012). The possibility of regulating the alginate gel degradability and maintaining mechanical properties during degradation should largely increase the number of their applications in biomedicine (Birdi et al., 2012).

The hydrogel pore size and their distribution is another important parameter that can be partly achieved by selecting and purifying the alginates, by controlling gelling ions and gelling kinetics, and by interacting with other polymers (Milivojevic et al., 2015). To be used as tissue engineering scaffolds biomaterials needs pores large enough for holding living cells and freeze-dried alginate gels possess such macroporous structure needed for cell growth and transplantation and are proved for tissue reconstruction, in vitro and in animals (Tığlı and Gumusderelioglu, 2009).

Gel matrices' surface to volume ratio (dimensions) and shape (sheet, bead, or cylinder) is very important, too, because the mass transfer through the matrix, that is diffusion limited and hence determined by diffusion lengths, may limit the alginate usage for cell and tissue immobilization (Milivojevic et al., 2015). It may be improved by using cell supports that have a small diameter (1 mm in diameter), such as microbeads, that have short diffusion lengths (Stojkovska et al., 2010).

The biggest hydrogels' disadvantages are their low mechanical strength since it is not strong enough to maintain the structural shape of the regenerated tissue and this makes handling very difficult (Hutmacher, 2001). One of the most used approaches to do this is their combination with other biomaterials in order to improve the mechanical properties (Zhao et al., 2010). The same approach is used to overcome their lack of cell adhesion ability (Park and Lee, 2014; Jaikumar et al., 2015). Another disadvantage is challenging sterilization that needs to be addressed before hydrogels become more useful in the tissue engineering.

One technique that has potential application in tissue engineering is the inkjet printing, which may be used for the construction of synthetic 3D biodegradable hydrogel scaffolds. Construction is simple and uses printing of cross-linkers onto liquid alginate/gelatin solutions (Boland et al., 2007).

Alginate gels' applications and researches for cell and tissue delivery and cultivation are various. They are mainly used for cell delivery to regenerate bone, cartilage, blood vessels, liver, pancreatic, neural, and other tissues.

2.6.2.2.1 Alginates for Bone Tissue Engineering

In the cases when some kind of trauma, osseous tumor, or other disease defect the bone, the tissue engineering may help to fill defects. The bone tissue is a highly vascularized and biomineralized tissue that possess extreme mechanical strength. In addition, natural bone structural complexity is hierarchical with the different structure at macrostructural, microstructural, and nanostructural levels. Almost all bone tissue engineering approaches use temporary scaffolds that are either seeded with cells prior to implantation or designed to induce the formation of bone from the surrounding tissue after implantation. This is done by the local release of bioactive agents such as growth factors, protein drugs, or others that potentially can accelerate bone regeneration process (Venkatesan et al., 2015). Bone injury's poor healing can be improved when bone-forming cells, osteoinductive factors, or both, entrapped in alginate gel, are used (Lee and Mooney, 2012). All those factors may be applied to improve regenerative characteristics such as osteogenesis, osteoinduction, osteoconduction, and osteointegration. Till date, many different alginate scaffolds (Abbah et al., 2006; Grellier et al., 2009; Man et al., 2012; Moshaverinia et al., 2013) and composites of alginates with various polymers (i.e., chitosan (Li et al., 2005; Lee et al., 2014; Jaikumar et al., 2015) and PLGA (Quinlan et al., 2015), proteins (i.e. gelatin (Petrenko et al., 2011; Xia et al., 2012; Yan et al., 2016) and collagen (Perez et al., 2014)), inorganic materials (i.e., ceramics (Florczyk et al., 2011), biosilica (Müller et al., 2014; Wang et al., 2014), bioglass (Mourino et al., 2010;

Luo et al., 2012; Zeng et al., 2014; Zhao et al., 2016b), HAp (Lin and Yeh, 2004; Jin et al., 2012; Xia et al., 2012; Yan et al., 2016), calcium phosphate (Zhao et al., 2010; Chen et al., 2012a; Park et al., 2014)), RGD peptides (Nakaoka et al., 2013), and others (Kolambkar et al., 2011; Ma et al., 2012; Park, 2014 et al.; Venkatesan et al., 2014) were investigated for use in bone tissue engineering. There is commercially available bone graft substitute Progenix™ DBM Putty composed of DBM in type1 bovine collagen and sodium alginate.

2.6.2.2.2 Alginates for Cartilage Tissue Engineering

Cartilages are tough but flexible tissues that serve as shock absorbers. The cartilage represents composite material, fiber-reinforced that is composed of chondrocytes surrounded by ECM. In addition cartilage unlike other tissues has no blood supply and limited capacity for intrinsic repair, so commonly it can suffer serious and progressive damage even after minor lesions or injuries. Therefore, it would be of primary interest to developing appropriate and functional 3D scaffold matrix for repairing cartilage tissues in clinical applications. However, it is not an easy and simple task. Therefore, there are numerous investigations in order to attain this goal and among them, various alginate-based hydrogel scaffolds have an important part.

For in vitro cartilage regeneration by chondrogenic cell transplantation, alginates are widely used (Lee et al., 2007; Stojkovska et al., 2010; Birdi et al., 2012; Dhollander et al., 2012; Lee and Mooney, 2012). Cells usually used for this purpose are chondrocytes (that are fully differentiated cells), and BMSC, that are osteochondral progenitor cells from bone marrow. The main problems for the former are that their use is limited by the amount that could be harvested, donor site morbidity, low proliferative capacity, and the gel strength decrease caused by the network structure irregularities when they are immobilized (Gilson et al., 1990; Junter and Vinet, 2009). The main problem for the latter is that they need additional and complex biochemical signals for regulation and induction of chondrogenic differentiation when compared to chondrocytes, although they have high proliferative and regenerative capacity (Milivojevic et al., 2015).

Cartilage repair or reconstruction is mostly based on cartilage cell regeneration and culturing. Mesenchymal stem cells (MSCs) can be cultured on many different scaffolds that facilitate chondrogenesis and cartilage but there are some limitations. Native cartilages properties are hard to achieve while generation of functional cartilage by MSCs is somewhat troublesome.

Only the uniform distribution of extracellular cartilage matrix generated by MSCs give the optimum mechanical strength of the tissue; consequently, 3D structured biomaterial used for distribution of formed tissue has an essential role in cartilage tissue formation. Besides, 3D scaffold used for cartilage tissue engineering should have a degradation rate equal to the ECM production. Therefore, a 3D scaffold for cartilage tissue regeneration must have highly tuned mechanical and physical properties (two most important are mechanical stability and the degradation rate). This cannot be easily achieved since those requirements are usually confronted making the development of hydrogels with desirable properties a challenging task. One among many methods that are expected to bring best results is 3D bioprinting. Alginate, having the fast cross-linking ability, may be very applicable for this method if its small mechanical stability is overcome. Therefore, alginates are combined with other materials or chemically modified.

The main approaches in cartilage tissue repair using alginates may be roughly divided as: immobilizing chondrocytes or chondrogenetic materials in alginate hydrogel scaffolds (Lee et al., 2007; Dhollander et al., 2012; Reppel et al., 2015), using different technology and modifications to produce appropriate hydrogel (Tan et al., 2009; Wang et al., 2011b) and using injectable hydrogels for in situ 3D printing (Yan et al., 2014; Kundu et al., 2015; Markstedt et al., 2015). Normally, those approaches may be also combined together (Markstedt et al., 2015). The injectable therapies have the advantage that the tissue regenerating implant is provided directly within the defect and immediate weight bearing is allowed because almost instantly obtained implant strength and stiffness (Sun and Tan, 2013).

2.6.2.2.3 Alginates for Myocardial and Blood Vessels Tissue Engineering

Regeneration and replacement of cardiovascular tissue are among the most challenging goals in the field of tissue engineering. Neovascularization (blood vessel regeneration) and cardiac tissue regeneration can be realized by transplantation of different cell types, delivery of various angiogenic molecules (recombinant proteins or genes) or by their combination, and alginates and their composites have been widely used for this (Liberski et al., 2016; Ruvinov and Choen, 2016).

The alginates were used as support in cardiac implants (Landa et al., 2008; Leor et al., 2009; Sabbah et al., 2013), as a vehicle for delivery of cells (i.e., cardiac (Dar et al., 2002), mesenchymal stem (Yu et al., 2010), endothelial (Nemati et al., 2017)), for the controlled delivery of multiple combinations of bioactive molecules and regenerative growth factors for angiogenesis (i.e., VEGF [Hao et al., 2007; Jeon et al., 2011; Lee and Mooney, 2012; Sun and Tan, 2013], HGF [Ruvinov et al., 2010], FGF [Perets et al., 2003], peptides [Shachar et al., 2011; Wang et al., 2017b] and others [Sapir et al., 2011; Dahlmann et al., 2013]). The 3D bioprinting of alginate-based hydrogels is a promising and powerful technique for regenerating cardiac and vascular tissue (Aljohani et al., 2017).

2.6.2.2.4   Alginates for Pancreatic Tissue Engineering

Among many different polymers used for the immune isolation of pancreatic cells, the vast majority is based on alginate (de Vos et al., 2014). The alginate gel beads after isolation of pancreatic cells can be further coated with different polycations such as PLL (Lim and Sun, 1980; Thu et al., 1996a), PLO (Calafiore et al., 1996), and poly-methylene co-guanidine (Wang et al., 1997). Alginate gel capsules coated with polycations were tested in clinical trials (Calafiore et al., 2006; Basta et al., 2011). However, polycations limit the oxygen and nutrients diffusion and may have the pro-inflammatory properties so newer capsules are based only on alginate (Strand et al., 2017). This type of capsules was also clinically tested (Tuch et al., 2009; Jacobs-Tulleneers-Thevissen et al., 2013).

(Lim and Sun, 1980; Wang et al., 1997; Chen et al., 1998; de Vos et al., 2006; Lee et al., 2012).

2.6.2.2.5   Alginates for Neural Tissue Engineering

Damaged neural tissue regeneration is a very demanding task since it has complex structure and functioning. Owing to the disadvantages of currently used approaches for treating physical injured or neurodegenerative disease neural tissue there is a growing need for a proper strategy to develop appropriate 3D scaffold. Generally, hydrogels with adequate mechanical properties are desirable for neural regeneration since they allow human neural stem cells to differentiate between neurons and glial cells and they should be preferably negatively charged (Khan et al., 2015). The usage of alginate gels for regeneration and engineering of nerve tissues was also widely investigated (Prang et al., 2006; Wang et al., 2013; Grulova et al., 2015; Wang et al., 2017a).

2.6.2.2.6   Alginates for Other Tissue Engineering Applications

The alginates were also used for regeneration and engineering of many other tissues and organs such as liver (Bierwolf et al., 2012; Jitraruch et al., 2014; Shteyer et al., 2014; Lin et al., 2015), muscle (Liu et al., 2012; Ansari et al., 2016; Baniasadi et al., 2016; Yi et al., 2017), skin (Chandika et al., 2015; Solovieva et al., 2017), adipose (Galateanu et al., 2012; Xiao et al., 2017), bladder (Xiao et al., 2017), and for many other, more specific, applications.

2.6.3   ALGINATES AS DENTAL MATERIALS

Alginates are among the most frequently used dental materials since their impression is a simple and cost-effective, and they have become a necessary part of dental practice (Nandini et al., 2008). Alginates as an elastic, irreversible hydrocolloid can be used for dental impressions (orthodontic models) and other applications in dental medicine such as scaffolds for periodontal tissue regeneration (Srinivasan et al., 2011; Soran et al., 2012), bleaching trays, sports mouth guards, and others (Ratnaweera et al., 2003; Ashley, 2005). Viscous and elastic properties of alginates are among main reasons for their use as impression material, as well as their ability to produce dental impressions by the reaction between a sparingly soluble calcium salt and a soluble alginate with a resulting irreversible hydrocolloid impression (Murata et al., 2004; King et al., 2008).

SUMMARY

Alginates as natural, anionic polymers have many properties that make them very attractive for applications in many different industries. Most advantageous characteristics that make alginates so widely used are their low cost, biocompatibility, low toxicity, and especially, easy gel forming in mild conditions. In addition, an abundance of carboxyl and hydroxyl groups enables easy chemical or biochemical modification which may give the further improvement of their properties to tailor some specific demands, or to eliminate some of their disadvantages. Biomedical applications of alginates mainly include encapsulations for drug delivery and controlled release, tablet formulation, wound healing, as a scaffold for tissue engineering, dental impression materials, water absorbents, chelators, and so on. Their use in this field is attributed to their nonimmunogenicity and hydrophilicity, the simple formulation in any form (such as capsule, film, bead, or fiber), and easy blending with other polymers. However, application of alginates for modern biomedical treatments demand a comprehensive understanding of their properties, broad knowledge about the relationship between their structure and their functions, as well as, clear insight in possibilities for their chemical or biochemical methods of modifications. This chapter is focused on recent advances related to the applications, research, and development of the biomedical use of alginate and survey of possible chemical and biochemical means for their modifications.

ACKNOWLEDGMENT

This research was funded by grant III46010 from the Ministry of Science and Environmental Protection, Republic of Serbia.

KEYWORDS

- **alginates**
- **properties**
- **modifications**
- **biomedical applications**
- **pharmaceutical applications**

REFERENCES

Aarstad, O.; Strand, B. L.; Klepp-Andersen, L. M.; Skjåk-Bræk, G. Analysis of G-block Distributions and their Impact on Gel Properties of in Vitro Epimerized Mannuronan. *Biomacromolecules* **2013,** *14,* 3409–3416.

Abbah, S. A.; Lu, W. W.; Chan, D.; Cheung, K. M.; Liu, W. G.; Zhao, F.; Li, Z. Y.; Leong, J. C. Y.; Luk, K. D. K. In Vitro Evaluation of Alginate Encapsulated Adipose-Tissue Stromal Cells for Use as Injectable Bone Graft Substitute. *Biochem. Biophys. Res. Commun.* **2006,** *347,* 185–191.

Agnihotri, S. A.; Kulkarni, R. V.; Mallikarjuna, N. N.; Kulkarni, P. V.; Aminabhavi, T. M. Electrically Modulated Transport of Diclofenac Salts through Hydrogels of Sodium Alginate, Carbopol, and their Blend Polymers. *J. Appl. Polym. Sci.* **2005,** *96,* 301–311.

Agren, M. S. Zinc in Wound Repair. *Arch. Dermatol.* **1999,** *135,* 1273–1274.

Ahmad, Z.; Sharma, S.; Khuller, G. K. Inhalable Alginate Nanoparticles as Antitubercular Drug Carriers Against Experimental Tuberculosis. *Int. J. Antimicrob. Agents* **2005,** *26,* 298–303.

Ahmad, Z.; Pandey, R.; Sharma, S.; Khuller, G. K. Pharmacokinetic and Pharmacodynamic Behaviour of Antitubercular Drugs Encapsulated in Alginate Nanoparticles at Two Doses. *Int. J. Antimicrob. Agents* **2006,** *27,* 409–416.

Ahmad, Z.; Sharma, S.; Khuller, G. K. Chemotherapeutic Evaluation of Alginate Nanoparticle-Encapsulated Azole Antifungal and Antitubercular Drugs Against Murine Tuberculosis. *Nanomedicine* **2007,** *3,* 239–243.

Alban, S.; Schauerte, A.; Franz, G. Anticoagulant Sulfated Polysaccharides: Part I. Synthesis and Structure-Activity Relationships of New Pullulan Sulphates. *Carbohydr. Polym.* **2002,** *47,* 267–276.

Aljohani, W.; Ullah, M. W.; Zhang, X.; Yang, G. Bioprinting and its Applications in Tissue Engineering and Regenerative Medicine. *Int. J. Biol. Macromol.* **2017,** *107,* 261–275.

Al-Shamkhani, A.; Duncan, R. Radioiodination of Alginate via Covalently-Bound Tyrosinamide Allows Monitoring of its Fate in Vivo. *J. Bioact. Compat. Polym.* **1995,** *10,* 4–13.

Anal, A. K.; Stevens, W. F. Chitosan-Alginate Multilayer Beads for Controlled Release of Ampicillin. *Int. J. Pharm.* **2005,** *290,* 45–54.

Angadi, S. C.; Manjeshwa, L. S.; Aminabhavi, T. M. Novel Composite Blend Microbeads of Sodium Alginate Coated with Chitosan for Controlled Release of Amoxicillin. *Int. J. Biol. Macromol.* **2012,** *51,* 45–55.

Ansari, S.; Chen, C.; Xu, X.; Annabi, N.; Zadeh, H. H.; Wu, B. M.; Khademhosseini, A.; Shi, S.; Moshaverinia, A. Muscle Tissue Engineering Using Gingival Mesenchymal Stem Cells Encapsulated in Alginate Hydrogels Containing Multiple Growth Factors. *Ann. Biomed. Eng.* **2016,** *44,* 1908–1920.

Arlov, O.; Skjak-Braek, G.; Rokstad, A. M. Sulfated Alginate Microspheres Associate with Factor H and Dampen the Inflammatory Cytokine Response. *Acta Biomater.* **2016,** *42,* 180–188.

Ashley, M.; et al. Making a Good Impression: A 'How to' Paper on Dental Alginate. *Dent. Update* 2005, 32, 169–175.

Azhdarinia, A.; Yang, D.; Yu, D.; Mendez, R.; Oh, C.; Kohanim, S.; Kim, E. Regional Radiochemotherapy Using in Situ Hydrogel. *Pharm. Res.* **2005,** *22,* 776–783.

Babu, V. R.; Sairam, M.; Hosamani, K. M.; Aminabhavi, T. M. Preparation of Sodium Alginate-Methylcellulose Blend Microspheres for Controlled Release of Nifedipine. *Carbohydr. Polym.* **2007,** *69,* 241–250.

Balakrishnan, B.; Jayakrishnan, A. Self-Cross-Linking Biopolymers as Injectable in Situ Forming Biodegradable Scaffolds. *Biomaterials* **2005,** *26,* 3941–3951.

Balakrishnan, B.; Mohanty, M.; Umashankar, P. R.; Jayakrishnan, A. Evaluation of an in Situ Forming Hydrogel Wound Dressing Based on Oxidized Alginate and Gelatine. *Biomaterials* **2005,** *26,* 6335–6342.

Balakrishnan, B.; Mohanty, M.; Fernandez, A. C.; Mohanan, P. V.; Jayakrishnan, A. Evaluation of the Effect of Incorporation of Dibutyryl Cyclic Adenosine Monophosphate in an in Situ-Forming Hydrogel Wound Dressing Based on Oxidized Alginate and Gelatin. *Biomaterials* **2006,** *27,* 1355–1361.

Baniasadi, H.; Mashayekhan, S.; Fadaoddini, S.; et al. Design, Fabrication and Characterization of Oxidized Alginate-Gelatin Hydrogels for Muscle Tissue Engineering Applications. *J. Biomater. Appl.* **2016,** *31,* 152–161.

Barnett, S.; Varley, S. The Effects of Calcium Alginate on Wound Healing. *Ann. R. Coll. Surg. Engl.* **1987,** *69,* 153–155.

Basta, G.; Montanucci, P.; Luca, G.; Boselli, C.; Noya, G.; Barbaro, B.; Qi, M.; Kinzer, K. P.; Oberholzer J.; Calafiore, R. Long-Term Metabolic and Immunological Follow-Up Of Nonimmuno Suppressed Patients with Type 1 Diabetes Treated with Microencapsulated Islet Allografts: Four Cases. *Diabetes Care* **2011,** *34,* 2406–2409.

Becherán-Marón, L. B.; Peniche, C.; Argüelles-Monal, W. A. Study of the Interpolyelectrolyte Reaction Between Chitosan and Alginate: Influence of Alginate Composition and Chitosan Molecular Weight. *Int. J. Biol. Macromol.* **2004,** *34,* 127–133.

Becker, T. A.; Preul, M. C.; Bichard, W. D.; Kipke, D. R.; McDougall, C. G. Calcium Alginate Gel as a Biocompatible Material for Endovascular Arteriovenous Malformation Embolization: Six-Month Results in an Animal Model. *Neurosurgery* **2005,** *56,* 793–801.

Belalia, F.; Djelali, N. Rheological Properties of Sodium Alginate Solutions. *Rev. Roum. Chim.* **2014,** *59,* 135–145.

Belščak-Cvitanović, A.; Stojanović, R.; Manojlović, V.; Komes, D.; Juranović-Cindrić, I.; Nedović, V.; Bugarski, B. Encapsulation of Polyphenolic Antioxidants from Medicinal Plant Extracts in Alginate-Chitosan System Enhanced with Ascorbic Acid by Electrostatic Extrusion. *Food Res. Int.* **2011,** *44,* 1094–1101.

Bernkop-Schnurch, A. Mucoadhesive Polymers. In *Polymer Biomaterial;* Dumitriu, S., Ed.; Marcel Dekker: New York, 2002; pp 147–165.

Bhattarai, N.; Li, Z.; Edmondson, D.; Zhang, M. Alginate-Based Nanofibrous Scaffolds: Structural, Mechanical, and Biological Properties. *Adv. Mater.* **2006,** *18,* 1463–1467.

Bidarra, S. J.; Barrias, C. C.; Barbosa, M. A.; Soares, R.; Granja, P. L. Immobilization of Human Mesenchymal Stem Cells within RGD-Grafted Alginate Microspheres and Assessment of their Angiogenic Potential. *Biomacromolecules* **2010,** *11,* 1956–1964.

Bidarra, S. J.; Barrias, C. C.; Granja, P. L. Injectable Alginate Hydrogels for Cell Delivery in Tissue Engineering. *Acta Biomater.* **2014,** *10,* 1646–1662.

Bierwolf, J.; Lutgehetmann, M.; Deichmann, S.; Erbes, J.; Volz T.; Dandri, M.; Cohen, S.; Nashan.; B, Pollok.; J. M. Primary Human Hepatocytes from Metabolic-Disordered Children Recreate Highly Differentiated Liver-Tissue-Like Spheroids on Alginate Scaffolds. *Tissue Eng. Part A* **2012,** *18,* 1443–1453.

Birdi, G.; Bridson, R. H.; Smith, A. M.; Bohari, S. P.; Grover, L. M. Modification of Alginate Degradation Properties Using Orthosilicic Acid. *J. Mech Behav. Biomed. Mater.* **2012,** *6,* 181–718.

Boanini, E.; Rubini, K.; Panzavolta, S.; Bigi, A. Chemico-Physical Characterization of Gelatin Films Modified with Oxidized Alginate. *Acta Biomater.* **2010,** *6,* 383–388.

Boateng, J. S.; Matthews, K. H.; Stevens, H. N. E.; Eccleston, G. M. Wound Healing Dressings and Drug Delivery Systems: A Review. *J. Pharm. Sci.* **2008,** *97,* 2892–2923.

Boland, T.; Tao, X.; Damon, B. J.; Manley, B.; Kesari, P.; Jalota, S.; Bhaduri, S.; Drop-on-Demand Printing of Cells and Materials for Designer Tissue Constructs. *Mater. Sci. Eng. C* **2007,** *27,* 372–376.

Boontheekul, T.; Kong, H. J.; Mooney, D. J. Controlling Alginate Gel Degradation Utilizing Partial Oxidation and Bimodal Molecular Weight Distribution. *Biomaterials* **2005,** *26,* 2455–2465.

Bouhadir, K. H.; Kruger, G. M.; Lee, K. Y.; Mooney, D. J. Sustained and Controlled Release of Daunomycin from Cross-Linked Poly (Aldehydes Guluronate) Hydrogels. *J. Pharm. Sci.* **2000,** *89,* 910–919.

Bouhadir, K. H.; Alsberg, E.; Mooney, D. J. Hydrogels for Combination Delivery of Antineoplastic Agents. *Biomaterials* **2001a,** *22,* 2625–2633.

Bouhadir, K. H.; Lee, K. Y.; Alsberg, E.; Damm, K. L.; Anderson, K. W.; Mooney, D. J. Degradation of Partially Oxidized Alginate and its Potential Application for Tissue Engineering. *Biotechnol. Prog.* **2001b,** *17,* 945–950.

Bu, H.; Nguyen, G. T. M.; Kjøniksen, A. L. Effects of the Quantity and Structure of Hydrophobes on the Properties of Hydrophobically Modified Alginates in Aqueous Solutions. *Polym. Bull.* **2006,** *57,* 563–574.

Cable, C. G. Sodium Alginate. In *Handbook of Pharmaceutical Excipient*, 6th ed.; Rowe, R. C., Sheskey, P. J., Quinn, M. E., Eds.; Pharmaceutical Press: London, UK, 2009; pp 622–624.

Calafiore, R.; Basta, G.; Sarchielli, P.; Luca, G.; Tortoioli, C.; Brunetti, P. A Rapid Qualitative Method to Assess in Vitro Immunobarrier Competence of Pancreatic Islets Containing Alginate/Polyaminoacidic Microcapsules. *Acta Diabetol.* **1996,** *33,* 150–153.

Calafiore, R.; Basta, G.; Luca, G.; Lemmi, A.; Montanucci, M. P.; Calabrese G.; Racanicchi, L.; Mancuso, F.; Brunetti, P. Microencapsulated Pancreatic Islet Allografts into Nonimmunosuppressed Patients with Type 1 Diabetes: First Two Cases. *Diabetes Care* **2006,** *29,* 137–138.

Chan, G.; Mooney, D. J. Ca^{2+} Released from Calcium Alginate Gels can Promote Inflammatory Responses in Vitro and in Vivo. *Acta Biomater.* **2013,** *9,* 9281–9291.

Chen, J. P.; Chu, I. M.; Shiao, M. Y.; Hsu, B. R.; Fu, S. H.; Microencapsulation of Islets in PEG-Amine Modified Alginate-Poly(l-Lysine)-Alginate Microcapsules for Constructing Bioartificial Pancreas. *J. Ferment. Bioeng.* **1998,** *86,* 185–190.

Chen, S. C.; Wu, Y. C.; Mi, F. L.; Lin, Y. H.; Yu, L. C.; Sung, H. W. A Novel pH-Sensitive Hydrogel Composed of *N,O*-Carboxymethyl Chitosan and Alginate Cross-Linked by Genipin for Protein Drug Delivery. *J. Controlled Release* **2004,** *96,* 285–300.

Chen, W.; Zhou, H.; Weir, M. D.; Bao, C.; Xu, H. Umbilical Cord Stem Cells Released from Alginate-Fibrin Microbeads Inside Macroporous and Biofunctionalized Calcium Phosphate Cement for Bone Regeneration. *Acta Biomater.* **2012a,** *8,* 2297–2306.

Chen, A. Z.; Chen, M. Y.; Wang, S. B.; Huang, X. N.; Liu, Y. G.; Chen, Z. X. Poly(L-Histidine)-Chitosan/Alginate Complex Microcapsule as a Novel Drug Delivery Agent. *J. Appl. Polym. Sci.* **2012b,** *124,* 3728–3736.

Chandika, P.; Ko, S. C.; Oh, G. W.; Heo, S. Y.; Nguyen, V. T.; Jeon, Y. J.; Lee, B.; Jang, C. H.; Kim, G.; Park, W. S.; Chang, W. Choi, I. W.; Jung, W. K. Fish Collagen/Alginate/Chitooligosaccharides Integrated Scaffold for Skin Tissue Regeneration Application. *Int. J. Biol. Macromol.* **2015,** *81,* 504–513.

Chevalier, P.; Consentino, G. P.; de la Noue, J.; Rakhit, S. Comparative Study on the Diffusion of an IgG from Various Hydrogel Beads. *Biotechnol. Tech.* **1987,** *1,* 201–206.

Chickering, D. E.; Mathiowitz, E. Bioadhesive Microspheres: A Novel Electrobalance-Based Method to Study Adhesive Interactions between Individual Microspheres and Intestinal Mucosa. *J. Controlled Release* **1995,** *34,* 251–261.

Choonara, Y. E.; Pillay, V.; Ndesendo, V. M.; du-Toit, L. C.; Kumar, P.; Khan, R. A.; Murphy, C. S.; Jarvis, D. L. Polymeric Emulsion and Cross Link-Mediated Synthesis of Super Stable Nanoparticles as Sustained Release Anti-Tuberculosis Drug Carriers. *Colloids Surf. B* **2011,** *87,* 243–254.

Cohen, S.; Lobel, E.; Trevgoda, A.; Peled, Y. A Novel in Situ Forming Ophthalmic Drug Delivery System from Alginates Undergoing Gelation in the Eye. *J. Controlled Release* **1997,** *44,* 201–208.

Coilent, I.; Dulong, V.; Mocanu, G.; Picton, L.; Le-Cerf, D. New Amphiphilic and pH-Sensitive Hydrogel for Controlled Release of Model Poorly Water Soluble Drug. *Eur. J. Pharm. Biopharm.* **2009a,** *73,* 345–350.

Colinet, I.; Dulong, V.; Hamaide, T.; Le Cerf, D.; Picton, L. New Amphiphilic Modified Polysaccharides with Original Solution Behaviour in Salt Media. *Carbohydr. Polym.* **2009b,** *75,* 454–462.

Comisar, W. A.; Kazmers, N. H.; Mooney, D. J.; Linderman, J. J. Engineering RGD Nanopatterned Hydrogels to Control Preosteoblast Behavior: A Combined Computational and Experimental Approach. *Biomaterials* **2007,** *28,* 4409–4417.

Cook, M. T.; Charalampopoulos, D.; Khutoryanskiy, V. V. Microencapsulation of Probiotic Bacteria into Alginate Hydrogels. In *Hydrogels in Cell-Based Therapies;* Connon, C. J., Hamley, I. W., Eds.; RSC, Cambridge, UK, 2014; pp 95–111.

Coppi, G.; Iannuccelli, V.; Leo, E.; Bernabei, M. T.; Cameroni, R. Chitosan-Alginate Microparticles as a Protein Carrier. *Drug Dev. Ind. Pharm.* **2001,** *27,* 393–400.

Coppi, G.; Iannuccelli, V. Alginate/Chitosan Microparticles for Tamoxifen Delivery to the Lymphatic System. *Int. J. Pharm.* **2009,** *367,* 127–132.

Dahlmann, J.; Krause, A.; Möller, L.; Kensah, G.; Möwes, M.; Diekmann, A.; Martin, U.; Kirschning, A.; Gruh, I.; Dräger, G. Fully Defined in Situ Cross-Linkable Alginate and Hyaluronic Acid Hydrogels for Myocardial Tissue Engineering. *Biomaterials* **2013,** *34,* 940–951.

Dang, J. M.; Leong, K. W. Natural Polymers for Gene Delivery and Tissue Engineering. *Adv. Drug Delivery Rev.* **2006,** *58,* 487–499.

Dar, A.; Shachar, M.; Leor, J.; Cohen, S. Optimization of Cardiac Cell Seeding and Distribution in 3D Porous Alginate Scaffolds. *Biotechnol. Bioeng.* **2002,** *80,* 305–312.

Davidovich-Pinhas, M.; Bianco-Peled, H. Alginate-PEGAc. A New Mucoadhesive Polymer. *Acta Biomater.* **2011,** *7,* 625–633.

De Boisseson, M. R.; Leonard, M.; Hubert, P.; Marchal, P.; Stequert, A.; Castel, C.; Favre, E.; Dellacherie, E. Physical Alginate Hydrogels Based on Hydrophobic or Dual Hydrophobic/Ionic Interactions: Bead Formation, Structure, and Stability. *J. Colloid Interface Sci.* **2004,** *273,* 131–139.

de Vos, P.; Faas, M. M.; Strand, B.; Calafiore, R. Alginate-Based Microcapsules for Immunoisolation of Pancreatic Islets. *Biomaterials* **2006,** *27,* 5603–5617.

de Vos, P.; Lazarjani, H. A.; Poncelet, D.; Faas, M. M. Polymers in cell Encapsulation from an Enveloped Cell Perspective. *Adv. Drug Delivery Rev.* **2014,** *67–68,* 15–34.

Degala, S.; Zipfel, W. R.; Bonassar, L. J. Chondrocyte Calcium Signaling in Response to Fluid Flow is Regulated by Matrix Adhesion in 3-D Alginate Scaffolds. *Arch. Biochem. Biophys.* **2011,** *505,* 112–117.

Deladino, L.; Anbinder, P. S.; Navarro, A. S.; Martino, M. N. Encapsulation of Natural Antioxidants Extracted from *Ilex paraguariensis. Carbohydr. Polym.* **2008,** *71,* 126–134.

Dhollander, A. A. M.; Verdonk, P. C. M.; Lambrecht, S.; Verdonk, R.; Elewaut, D.; Verbruggen, G.; Almqvist, K. F. Midterm Results of the Treatment of Cartilage Defects in the Knee Using Alginate Beads Containing Human Mature Allogenic Chondrocytes. *Am. J. Sports Med.* **2012,** *40,* 75–82.

Díaz-Barrera, A.; Silva, P.; Berrios, J.; Acevedo, F. Manipulating the Molecular Weight of Alginate Produced by *Azotobacter vinelandii* in Continuous Cultures. *Bioresour. Technol.* **2010,** *101,* 9405–9408.

Donati, I.; Draget, K. I.; Borgogna, M.; Paoletti, S.; Skjåk-Bræk, G. Tailor-Made Alginate Bearing Galactose Moieties on Mannuronic Residues: Selective Modification Achieved by a Chemoenzymatic Strategy. *Biomacromolecules* **2005**, *6*, 88–98.

Donati, I.; Vetere, A.; Gamini, A.; Skjåk-Bræk, G.; Coslovi, A.; Campa, C.; Paoletti, S. Galactose-Substituted Alginate: Preliminary Characterization and Study of Gelling Properties. *Biomacromolecules* **2003**, *4*, 624–631.

Donati, I.; Paoletti, S. Material Properties of Alginates. In *Alginates: Biology and Applications;* Rehm, B. H. A., Ed.; Springer: Berlin, Heidelberg, Genmany, 2009; pp 1–53.

Douglas, K. L.; Piccirillo, C. A.; Tabrizian, M.; Effects of Alginate Inclusion on the Vector Properties of Chitosan-Based Nanoparticles. *J. Controlled Release* **2006**, *115*, 354–361.

Doyle, J. W.; Roth, T. P.; Smith, R. M.; Li, Y. Q.; Dunn, R. M. Effects of Calcium Alginate on Cellular Wound Healing Processes Modeled in Vitro. *J. Biomed. Mater. Res.* **1996**, *32*, 561–568.

Draget, K. I.; Skjåk-Bræk, G.; Smidsrød, O. Alginic Acid Gels: The Effect of Alginate Chemical Composition and Molecular Weight. *Carbohydr. Polym.* **1994**, *25*, 31–38.

Draget, K. I.; Skjåk-Bræk G.; Smidsrød, O. Alginate Based New Materials. *Int. J. Biol. Macromol.* **1997**, *21*, 47–55.

Draget, K. I.; Gaserod, O.; Aune, I.; Andersen, P. O.; Storbakken, B.; Stokke, B. T.; Smidsrød, O. Effects of Molecular Weight and Elastic Segment Flexibility on Syneresis in Ca-Alginate Gels. *Food Hydrocolloids* **2001**, *15*, 485–490.

Draget, K. I. Alginates. In *Handbook of Hydrocolloids,* 2nd ed.; Phillips, G. O., Williams, P. A., Ed.; CRC Press and Woodhead Publishing: Boca ratón, FL, 2009; pp 807–828.

Drury, J. L.; Mooney, D. L. Hydrogels for Tissue Engineering: Scaffold Design Variables and Applications. *Biomaterials* **2003**, *24*, 4337–4351.

Dusseault, J.; Langlois, G.; Meunier, M. C.; Ménard, M.; Perreault C.; Hallé, J. P. The Effect of Covalent Cross-Links between the Membrane Components of Microcapsules on the Dissemination of Encapsulated Malignant Cells. *Biomaterials* **2008**, *29*, 917–924.

Edelman, E. R.; Nathan, A.; Katada, M.; Gates, J.; Karnovsky, M. J. Perivascular Graft Heparin Delivery Using Biodegradable Polymer Wraps. *Biomaterials* **2000**, *21*, 2279–2286.

Eiselt, P.; Yeh, J.; Latvala, R. K.; Shea, L. D.; Mooney, D. J. Porous Carriers for Biomedical Applications Based on Alginate Hydrogels. *Biomaterials* **2000**, *21*, 1921–1927.

Ekerdt, B. L.; Segalman, R. A.; Schaffer, D. V. Spatial Organization of Cell-Adhesive Ligands for Advanced Cell Culture. *Biotechnol. J.* **2013**, *8*, 1411–1423.

Elnashar, M. M.; Yassin, M. A.; Moneim, A. E.; Bary, E. M. Surprising Performance of Alginate Beads for the Release of Low-Molecular-Weight Drugs. *J. Appl. Polym. Sci.* **2010**, *116*, 3021–3026.

El-Sherbiny, I. M.; Abdel-Mogib, M.; Dawidar, A. A. M.; Elsayed, A.; Smyth, H. D. Biodegradable pH-Responsive Alginate-Poly (Lactic-co-Glycolic Acid) Nano/Micro Hydrogel Matrices for Oral Delivery of Sylimarin. *Carbohydr. Polym.* **2011**, *83*, 1345–1354.

Eroglu, M.; Oeztuerk, E.; Oezdemyr, N.; Denkbap, E.; Dogan, I.; Acar, A.; Guezel, M. Mitomycin-C-Loaded Alginate Carriers for Bladder Cancer Chemotherapy: In Vivo Studies. *J. Bioact. Compat. Polym.* **2005**, *20*, 197–208.

Ertesvåg, H. Alginate-Modifying Enzymes: Biological Roles and Biotechnological Uses. *Front. Microbiol.* **2015**, *6*, 523.

Ertesvåg, H.; Høidal, H. K.; Hals, I. K.; Rian, A.; Doseth, B.; Valla, S. A Family of Modular Type Mannuronan C-5-Epimerase Genes Controls Alginate Structure in *Azotobacter vinelandii. Mol. Microbiol.* **1995**, *16*, 719–731.

Espevik, T.; Otterlei, M.; Skjak-Bræk, G.; Ryan, L.; Wright, S. D.; Sundan, A. The Involvement of CD14 in Stimulation of Cytokine Production by Uronic Acid Polymers. *Eur. J. Immunol.* **1993**, *23,* 255–261.

Facchi, D. P.; Lima, A. C.; de Oliveira, J. H.; Lazarin-Bidóia, D.; Nakamura, C. V.; Canesin, E. A.; Bonafé, E. G.; Monteiro, J. P.; Visentainer, J. V.; Muniz, E. C.; Martins, A. F. Polyelectrolyte Complexes Based on Alginate/Tanfloc: Optimization, Characterization and Medical Application. *Int. J. Biol. Macromol.* **2017**, *103,* 129–138.

Fang, X.; Lei, L.; Jiang, T.; Chen, Y.; Kang, Y. Injectable Thermosensitive Alginate/β-Tricalcium Phosphate/Aspirin Hydrogels for Bone Augmentation. *J. Biomed. Mater. Res. B* **2017**, DOI: 10.1002/jbm.b.33982.

Fernandez, I. F.; Norton, I. Formation Kinetics and Rheology of Alginate Fluid Gels Produced by in-Situ Calcium Release. *Food Hydrocolloids* **2014**, *40,* 76–84.

Ferreiro, M. G.; Tillman, L. G.; Hardee, G.; Bodmeier, R. Alginate/Poly-L-Lysine Microparticles for the Intestinal Delivery of Antisense Oligonucleotides. *Pharm. Res.* **2002**, *19,* 755–764.

Florczyk, S. J.; Kim, D. J.; Wood, D. L.; Zhang, M. Influence of Processing Parameters on Pore Structure of 3D Porous Chitosan-Alginate Polyelectrolyte Complex Scaffolds. *J. Biomed. Mater. Res. A* **2011**, *98,* 614–620.

Franklin, M. J.; Douthit, S. A.; McClure, M. A. Evidence that the AlgI/AlgJ Gene Cassette, Required for O Acetylation of *Pseudomonas aeruginosa* Alginate, Evolved by Lateral Gene Transfer. *J. Bacteriol.* **2004**, *186,* 4759–4773.

Galant, C.; Kjøniksen, A. L.; Nguyen, G. T. M.; Knudsen, K. D.; Nyström, B. Altering Associations in Aqueous Solutions of a Hydrophobically Modified Alginate in the Presence of Beta-Cyclodextrin Monomers. *J. Phys. Chem. B* **2006**, *110,* 190–195.

Galateanu, B.; Dimonie, D.; Vasile, E.; Nae, S.; Cimpean, A.; Costache, M. Layer-Shaped Alginate Hydrogels Enhance the Biological Performance of Human Adipose-Derived Stem Cells. *BMC Biotechnol* **2012**, *12,* 35.

Gao, C.; Liu, M.; Chen, J.; Chen, C. pH-and Temperature-Responsive P(DMAEMAGMA)-AlginateSemi-IPN Hydrogels Formed by Radical and Ring-Opening Polymerization for Aminophylline. *J. Biomater. Sci. Polym.* **2012**, *23,* 1039–1054.

George, M.; Abraham, T. E. Polyionic Hydrocolloids for the Intestinal Delivery of Protein Drugs: Alginate and Chitosan-A Review. *J. Controlled Release* **2006**, *114,* 1–14.

Gilson, C. D.; Hawkes, F. R.; Thomas, A. Gelling Mechanism of Alginate Beads with and without Immobilised Yeast. *Process Biochem.* **1990**, *25,* 104–108.

Giovagnoli, S.; Tsai, T.; Deluca, P. P. Formulation and Release Behaviour of Doxycycline-Alginate Hydrogel Microparticles Embede into Pluronic F127 Thermogels as a Potential New Vehicle for Doxycycline Intradermal Sustained Delivery. *AAPS PharmSciTech* **2010**, *11,* 212–220.

Giri, T. K.; Thakur, D.; Alexander, A.; Ajazuddin; Badwaik, H.; Tripathi, D. K. Alginate Based Hydrogel as a Potential Biopolymeric Carrier for Drug Delivery and Cell Delivery Systems: Present Status and Applications. *Curr. Drug Delivery* **2012**, *9,* 539–555.

Gómez, C. G.; Chambat, G.; Heyraud, A.; Villar, M. A.; Auzély-Velty, R. Synthesis and Characterization of a b-CD-Alginate Conjugate. *Polymer* **2006**, *47,* 8509–8516.

Gómez, C. G.; Rinaudo, M.; Villar, M. A. Oxidation of Sodium Alginate and Characterization of the Oxidized Derivatives. *Carbohydr. Polym.* **2007**, *67,* 296–304.

Gong, J. P.; Katsuyama, Y.; Kurokawa, T.; Osada, Y. Double Network Hydrogels with Extremely High Mechanical Strength. *Adv. Mater.* **2003**, *15,* 1155–1158.

Gray, C. J.; Dowsett, J. Retention of Insulin in Alginate Gel Beads. *Biotechnol. Bioeng.* **1988,** *31,* 607–612.

Grellier, M.; Granja, P. L.; Fricain, J. C.; Bidarra, S. J.; Renard, M.; Bareille, R.; Bourget, C.; Amédée, J.; Barbosa, M. A. The Effect of the Co-Immobilization of Human Osteoprogenitors and Endothelial Cells within Alginate Microspheres on Mineralization in a Bone Defect. *Biomaterials* **2009,** *30,* 3271–3278.

Grulova, I.; Slovinska, L.; Blasko, J.; Devaux, S.; Wisztorski, M.; Salzet, M.; Fournier, I.; Kryukov, O.; Cohen, S.; Cizkova, D. Delivery of Alginate Scaffold Releasing Two Trophic Factors for Spinal Cord Injury Repair. *Sci. Rep.* **2015,** *5,* 13702.

Guo, S.; Dipietro, L. A. Factors Affecting Wound Healing. *J. Dent. Res.* 2010, 89, 219–229.

Gürsoy, A.; Kalkan, F.; Okar, I. Preparation and Tabletting of Dipyridamole Alginate-Eudragit Microspheres. *J. Microencapsulation* **1998,** *15,* 621–628.

Guzman, M.; Dille, J.; Godet, S. Synthesis and Antibacterial Activity of Silver Nanoparticles Against Gram-Positive and Gram-Negative Bacteria. *Nanomedicine* **2012,** *8,* 37–45.

Hamidi, M.; Azadi, A.; Rafiei, P. Hydrogel Nanoparticles in Drug Delivery. *Adv. Drug Delivery Rev.* **2008,** *60,* 1638–1649.

Hampson, F. C.; Farndale, A.; Strugala, V.; Sykes, J.; Jolliffe, I. G.; Dettmar, P. W. Alginate Rafts and their Characterisation. *Int. J. Pharm.* **2005,** *294,* 137–147.

Hao, X.; Silva, E. A.; Månsson-Broberg, A.; Grinnemo, K. H.; Siddiqui, A. J.; Dellgren, G.; Wärdell, E.; Brodin, L. A.; Mooney, D. J.; Sylvén, C. Angiogenic Effects of Sequential Release of VEGF-A165 and PDGF-BB with Alginate Hydrogels After Myocardial Infarction. *Cardiovasc. Res.* **2007,** *75,* 178–185.

Hari, P. R.; Chandy, T.; Sharma, C. P. Chitosan/Calcium–Alginate Beads for Oral Delivery of Insulin. *J. Appl. Polym. Sci.* **1996,** *59,* 1795–1801.

Hartmann, M.; Dentini, M.; Draget, K. I.; Skjak-Braek, G. Enzymatic Modification of Alginates with the Mannuronan C-5 Epimerase AlgE4 Enhances their Solubility at Low pH. *Carbohydr. Polym.* **2006,** *63,* 257–262.

Hay, I. D.; Ur Rehman, Z.; Moradali, M. F.; Wang, Y.; Rehm, B. H. Microbial Alginate Production, Modification and its Applications. *Microb. Biotechnol.* **2013,** *6,* 637–650.

Hoffman, A. S. Hydrogels for Biomedical Applications. *Adv. Drug. Delivery Rev.* **2012,** *64,* 18–23.

Holte, Ø.; Tønnesen, H. H.; Karlsen, J. Measurement of Diffusion through Calcium Alginate Gel Matrices. *Pharmazie* 2006, *61,* 30–34.

Hooper, S. J.; Percival, S. L.; Hill, K. E.; Thomas, D. W.; Hayes, A. J.; Williams, D. W. The Visualisation and Speed of Kill of Wound Isolates on a Silver Alginate Dressing. *Int. Wound J.* **2012,** *9,* 633–642.

Huang, L.; Shen, M.; Li, R.; Zhang, X.; Sun, Y.; Gao, P.; Fu, H.; Liu, H.; He, Y.; Du, Y.; Cao, J.; Duan, Y. Thermo-Sensitive Composite Hydrogels Based on Poloxamer 407 and Alginate and their Therapeutic Effect in Embolization in Rabbit VX2 Liver Tumors. *Oncotarget* **2016,** *7,* 73280–73291.

Huang, S.-L.; Lin, Y.-S. The Size Stability of Alginate Beads by Different Ionic Crosslinkers. *Adv. Mater. Sci. Eng.* **2017,** *2017,* 9304592.

Huguet, M. L.; Groboillot, A.; Neufeld, R. J.; Poncelet, D.; Dellacherie, E. Hemoglobin Encapsulation in Chitosan/Calcium Alginate Beads. *J. Appl. Polym. Sci.* **1994,** *51,* 1427–1432.

Huguet, M. L.; Neufeld, R. J.; Dellacherie, E. Calcium Alginate Beads Coated with Chitosan: Effect of the Structure of Encapsulated Materials on their Release. *Process Biochem.* **1996,** *31,* 347–353.

Hunt, N. C.; Grover, L. M. Cell Encapsulation Using Biopolymer Gels for Regenerative Medicine. *Biotechnol. Lett.* **2010a,** *32,* 733–742.

Hunt, N. C.; Smith, A. M.; Gbureck, U.; Shelton, R. M.; Grover, L. M. Encapsulation of Fibroblasts Causes Accelerated Alginate Hydrogel Degradation. *Acta Biomater.* **2010b,** *6,* 3649–3656.

Hurteaux, R.; Edwards-Lévy, F. E.; Laurent-Maquin, D.; Lévy, M. C. Coating Alginate Microspheres with a Serum Albumin-Alginate Membrane: Application to the Encapsulation of a Peptide. *Eur. J. Pharm. Sci.* **2005,** *24,* 187–197.

Hutmacher, D. W. Scaffold Design and Fabrication Technologies for Engineering Tissues—State of the Art and Future Perspectives. *J. Biomater. Sci. Polym. Ed.* **2001,** *12,* 107–124.

Iannuccelli, V.; Montanari, M.; Bertelli, D.; Pellati, F.; Coppi, G. Microparticulate Polyelectrolyte Complexes for Gentamicin Transport Across Intestinal Epithelia. *Drug Delivery* **2011,** *18,* 26–37.

Imeson, A. *Food Stabilisers, Thickeners and Gelling Agents*; John Wiley & Sons: Sussex, UK, 2009.

Isiklan, N.; Inal, M.; Kursun, F.; Ercan, G. pH Responsive Itaconic Acid Grafted Alginate Microspheres for the Controlled Release of Nifedipine. *Carbohydr. Polym.* **2011,** *84,* 933–943.

Ivancic, A.; Macaev, F.; Aksakal, F.; Boldescu, V.; Pogrebnoi, S.; Duca, G. Reparation of Alginate–Chitosan–Cyclodextrin Micro- and Nanoparticles Loaded with Anti-Tuberculosis Compounds. *Beilstein J. Nanotechnol.* **2016,** *7,* 1208–1218.

Izawa, H.; Kawakami, K.; Sumita, M.; Tateyama, Y.; Hill, J. P.; Ariga, K. β-Cyclodextrin-Crosslinked Alginate Gel for Patient-Controlled Drug Delivery Systems: Regulation of Host-Guest Interactions With Mechanical Stimuli. *J. Mater. Chem. B* **2013,** *1,* 2155–2161.

Jacobs-Tulleneers-Thevissen, D.; Chintinne, M.; Ling, Z.; Gillard, P.; Schoonjans, L.; Delvaux, G. B.; Strand, L.; Gorus, F.; Keymeulen, B. Sustained Function of Alginate-Encapsulated Human Islet Cell Implants in the Peritoneal Cavity of Mice Leading to a Pilot Study in a Type 1 Diabetic Patient. *Diabetologia* **2013,** *56,* 1605–1614.

Jaikumar, D.; Sajesh, K. M.; Soumya, S.; Nimal, T. R.; Chennazhi, K. P.; Nair, S. V.; Jayakumar, R. Injectable Alginate-O-Carboxymethyl Chitosan/Nano Fibrin Composite Hydrogels for Adipose Tissue Engineering. *Int. J. Biol. Macromol.* **2015,** *74,* 318–326.

Jamstorp, E.; Bodin, A.; Gatenholm, P.; Jeppsson, A.; Stromme, M. Release of Antithrombotic Drugs from Alginate Gel Beads. *Curr. Drug Delivery* **2010,** *7,* 297–302.

Jay, S. M.; Saltzman, W. M. Controlled Delivery of VEGF via Modulation of Alginate Microparticle Ionic Crosslinking. *J. Control Release* **2009,** *134,* 26–34.

Jeon, O.; Bouhadir, K. H.; Mansour, J. M.; Alsberg, E. Photocrosslinked Alginate Hydrogels with Tunable Biodegradation Rates and Mechanical Properties. *Biomaterials* **2009,** *30,* 2724–2734.

Jeon, O.; Powell, C.; Solorio, L. D.; Krebs, M. D.; Alsberg, E. Affinity-Based Growth Factor Delivery using Biodegradable, Photocrosslinked Heparin-Alginate Hydrogels. *J. Control. Release* **2011,** *154,* 258–266.

Jin, H.-H.; Kim, D.-H.; Kim, T.-W.; Shin, K.-K.; Jung, J.-S.; Park, H. C.; Yoon, S.-Y. In Vitro Evaluation of Porous Hydroxyapatite/Chitosan-Alginate Composite Scaffolds for Bone Tissue Engineering. *Int. J. Biol. Macromol.* **2012,** *51,* 1079–1085.

Jitraruch, S.; Dhawan, A.; Hughes, R. D.; Filippi, C.; Soong, D.; Philippeos, C.; Lehec, S. C.; Heaton, N. D.; Longhi, M. S.; Mitry, R. R. Alginate Microencapsulated Hepatocytes Optimised for Transplantation in Acute Liver Failure. *PLoS One* **2014,** *9,* 113609.

Junter, G.-A.; Vinet, F. Compressive Properties of Yeast Cell-Loaded Ca-Alginate Hydrogel Layers: Comparison with Alginate-CaCO₃ Microparticle Composite Gel Structures. *Chem. Eng. J.* **2009**, *145*, 514–521.

Kajjari, P. B.; Manjeshwar, L. S.; Aminabhavi, T. M. Novel pH- and Temperature-Responsive Blend Hydrogel Microspheres of Sodium Alginate and PNIPAAm-g-GG for Controlled Release of Isoniazid. *AAPS PharmSciTech.* **2012**, *13*, 1147–1157.

Kamitakahara, M.; Ohtsuki, C.; Miyazaki, T. Review Paper: Behaviour of Ceramic Biomaterials Derived from Tricalcium Phosphate in Physiological Condition. *Curr. Opin. Biotechnol.* **2008**, *23*, 197–212.

Kashyap, N.; Kumar, N.; Kumar, M. N. Hydrogels for Pharmaceutical and Biomedical Applications. *Crit. Rev. Ther. Drug Carrier Syst.* **2005**, *22*, 107–149.

Khan, F.; Ahmad, S. R.; Polysaccharides and their Derivatives for Versatile Tissue Engineering Application. *Macromol. Biosci.* **2013**, *13*, 395–421.

Khan, F.; Tanaka, M.; Ahmad, S. R. Fabrication of Polymeric Biomaterials: A Strategy for Tissue Engineering and Medical Devices. *J. Mater. Chem. B* 2015, 3, 8224–8249.

Kim, B.; Bowersock, T.; Griebel, P.; Kidane, A.; Babiuk, L. A.; Sanchez, M.; Attah-Poku, S.; Kaushik, R. S.; Mutwiri, G. K. Mucosal Immune Responses Following Oral Immunization with Rotavirus Antigens Encapsulated in Alginate Microspheres. *J. Control Release* **2002a,** *85*, 191–202.

Kim, J. H.; Lee, S. B.; Kim, S. J.; Lee, Y. M. Rapid Temperature/pH Response of Porous Alginate-g-poly(N-isopropylacrylamide) Hydrogels. *Polymer* 2002b, *43*, 7549–7558.

King, S.; See, H.; Thomas, G.; Swain, M. Determining the Complex Modulus of Alginate Irreversible Hydrocolloid Dental Material. *Dent. Mater.* **2008**, *24*, 1545–1548.

Kirzhanova, E. A.; Pechenkin, M. A.; Demina, N. B.; Balabushevich, N. G. Alginate–Chitosan Micro- and Nanoparticles for Transmucosal Delivery of Proteins. *Moscow Univ. Chem. Bull.* **2016**, *71*, 127–133.

Kolambkar, Y. M.; Dupont, K. M.; Boerckel, J. D.; Huebsch, N.; Mooney, D. J.; Hutmacher, D. W.; Guldberg, R. E. An Alginate-Based Hybrid System for Growth Factor Delivery in the Functional Repair of Large Bone Defects. *Biomaterials* **2011**, *32*, 65–74.

Kong, H.-J.; Lee, K. Y.; Mooney, D. J. Decoupling the Dependence of Rheological/Mechanical Properties of Hydrogels from Solids Concentration. *Polymer* **2002**, *43*, 6239–6246.

Krebs, M. D.; Salter, E.; Chen, E.; Sutter, K. A.; Alsberg, E. Calcium Phosphate–DNA Nanoparticle Gene Delivery from Alginate Hydrogels Induces in Vivo Osteogenesis. *J. Biomed. Mater. Res. A* **2010**, *92*, 1131–1138.

Kreeger, P. K.; Deck, J. W.; Woodruff, T. K.; Shea, L. D. The in Vitro Regulation of Ovarian Follicle Development using Alginate-Extracellular Matrix Gels. *Biomaterials* **2006**, *27*, 714–723.

Kulkarni, A. R.; Soppimath, K. S.; Aminabhavi, T. M.; Rudzinski, W. E. In-Vitro Release Kinetics of Cefadroxil-Loaded Sodium Alginate Interpenetrating Network Beads. *Eur. J. Pharm. Biopharm.* **2001**, *51*, 127–133.

Kulkarni, R. V.; Sa, B. Polyacrylamide -grafted-Alginate-Based pH-Sensitive Hydrogel Beads for delivery of Ketoprofen to the Intestine: in Vitro and in Vivo Evaluation. *J. Biomater. Sci. Polym.* **2009**, *20*, 235–251.

Kulkarni, R. V.; Sreedhar, V. Srinivas, M.; Setty, C. M.; Sa, B. Interpenetrating network Hydrogel Membranes of Sodium Alginate and Poly(inyl Alcohol) for Controlled Release of Prazosin Hydrochloride Through Skin. *Int. J. Biol. Macromol.* **2010**, *47*, 520–527.

Kundu, J.; Shim, J. H.; Jang, J.; Kim, S. W.; Cho, D. W. An Additive Manufacturing-Based PCL-Alginate-Chondrocyte Bioprinted Scaffold for Cartilage Tissue Engineering. *J. Tissue Eng. Regener. Med.* **2015,** *9,* 1286–1297.

Kuo, C. K.; Ma, P. X. Ionically Crosslinked Alginate Hydrogels as Scaffolds for Tissue Engineering: Part 1. Structure, Gelation Rate and Mechanical Properties. *Biomaterials* **2001,** *22,* 511–521.

Kuo, C. K.; Ma, P. X. Maintaining Dimensions and Mechanical Properties of Ionically Crosslinked Alginate Hydrogel Scaffolds in Vitro. *J. Biomed. Mater. Res. A* **2008,** *84,* 899–907.

Kwok, K. K.; Groves, M. J.; Burgess, D. J. Sterile Microencapsulation of BCG in Alginate-Poly-L-Lysine by an Air Spraying Technique. *Proc. Int. Symp. Control Release Bioact. Mater.* **1989,** *16,* 170–171.

Lalau, J. D.; Bresson, R.; Charpentier, P.; Coliche, V.; Erlher, S.; Van, G. H.; Magalon, G.; Martini, J.; Moreau, Y.; Pradines, S.; Rigal, F.; Wemeau, J. L.; Richard, J. L. Efficacy and Tolerance of Calcium Alginate Versus Vaseline Gauze Dressings in the Treatment of Diabetic Foot Lesions. *Diabetes Metab.* **2002,** *28,* 223–229.

Lambert, G.; Fattal, E.; Couvreur, P. Nanoparticulate Systems for the Delivery of Antisense Oligonucleotides. *Adv. Drug Delivery Rev.* **2001,** *47,* 99–112.

Lan, Q.; Wang, Y.; Wang, S.; Liu, Y. In Vitro Study of Alginate/poly-L-Arginine Microcapsules as a Protein or Anticancer Drug Carrier. *IFMBE Proc.* **2008,** *19,* 32–35.

Landa, N.; Miller, L.; Feinberg, M. S.; Holbova, R.; Shachar, M.; Freeman, I.; Cohen, S.; Leor, J. Effect of Injectable Alginate Implant on Cardiac Remodeling and Function After Recent and Old Infarcts in Rat. *Circulation* **2008,** *117,* 1388–1396.

Lansdown, A. B. G. Calcium: A Potential Central Regulator in Wound Healing in the Skin. *Wound Repair Regener.* **2002,** *10,* 271–285.

Larsen, B. E.; Bjørnstad, J.; Pettersen, E. O.; Tønnesen, H. H.; Melvik, J. E. Rheological Characterization of an Injectable Alginate Gel System. *BMC Biotechnol.* **2015,** *15,* 29.

Laurienzo, P.; Malinconico, M.; Motta, A.; Vicinanza, A. Synthesis and Characterization of a Novel Alginate–poly(Ethylene Glycol) Graft Copolymer. *Carbohydr. Polym.* **2005,** *62,* 274–282.

Lawuyi, B.; Chen, H.; Afkhami, F.; Kulamarva, A.; Prakash, S. Microencapsulated Engineered *Lactococcus Lactis* Cells for Heterologous Protein Delivery: Preparation and in Vitro Analysis. *Appl. Biochem. Biotechnol.* **2007,** *142,* 71–80.

Lee, K. Y.; Park, W. H. Polyelectrolyte Complexes of Sodium Alginate with Chitosan or its Derivatives for Microcapsules. *J. Appl. Polym. Sci.* 1996a, *63,* 425–432.

Lee, B.-J.; Min, G.-H. Oral Controlled Release of Melatonin Using Polymer-Reinforced and Coated Alginate Beads. *Int. J. Pharm.* 1996b, *144,* 37–46.

Lee, K. Y.; Kong, H. J.; Larson, R. G.; Mooney, D. J. Hydrogel Formation via Cell Crosslinking. *Adv. Mater.* **2003,** *15,* 1828–1832.

Lee, C. S. D.; Gleghorn, J. P.; Choi, N. W.; Cabodi, M.; Stroock, A. D.; Bonassar, L. J. Integration of Layered Chondrocyte-Seeded Alginate Hydrogel Scaffolds. *Biomaterials* **2007,** *28,* 2987–2993.

Lee, K. Y.; Mooney, D. J. Alginate: Properties and Biomedical Applications. *Prog. Polym. Sci.* **2012,** *37,* 106–126.

Lee, B. R.; Hwang, J. W.; Choi, Y. Y.; Wong, S. F.; Hwang, Y. H.; Lee, D. Y.; Lee, S. H. In Situ Formation and Collagen-Alginate Composite Encapsulation of Pancreatic Islet Spheroids. *Biomaterials* **2012,** *33,* 837–845.

Lee, S. H.; Chung, H. Y.; Shin, H. I.; Park, D. J.; Choi, J. H. Osteogenic Activity of Chitosan-Based Hybrid Scaffold Prepared by Polyelectrolyte Complex Formation with Alginate. *Tissue Eng. Regener. Med.* **2014**, *11*, 1–7.

Leonard, M.; De Boisseson, M. R.; Hubert, P.; Dalencon, F.; Dellacherie, E. Hydrophobically Modified Alginate Hydrogels as Protein Carriers with Specific Controlled Release Properties, *J. Control Release* **2004**, *98*, 395–405.

Leor, J.; Amsalem, Y.; Cohen, S. Cells, Scaffolds, and Molecules for Myocardial Tissue Engineering. *Pharmacol. Ther.* **2005**, *105*, 151–163.

Leor, J.; Tuvia, S.; Guetta, V.; Manczur, F.; Castel, D.; Willenz, U.; Petneházy, O.; Landa, N.; Feinberg, M. S.; Konen, E.; Goitein, O.; Tsur-Gang, O.; Shaul, M.; Klapper, L.; Cohen, S. Intracoronary Injection of in Situ Forming Alginate Hydrogel Reverses Left Ventricular Remodeling After Myocardial Infarction in Swine. *J. Am. Coll. Cardiol.* **2009**, *54*, 1014–1023.

Lévy, M. C.; Edwards-Lévy, F. Coating Alginate Beads with Cross-Linked Biopolymers: A Novel Method Based on a Transacylation Reaction. *J. Microencapsulation* **1996**, *13*, 169–183.

Li, Z.; Ramay, H. R.; Hauch, K. D.; Xiao, D.; Zhang, M. Chitosan-Alginate Hybrid Scaffolds for Bone Tissue Engineering. *Biomaterials* **2005**, *26*, 3919–3928.

Li, T.; Shi, X. W.; Du, Y. M.; Tang, Y. F. Quaternized Chitosan/Alginate Nanoparticles for Protein Delivery. *J. Biomed. Mater. Res.* A. **2007**, *83*, 383–390.

Li, Q.; Liu, C. G.; Huang, Z. H.; Xue, F. F. Preparation and Characterization of Nanoparticles Based on Hydrophobic Alginate Derivative as Carriers for Sustained Release of Vitamin D3. *J. Agric. Food Chem.* **2011**, *59*, 1962–1967.

Li, X.; Chen, S.; Zhang, B.; Li, M.; Diao, K.; Zhang, Z.; Li, J.; Xu, Y.; Wang, X.; Chen, H. In Situ Injectable Nano-Composite Hydrogel Composed of Curcumin, N, O-Carboxymethyl Chitosan and Oxidized Alginate for Wound Healing Application. *Int. J. Pharm.* **2012**, *437*, 110–119.

Liberski, A.; Latif, N.; Raynaud, C.; Bollensdorff, C.; Yacoub, M. Alginate for Cardiac Regeneration: from Seaweed to Clinical Trials. *Global. Cardiol. Sci. Pract.* **2016**, *2016*, 201604.

Lim, F.; Sun, A. M. Microencapsulated Islets as Bioartificial Endocrine Pancreas. *Science* **1980**, *210*, 908–910.

Lin, H. R.; Yeh, Y. J. Porous Alginate/Hydroxyapatite Composite Scaffolds for Bone Tissue Engineering: Preparation, Characterization, and in Vitro Studies. *J. Biomed. Mater. Res.* B **2004**, *71*, 52–65.

Lin, S. S.; Ueng, S. W. N.; Lee, S. S.; Chan, E. C.; Chen, K. T.; Yang, C. Y.; Chen, C. Y.; Chan, Y. S. In Vitro Elution of Antibiotic from Antibiotic-Impregnated Biodegradable Calcium Alginate Wound Dressing. *J. Trauma* **1999**, *47*, 136–141.

Lin, Y.-H.; Liang, H.-F.; Chung, C.-K.; Chen, M.-C.; Sung, H.-W. Physically Crosslinked Alginate/N,O-Carboxymethyl Chitosan Hydrogels with Calcium for Oral Delivery of Protein Drugs. *Biomaterials* **2005**, *26*, 2105–2113.

Lin, J.; Meng, L.; Yao, Z.; Chen, S.; Yang J.; Tang, Z.; Lin, N.; Xu, R. Use an Alginate Scaffold-Bone Marrow Stromal Cell (BMSC) Complex for the Treatment of Acute Liver Failure in Rats. *Int. J. Clin. Exp. Med.* **2015**, *8*, 12593–12600.

Liu, P.; Krishnan, T. R. Alginate-Pectin-Poly-L-Lysine Particulate as a Potential Controlled Release Formulation. *J. Pharm. Pharmacol.* **1999**, *51*, 141–149.

Liu, H.-J.; Li, P.; Wei, Q. Magnetic N-Succinyl Chitosan/Al Beads for Carbamazepine Delivery. *Drug Dev. Ind. Pharm.* **2010**, *36*, 1286–1294.

Liu, J.; Zhou, H.; Weir, M. D.; Xu, H.; Chen, Q.; Trotman, C. A. Fast-Degradable Microbeads Encapsulating Human Umbilical Cord Stem Cells in Alginate for Muscle Tissue Engineering. *Tissue Eng. Part A* **2012**, *18*, 2303–2314.

Lum, L.; Elisseeff, J. Injectable Hydrogels for Cartilage Tissue Engineering. In *Topics in Tissue Engineering;* Ashammakhi, N., Ferretti, P., Eds.; University of Oulu: Oulu, 2003; pp 1–25.

Luo, Y.; Wu, C.; Lode, A.; Gelinsky, M. Hierarchical Mesoporous Bioactive Glass/Alginate Composite Scaffolds Fabricated by Three-Dimensional Plotting for Bone Tissue Engineering. *Biofabrication* 2012, 5, 015005.

Ma, P.; Xiao, C.; Li, L.; Shi, H.; Zhu, M. Facile Preparation of Ferromagnetic Alginate-g-poly(Vinyl Alcohol) Microparticles. *Eur. Polym. J.* **2008**, *44*, 3886–3889.

Ma, K.; Titan, A. L.; Stafford, M.; Zheng, C.; Levenston, M. E. Variations in Chondrogenesis of Human Bone Marrow-Derived Mesenchymal Stem Cells in Fibrin/Alginate Blended Hydrogels. *Acta Biomater.* **2012**, *8*, 3754–3764.

Mahou, R.; Meier, R. P. H.; Bühler, L. H.; Wandrey, C. Alginate-Poly(Ethylene Glycol) Hybrid Microspheres for Primary Cell Microencapsulation. *Materials (Basel)* **2014**, *7*, 275–286.

Makai, Z.; Bajdik, J.; Erős, I.; Pintye-Hódi, K. Evaluation of the Effects of Lactose on the Surface Properties of Alginate Coated Trandolapril Particles Prepared by a Spray-Drying Method. *Carbohydr. Polym.* **2008**, *74*, 712–716.

Man, Y.; Wang, P.; Guo, Y.; Xiang, L.; Yang, Y.; Qu, Y.; Gong, P.; Deng, L. Angiogenic and Osteogenic Potential of Platelet-Rich Plasma and Adipose-Derived Stem Cell Laden Alginate Microspheres. *Biomaterials* **2012**, *33*, 8802–8811.

Mandal, S.; Basu, S. K.; Sa, B. Ca2+ ion Cross-Linked interpenetrating Matrix Tablet of polyacrylamide-grafted-grafted-sodium Alginate and sodium alginate for Sustained Release of Diltiazem Hydrochloride. *Carbohydr. Polym.* **2010**, *82*, 867–873.

Marijnissen, W. J. C. M.; van Osch, G. J. V. M.; Aigner, J.; van der Veen, S. W.; Hollander, A. P.; Verwoerd-Verhoef, H. L.; Verhaar, J. A. N. Alginate as a Chondrocyte-Delivery Substance in Combination with a Non-Woven Scaffold for Cartilage Tissue Engineering. *Biomaterials* **2002**, *23*, 1511–1517.

Markstedt, K.; Mantas, A.; Tournier, I.; Martínez Ávila, H.; Hägg, D.; Gatenholm, P. 3D Bioprinting Human Chondrocytes with Nanocellulose-Alginate Bioink for Cartilage Tissue Engineering Applications. *Biomacromolecules* **2015**, *16*, 1489–1496.

Martins, S.; Sarmento, B.; Souto, E. B.; Ferreira, D. C. Insulin-Loaded Alginate Microspheres for Oral Delivery – Effect of Polysaccharide Reinforcement on Physicochemical Properties and Release Profile. *Carbohydr. Polym.* **2007**, *69*, 725–731.

Matricardi, P. Onorati, I.; Coviello, T.; Alhaique, F. Drug Delivery Matrices Based on Scleroglucan/Alginate/Borax Gels. *Int. J. Pharm.* **2006**, *316*, 21–28.

Mazur, K.; Buchner, R.; Bonn, M.; Hunger, J. Hydration of Sodium Alginate in Aqueous Solution. *Macromolecules* **2014**, *47*, 771–776.

McQuilling, J. P.; Arenas-Herrera, J.; Childers, C.; Pareta, R. A.; Khanna, O. Jiang, B. Brey, E. M.; Farney, A. C.; Opara, E. C. New Alginate Microcapsule System for Angiogenic Protein Delivery and Immunoisolation of Islets for Transplantation in the Rat Omentum Pouch. *Transplant. Proc.* 2011, 43, 3262–3264.

Mennini, N.; Furlanetto, S.; Cirri, M.; Mura, P. Quality by Design Approach for Developing Chitosan-Ca-alginate Microspheres for Colon Delivery of Celecoxib-Hydroxypropyl-β-Cyclodextrin-PVP Complex. *Eur. J. Pharm. Biopharm.* **2012**, *80*, 67–75.

Milivojevic, M.; Pajić-Lijaković, I.; Levic, S.; Nedovic, V.; Bugarski, B. Alginic Acid: Sources, Modifications and Main Applications. In: *Alginic Acid: Chemical Structure, Uses and Health Benefits;* Moore, A., Ed.; Nova Science Publishers, Inc.: New York, 2015; pp 45–88.

Mitchell, J. R.; Blanshard, J. M. V. Viscoelastic Behaviour of Alginate Gels. *Rheol. Acta.* **1974,** *13,* 180–184.

Mohan, N.; Nair, P. D. Novel Porous, Polysaccharide Scaffolds for Tissue Engineering Applications. *Trends Biomater. Artif. Organs* **2005,** *18,* 219–224.

Monteiro, D. R.; Gorup, L. F.; Takamiya, A. S.; Ruvollo-Filho, A. C.; Camargo, E. R.; Barbosa, D. B. The Growing Importance of Materials that Prevent Microbial Adhesion: Antimicrobial Effect of Medical Devices Containing Silver. *Int. J. Antimicrob. Agents* **2009,** *34,* 103–110.

Mørch, Y. A.; Donati, I.; Strand, B. L.; Skjåk-Braek, G. Molecular Engineering as an Approach to Design New Functional Properties of Alginate. *Biomacromolecules* **2007,** *8,* 2809–2814.

Moshaverinia, A.; Ansari, S.; Chen, C.; Xu, X.; Akiyama, K.; Snead, M. L.; Zadeh, H. H.; Shi, S. Co-Encapsulation of Anti-BMP2 Monoclonal Antibody and Mesenchymal Stem Cells in Alginate Microspheres for Bone Tissue Engineering. *Biomaterials* **2013,** *34,* 6572–6579.

Mourino, V.; Newby, P.; Boccaccini, A. R. Preparation and Characterization of Gallium Releasing 3-D Alginate Coated 45S5 Bioglass® Based Scaffolds for Bone Tissue Engineering. *Adv. Eng. Mater.* **2010,** *12,* 283–291.

Müller, W. E.; Schröder, H. C.; Feng, Q.; Schlossmacher, U.; Link, T.; Wang, X. Development of a Morphogenetically Active Scaffold for Three-Dimensional Growth of Bone Cells: Biosilica-Alginate Hydrogel for SaOs-2 Cell Cultivation. *J. Tissue. Eng. Regener. Med.* **2015,** *9,* 39–50.

Murakami, K.; Aoki, H.; Nakamura, S.; Nakamura, S.; Takikawa, M.; Hanzawa, M.; Kishimoto, S.; Hattori, H.; Tanaka, Y.; Kiyosawa, T.; Sato, Y.; Ishihara, M. Hydrogel Blends of Chitin/Chitosan, Fucoidan and Alginate as Healing-Impaired Wound Dressings. *Biomaterials* **2010,** *31,* 83–90.

Murata, H.; Kawamura, M.; Hamada, T.; Chimori, H.; Nikawa, H. Physical Properties and Compatibility with Dental Stones of Current Alginate Impression Materials. *J. Oral Rehabil.* 2004, 31, 1115–1122.

Nakaoka, R.; Hirano, Y.; Mooney, D. J.; Tsuchiya, T.; Matsuoka, A. Study on the Potential of RGD- and PHSRN-Modified Alginates as Artificial Extracellular Matrices for Engineering Bone. *J. Artif. Organs* **2013,** *16,* 284–293.

Nandini, V. V.; Venkatesh, K. V.; Nair, K. C. Alginate Impressions: A Practical Perspective. *J. Conservative Dent.* **2008,** *11,* 37–41.

Narayanan, R. P.; Melman, G.; Letourneau, N. J.; Mendelson, N. L.; Melman, A. Photodegradable Iron(III) Cross-Linked Alginate Gels. *Biomacromolecules* **2012,** *13,* 2465–2471.

Nause, R. G.; Reddy, R. D.; Soh, J. L. P. *Propyleneglycol Alginate,* 6th ed., Pharmaceutical Press: London, UK, 2009; pp 594–595.

Nemati, S.; Rezabakhsh, A.; Khoshfetrat, A. B.; Nourazarian, A.; Biray Avci, Ç.; Goker Bagca, B.; Alizadeh Sardroud, H.; Khaksar, M.; Ahmadi, M.; Delkhosh, A.; Sokullu, E.; Rahbarghazi, R. Alginate-Gelatin Encapsulation of Human Endothelial Cells Promoted Angiogenesis in in Vivo and in Vitro Milieu. *Biotechnol. Bioeng.* **2017,** *114,* 2920–2930.

Nograles, N.; Abdullah, S.; Shamsudin, M. N.; Billa, N.; Rosli, R. Formation and Characterization of pDNA-Loaded Alginate Microspheres for Oral Administration in Mice. *J. Biosci. Bioeng.* **2012,** *113,* 133–140.

Nunamaker, E. A.; Purcell, E. K.; Kipke, D. R. In Vivo Stability and Biocompatibility of Implanted Calcium Alginate Disks. *J. Biomed. Mater. Res. A* **2007,** *83,* 1128–1137.

O'Sullivan, L.; Murphy, B.; McLoughlin, P.; Duggan, P.; Lawlor, P. G.; Hughes, H.; Gardiner, G. E. Prebiotics from Marine Macroalgae for Human and Animal Health Applications. *Mar. Drugs* **2010,** 8, 2038–2064.

Omagari, Y.; Kaneko, Y.; Kadokawa, J.-I. Chemoenzymatic Synthesis of Amylose- Grafted Alginate and its Formation of Enzymatic Disintegratable Beads. *Carbohydr. Polym.* **2010,** *82,* 394–400.

Onsøyen, E. Alginate Production, Composition, Physicochemical Properties, Physiological Effects, Safety, and Food Applications. *Handbook of Dietary Fiber,* 1st ed.; Taylor and Francis: Boca Raton, 2001; pp 659–674.

Orive, G.; Hernandez, R. M.; Gascon, A. R.; Calafiore, R.; Chang, T. M. S.; de Vos, P.; Hortelano, G.; Hunkeler, D.; Lacik, I.; Pedraz, J. L. History, Challenges and Perspectives of Cell Microencapsulation. *Trends Biotechnol.* **2004,** *22,* 87–92.

Orive, G.; Carcaboso, A. M.; Hernández, R. M.; Gascón, A. R.; Pedraz, J. L. Biocompatibility Evaluation of Different Alginates and Alginate-Based Microcapsules. *Biomacromolecules* **2005,** *6,* 927–931.

Otterlei, M.; Østgaard, K.; Skjåk-Braek, G.; Smidsrød, O.; Soon-Shiong, P.; Espevik, T. Induction of Cytokine Production from Human Monocytes Stimulated with Alginate. *J. Immunother.* **1991,** *10,* 286–291.

Ouwerx, C.; Velings, N. M.; Mestdagh, M. M.; Axelos, M. A. V. Physico-Chemical Properties and Rheology of Alginate Gel Beads Formed with Various Divalent Cations. *Polym. Gels. Networks* **1998,** *6,* 393–408.

Pajic-Lijakovic, I.; Plavsic, M. B.; Nedovic, V.; Bugarski, B. Ca-Alginate Hydrogel Rheological Changes Caused by Yeast Cell Growth Dynamics. In *Current Research, Technology and Education Topics in Applied Microbiology and Biotechnology, Microbiology,* Mendez-Vilas A., Ed.; Book Series No 2; Formatex Research Center: Badajoz, 2010; pp 1486–1493.

Panácek, A.; Kolár, M.; Vecerová, R.; Prucek, R.; Soukupová, J.; Krystof, V.; Hamal, P.; Zboril, R.; Kvítek, L. Antifungal Activity of Silver Nanoparticles Against *Candida* spp. *Biomaterials* **2009,** *30,* 6333–6340.

Park, H.; Kim, P. H.; Hwang, T.; Kwon, O. J.; Park, T. J.; Choi, S. W.; Yun, C. O.; Kim, J. H. Fabrication of Cross-Linked Alginate Beads Using Electrospraying for Adenovirus Delivery. *Int. J. Pharm.* **2012,** *427,* 417–425.

Park, H.; Lee, K. Y. Cartilage Regeneration Using Biodegradable Oxidized Alginate/ Hyaluronate Hydrogels. *J. Biomed. Mater. Res. A* **2014,** *102,* 4519–4525.

Park, J. H.; Um, J. I.; Lee, B. J.; Goh, J. S.; Park, S. Y.; Kim, W. S.; Kim, P. H. Encapsulated Bifidobacterium Bifidum Potentiates Intestinal IgA Production. *Cell. Immunol.* **2002,** *219,* 22–27.

Park, J.-H.; Lee, E.-J.; Knowles, J. C.; Kim, H.-W. Preparation of in Situ Hardening Composite Microcarriers: Calcium Phosphate Cement Combined with Alginate for Bone Regeneration. *J. Biomater. Appl.* **2014,** *28,* 1079–1084.

Paul, W.; Sharma, C. P. Chitosan and Alginate Wound Dressings: A Short Review. *Trends Biomater. Artif. Organs* **2004,** *18,* 18–23.

Pawar, S. N.; Edgar, K. J. Chemical Modification of Alginates in Organic Solvent Systems. *Biomacromolecules* **2011,** *12,* 4095–4103.

Pelletier, S.; Hubert, P.; Payan, E.; Choplin, L.; Marchal, P.; Dellacherie, E. Amphiphilic Derivatives of Sodium Alginate and Hyaluronate for Cartilage Repair: Rheological Properties. *J. Biomed. Mater. Res.* **2001,** *54,* 102–108.

Peppas, N. A. Physiologically-Responsive Hydrogels. *J. Bioact. Compat. Polym.* **1991,** *6,* 241–246.

Perets, A.; Baruch, Y.; Weisbuch, F.; Shoshany, G.; Neufeld, G.; Cohen, S. Enhancing the Vascularization of Three-Dimensional Porous Alginate Scaffolds by Incorporating Controlled Release Basic Fibroblast Growth Factor Microspheres. *J. Biomed. Mater. Res.* **2003,** *65A,* 489–497.

Perez, R. A.; Kim, M.; Kim, T. H.; Kim, J. H.; Lee, J. H.; Park, J. H.; Knowles, J. C.; Kim, H. W. Utilizing Core-Shell Fibrous Collagen-Alginate Hydrogel Cell Delivery System for Bone Tissue Engineering. *Tissue Eng. Part A* **2014,** *20,* 103–114.

Petrenko, Y. A.; Ivanov, R. V.; Petrenko, A. Y.; Lozinsky, V. I. Coupling of Gelatin to Inner Surfaces of Pore Walls in Spongy Alginate-Based Scaffolds Facilitates the Adhesion, Growth and Differentiation of Human Bone Marrow Mesenchymal Stromal Cells. *J. Mater. Sci. Mater. Med.* **2011,** *22,* 1529–1540.

Polk, A.; Amsden, B. De Yao, K.; Peng, T.; Goosen, M. F. Controlled Release of Albumin from Chitosan-Alginate Microcapsules. *J. Pharm. Sci.* **1994,** *83,* 178–185.

Polyzois, G. L.; Andreopoulos, A. G. Stability of Some Soluble Alginate Solutions. *Biomaterials* **1985,** *6,* 68–69.

Prang, P.; Muller, R.; Eljaouhari, A.; Heckmann, K.; Kunz, W.; Weber, T.; Faber, C.; Vroemen, M.; Bogdahn, U.; Weidner, N. The Promotion of Oriented Axonal Regrowth in the Injured Spinal Cord by Alginate-Based Anisotropic Capillary Hydrogels. *Biomaterials* **2006,** *27,* 3560–3569.

Priddy, L. B.; Chaudhuri, O.; Stevens, H. Y.; Krishnan, L.; Uhrig, B. A.; Willett, N. J.; Guldberg, R. E. Oxidized Alginate Hydrogels for Bone Morphogenetic Protein-2 Delivery in Long Bone Defects. *Acta Biomater* **2014,** *10,* 4390–4399.

Qin, Y. Alginate Fibres: An Overview of the Production Processes and Applications in Wound Management. *Polym. Int.* **2008a,** *57,* 171–180.

Qin, Y. The Gel Swelling Properties of Alginate Fibers and their Applications in Wound Management. *Polym. Adv. Technol.* **2008b,** *19,* 6–14.

Quinlan, E.; López-Noriega, A.; Thompson, E.; Kelly, H. M.; Cryan, S. A.; O'Brien, F. J. Development of Collagen-Hydroxyapatite Scaffolds Incorporating PLGA and Alginate Microparticles for the Controlled Delivery of rhBMP-2 for Bone Tissue Engineering. *J. Control Release* 2015, *198,* 71–79.

Quong, D.; Neufeld, R. J. Electrophoretic Extraction and Analysis of DNA from Chitosan or Poly-L-lysine-coated Alginate Beads. *Appl. Biochem. Biotechnol.* **1999,** *81,* 67–77.

Rabbany, S. Y.; Pastore, J.; Yamamoto, M.; Miller, T.; Rafii, S.; Aras, R.; Penn, M. Continuous Delivery of Stromal Cell-Derived Factor-1 from Alginate Scaffolds Accelerates Wound Healing. *Cell Transplant.* **2010,** *19,* 399–408.

Radzig, M. A.; Nadtochenko, V. A.; Koksharova, O. A.; Kiwi, J.; Lipasova, V. A.; Khmel, I. A. Antibacterial Effects of Silver Nanoparticles on Gram-Negative Bacteria: Influence on the Growth and Biofilms Formation, Mechanisms of Action. *Colloid. Surf. B* **2013,** *102,* 300–306.

Rahmani, V.; Sheardown, H. Protein-Alginate Complexes as pH-/Ion-Sensitive Carriers of Proteins. *Int. J. Pharm.* **2017,** *535,* 452–461.

Rajaonarivony, M.; Vauthier, C.; Couarraze, G.; Puisieux, F.; Couvreur, P. Development of a New Drug Carrier Made from Alginate. *J. Pharm. Sci.* **1993,** *82,* 912–917.

Rath, G.; Johal, E. S.; Goyal, A. K. Development of Serratiopeptidase and Metronidazole Based Alginate Microspheres for Wound Healing. *Artif. Cells Blood Substitutes Immobilization. Biotechnol.* **2011,** *39,* 44–50.

Ratnaweera, P. M.; Yoshida, K.; Miura, H.; Kohta, A.; Tsuchihira, K. A Clinical Evaluation of Agar Alginate Combined Impression: Dimensional Accuracy of Dies with a New Master Crown Technique. *J. Med. Dent. Sci.* 2003, 50, 231–238.

Reakasame, S.; Boccaccini, A. R. Oxidized Alginate-Based Hydrogels for Tissue Engineering Applications: A Review. *Biomacromolecules* **2017,** DOI: 10.1021/acs.biomac.7b01331.

Rehm, B. H. A. *Alginates: Biology and Applications, Microbiology Monographs*; Springer-Verlag: Berlin Heidelberg, 2009; Vol. 13, pp 55–71.

Reis, C. P.; Ribeiro, A. J.; Neufeld, R. J.; Veiga, F. Alginate Microparticles as Novel Carrier for Oral Insulin Delivery. *Biotechnol. Bioeng.* **2007,** *96,* 977–989.

Reis, R. L.; Neves, N. M.; Mano, J. F.; Gomes, M. E.; Marques A. P.; Azevedo, H. S. *Natural-Based Polymers for Biomedical Applications,* 1st ed.; Woodhead Publishing: Cambridge, UK, 2008.

Repka, M. A.; Singh, A. Alginic Acid. In *Handbook of Pharmaceutical Excipients,* 6th ed.; Rowe, R. C., Sheskey, P. J., Quinn, M. E., Eds.; Pharmaceutical Press: London, UK, 2009; pp 20–22.

Reppel, L.; Schiavi, J.; Charif, N.; Leger, L.; Yu, H.; Pinzano, A.; Henrionnet, C.; Stoltz, J. F.; Bensoussan, D.; Huselstein, C. Chondrogenic Induction of Mesenchymal Stromal/Stem Cells from Wharton's Jelly Embedded in Alginate Hydrogel and Without Added Growth Factor: An Alternative Stem Cell Source for Cartilage Tissue Engineering. *Stem Cell Res. Ther.* **2015,** *6,* 260.

Rigo, M. V.; Allemandi, D. A.; Manzo, R. H. Swellable Drug-Polyelectrolyte Matrices (SDPM) of Alginic Acid Characterization and Delivery Properties. *Int. J. Pharm.* **2006,** *322,* 36–43.

Rokstad, A. M.; Holtan, S.; Strand, B.; Steinkjer, B.; Ryan, L.; Kulseng, B.; Skjak-Braek, G.; Espevik, T. Microencapsulation of Cells Producing Therapeutic Proteins: Optimizing Cell Growth and Secretion. *Cell Transplant.* **2002,** *11,* 313–324.

Rokstad, A. M. Donati, I.; Borgogna, M.; Oberholzer, J.; Strand, B. L.; Espevik, T.; Skjåk-Bræk, G. Cell-Compatible Covalently Reinforced Beads Obtained from a Chemoenzymatically Engineered Alginate. *Biomaterials* **2006,** *27,* 4726–4737.

Rokstad, A. M.; Brekke, O. L.; Steinkjer, B.; Ryan, L.; Kollarikova, G.; Strand, B. L.; Skjåk-Bræk, G.; Lacik, I.; Espevik, T.; Mollnes, T. E. Alginate Microbeads are Complement Compatible, in Contrast to Polycation Containing Microcapsules, as Revealed in a Human Whole Blood Model. *Acta Biomater.* **2011,** *7,* 2566–2578.

Romalde, J. L.; Alvarez, A. L.; Ravelo, C.; Toranzo, A. E.; Mendez, J. B. Oral Immunisation Using Alginate Microparticles as a Useful Strategy for Booster Vaccination Against Fish Lactoccocosis. *Aquaculture* **2004,** *236,* 119–129.

Rowley, J. A.; Mooney, D. J. Alginate Type and RGD Density Control Myoblast Phenotype. *J. Biomed. Mater. Res.* **2002,** *60,* 217–223.

Rowley, J. A.; Sun, Z. X.; Goldman, D.; Mooney, D. J. Biomaterials to Spatially Regulate Cell Fate. *Adv. Mater.* **2002,** *14,* 886–889.

Ruvinov, E.; Cohen, S. Alginate Biomaterial for the Treatment of Myocardial Infarction: Progress, Translational Strategies, and Clinical Outlook: from Ocean Algae to Patient Bedside. *Adv. Drug Delivery Rev.* **2016,** *96,* 54–76.

Ruvinov, E.; Leor, J.; Cohen, S. The Effects of Controlled HGF Delivery from an Affinity-Binding Alginate Biomaterial on Angiogenesis and Blood Perfusion in a Hindlimb Ischemia Model. *Biomaterials* **2010**, *31,* 4573–4582.

Rzaev, Z. M. O.; Dincer, S.; Piskin, E. Functional Copolymers of *N*-Isopropylacrylamide for Bioengineering Applications. *Prog. Polym. Sci.* **2007**, *32,* 534–595.

Sabbah, H. N.; Wang, M.; Gupta, R. C.; Rastogi, S.; Ilsar, I.; Sabbah, M. S.; Kohli, S.; Helgerson, S.; Lee, R. J. Augmentation of Left Ventricular Wall Thickness with Alginate Hydrogel Implants Improves Left Ventricular Function and Prevents Progressive Remodeling in Dogs with Chronic Heart Failure. *JACC Heart Failure* **2013**, *1,* 252–258.

Saez, V.; Ramón, J.; Peniche, C.; Hardy, E. Microencapsulation of Alpha Interferons in Biodegradable Microspheres. *J. Interferon Cytokine Res.* **2012**, *32,* 299–311.

Sanchez, C.; Mathy-Hartert, M.; Deberg, M. A.; Ficheux, H.; Reginster, J.-Y. L.; Henrotin, Y. E. Effects of Rhein on Human Articular Chondrocytes in Alginate Beads. *Biochem. Pharmacol.* **2003**, *65,* 377–388.

Sand, A.; Yadav, M.; Behari, K. Synthesis and Characterization of Alginate-g-vinyl Sulfonic Acid with a Potassium Peroxydiphosphate/Thiourea System. *J. Appl. Polym. Sci.* **2010**, *118,* 3685–3694.

Sankalia, M. G.; Mashru, R. C.; Sankalia, J. M.; Sutariya, V. B. Papain Entrapment in Alginate Beads for Stability Improvement and Site-Specific Delivery: Physicochemical Characterization and Factorial Optimization Using Neural Network Modeling. *AAPS PharmSciTech.* **2005**, *6,* 209–222.

Sapir, Y.; Kryukov, O.; Cohen, S. Integration of Multiple Cell-Matrix Interactions into Alginate Scaffolds for Promoting Cardiac Tissue Regeneration. *Biomaterials* **2011**, *32,* 1838–1847.

Sarmento, B.; Ribeiro, A. J.; Veiga, F.; Ferreira, D. C.; Neufeld, R. J. Insulin-Loaded Nanoparticles are Prepared by Alginate Ionotropic Pre-Gelation Followed by Chitosan Polyelectrolyte Complexation. *J. Nanosci. Nanotechnol.* **2007**, *7,* 2833–2841.

Scott, J. E.; Tigwell, M. J.; Phelps, C. F.; Nieduszynski, I. A. On the Mechanism of Scission of Alginate Chains by Periodate. *Carbohydr. Res.* **1976**, *47,* 105–117.

Séchoyo, O.; Tissie, G.; Sebastian, C.; Maurin, F.; Driot, J. Y.; Trinquand, C. A New Long Acting Ophthalmic Formulation of Carteolol Containing Alginic Acid. *Int. J. Pharm.* **2000**, *207,* 109–116.

Sen, G.; Singh, R. P.; Pal, S. Microwave-Initiated Synthesis of Polyacrylamide Grafted Sodium Alginate: Synthesis and Characterization. *J. Appl. Polym. Sci.* **2010**, *115,* 63–71.

Sezer, A. D.; Akbuğa, J. Release Characteristics of Chitosan Treated Alginate Beads: I. Sustained Release of a Macromolecular Drug from Chitosan Treated Alginate Beads. *J. Microencapsulation* **1999**, *16,* 195–203.

Shachar, M.; Tsur-Gang, O.; Dvir, T.; Leor, J.; Cohen, S. The Effect of Immobilized RGD Peptide in Alginate Scaffolds on Cardiac Tissue Engineering. *Acta Biomater.* **2011**, *7,* 152–162.

Shah, S. A.; Thassu, D. *Ammonium Alginate,* 6th ed.; Pharmaceutical Press: London, UK, 2009; p 41.

Shah, S. B.; Patel, C. P.; Trivedi, H. C. Ceric-Induced Grafting of Acrylate Monomers onto Sodium Alginate. *Carbohydr. Polym.* **1995**, *26,* 61–67.

Shteyer, E.; Ben Ya'acov, A.; Zolotaryova, L.; Sinai, A.; Lichtenstein, Y.; Pappo, O.; Kryukov, O.; Elkayam, T.; Cohen, S.; Ilan, Y. Reduced Liver Cell Death Using an Alginate Scaffold Bandage: A Novel Approach for Liver Reconstruction After Extended Partial Hepatectomy. *Acta Biomater.* **2014**, *10,* 3209–3216.

Silva, E. A.; Mooney, D. J. Effects of VEGF Temporal and Spatial Presentation on Angiogenesis. *Biomaterials* **2010,** *31,* 1235–1241.

Silva, C. M.; Ribeiro, A. J.; Figueiredo, M.; Ferreira, D.; Veiga, F. Microencapsulation of Hemoglobin in Chitosan-Coated Alginate Microspheres Prepared by Emulsification/ Internal Gelation. *AAPS J.* **2005,** *7,* 903–913.

Silva, C. M.; Ribeiro, A. J.; Ferreira, D.; Veiga, F. Insulin Encapsulation in Reinforced Alginate Microspheres Prepared by Internal Gelation. *Eur. J. Pharm. Sci.* **2006,** *29,* 148–159.

Silva, G. A.; Ducheyne, P.; Reis, R. L. Materials in Particulate form for Tissue Engineering. 1. Basic Concepts. *J. Tissue Eng. Regener. Med.* **2007,** *1,* 4–24.

Simi, C. K.; Abraham, T. E. Encapsulation of Crosslinked Subtilisin Microcrystals in Hydrogel Beads for Controlled Release Applications. *Eur. J. Pharm. Sci.* **2007,** *32,* 17–23.

Singh, O. N.; Burgess, D. J. Characterization of Albumin-Alginic Acid Complex Coacervation. *J. Pharm. Pharmacol.* **1989,** *41,* 670–673.

Skjåk-Bræk, G.; Flo, T.; Halaas, Ø.; Espevik, T. Immune stimulating properties of di-equatorially Beta (1→4) Linked Poly-Uronides. In *Bioactive Carbohydrate Polymers;* Paulsen, B. S., Ed.; Kluwer Academic Publishers: Dordrecht, 2000; pp 85–93.

Smidsrød, O.; Glover, R. M.; Whittington, S. G. The Relative Extension of Alginates Having Different Chemical Composition. *Carbohydr. Res.* **1973,** *27,* 107–118.

Smidsrød, O.; Haug, A.; Larsen, B. The Influence of pH on the Rate of Hydrolysis of Acidic Polysaccharides. *Acta Chem. Scand.* **1966,** *20,* 1026–1034.

Solovieva, E. V.; Fedotov, A. Y.; Mamonov, V. E.; Komlev, V. S.; Panteleyev, A. A. Fibrinogen-Modified Sodium Alginate as a Scaffold Material for Skin Tissue Engineering. *Biomed. Mater.* **2017.** DOI: 10.1088/1748-605X/aa9089.

Soon-Shoing, P.; Desai, N.; Sandford, P.; Heintz, R. Crosslinkable polysaccharides, polycations and lipids useful for encapsulation and drug release. PCT/US/1992/09364.

Soran, Z.; Aydın, R. S.; Gümüşderelioğlu, M. Chitosan Scaffolds with BMP-6 Loaded Alginate Microspheres for Periodontal Tissue Engineering. *J. Microencapsulation* **2012,** *29,* 770–780.

Srinivasan, S.; Jayasree, R.; Chennazhi, K. P.; Nair, S. V.; Jayakumar, R. Biocompatible Alginate/Nano Bioactive Glass Ceramic Composite Scaffolds for Periodontal Tissue Regeneration. *Carbohydr. Polym.* **2011,** *87,* 274–283.

Stojkovska, J.; Bugarski, B.; Obradovic, B. Evaluation of Alginate Hydrogels Under in Vivo-Like Bioreactor Conditions for Cartilage Tissue Engineering. *J. Mater. Sci. Mater. Med.* **2010,** *21,* 2869–2879.

Stojkovska, J.; Kostić, D.; Jovanović, Z.; Vukašinović-Sekulić, M.; Mišković-Stanković, V.; Obradović, B. A Comprehensive Approach to in Vitro Functional Evaluation of Ag/ Alginate Nanocomposite Hydrogels. *Carbohydr. Polym.* **2014,** *111,* 305–314.

Stokke, B. T.; Smidsrød, O.; Brant, D. A. Predicted Influence of Monomer Sequence Distribution and Acetylation on the Extension of Naturally Occurring Alginates. *Carbohydr. Polym.* **1993a,** *22,* 57–66.

Stokke, B. T.; Smidsrød, O.; Zanetti, F.; Strand, W.; Skjåk-Bræk, G. Distribution of Uronate Residues in Alginate Chains in Relation to Alginate Gelling Properties—2: Enrichment of β-D-mannuronic Acid and Depletion of α–L-Guluronic acid in Sol Fraction. *Carbohydr. Polym.* **1993b,** *21,* 39–46.

Straccia, M. C.; d'Ayala, G. G.; Romano, I.; Oliva, A.; Laurienzo, P. Alginate Hydrogels Coated with Chitosan for Wound Dressing. *Mar Drugs* **2015,** *13,* 2890–2908.

Strand, B. L.; Coron, A.E.; Skjak-Braek, G. Current and Future Perspectives on Alginate Encapsulated Pancreatic Islet. *Stem Cells Transl Med.* **2017,** *6,* 1053–1058.

Sun, J.; Tan, H. Alginate-Based Biomaterials for Regenerative Medicine Applications. *Materials (Basel)* **2013,** *6,* 1285–1309.

Szekalska, M.; Pucilowska, A.; Szymanska, E.; Ciosek, P.; Winnicka, K. Alginate: Current Use and Future Perspectives in Pharmaceutical and Biomedical Applications. *Int. J. Polym. Sci.* **2016,** *2016,* 7697031.

Takeuchi, H.; Yasuji, T.; Hino, T.; Yamamoto, H.; Kawashima, Y. Spray-Dried Composite Particles of Lactose and Sodium Alginate for Direct Tableting and Controlled Releasing. *Int. J. Pharm.* **1998,** *174,* 91–100.

Takka, S.; Acarturk, F. Calcium Alginate Microparticles for Oral Administration. I: Effect of Sodium Alginate Type on Drug Release and Drug Entrapment Efficiency. *J. Microencapsulation* **1999,** *16,* 275–290.

Tan, H.; Wu, J.; Lao, L.; Gao, C. Gelatin/Chitosan/Hyaluronan Scaffold Integrated with PLGA Microspheres for Cartilage Tissue Engineering. *Acta Biomater.* **2009,** *5,* 328–337.

Tan, R.; She, Z.; Wang, M.; Fang, Z.; Liu, Y.; Feng, Q. Thermo-Sensitive Alginate-Based Injectable Hydrogel for Tissue Engineering. *Carbohydr. Polym.* **2012,** *87,* 1515–1521.

Tanaka, H.; Sato, Y. Photosensitivity of Polyvinylesters of Substituted Cinnamylideneacetic Acids. *J. Polym. Sci.* **1972,** *10,* 3279–3287.

Tanaka, H.; Matsumura, M.; Veliky, I. A. Diffusion Characteristics of Substrates in Ca-Alginate Gel Beads. *Biotechnol. Bioeng.* **1984a,** *26,* 53–58.

Tanaka, H.; Kurosawa, H.; Kokufuta, E. Preparation of Immobilized Glucoamylase using Ca-alginate Gel Coated with Partially Quaternized Poly(Ethyleneimine). *Biotechnol. Bioeng.* **1984b,** *26,* 1393–1394.

Tanihara, M.; Suzuki, Y.; Yamamoto, E.; Mizushima, Y. Sustained Release of Basic Fibroblast Growth Factor and Angiogenesis in a Novel Covalently Crosslinked Gel of Heparin and Alginate. *J. Biomed. Mater. Res.* **2001,** *56,* 216–221.

Thakral, N. K.; Ray, A. R.; Bar-Shalom, D.; Eriksson, A. H.; Majumdar, D. K. The Quest for Targeted Delivery in Colon Cancer: Mucoadhesive Valdecoxib Microspheres. *Int. J. Nanomed.* **2011,** *6,* 1057–1068.

Thomas, S. Alginate Dressings in Surgery and Wound Management—Part 1. *J. Wound Care* **2000,** *9,* 56–60.

Thomas, A.; Harding, K. G.; Moore, K. Alginates from Wound Dressings Activate Human Macrophages to Secret Tumour Necrosis Factor-α. *Biomaterials* **2000,** *21,* 1797–1802.

Thu, B.; Bruheim, P.; Espevik, T.; Smidsrød, O.; Soon-Shiong P.; Skjak-Braek, G. Alginate Polycation Microcapsules. I. Interaction between Alginate and Polycation. *Biomaterials* **1996a,** *17,* 1031–1040.

Thu, B.; Bruheim, P.; Espevik, T.; Smidsrød, O.; Soon-Shiong P.; Skjåk-Bræk, G. Alginate Polycation Microcapsules. II. Some Functional Properties. *Biomaterials* **1996b,** *17,* 1069–1079.

Thu, B.; Gaserod, O.; Paus, D.; Mikkelsen, A.; Skak-Braek, G.; Toffanin, R.; Vittur, F.; Rizzo, R. Inhomogeneous Alginate Gel Spheres: An Assessment of the Polymer Gradients by Synchroton Radiation-Induced X-ray Emission, Magnetic Resonance, Microimaging, and Mathematical Modeling. *Biopolymers* **2000,** *53,* 60–71.

Tıglı, R. S.; Gumusderelioglu, M. Evaluation of Alginate-Chitosan Semi IPNs as Cartilage Scaffolds. *J. Mater. Sci: Mater. Med.* **2009,** *20,* 699–709.

Tripathi, R.; Mishra, B. Development and Evaluation of Sodium Alginate-Polyacrylamide Graft-Co-Polymer-Based Stomach Targeted Hydrogels of Famotidine. *AAPS PharmSciTech.* **2012,** *13,* 1091–1102.

Tuch, B. E.; Keogh, G. W.; Williams, L. J.; Wu, W.; Foster, J. L.; Vaithilingam, V.; Philips, R. Safety and Viability of Microencapsulated Human Islets Transplanted into Diabetic Humans. *Diabetes Care* **2009,** *32,* 1887–1889.

Ugi, I. The α-Addition of Immonium Ions and Anions to Isonitriles Accompanied by Secondary Reactions. *Angew. Chem. Int. Ed. Engl.* **1962,** *1,* 8–21.

Valla, S.; Ertesvåg, H.; Skjåk-Bræk, G. Genetics and Biosynthesis of Alginates. *Carbohydr. Eur.* **1996,** *14,* 14–18.

Vandenberg, G. W.; Drolet, C.; Scott, S. L.; de la Noüe, J. Factors Affecting Protein Release from Alginate-Chitosan Coacervate Microcapsules During Production and Gastric/Intestinal Simulation. *J. Control Release* **2001,** *77,* 297–307.

Venkatesan, J.; Pallela, R.; Kim, S.-K. Dispersion of Single Walled Carbon Nanotubes in Marine Polysaccharides for Bone Tissue Engineering. *J. Biomater. Tissue Eng.* **2014,** *4,* 501–505.

Venkatesan, J.; Bhatnagar, I.; Manivasagan, P.; Kang, K. H.; Kim, S. K. Alginate Composites for Bone Tissue Engineering: A Review. *Int. J. Biol. Macromol.* **2015,** *72,* 269–281.

Vold, I. M. N.; Kristiansen, K. A.; Christensen, B. E. A Study of the Chain Stiffness and Extension of Alginates, in Vitro Epimerized Alginates, and Periodate-Oxidized Alginates Using Size-Exclusion Chromatography Combined with Light Scattering and Viscosity Detectors. *Biomacromolecules* **2006,** *7,* 2136–2146.

Voo, W.-P.; Ooi, C.-W.; Islam, A.; Tey, B.-T.; Chan, E.-S. Calcium Alginate Hydrogel Beads with High Stiffness and Extended Dissolution Behaviour. *Eur. Polym. J.* **2016,** 75, 343–353.

Wang, T.; Lacik, I.; Brissova, M.; Prokop, A.; Hunkeler, D.; Anilkumar, A. V.; Green, R.; Shahrokhi, K.; Powers, A. C. An Encapsulation System for the Immunoisolation of Pancreatic Islets. *Nat. Biotechnol.* **1997,** *15,* 358–362.

Wang, L.; Shelton, R. M.; Cooper, P. R.; Lawson, M.; Triffitt, J. T.; Barralet, J. E. Evaluation of Sodium Alginate for Bone Marrow Cell Tissue Engineering. *Biomaterials* **2003,** *24,* 3475–3481.

Wang, S. B.; Xu, F. H.; He, H. S. Weng, L. J. Novel Alginate-poly(L-histidine) Microcapsules as Drug Carriers: In Vitro Protein Release and Short Term Stability. *Macromol. Biosci.* **2005,** *5,* 408–414.

Wang, Q.; Zhang, J.; Wang, A. Preparation and Characterization of a Novel pH- Sensitive Chitosan-g-poly (Acrylic Acid)/Attapulgite/Sodium Composite Hydrogel Bead for Controlled Release of Diclofenac Sodium. *Carbohydr. Polym.* **2008,** *78,* 731–737.

Wang, C. C.; Yang, K. C.; Lin, K. H.; Liu, H. C.; Lin, F. H. A Highly Organized Three-Dimensional Alginate Scaffold for Cartilage Tissue Engineering Prepared by Microfluidic Technology. *Biomaterials* **2011a,** *32,* 7118–7126.

Wang, F. Q.; Li, P.; Zhang, J. P.; Wang, A. Q.; Wei, Q. pH-Sensitive Magnetic Alginate-Chitosan Beads for Albendazole Delivery. *Pharm. Dev. Technol.* **2011b,** *16,* 228–236.

Wang, M.-D.; Zhai, P.; Schreyer, D. J.; Zheng, R.-S.; Sun, X. D.; Cui, F.-Z.; Chen, X. B.; Novel Crosslinked Alginate/Hyaluronic Acid Hydrogels for Nerve Tissue Engineering. *Front Mater. Sci.* **2013,** *7,* 269–284.

Wang, X.; Schröder, H. C.; Grebenjuk, V.; Diehl-Seifert, B.; Mailänder, V.; Steffen, R.; Schloßmacher, U.; Müller, W. E. The Marine Sponge-Derived Inorganic Polymers, Biosilica and Polyphosphate, as Morphogenetically Active Matrices/Scaffolds for the Differentiation of Human Multipotent Stromal Cells: Potential Application in 3D Printing and Distraction Osteogenesis. *Mar Drugs* **2014,** *12,* 1131–1147.

Wang, B.; Wang, W.; Yu, Y.; Zhang, Y.; Zhang, J.; Yuan, Z. The Study of Angiogenesis Stimulated by Multivalent Peptide Ligand-Modified Alginate. *Colloids Surf. B* **2017a,** *154,* 383–390.

Wang, G.; Wang, X.; Huang L. Feasibility of Chitosan-Alginate (Chi-Alg) Hydrogel used as Scaffold for Neural Tissue Engineering: A Pilot Study in Vitro. *Biotechnol. Biotechnol. Equip.* **2017b,** *31,* 766–773.

Wasikiewicz, J. M.; Yoshii, F.; Nagasawa, N.; Wach, R. A.; Mitomo, H. Degradation of Chitosan and Sodium Alginate by Gamma Radiation, Sonochemical and Ultraviolet Methods. *Radiat. Phys. Chem.* **2005,** *73,* 287–295.

Wee, S.; Gombotz, W. R. Protein Release from Alginate Matrices. *Adv. Drug Delivery Rev.* **1998,** *31,* 267–285.

Wells, L. A.; Sheardown, H. Extended Release of High pI Proteins from Alginate Microspheres via a Novel Encapsulation Technique. *Eur. J. Pharm. Biopharm.* **2007,** *65,* 329–335.

Wiegand, C.; Heinze, T.; Hipler, U. C. Comparative in Vitro Study on Cytotoxicity, Antimicrobial Activity, and Binding Capacity for Pathophysiological Factors in Chronic Wounds of Alginate and Silver-Containing Alginate. *Wound Repair Regener.* **2009,** *17,* 511–521.

Williams, D. F. On the Nature of Biomaterials. *Biomaterials* **2009,** *30,* 5897–5909.

Wu, W.; Liu, W.; Wang, S.; Liu, Y. Drug Controlled Release of Novel Alginate/Poly-L-Arginine Microcapsules. *IFMBE Proc.* **2008,** 19, 26–28.

Xia, Y.; Mei, F.; Duan, Y.; Gao, Y.; Xiong, Z.; Zhang, T.; Zhang, H. Bone Tissue Engineering using Bone Marrow Stromal Cells and an Injectable Sodium Alginate/Gelatin Scaffold. *J. Biomed. Mater. Res. A* **2012,** *100,* 1044–1050.

Xiang, D. X.; Chen, Q.; Pang, L.; Zheng, C. L. Inhibitory Effects of Silver Nanoparticles on H1N1 Influenza a Virus in Vitro. *J. Virol. Methods* **2011,** *178,* 137–142.

Xiao, D.; Yan, H.; Wang, Q.; Lv, X.; Zhang, M.; Zhao, Y.; Zhou, Z.; Xu, J.; Sun, Q.; Sun, K.; Li, W.; Lu, M. Trilayer Three-Dimensional Hydrogel Composite Scaffold Containing Encapsulated Adipose-Derived Stem Cells Promotes Bladder Reconstruction via SDF-1α/CXCR4 Pathway. *ACS Appl. Mater. Interfaces* **2017,** *9,* 38230–38241.

Xin, J.; Guo, Z.; Chen, X.; Jiang, W.; Li, J.; Li, M. Study of Branched Cationic Beta-Cyclodextrin Polymer/Indomethacin Complex and its Release Profile from Alginate Hydrogel. *Int. J. Pharm.* **2010,** *386,* 221–228.

Yadav, M.; Sand, A.; Behari, K. Synthesis and Characterization of Graft Copolymer (Alginate-g-poly(N,N-dimethylacrylamide)). *Chin. J. Polym. Sci.* **2010,** *28,* 673–683.

Yan, S.; Wang, T.; Feng L.; Zhu, J.; Zhang, K.; Chen X.; Cui, L.; Yin, J. Injectable in Situ Self-Cross-Linking Hydrogels Based on Poly(L-glutamic acid) and Alginate for Cartilage Tissue Engineering. *Biomacromolecules* **2014,** *15,* 4495–4508.

Yan, J.; Miao, Y.; Tan, H.; Zhou, T.; Ling, Z.; Chen, Y.; Xing, X.; Hu, X. Injectable Alginate/Hydroxyapatite Gel Scaffold Combined with Gelatin Microspheres for Drug Delivery and Bone Tissue Engineering. *Mater. Sci. Eng. C* **2016,** *63,* 274–284.

Yang, J.; Goto, M.; Ise, H.; Cho, C. S.; Akaike, T. Galactosylated Alginate as a Scaffold for Hepatocytes Entrapment. *Biomaterials* **2002,** *23,* 471–479.

Yang, W.; Zhang, L.; Wu, L.; Li, J.; Wang, J.; Jiang, H.; Li, Y. Synthesis and Characterization of MMA-NaAlg/Hydroxyapatite Composite and the Interface Analyse with Molecular Dynamics. *Carbohydr. Polym.* **2009,** *77,* 331–337.

Yang, J. S.; Ren, H. B.; Xie, Y. J. Synthesis of Amidic Alginate Derivatives and their Application in Microencapsulation of λ-cyhalothrin. *Biomacromolecules* **2011,** *12,* 2982–2987.

Ye, S.; Wang, C.; Liu, X.; Tong, Z.; Ren, B.; Zeng, F. New Loading Process and Release Properties of Insulin from Polysaccharide Microcapsules Fabricated through Layer-By-Layer Assembly. *J. Controlled Release* **2006**, *112*, 79–87.

Yi, H.; Forsythe, S.; He, Y.; Liu, Q.; Xiong, G.; Wei, S.; Li, G.; Atala, A.; Skardal, A.; Zhang, Y. Tissue-Specific Extracellular Matrix Promotes Myogenic Differentiation of Human Muscle Progenitor Cells on Gelatin and Heparin Conjugated Alginate Hydrogels. *Acta Biomater.* **2017**, *62*, 222–233.

Yin, M.; Xu, F.; Ding, H.; Tan, F.; Song, F.; Wang, J. Incorporation of Magnesium Ions into Photo-Crosslinked Alginate Hydrogel Enhanced Cell Adhesion Ability. *J. Tissue Eng. Regener. Med.* **2015**, *9*, 1088–1092.

Yu, J.; Du, K. T.; Fang, Q. The use of Human Mesenchymal Stem Cells Encapsulated in RGD Modified Alginate Microspheres in the Repair of Myocardial Infarction in the Rat. *Biomaterials* **2010**, *31*, 7012–7020.

Yuk, S. H.; Cho, S. H.; Lee, H. B. Electric Current-Sensitive Drug Delivery Systems using Sodium Alginate/Polyacrylic Acid Composites. *Pharm. Res.* **1992**, *9*, 955–957.

Yuvarani, I.; Kumar, S. S.; Venkatesan, J.; Kim, S.-K.; Sudha P. N. Preparation and Characterization of Curcumin Coated Chitosan-Alginate Blend for Wound Dressing Application. *J. Biomater. Tissue Eng.* **2012**, *2*, 54–60.

Zeng, Q.; Han, Y.; Li, H. Chang, J. Bioglass/Alginate Composite Hydrogel Beads as Cell Carriers for Bone Regeneration. *J. Biomed. Mater. Res. B* **2014**, *102*, 42–51.

Zhai, P.; Chen, X. B.; Schreyer, D. J. PLGA/Alginate Composite Microspheres for Hydrophilic Protein Delivery. *Mater. Sci. Eng. C* **2015**, *56*, 251–259.

Zhang, Y.; Wei, W.; Lu, P.; Wang, L.; Ma, G. Preparation and Evaluation of Alginate-Chitosan Microspheres for Oral Delivery of Insulin. *Eur. J. Pharm. Biopharm.* **2011**, *77*, 11–19.

Zhao, Y.; Shen, W.; Chen, Z.; Wu, T. Freeze-Thaw Induced Gelation of Alginates. *Carbohydr. Polym.* **2016a**, *148*, 45–51.

Zhao, F.; Zhang, W.; Fu, X.; Xie, W.; Chen, X. Fabrication and Characterization of Bioactive Glass/Alginate Composite Scaffolds by a Self-Crosslinking Processing for Bone Regeneration. *RSC Adv.* **2016b**, *6*, 91201–91208.

Zhao, L.; Weir, M. D.; Xu, H. H. An Injectable Calcium Phosphate-Alginate Hydrogel-Umbilical Cord Mesenchymal Stem Cell Paste for Bone Tissue Engineering. *Biomaterials* **2010**, *31*, 6502–6510.

Zhao, J.; Zhao, X.; Guo, B.; Ma, P. X. Multifunctional Interpenetrating Polymer Network Hydrogels Based on Methacrylated Alginate for the Delivery of Small Molecule Drugs and Sustained Release of Protein. *Biomacromolecules* **2014**, *15*, 3246–3252.

Zhiyong, L.; Caihua, N.; Cheng, X.; Qian, L. Preparation and Drug Release of Hydrophobically Modified Alginate. *Chemistry* **2009**, *1*, 93–96.

Zhou, Y.; Kajiyama, S.; Masuhara, H.; Hosokawa, Y.; Kaji, T.; Fukui, K. A New Size and Shape Controlling Method for Producing Calcium Alginate Beads with Immobilized Proteins. *J. Biomed. Sci. Eng.* **2009**, *2*, 287–293.

Zhu, Y. Immobilized Cell Fermentation for Production of Chemicals and Fuels. In *Bioprocessing for Value-Added Products from Renewable Resources: New Technologies and Applications;* Yang, S. T., Ed.; Elsevier: Amsterdam, 2007; pp 373–396.

Zhu, A. M.; Chen, J. H.; Liu, Q. L.; Jiang, Y. L. Controlled Release of Berberine Hydrochloride from Alginate Microspheres Embedded within Carboxymethyl Chitosan Hydrogels. *J. Appl. Polym. Sci.* **2011**, *120*, 2374–2380.

Zhuang, Y.; Yu, F.; et al. Alginate/Graphene Double-Network Nanocomposite Hydrogel Beads with Low-Swelling, Enhanced Mechanical Properties, and Enhanced Adsorption Capacity. *J. Mater. Chem. A* **2016,** *4,* 10885–10892.

Zimmermann, U.; Klock, G.; Federlin, K.; Hannig, K.; Kowalski, M.; Bretzel, R. G.; Horcher, A.; Entenmann, H.; Sieber, U.; Zekorn, T. Production of Mitogen-Contamination Free Alginates with Variable Ratios of Mannuronic Acid to Guluronic Acid by Free Flow Electrophoresis. *Electrophoresis* **1992,** *13,* 269–274.

Zorzin, L.; Cocchietto, M.; Voinovich, D.; Marcuzzi, A.; Filipovic-Grcic, J.; Mulloni, C.; Crembiale, G.; Casarsa, C.; Bulla, R.; Sava, G. Lysozyme-Containing Chitosan-Coated Alginate Microspheres for Oral Immunisation. *J. Drug Delivery Sci. Technol.* **2006,** *16,* 413–420.

CHAPTER 3

ALGINATES: HYDROGELS, THEIR CHEMISTRY, AND APPLICATIONS

VERÓNICA ELENA MANZANO,[1,2] MARÍA NATALIA PACHO,[2] JOANA ELISA TASQUÉ,[2] and NORMA BEATRIZ D'ACCORSO[1,2,*]

[1]*Universidad de Buenos Aires, Facultad de Ciencias Exactas y Naturales, Departamento de Química Orgánica, Pabellón 2, Ciudad Universitaria, C1428EHA, Buenos Aires, Argentina*

[2]*CONICET, Centro de Investigaciones en Hidratos de Carbono (CIHIDECAR), Universidad de Buenos Aires, Buenos Aires, Argentina*

Corresponding author. E-mail: norma@qo.fcen.uba.ar

3.1 INTRODUCTION OF HYDROGELS: DEFINITION, CLASSIFICATION, AND USES

Over the past decades, special attention has been placed in hydrogels because as natural tissue, they have a large degree of flexibility and can retain a large amount of water and possesses a soft rubbery consistency (Ullah et al., 2015) which makes them attractive materials in many applications that range from industrial to biological. Due to their unique properties which include not only high water content but also softness, flexibility, biocompatibility, reversibility, and sterilizability, they are widely used in the biomedical field as a promising biomaterial. It is worth to mention that for a material to be considered as a biomaterial it must meet certain criteria such as biocompatibility, biostability, biofunctionality during the implantation; mechanical, electrical, and physical compatibility; morphological or topographical aspects; and adequate manufacturing (Parisi et al., 2015). Hydrogels satisfied those requirements and more and that is the reason why they are usually used in biomedicine. For instance, some applications include uses in contact lenses, membranes for biosensors, linings for artificial hearts, hygiene products, tissue engineering scaffolds, drug delivery systems, and wound dressings among others (Caló et al., 2015; Peppas et al., 2000; Kamoun et al., 2017; Chirani et al., 2015). Also, hydrogels serve as scaffolds for microfluidic control, biomimetic, biosensor/bioactuator, bioseparation, and artificial skin and muscles in view of its high environmental sensitivity, ionic conductivity, permeability, and novel mechanical properties and sorption capacity (Ullah et al., 2015).

It is interesting to note that the properties of a hydrogel can be tailored in order to have a material that may be chemically stable or may degrade and eventually disintegrate and dissolve (Calo et al., 2015). As mention before, hydrogels can swell and deswell water in a reversible direction in response to changes in temperature, pH, and ionic strength which are promising smart materials (Buwalda et al., 2014).

Taking into account the definition, hydrogel is a polymeric material, either natural or synthetic, which is capable of holding large amounts of water (at least 10% of the total weight or volume) in its three-dimensional networks but will not dissolve in it. These hydrophilic gels are sometimes found as colloids in which water is the dispersion medium. The networks are composed of homopolymers or copolymers which have cross-links (tie-points, junctions), joined together in either chemical or physical way (Peppas et al., 2000). The reason why hydrogels have this characteristic ability relies on the fact that hydrogels have hydrophilic groups attached to the polymeric backbone. The fact that the polymer is cross-linked confers great resistance to dissolution. Nowadays, this definition has evolved and hydrogels are defined as a natural or synthetic system, either of two- or multicomponent, which forms a three-dimensional network of polymer material in which the spaces between the chains is filled with water (Ahmed et al., 2015).

Natural hydrogels from the biomass include collagen, fibrin, hyaluronic acid, matrigel, and derivatives of natural materials such as chitosan, alginate, and fibers of silk. Generally, they are biopolymers or polyelectrolytes. Many hydrogel scaffolds based on alginate, chitosan, and collagen showed potential use as general bulking agents. Although physiological gels are components of the extracellular matrix, their properties and reproducibility in different experiments are difficult to control due to the diversity of composition derived from their natural origin. The search of new and varied properties led to the modification of natural hydrogels or to the replacement by synthetic polymers, which has a long service life, more flexibility, high capacity of water absorption, and high gel strength. They can also be selected or tuned to be hydrolyzable or biodegradable over variable periods of time.

Therefore, the development of synthetic hydrogels (poly(ethylene glycol) diacrylate, poly(acrylamide), poly(vinyl alcohol)) makes reproducibility easier to control despite the fact that their final structure depends on polymerization (Chirani et al., 2015). In order to fit the new requirements and properties for different applications, smart hydrogel systems, with various chemically and structurally responsive moieties, were synthesized. These types of gels are characterized for exhibiting a response to certain external stimuli as temperature, pressure, pH, ionic concentration, light intensity, magnetic or electrical fields, solvent composition, and chemicals (Bahram et al., 2016). When exposed to certain stimuli, the polymer hydrogel changes their structural and volume phase transition, expanding its application in many new technological areas (Chirani et al., 2015). Generally, such conformational transitions are reversible and gels recover from the initial state.

As mention before, hydrogels attract the attention of many material scientists and biomedical researchers as these gels are promising materials. In this sense, a considerable number of advances have been made in terms of their formulations and applications.

3.1.1 CLASSIFICATION OF HYDROGELS

There are many classifications for hydrogels but the most common is the one that divides them into *physical* or *chemical* gels, depending on the type of cross-linking (Akhta et al., 2016). It is observed that hydrogels are "physical" or "reversible" if the chains of polymer are held together by ionic, hydrogen bonding or hydrophobic interactions as represented in Figure 3.1. This means that it is possible to dissolve them by changing environmental conditions, such as pH, and the ionic strength of solution or temperature (Caló et al., 2015). These gels tend to have inhomogeneity due to the clusters of molecular entanglements or hydrophobically or ionically associated domains. Among the physically cross-linked gels, we can mention the ones held together by hydrogen bonds, the amphiphilic graft, and block polymers, the cross-linking by crystallization and due to the ionic and protein interaction (Akhta et al., 2016). Depending on the nature of the groups present in the structure, the gels may be charged or non-charged. Charged hydrogels usually exhibit changes in swelling upon variations in pH, and when exposed to electric fields, they may show changes in shape (Rosiak et al., 1999).

On the contrary, in "permanent" or "chemical" gels, covalent bonds are the responsible for joining the chains together. Similarly, in physical gels, chemical hydrogels are not homogeneous and also contain regions of low water swelling (high cross-link also called "clusters") that are dispersed within regions of high swelling (low cross-link) (Hoffman et al., 2012).

Chemical cross-linked gels involve the linking reaction by complementary groups, for instance, amine-carboxylic acid or isocyanate-OH/NH$_2$ reaction or Schiff base formation. It is also found that the chemical cross-linking may be produced by high-energy radiation, by free-radical polymerization, or by the use of enzymes (Akhta et al., 2016).

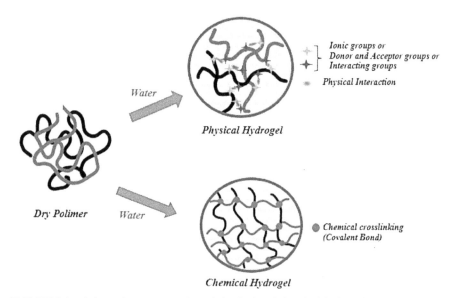

FIGURE 3.1   Schematic representation of physical and chemical hydrogels.

As mention before, hydrogels may be classified on different basis depending on the characteristic emphasized or highlighted (Ahmed et al., 2015; Ullah et al., 2015; Bahram et al., 2016). For instance, the following must be taken into account:

a) *Source:* They are natural, synthetic, or hybrids gels
b) *Preparation or polymeric composition*: In this, we found the *homopolymeric, copolymeric,* and *multipolymer interpenetrating polymeric* hydrogels or *interpenetrating polymer networks* (IPNs). This classification depends on whether the monomer is a single- or is multi-composed.

   Copolymeric hydrogels are composed of two types of monomers, of which at least one is hydrophilic in nature.

   When a linear polymer penetrates into another cross-linked network without any other chemical bonds, it is called semi-IPN forms.

c) *Configuration*: It depends on their physical structure and chemical composition, for instance, hydrogels may be subclassified depending on their nature, that is, amorphous, semicrystalline, or crystalline.
d) *Physical appearance:* Matrix, film, or microsphere
e) *Ionic charge*: Subcategorized in four groups depending on the electrical charge, that is, nonionic, ionic, amphotheric (which contains acidic and basic groups) and zwitterionic (which have both anionic and cationic groups in equal amounts).
f) *Response*: Chemical (pH, glucose, oxidant responsive), physical (temperature, pressure, light, magnetic and electric field responsive), or biochemical (enzymes, antigens, and ligands responsive).
g) *Physical properties*: Smart or conventional hydrogels. Smart gels are environment-sensitive, which means that they show a response to a certain stimulus, as mention before.
h) *Degradability*

3.1.2 SYNTHESIS OF HYDROGELS

There are different methods for modifying the properties of a polymer with tailor-made specifications. Blending, grafting/cross-linking, and curing the polymers are some of the types of modifications. In a blend, the interaction is only physical in contrast to the grafting or cross-linking in which a covalent bond is formed (Figure 3.2). The difference between grafting and cross-linking is that, in the first one, some monomers are covalently linked to the polymer chain, while in the chemical cross-linking, two chains are linked together by a reactive group or monomer. Finally, the curing involves the formation of a coating on the polymer backbone which is held together by physical forces.

The most common ways to synthesize hydrogels are the three-dimensional polymerization or the direct cross-linking of water-soluble polymers (Caló et al., 2015). The first type of polymerization involves the use of a hydrophilic monomer in the presence of a polyfunctional cross-linking agent and the second one, as mention before, consists of the formation of new covalent bonds between polymer chains. In all cases, they are usually radical polymerizations initiated by compounds such as benzoyl peroxide, 2,2-azoisobutyronitrile (AIBN), and ammonium peroxodisulfate. Sometimes the polymerization may be started by ultraviolet (UV), gamma, or electron beam radiation (Buwalda et al., 2014). The main problem of three-dimensional polymerization is the content of residual monomers which complicates the purification. It is worth to mention that unreacted monomers are usually toxic.

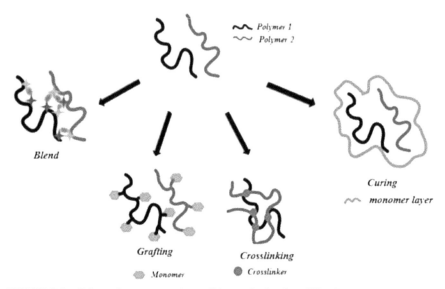

FIGURE 3.2   Schematic representations of the methods of modification.

3.1.3   BIOPOLYMER-BASED HYDROGELS

Over the last years, there has been an increasing interest in the uses of biopolymers in biomedical and technological applications. The use of biopolymers in many biomedical areas, for instance, as drug delivery matrices or regenerative medicine, is based on the good biocompatibility, biodegradability, nontoxicity, water solubility, or high capability for swelling and low disposal costs. They also served as scaffolds for the synthesis of advanced modified materials (Das et al., 2015).

In the technological field, the biopolymer-based hydrogels such as chitosan, alginate, starch, and cellulose were used to remove heavy metal ions from aqueous media. It has been shown that the mechanism and capacity of sorption of heavy metal ions were both influenced by the functional groups of the hydrogel (Bahram et al., 2016).

Natural polysaccharides may be formed of one or more different monomers (monosaccharides). These repeating units may be or not charged. The polyelectrolytes can be either positively or negatively charged, defining the properties and fields of application of the polymer. Microbial contamination, uncontrolled rate of hydration, and drop in viscosity on storing are some of the limitations of these biopolymers. In order to overcome these drawbacks, several suitable chemical modifications, such as grafting/cross-linking of synthetic polymer chains, were developed (Das et al., 2015). Thus, the use of these modified biopolymer-based hydrogels, specifically for drug delivery applications, is advantageous than that of neat polysaccharides. The modifications applied to the natural polysaccharides make them suitable for the application in diverse areas, just as agricultural, biomedical, and industrial (Table 3.1).

TABLE 3.1 Some Applications of Biopolymer Hydrogels.

Area	Application as
Biomedical	Coatings
	Drug delivery
	Biosensor
	Implantable devices
	Wound dressing
	Ophthalmologic
	Dental impression
	Stabilizer or plasticizer
Agricultural	Controlled release of pesticides
	Sorption of heavy metals
	Water storage granules
Industrial	Cosmetic
	Food industry
	Electrophoresis
	Wastewater treatments or bioremediation
	Corrosion inhibitor
	Textile
	Hygiene products

Among the most popular and promising hydrogel biopolymers is alginate. Alginate hydrogels have been used in several areas including industrial applications and biomedical science. The use is based in their favorable properties, including biocompatibility and ease of gelation. In the next paragraphs, we will explore the structure, properties, chemical modifications, and applications of this interesting biopolymer.

3.2 ALGINATES

3.2.1 SOURCES OF ALGINATE

"Alginate" is the term usually used for the salts of alginic acid but it can also refer to all the derivatives of alginic acid and alginic acid itself; in some publications, the term "algin" is used instead of alginate. Alginic acid is a chemical compound found in the cell wall of brown algae (*Phaeophyceae*). Alginates are salts of alginic acid that can be formed with Na, Ca, Mg, K, among others, forming salts with different degrees of solubility in water, which confers varying degrees of viscosity. They comprise up to 40% of their dry weight, and after further purification and conversion, the alginate content is 22–30% for *Ascophyllum nodosum* and 25–44% for *Laminaria digitata* (Qin et. al., 2008). Alginates are the structural components of the cell wall of algae, whose main function is to give rigidity, elasticity, flexibility, and ability to bind to water (Hernández et al., 2005).

The first studies related to the extraction of alginates from brown algae were made by the British chemist E. C. Stanford in 1883. Stanford observed that through digestion procedures of brown algae with sodium carbonate, a substance was formed gelatinous to which he denominated "algina," for being a substance derived from algae (Medina and Ledo, 2010).

Currently, the major alginate-producing countries are the United States and England, followed by Norway, France, Russia, and Japan (Luna and Villegas, 1989). There are two basic processes for obtaining sodium alginate. In both processes, water or alcohol is used as a solvent during the conversion of alginic acid to sodium alginate, obtaining very different results. Some patents describe processes but do not give details of the concentration or volume of solvent employed (Arvizu et al., 2002). In the first, the main intermediaries are calcium alginate and alginic acid. In the second, calcium alginate is not formed—only alginic acid is formed.

As mention before, commercially available alginate is typically extracted from brown algae (*Phaeophyceae*), including *Laminaria hyperborea*, *L. digitata*, *Laminaria japonica*, *A. nodosum*, and *Macrocystis pyrifera* (Smidsrod and Skjak-Bræk, 1990) by the treatment with aqueous alkali solutions, typically with NaOH (US Patent 2036922). The extract is filtered, and either sodium or calcium chloride is added to the filtrate in order to precipitate alginate. This alginate salt can be transformed into alginic acid by treatment with dilute hydrochloride acid.

Bacterial biosynthesis, carried out by *Azotobacter* and *Pseudomonas*, can provide alginate with more definite chemical structures and physical properties that can be obtained from alginate derived from seaweed. The biosynthesis pathway of alginate is generally divided into (i) precursor substrate synthesis, (ii) cytoplasmic membrane polymerization and transfer, (iii) periplasmic transfer and modification, and (iv) export through the outer membrane (Remminghorst and Rehm, 2006).

In *Azotobacter vinelandii*, the alginate is synthesized from fructose-6-phosphate, which is converted by phosphomannose isomerase to mannose-6-phosphate; this, in turn, is converted to mannose-1-phosphate by the phospho-mano-mutasa. The next step is the activation of mannose-1-phosphate by GDP-mannose pyrophosphorylase, resulting in the formation of GDP-mannose, which is oxidized to GDP-mannuronic acid by GDP-mannose dehydrogenase. GDP-mannuronic acid is the substrate that is polymerized at the level of the inner membrane to form polymannuronic acid. In the periplasm, some of the mannuronic residues of the polymannuronic acid are acetylated by an acetylase (Pindar and Bucke, 1975). The polymer is exported out of the cell where some non-acetylated mannuronic residues are epimerized to guluronic residues by multiple extracellular epimerases, thus giving the final product alginate.

3.2.2   CHEMISTRY OF ALGINATES

From a chemical point of view, alginate is an unbranched anionic polysaccharide composed of the two monomers, β-D-mannuronate (M) and α-L-guluronate (G) (Figure 3.3), linked 1→4. The polyanionic character that appears along the chain is due to carboxyl groups.

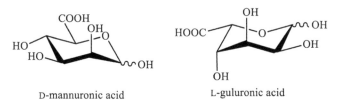

D-mannuronic acid   L-guluronic acid

FIGURE 3.3   Structure of monomers components of the alginates.

The alginates are grouped or distributed in sections constituting homopolymers of G-blocks (GGGGGG), M-blocks (MMMMMM), or heteropolymers in which the M- and G-blocks alternate (MGMGMG) (Figure 3.4). The blocks of MM and MG sequences are linked by glycosidic bonds β (1→4), whereas the GG- and GM-blocks by bonds α (1→4) (Lupo et al., 2012).

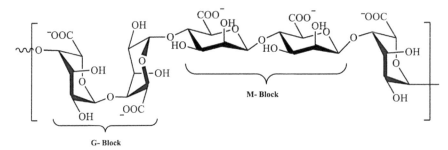

FIGURE 3.4   Sodium alginate sequences [G=guluronic acid, M=mannuronic acid].

The fact that G and M are C-5 epimers results in a switchover of the monomer chair conformation, giving rise to all four possible glycosidic linkages at the molecular level. The distribution of the monomers in the polymer chain and the charge and volume of the carboxyl groups give the gel formed the characteristics of flexibility or rigidity, depending on the content of guluronic acid.

The M and G units in the alginates may be randomly or nonrandomly arrayed as heterogeneous or homogeneous sequences (Figure 3.5). The stiffness of the sequences in aqueous solution increases in the order MG<M<G (Smidsroed et al., 1973; Stokke et al., 1993; Dentini et al., 2005). As we mentioned earlier, the content of units G or M depends on the species that produces the alginate. Table 3.2 exemplifies this variation of alginate as a function of the type of synthesizing species.

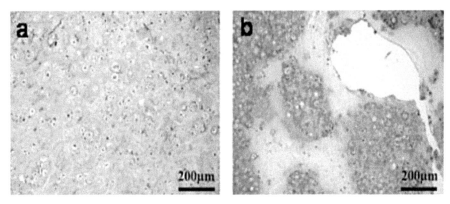

FIGURE 3.5   Chemical structures of G-block, M-block, and alternating block in alginate.
Source: Reprinted with permission from Lee and Mooney. © 2012 Elsevier.

TABLE 3.2   Typical M- and G-Block Profiles for Different Seaweeds as Measured by Nuclear Magnetic Resonance Spectroscopy.

Type of seaweed	%MM	%(MG–GM)	%GG
Laminaria hyperborea (stem)	17	26	57
Laminaria hyperborea (leaf)	36	38	26
Lessonia nigrescens	40	38	22
Lessonia trabeculata	25	26	49
Durvillaea antarctica	56	26	18
Laminaria digitata	43	32	25
Ecklonia maxima	38	24	28
Macrocystis pyrifera	38	46	16
Ascophyllum nodosum	44	40	16
Laminaria japonica	48	36	16

3.2.3   PROPERTIES OF ALGINATES

3.2.3.1   MOLECULAR WEIGHT

The molecular weight of commercially available sodium alginates is in a range between 32,000 and 400,000 g/mol. The viscosity of the alginate solutions depends on the length of the molecules—the longer the molecules, the higher the viscosity. Increasing the molecular weight of alginate can improve the physical properties of resultant gels. However, an alginate solution formed from high-molecular-weight polymer becomes greatly viscous, which is often undesirable in processing (LeRoux et al., 1999). For example, proteins or cells mixed with an alginate solution of high viscosity risk damage due to the high shear forces generated during mixing and injection into the body (Kong et al., 2005).

3.2.3.2   VISCOSITY

The viscosity of an alginate solution depends on the alginate concentration and length of the alginate molecules, or the number of monomer units in the chains (i.e., average molecular weight), with longer chains resulting in higher viscosities at similar concentrations. On the other hand, the complete hydration of alginates is necessary to obtain full functionality of the polymer. Aqueous solutions of alginates have shear-thinning character-istics, meaning that viscosity decreases as the shear rate, or stirrer speed, increases. This property is known as pseudoplasticity or non-Newtonian flow. The temperature will influence viscosity as well, with increasing temperature resulting in decreased viscosity. Such a phenomenon is more apparent for high viscosity alginates. The viscosity increases and flow properties decrease if the concentration of polyvalent metal ion is increased. Sodium alginate solution decreases in apparent viscosity with increasing shear rate. Low-molecular-weight alginate exhibits the Newto-nian behavior. At low levels of calcium ion, the effect of calcium increasing viscosity is particularly apparent in the case of alginates with higher content of D-mannuronic acid. In addition, the viscosity of the alginate solutions increases as the pH decreases and reaches a maximum around pH 3–3.5 as the carboxylate groups in the alginate backbone protonate and form hydrogen bonds.

3.2.3.3   SOLUBILITY

Only alginic acid and its polyvalent metal salts are insoluble in water, the rest of the alginic acid salts with alkali metal (Na^+, K^+, etc.) and ammo-nium and quaternary ammonium compounds are water soluble. Alginate is soluble in alcohols and ketones but not soluble in hard water and milk because both of them contain Ca^{2+}. If sodium alginate needs to be added in such solution, a chelant agent such as ethylenediaminetetraacetic acid (EDTA) or sodium hexametaphosphate can be used to sequester Ca^{2+}. Propylene glycol alginate (PGA) (80–85% esterified) is less affected by calcium ions and can be used in milk. It is acid resistant, remaining soluble when pH downs to about pH 2.

3.2.3.4   STABILITY

Like many natural polysaccharides, dried alginates are not resistant to heat, oxygen, or metallic ions. Alginates will be degraded naturally if stored in such circumstances. The order of stability in storage is as follows: sodium alginate > ammonium alginate > alginic acid.

   Different kinds of alginate salt give different stability, so does the different grade product. The industrial grade alginate solution is more easily degraded by a microbe in the air because such products contain much algal particles and nitrogenous matter which offer plenty of nutrition for the microbe. The pure sodium alginate solution can be kept at room temperature for several months without an obvious change in viscosity. When the temperature increases, all alginate solutions will depolymerize. Alginate solutions are stable in the pH range of 5.5–10 at room temperature for a long time but will form the gel below pH 5.5. PGA solution is relatively stable at room temperature at pH 3–4 but it will lose the viscosity rapidly below pH 2 and above pH 6. On the other hand, it is known that the high-viscosity alginate is more rapidly degraded than the medium-or low- viscosity ones.

3.2.3.5   ION EXCHANGE

Alginate matrix can be prepared through physical and/or chemical cross-linking of the polymer chains. The ionic cross-linking generates a three-dimensional network mainly by the interaction of the carbonyl groups of guluronate moieties with multivalent cations, giving rise to the well-known "egg-box" conformation (Braccini and Pérez, 2012), which we will later explain in Section 3.2.3.6. The interaction strength of important alginate cross-linking cations follows the order: trivalent cations $> Pb^{2+} > Cu^{2+} > Cd^{2+} > Ba^{2+} > Sr^{2+} > Ca^{2+}$ (Mørch et al., 2006). Although Ca^{2+} ion does not show the highest interaction strength, it is the most used (Sun and Tan, 2013). This preference could be associated to the adequate network of Ca–alginate gel and the acceptability of calcium by human organism because of its role as a major component of the skeletal system as well as in the regulation of several physiological processes. Sr^{2+} and Ba^{2+} cations are also considered as cross-linking agents but the use of Pb^{2+}, Cu^{2+} and Cd^{2+} is limited because of their toxicity (Gombotz and Wee, 2012).

Physical entanglements obtained by ionic cross-linking lead to a limited long-term stability in physiological conditions because of the di- and trivalent cations exchange with monovalent ions, causing destabilization and rupture of the three-dimensional matrix (Straccia et al., 2015). For example, Yang et al. (2013) found that trivalent cations produce alginate/polyacrylamide hydrogels with significantly higher strength and elastic modulus than divalent cations, leading the alternative simple way to prepare hydrophilic materials with exceptional mechanical properties for biomedical applications.

On the other hand, the insoluble alginate salt behaves like typical ion-exchange resin. The affinities of divalent metal ions are dependent on the relative amounts of D-mannuronic acid and L-guluronic acid units in the alginate. The affinity of alginates for divalent ions decreases in the following order:

a) For the alginate rich in M from *L. digitata:*
    Pb>Cu>Cd>Ba>Sr>Ca>Co, Ni, Zn, Mn>Mg

b) For the alginate rich in G from *L. hyperborea:*
    Pb>Cu>Ba>Sr>Cd>Ca>Co, Ni, Zn, Mn>Mg

The concentration of divalent cations required for gel formation and precipitation of sodium alginate from two type seaweeds is the same, and increases in the order:

$$Ba<Pb<Cu<Sr<Cd<Ca<Zn<Ni<Co<Mn, Fe<Mg$$

Aside from the interaction of metal ions with carboxyl groups of alginate, the hydroxyl groups on the polymer also play some role in ion binding.

3.2.3.6   GELATION OF ALGINATES

Gelation of alginates is based on the affinity of alginates toward certain ions and the ability to bind these ions selectively and cooperatively. Ion binding is selectively linked to the content of guluronate residues (G), or more precisely, the length of the G-blocks. The composition (i.e., M/G ratio), sequence, G-block length, and molecular weight are thus critical factors affecting the physical properties of alginate and its resultant hydrogels.

When two chains of G blocks are aligned, coordination sites are formed. Due to the looping of these chains, there are cavities between them that are sized to accommodate the calcium ion and are also coated with carboxylic groups and other electronegative oxygen atoms. After the addition of calcium ions, the alginate undergoes conformational changes, giving rise to what is known as "egg box" (Figure 3.6). This is based on the dimerization of the chain and, finally, on the greater aggregation of the dimers.

Then, alginates having large G-block regions form a high-strength gel and exhibit high porosity, while those with large M-blocks form a medium force gel but with a high resistance to syneresis and exhibit more small pores that make them softer (Hernández et al., 2005).

Present and future applications of alginates are mainly linked to the most striking feature of the alginate molecule; that is, a solgel transition in the presence of multivalent cations, for example, Ca^{2+}, almost independent of temperature. These very mild conditions, combined with the fact that alginates are highly characterized and understood both in the liquid and in the gel phase, make this biopolymer unique compared to other gelling polysaccharides.

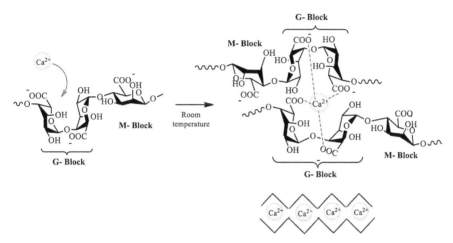

FIGURE 3.6 Schematic representation of the "egg-box" structure by major ionic interaction of carboxylate ions of alginate guluronate units and Ca²⁺ ions.

In addition to ionic gels, alginates can form acid gels at pH below the pKa value of the uronic acid residues. Some publications (Draget et al., 1994 and 1996) have shown that, as in the case of cross-linked ionized gels, the most important element in the stabilization of such gels are the G-blocks because at low pH the carboxyl groups of uronic acids accept protons favoring the formation of bonds. However, M-blocks also support acid gel formation and the acid gel, contrary to the ionic gel, seems to be more of an equilibrium type.

Important technological properties are gel strength, porosity/diffusion, alginate distribution, swelling/shrinking, transparency, leaching of alginate from the gels, and immunology of the leached material. In this way, alginate has demonstrated great utility and potential as a biomaterial for many biomedical applications, particularly in the areas of wound healing, drug delivery, in vitro cell culture, and tissue engineering. Like other hydrogels, however, alginate gels have very limited mechanical stiffness, and more general physical properties. A continuing challenge is matching the physical properties of alginate gels to the need in a particular application. Consideration of the range of different available cross-linking strategies, using molecules with various chemical structures, molecular weights, and cross-linking functionality will often yield gels suitable for each application.

Alginates extracted from different sources differ in M and G contents as well as the length of each block, and more than 200 different alginates are currently being manufactured. The only derivative of alginates today having a commercial value is the PGA. This product is processed by an esterification of alginate with propylene oxide. PGA is used in beers and salad dressings due to its higher solubility at low pH.

3.2.3.6.1   Ionic Cross-Linking

As mention before, one of the most common methods to prepare hydrogels from an aqueous alginate solution is to combine the solution with ionic cross-linking agents, such as divalent cations (i.e., Ca^{2+}). The divalent cations are believed to bind solely to guluronate blocks of the alginate chains as the structure of the guluronate blocks allows a high degree of coordination of the divalent ions. The guluronate blocks of one polymer then form junctions with the guluronate blocks of adjacent polymer chains in what is termed the egg-box model of cross-linking, resulting in a gel structure (Grant et al., 1973). Calcium chloride ($CaCl_2$) is one of the most frequently used agents to ionically cross-link alginate. However, it typically leads to rapid and poorly controlled gelation due to its high solubility in aqueous solutions. One approach to slow and control gelation is to utilize a buffer containing phosphate (e.g., sodium hexametaphosphate) as phosphate groups in the buffer compete with carboxylate groups of alginate in the reaction with calcium ions and retard gelation. Calcium sulfate ($CaSO_4$) and calcium carbonate ($CaCO_3$), due to their lower solubilities, can also slow the gelation rate and widen the working time for alginate gels. For example, an alginate solution can be mixed with $CaCO_3$ which is not soluble in water at neutral pH. Glucono-delta-lactone (GDL) is then added to the alginate/$CaCO_3$ mixture in order to dissociate Ca^{2+} from the $CaCO_3$ by lowering the pH. The released Ca^{2+} subsequently initiates the gelation of the alginate solution in a more gradual manner (Crow and Nelson, 2006).

The gelation rate is a critical factor in controlling gel uniformity and strength when using divalent cations, and slower gelation produces more uniform structures and greater mechanical integrity (Kuo and Ma, 2001). The gelation temperature also influences gelation rate, and the resultant mechanical properties of the gels. At lower temperatures, the reactivity of ionic cross-linkers (e.g., Ca^{2+}) is reduced, and cross-linking becomes slower. The resulting cross-linked network structure has greater order, leading to enhanced mechanical properties (Augst et al., 2006). The ionic gelation mechanisms have been carried out mainly by two processes: external and internal gelation.

The external gelation process occurs with the diffusion of the calcium ion from a source that surrounds the hydrocolloid to the neutral pH alginate solution. Gel formation starts at the interface and proceeds inwardly as the surface is saturated with calcium ions, so that the sodium ion from the alginate salt is displaced by the divalent cation solubilized in water. It interacts with the G-blocks of different polymer molecules, linking them together. Although the most commonly used calcium source is calcium chloride because of its higher percentage of available calcium, there are other less commonly used salts such as acetate monohydrate and calcium lactate (Helgerud et al., 2010).

The internal gelation process consists of the controlled release of the calcium ion from an internal source of insoluble or partially soluble calcium salt dispersed in the sodium alginate solution. The release of the calcium ion can occur in two ways depending on the solubility of the salt. In the case that the salt is insoluble at neutral pH but soluble at acidic pH, it is necessary to add an organic acid. In this case, the most commonly used calcium salts are calcium carbonate and tricalcium phosphate, and in specific cases, dicalcium phosphate and tricalcium citrate. For the acidification of the medium, there are organic acids such as acetic, adipic, and GDL.

If the calcium salt is partially soluble, the internal gelation process consists of the addition to the calcium alginate–salt mixture, a sequestering agent such as sodium phosphate, sulfate, or citrate. By adding a sequestrated agent, this binds to free calcium, thus retarding the gelation process; sodium sulfate has been commonly used because of its low cost and convenient solubility. The mechanisms of ionic gelling are described in Figure 3.7 (Helgerud et al., 2010).

The main difference between the external and internal gelation mechanism is the process kinetics. If the control of the solgel transition is intended, in the external gelation process, the factors to be manipulated are the calcium concentration and the composition of the polymer. However, for the internal gelation process, the solubility and concentration of the calcium salt, concentration of the sequestering agent and the organic acid used should be considered (Draget, 2000).

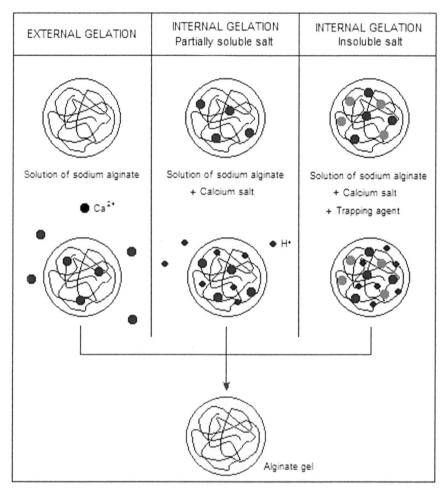

FIGURE 3.7   Ionic gelation mechanisms.

3.2.3.6.2   Covalent Cross-Linking

Covalent cross-linking has been widely investigated in an effort to improve the physical properties of gels for many applications, including tissue engineering. The stress applied to an ionically cross-linked alginate gel relaxes as the cross-links dissociate and reform elsewhere, and water is lost from the gel, leading to plastic deformation. While water migration also occurs in covalently cross-linked gels, leading to stress relaxation, the inability to dissociate and reform bonds leads to significant elastic deformation (Zhao et al., 2010). However, covalent cross-linking reagents may be toxic, and the unreacted chemicals may need to be removed thoroughly from gels.

It was subsequently demonstrated that the mechanical properties and swelling of alginate hydrogels can be tightly regulated by using different kinds of cross-linking molecules, and by controlling the cross-linking densities. Hydrogel swelling is also significantly influenced by the chemistry of the cross-linking molecules, as would be expected. The introduction of hydrophilic cross-linking molecules as a second macromolecule (e.g. PEG) can compensate for the loss of hydrophilic character of the hydrogel resulting from the cross-linking reaction (Lee et al., 2000).

The use of multi-functional cross-linking molecules to form hydrogels provides a wider range and tighter control over degradation rates and mechanical stiffness than bifunctional cross-linking molecules.

Photo-cross-linking is an exciting approach to in situ gelation that exploits covalent cross-linking. Photo-cross-linking can be carried out in mild reaction conditions, even in direct contact with drugs and cells, with the appropriate chemical initiators (Lee and Mooney, 2012).

3.2.3.6.3 Thermal Gelation

Thermosensitive hydrogels have been widely investigated for their adjustable swelling properties in response to temperature changes, leading to on-demand modulation of drug release from the gels (Roy et al., 2010). A few systems using alginate have been reported as alginate is not inherently thermosensitive. However, the transition temperature can be altered by copolymerization. semi-IPN structures were prepared through in situ copolymerization of N-isopropylacrylamide (NIPAAm) with PEG-co-poly(ε-caprolactone) (PEG-co-PCL) macromere in the presence of sodium alginate by UV irradiation. The swelling ratio of the gels increased with the concentration of sodium alginate at a constant temperature, and decreased with an increase in temperature. The use of sodium alginate in semi-IPN structures improved the mechanical strength and the cumulative release of bovine serum albumin from the gels, indicating potential in drug delivery applications (Zhao, et al., 2010). Graft copolymerization of NIPAAm onto the alginate backbone after reaction with ceric ions also provided a useful means to prepare temperature-responsive alginate gels, with sensitivity near body temperature.

3.2.3.6.4   Cell Cross-Linking

While a number of chemical and physical methods have been reported to form alginate gels, the ability of cells to contribute to gel formation has been largely ignored. When alginate is modified with cell adhesion ligands, the ability of cells to bind multiple polymer chains can lead to long-distance, reversible network formation even in the absence of chemical cross-linking agents. Cells added to modified alginate solution form a uniform dispersion within the solution, and this system subsequently generates the cross-linked network structure through specific receptor–ligand interactions without using any additional cross-linking molecules (Lee et al., 2003). In contrast, cells added to nonmodified alginate solutions aggregate and form a nonuniform structure due to the dominance of cell–cell interactions in that system. This gelation behavior is shear reversible and can be repeated multiple times. Once the gel structure is broken down by applying shear forces, cross-linked structures are recovered within a few minutes. This behavior is governed by the weak and reversible ligand–receptor interactions in the system. This system might be ideal for cell delivery in tissue engineering because a gel can flow like a liquid during injection into the body, but solidify once it is placed in the body (Drury et al., 2005).

3.2.3.7   MICROENCAPSULATION TECHNIQUES

Microencapsulation of small molecules such as enzymes into cells and microorganisms can be performed by different techniques. The selection of the suitable encapsulation technique is determined by the physicochemical properties of the carrier material and the desired final application is done in order to ensure the bioavailability of the compounds, their functionality, and even their easy incorporation into the food without the alteration of their sensory properties (Pal et al., 2009). By employing alginate as a polymeric matrix, microencapsulation techniques in food applications are reduced to extrusion, emulsion, and spray-drying.

3.2.3.7.1   Encapsulation by Extrusion

The technique consists of forming drops of the alginate solution containing the component to be encapsulated by passing said solution through an extruder device of size and controlled drip speed. These drops fall on a bath containing the source of the divalent ion, which induces gelation through the external gelation mechanism (Chan et al., 2009). The main limitation presented by this technique is the large size of the microcapsules, which depends on the diameter of the nozzle of the extruder device. Among other drawbacks, the difficulty of large-scale production is due to the formation of the microcapsules one by one, which results in long gelation times (Mofidi et al., 2000). Additionally, it is necessary to consider aspects that influence its spherical shape and size, such as the separation distance from the nozzle to the bath, the effect of gravity, and the surface tension of the solution that induces gelation (Chan et al., 2009). Despite all these factors, the microencapsulation technique by extrusion has traditionally been used to allow the production of microcapsules with uniform sizes.

In Figure 3.8, different types of extruder devices are shown for the preparation of microcapsules (Zuidam and Shimoni, 2010).

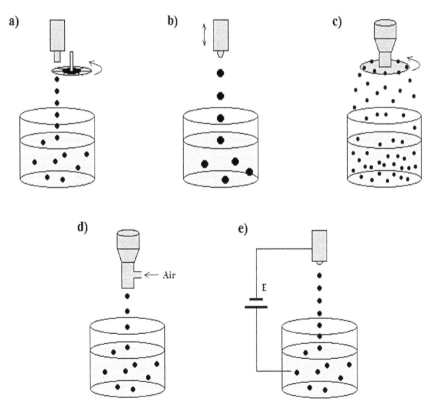

FIGURE 3.8 Types of extruder devices. (a) Atomizer with systematic jet cutting. (b) Vibratory nozzle. (c) Atomizing disk. (d) Coaxial airflow. (e) Electrostatic potential.

3.2.3.7.2   Emulsion Encapsulation

The emulsion encapsulation technique has been defined as the process of dispersing a liquid into another immiscible liquid where the dispersed phase consists of the matrix including the component to be encapsulated. The addition of a surfactant improves the formation and stability of the emulsion as well as the size distribution of the droplets (Poncelet, 2001; de Vos et al., 2010). In this regard, the preparation of microcapsules by emulsification can be carried out using the external or internal gelation mechanism. For the first case, the external gelation in emulsion consists of the dispersion of a solution mixture of alginate component in a continuous nonaqueous phase, followed by the addition of a source of calcium which upon diffusion to the dispersed phase initiates the gelation, allowing the encapsulation, and in turn, the destabilization of the emulsion for the separation of the capsules formed. While the internal gelation emulsion technique is based on the release of the calcium ion from an insoluble or partially soluble complex wherein a sequestering agent contained in an alginate-component solution is added which is dispersed in a continuous phase nonaqueous emulsion generating a water-in-oil (w/o) emulsion (Gouin 2004; Chan et al., 2006). The release of the calcium ion occurs with the addition of a soluble organic acid in the continuous phase which upon diffusion decreases the pH of the medium by solubilizing the salt and causing the gelation. Emulsion microencapsulation techniques are described in Figure 3.9 (Champagne and Fustier, 2007).

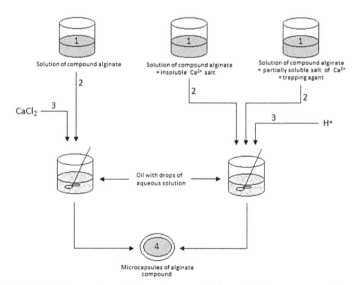

FIGURE 3.9   Techniques of emulsion microcapsulation of alginate compounds.

3.2.3.7.3   Encapsulation by Spray-Drying

Spray-drying has been a technology widely used by industry because of its reproducibility and economy. Its main application has been used to mask flavors, aromas and the encapsulation of vitamins. The process consists of the preparation of an emulsion or suspension containing the compound to be encapsulated and the polymeric material, which is sprayed onto a hot gas which is generally air, thus promoting the instantaneous evaporation of the water, allowing the present active principle to be trapped within a film of encapsulating material. The obtained microparticles are separated from the gas at low temperatures. One of the great advantages of this process is, in addition to its simplicity, that it is appropriate for materials sensitive to high temperatures because the exposure times are very short (5–30 s) (Martín Villena et al., 2009; de Vos et al., 2010; López-Hernández, 2010).

The preparation of microcapsules with this technique requires first the selection of the type of atomizer considering the viscosity of the solution as well as the desired drop size in order to generate the largest contact surface between hot air and liquid, contact between droplets and hot air depending on the heat sensitivity of the product, drop-air contact time, air temperature, and finally the type of dry solids separation method (Gharsallaoui et al., 2007). Basically, its application with alginate is summarized in three stages: dispersion of the active principle in the alginate, atomization of the mixture, and dehydration (Zuidam and Shimoni, 2010).

3.2.3.8   pH SENSITIVENESS

The pH plays an important role in different processes such as preparation, purification, hydrogel device formation, swelling, release, and degradation rate. The presence of carboxylic groups in alginate structure confers to the polymer a remarkable sensitivity to external pH stimuli. For a pH below its pKa (pH < 3.4), the carboxylic acid groups are in the nonionized form (COOH), leading to an insoluble structure. At pH > 4.4, the carboxylic group became ionized (COO⁻), resulting in an increase of electrostatic repulsion of these negative charges causing polymer chain expansion and swelling of the hydrophilic matrix, being highest around pH 7.4 (Fig 3.10). Therefore, approaches on pH variations along the gastrointestinal tract and alginate pH responsiveness of this biopolymer have been exploited for development oral colon-specific drug delivery devices (Agüero et al., 2017, 2015; Alvarez-Lorenzo et al., 2013; Bajpai and Sharma, 2004).

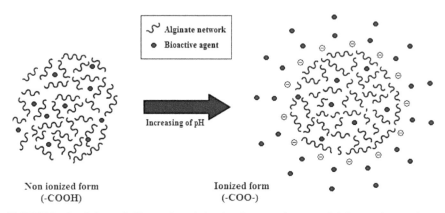

FIGURE 3.10   Schematic illustration of pH stimuli responsiveness of alginate microparticles.

3.2.3.9   FILM FORMATION

Another attribute of alginates which presents exciting possibilities is its film-forming capability. While several biopolymers can be used for film formation, alginate's inherent properties give it some distinct advantages. The films formed using alginates in combination with a plasticizer are generally strong oxygen barrier. Alginate films also offer excellent transparency and can be either soluble or insoluble. Soluble film of sodium alginate are made by casting and drying, while insoluble or gelled alginate films are produced by applying a layer of alginate solution followed by cross-linking with calcium salt and then drying.

3.2.3.10   RHEOLOGICAL PROPERTIES

Rheology is the study of the flow and deformation of matter. A certain material can behave as a solid or a liquid depending on the stress applied to it and the timescale used in the deformation process. There are two types of flow: shear flow and extensional flow (Figure 3.11). In shear flow, adjacent particles move over and past each other, while in extensional flow, adjacent particles move away from or toward each other (Handbook of Elementary Rheology. A. Barnes). We can visualize shear flow alternatively due to the movement of hypothetical layers sliding over each other. In the simplest case, the velocity of each layer increases linearly with respect to its neighbor below. The gradient of the velocity in the direction at right angles to the flow is called the shear rate and the force per unit area (F/A) created or produced by the flow is called the shear stress. In a simple example, the shear rate is described by the symbol γ, while the shear stress is given by *F/A* and is given the symbol σ (sigma).

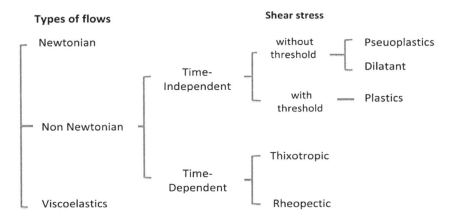

FIGURE 3.11   Classification of fluids.

The behavior of the material can be measured as a function of time, temperature, amplitude of applied stress or strain, and frequency. The results obtained give information on the structural properties of the material.

Rheological methods have many advantages over other methodologies for the characterization of polymer solutions: simple sample preparation, short time duration required for tests, and direct measurement of polymer behavior under conditions expected to be encountered during formulation processing or product storage or use. Nonetheless, the rheological properties of sodium alginate solutions are not specified in the United States Pharmacopeia.

The typical rheological behavior of many polymer solutions is highly sheared and concentration dependent, encompassing the range from Newtonian to shear-thinning non-Newtonian to viscoelastic behavior (Ikeda and Nishinari, 2001; Chronakis et al., 1996). The shear rates encountered in pharmaceutical manufacturing and in product use can vary considerably, ranging from 10^{-4} to 104 s^{-1} (Schnaare et al., 2005).

Most of the studies were limited to the rheological characterization of sodium alginate solutions at concentrations lower than 5%·w/v. Sodium alginate solutions at these low concentrations exhibit fluid-like behavior, whereas sodium alginate solutions at higher concentrations display a more substantial viscoelastic character.

Sodium alginate, extracted from seaweed using the calcium alginate method, may have residual calcium that could influence the rheological properties of the resultant sodium alginate solution. In some instances, calcium salts are added to sodium alginate to increase the viscosity of the corresponding polymer solutions (McHugh, 1988).

Rheological evaluations of multiple batches of one grade of sodium alginate produced over the course of 1 year showed significant variability between different batches in both rheological behavior at low solution concentration and viscoelastic behavior at high solution concentration (Fu et al., 2010, 2011).

3.2.3.11   BIOCOMPATIBILITY

Although the biocompatibility of alginate has been widely evaluated both in vitro and in vivo, there is still debate due to the presence of impurities. Since alginate is obtained from natural sources, potentially different impurities such as heavy metals, endotoxins, proteins, and polyphenolic compounds may be present, and it is believed that the immunogenic response at the sites of injection or implantation can be attributed to these impurities and not alginate. Alginate purified by a multistep extraction procedure at a very high purity does not induce any significant foreign body reaction when implanted or injected into animals (Orive et al., 2002; Lee and Lee et al., 2009).

Dusseault et al. (2006) evaluated the biocompatibility of alginate by quantification of the contaminants levels mentioned before. A comparative study about the efficiencies of various purification process previously reported in the literature was performed, but based on practical and economical aspects, free-flow electrophoresis was not included. Despite the differences in the efficiencies between methods, it could be concluded that all of them decreased the level of polyphenols, endotoxins, and proteins as common impurities in alginate.

It is important to mention that the oral administration of alginate has not shown to provoke a much immune response and is considered by the United States Food and Drug Administration (US FDA) as a Generally Regarded as Safe materials (George and Abraham, 2006).

On the other hand, there are different studies indicating the safety of the use of alginates in food. Sodium, magnesium, potassium and ammonium alginates, alginic acid, and PGA are food additives recognized as safe and safe according to the US FDA in the *Codex Alimentarius* that provides the Food and Agriculture Organization and the World Health Organization of the United Nations, which established that the daily intake limits of alginic acid and its derived salts for humans is 50 mg/kg body weight and of PGA is 25 mg/kg body weight (FAO/WHO, 2001).

3.3 CHEMICAL MODIFICATION OF ALGINATES

3.3.1 *DERIVATIZATION OF ALGINATES*

As mention before, alginate can be obtained from algal and bacterial sources. As a result of the great abundance of algae in water bodies, a large amount of alginate is obtained. Due to its potential uses as biomaterials, many researches focused their attention on the modification of alginate in order to design new materials with different properties. A chemical modification or derivatization of an alginate is performed in order to obtain either enhanced existing properties, for instance, ionic gel strength improved or more hydrophobicity, or to introduce new properties such as anticoagulant properties or the use as chemical/biochemical anchors (Pawar et al., 2012).

There are three parameters that govern the derivatization for alginates: solubility, reactivity, and characterization. When it comes to solubility, it means that the media or solvent chosen will govern the type of reagents to be used as well as the derivative substitution pattern. It is also important to mention that the reactivity of the hydroxyls is not the same in the alginate molecule. For instance, the more reactive ones are the hydroxyls of C-2 and C-3, and derivatization can be selectively made in these positions. It is also very reactive and easy to derivatize the acid group at C-6. Finally, characterization is very important and it is essential to have multiple alginate samples with a range of M/G ratios (Pawar et al., 2012).

Acetylation, phosphorylation, sulfation, among others, are the most common derivatization reactions made in the alginate polymer. Generally, acetylation is performed in classical conditions, which is acetic anhydride in pyridine. One of the first reports of modification by acetylation is the one by Schweiger et al. (1962) in which they synthesized partially and fully acetylated alginic acid derivatives using an acid-catalyzed esterification technique. These derivatives were used for understanding the chelate structure formed in ionically cross-linked alginate gels. Schweiger demonstrated that aqueous solutions of ammonium mono- and diacetylated alginates do not change the consistency in the presence of divalent ions. These results allowed them to suggest that the gelation or precipitation of calcium alginates occurred through a complex that involved the two carboxylic groups of neighboring units and that the free hydroxyls did not participate in the complex formation. Skjåk-Bræk et al. (1989) demonstrated that acetylation intensifies the swelling ability of calcium gels made from these polymers. Acetylation of the alginate diminished the affinity of alginate for calcium ions and caused an expansion of the molecular chain as reflected in the viscosity data.

Phosphorylation of alginate was achieved by Coleman et al. (2011) using urea/phosphate reaction in heterogeneous conditions. They demonstrated that the phosphorylation occurred predominantly at the C-3 of the polysaccharide (Fig 3.12). The hydrogel formed between phosphorylated alginate and alginate were ionically cross-linked and showed an enhanced resistance to degradation by chelating.

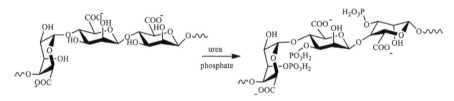

FIGURE 3.12   Phosphorylation of alginate.

In the search of new anticoagulants, Freeman et al. (2008) sulfated the uronic acids alginate and hydrogels of mixed alginate/alginate–sulfate were manufactured. They showed that the mixed hydrogels continued the release of basic fibroblast growth factors (FGF) and the release rate was dependent on the percentage of bFGF bound to the hydrogels.

Another type of derivatization involved the hydrophobic modification, which means that alginates must be transformed from its predominantly hydrophilic nature to amphiphilic or hydrophobic characteristics. The easier way to achieve this transformation involves covalent attachment of hydrophobic moieties such as long alkyl chains or aromatic groups to the polymer backbone (Pawar et al., 2012). In this sense, a new procedure for the preparation of microparticles of amphiphilic alginate derivative (modified with dedecyl chains) was developed by Leonard et al. (2004). The microparticles showed better stability than that of plain Ca²⁺–alginate hydrogels. The attachment of cell signaling molecules is also an interesting modification of alginates and a clear example of this is presented by Yang et al. (2002). In this report, alginate was modified by the addition of galactose moieties covalently coupled with ethylenediamine as the spacer in order to get an improved performance in the interaction with hepatocytes. The adhesion of hepatocytes was enhanced in an 18-fold and the number of hepatocytes attached was greater when the density of galactose residues on the galacto-sylated alginate-coated surface was higher.

3.3.2 MODIFICATION AND DERIVATIZATION OF ALGINATES

There are many ways in which alginate can be modified in order to get new compounds with improved properties. For instance, Amer et al. (2014) reported a new hybrid material based on brushite-alginate and monetite-alginate. The material was built by self-assembling through a gelation process within the alginate chains, the phosphate source, and the calcium ions. Due to the unique properties of the alginate (gelling and swelling), the gel served as a point for nucleation and growth of brushite and monetite. They reported that the properties of the new hybrid material are dependent on the concentration of the phosphate precursors.

3.4 APPLICATIONS OF ALGINATE

The uses of alginates are based on three main properties. The first is their ability, when dissolved in water, to increase the viscosity of aqueous solutions. The second is their ability to form gels. And the third property of alginates is the ability to form films of sodium or calcium alginate and fibers of calcium alginates.

As we observed earlier, these properties depend on the type of alginate, the chain length, the composition, and the species that synthesizes alginate. Some examples: *Macrocystis* can give a medium-viscosity alginate, or a high viscosity with a careful extraction procedure (lower temperature for the extraction); *Sargassum* usually gives a low-viscosity product; *L. digitata* gives a soft to medium strength gel, while *L. hyperborea* and *Durvillaea* give strong gels.

They also offer benefits as viscosifiers and disintegrants, and can be customized so that their gel-forming characteristics facilitate matrix and structural building properties. Alginates have a wide range of gel strengths so they could be used as dental impression and denture-adhesive markets for decades. These alginates hydrogels could create films, foams, and fibers, offering a wide range of potential uses in the areas of wound care and dermatology. A list of different products and main applications of alginates are listed in Table 3.3.

TABLE 3.3   List of Different Products and Main Application of Alginates.

Type of alginate	Main applications
Alginic acid	Anti-reflux tablets, natural disintegrant
Sodium alginate	Anti-reflux suspensions, controlled release tablets, wound dressing, dental impression material, denture fixatives, viscosifier, encapsulation, films, foams
Magnesium alginate	Anti-reflux suspensions for infants
Potassium alginate	Dental impression material
Triethanolamine alginate	Dental impression material
Propylene glycol alginate	Suspending agent/stabilizer, plasticizer, emulsifier

3.4.1   PHARMACEUTICAL AND MEDICAL USES

Alginates possess a valuable functionality in esophageal anti-reflux suspensions and tablets, and have demonstrated to be promising in the area of controlled release medications. Calcium alginate is widely investigated for its potential to control drug delivery in the intestinal tract due to its ability to shrink at acidic pH and swell at neutral or basic pH, joined to excellent mucoadhesion properties, biodegradability, biocompatibility, and the absence of toxicity (González-Rodríguez et al., 2002; George and Abraham, 2006; Patel et al., 2008; Agarwal et al., 2015). Alginate beads have been successfully used as a vehicle for liposomes (Xing et al., 2003; Bansal et al., 2016) to protect the entrapped hydrophilic drugs and release them to the fourth lower bowel after specific local biodegradation of the polymer.

Such an effect could be particularly beneficial in the case of metformin since it has been recently proved to be important for the lower bowel-mediated mechanism in the primary glucose-lowering effect of the drug, especially used for patients with type 2 diabetes (Buse et al., 2016). The drug presents few side effects even though problems of gastrointestinal intolerance may limit its use; moreover, chronic administration may cause hyperlactatemia due to drug accumulation, resulting in lactic acidosis (Page, 2011). The poor bioavailability and short half-life of this drug (Dunn and Peters, 1995; Scheen, 1996), make the development of extended-release formulations desirable in order to improve patient compliance and reduce the dosing frequency, resulting in better glycemic control and less side effects appearance (Di Colo et al., 2002; Hu et al., 2006; Corti et al., 2008, 2008; Momoh et al., 2013; Nayak et al., 2013, Li et al., 2014; Kim and Park, 2015).

Maestreli et al. (2017) prepared different types of metformin hydrochloride (MTF)-loaded colloidal systems (chitosomal and niosomal dispersions) as potential carriers for a prolonged drug release along the gastrointestinal tract. The entrapment of both kinds of colloidal dispersions in calcium alginate beads enabled to strongly limit the amount of drug released and to obtain a sustained release in a simulated intestinal fluid, which can be suitably tuned by varying the percentage of calcium alginate in the beads. In vivo studies on rats revealed the significant improvement of MTF hypoglycemic effect when administered as chitosomal and even more as niosomal dispersion entrapped in alginate beads not only with respect to the simple MTF solution but also with respect to the beads loaded with the plain drug. The more intense and more sustained therapeutic effect across time provided by the MTF-niosomes system in alginate beads formulation could be very profitable for maintaining tight blood glucose levels over prolonged period after oral administration, and improving patient compliance.

Ferreira et al. (2017) designed a delivery system for controlled and anti-angiogenic therapy under tumor microenvironmental conditions developing a bevacizumab (BVZ)-loaded alginate hydrogel by electrostatic interactions. The tridimensional hydrogel provides drug stability and a system that is able to introduce the drug as a flowable solution, stabilizing a depot after local administration. This kind of therapy is a promising strategy to be applied to solid tumors.

To enable an intratumoral application, the developed formulations must be able to be delivered by a syringe or through a needle. As an injectable system, the formation of aggregates cannot be allowed during the injection process to avoid needle clogging. Comparing the use of two different cross-linking agent concentrations, higher concentration promotes a significant increase in the work required for hydrogel ejection. Moreover, the addition of BVZ also promoted a higher syringeability value. A decreased viscosity might be observed due to the increased shear rates. This condition leads to temporary network destruction against molecular alignment in the flow direction. A typical non-Newtonian, shear thinning behavior was observed for all samples regardless of drug load or pH value.

In the study of Sangeetha and Girija (2017), alginate is tailored to control its swelling, entrapment, and release of ciprofloxacin (antibiotic) through the formation of IPN and composite matrices using gelatin and hydroxyapatite (HAP). Drug release prolonged from 5 to 240 h for composite matrix as compared with alginate matrix showing that alginate combined with gelatin and HAP sustained the release for longer periods. This matrix revealed excellent biocompatibility with osteoblast like MG-63 cell lines and showed good antibacterial activity against *Staphylococcus aureus* and *Escherichia coli* (Sangeetha et al., 2017).

Brady et al. (2017) have developed a novel hydrogel to treat aneurysms. An intracranial aneurysm is an irregular outpouching of a cerebral artery, and its rupture can lead to stroke, resulting in disability or death. The hydrogel developed is composed of a polymeric alginate, a novel ion-releasing glass and GDL. The last compound is a lactone that hydrolyzes in water to form a gluconic acid; its role in the novel hydrogel is to acidify the solution. The role of the glass in this hydrogel is to deliver a steady release of multivalent ions, controlling the rate of gelation and the strength of the hydrogel. This is an internally setting alginate hydrogel, wherein the setting rate can be controlled by both the glass and the alginate chemistry.

The hydrogel will fill the aneurysm more completely and prevent rupture. Alginate concentration, chemical composition, and molecular weight affect the compressive strength, working time, hardening time, and deliverability of the hydrogel. Gamma irradiation of the alginate for sterilization reduces the molecular weight, which has a negative effect on the usability of this hydrogel, which decreases the alginate's viscosity and strength, and increases the hydrogel's working and hardening time.

The main aim of this study was to obtain porous antimicrobial composites consisting of chitosan, alginate, and biosynthesized silver nanoparticles (AgNPs). Chitosan and alginate were used owing to their pore-forming capacity, while AgNPs were used for their antimicrobial property. Antimicrobial activity of the composites was checked with *E. coli* and *S. aureus*. The bacterial filtration efficiency of chitosan–alginate–AgNPs was 1.5 times higher than that of the chitosan–alginate composite. The developed chitosan–alginate–AgNPs composite showed a huge potential for its applications in antimicrobial filtration and cancer treatment.

Other researchers have used the chitosan–alginate polyelectrolyte complex for wound dressing. Some experiments show that chitosan–alginate polyelectrolyte complex hydrogels are highly biocompatible, degradable, nontoxic, antimicrobial, and can effectively enhance the wound healing. Various chitosan–alginate-based composites with Ag and drugs are utilized for wound dressing, sensor, bone tissue engineering, antimicrobial, anticancer, and dental applications. In addition to the strong antibacterial activity of AgNPs (Messaoud et al., 2014), they can also induce apoptosis in cancer cells, leading to efficient anticancer activity (Mihailović et al., 2010).

They proposed that chitosan–alginate–AgNPs composites can also be used as an antimicrobial filtration system. Recent studies revealed that air conditioners are breeding grounds for bacteria in hot conditions and rainy days. Even health officials warn that potential pathogenic bacteria can grow in the air conditioner. These bacteria can cause fever and ache. Installing an efficient microbial filter in the air-conditioning system is the only option to prevent these harmful microbes.

Reversal of intervertebral disc degeneration can have a potential effect on spinal health. The goal of the research of Growney Kalaf et al. (2016) was to create an injectable, cellularized alginate-based nucleus pulposus that would restore disc function, with the primary goal of creating an alginate gel with tailorable rates of gelation to improve functionality over standard $CaCl_2$ cross-linking techniques. Gelation characteristics of 1% sodium alginate were analyzed over various molar concentrations in a relation between $CaCO_3$:GDL with 10% $CaCl_2$ as the control cross-linker. Dehydration, swelling tests, and albumin release kinetics were determined, and cytotoxicity and cell homogeneity tests showed promising for cellularization strategies.

Another application of alginate hydrogels is for immobilizing enzymes into microfluidic systems. For instance, Akay et al. (2017) reported a system in which gelation was induced upon lowering the pH and by addition of D- GDL. They also studied the relationship between GDL concentration on enzymatic activity and gelation time, and concluded that the increased GDL concentration led to an increased in both surface area and enzymatic activity.

In the last years, synthetic bone substitutes, mainly based on HAP and tricalcium phosphate, have been developed as the treatment for bone disorder or injury. Glass-reinforced hydroxyapatite (GR-HAP) composites have been developed to improve the chemical similarity between bioceramics and bone inorganic part. The use of injectable form, by association with hydrogels working as a vehicle, should present a suitable viscosity to enable the bone substitute granules injectability. Morais et al. (2013) studied different hydrogels as vehicles for bone substitutes, potential vehicles to associate with GR-HAP granules so as to well aggregate them, maintaining the injectable system entirety and allowing a good handling of the injectable bone substitutes (IBSs) with low and stable injectability forces. Through rheology studies, it is demonstrated that all hydrogels are non-Newtonian viscoelastic fluids, and injectability tests showed that IBSs presented low maximum extrusion forces, as well as quite stable average forces (Morais et al., 2013).

In this same sense, Park et al. (2017) developed a hybrid structure of alginate and hyaluronate for cartilage regeneration. In this work, the alginate was used as a backbone and the hybrid coupling of hyaluronate and alginate was achieved with ethylenediamine. The characteristics of hybrid hydrogels containing various composition ratios of hyaluronate to alginate were studied and were successfully used to regulate chondrogenic differentiation and to maintain the chondrocytic cell phenotype, which may lead to many useful applications in cartilage regeneration.

3.4.2 FOOD

The application of alginates in the food industry is based on four main properties: (i) related to its ability as a thickener to be dissolved in water, increasing the viscosity of the solution in which it dissolves, (ii) the ability to retain water, (iii) the ability to form a gel from a series of ion-exchange chemical reactions (particularly an exchange of sodium ions by divalent or trivalent cations), leading to the formation of bonds between the adjacent chains of the alginate polymer, and (iv) ability to form films.

The ability of the alginate as a stabilizer is measured as a function of its degree of polymerization, which is a measure of the average molecular weight of the chains that constitute it and is directly related to the viscosity of its solutions. Loss of viscosity in storage is a measure of the degree of depolymerization of alginate (McHugh, 1987). Then, alginates with high PD are less stable than those with low PD.

One of the interesting characteristics of alginates is their water-holding capacity or absorbent, which is of such magnitude that they are called superabsorbents. That is, they can form three-dimensional polymeric reticules having hydrophilic groups capable of absorbing large volumes of water or biological fluids, from ten to a thousand times their own weight, and are capable of holding them under pressure. It may be mentioned as a disadvantage that the gels which are formed by absorbing the water can be blocked, and therefore lose the absorption capacity or decrease the rate of absorption. This problem can be minimized by the increase of carboxyl groups per unit of uronic acid through esterification reactions of the hydroxyl groups (Hernández et al., 2005).

The gel formation process is initiated from an alginate salt solution and an external or internal calcium source from where the calcium ion diffuses to reach the polymer chain, as a consequence of this union there is a structural rearrangement in the space resulting in a solid material with the characteristics of a gel. The degree of gelation depends on the hydration of the alginate, the concentration of the calcium ion, and the content of the G-blocks (Funami et al., 2009). The solgel transition has been essentially controlled by the ability to introduce the binding ion to the alginate. It has also been observed that the gelation kinetics and gel properties may depend on the type of counterion, for example, the monovalent ion of the alginate (K^+ or Na^+) salt. In fact, it has been found that potassium alginates have a faster solgel transition process than sodium alginates prepared at low calcium concentrations (Draget, 2000).

The thickening property of alginate is useful in sauces and in syrups and toppings for ice cream. By thickening pie fillings with alginate, softening of the pastry by liquid from the filling is reduced. The addition of alginate can make icings nonsticky and allow the baked goods to be covered with plastic wrap. W/O emulsions such as mayonnaise and salad dressings are less likely to separate into their original oil and water phases if thickened with alginate. Sodium alginate is not useful when the emulsion is acidic because insoluble alginic acid forms; for these applications, PGA is used since this is stable in mild acid conditions. Alginate improves the texture, body, and sheen of yogurt, but PGA is also used in the stabilization of milk proteins under acidic conditions as found in some yogurts. Some fruit drinks have fruit pulp added and it is preferable to keep this in suspension; addition of sodium alginate, or PGA in acidic conditions, can prevent sedimentation of the pulp. In chocolate milk, the cocoa can be kept in suspension by an alginate/phosphate mixture, although in this application, it faces strong competition from carrageenan. Small amounts of alginate can thicken and stabilize whipped cream.

Alginates have some applications that are not related to either their viscosity or gel properties. They act as stabilizers in ice cream; addition of alginate reduces the formation of ice crystals during freezing, giving a smooth product. Without alginate or similar stabilizer the refrozen ice cream develops large ice crystals, giving it an undesirable crunchy mouth feel. Alginate also reduces the rate at which the ice cream will melt. Beer drinkers prefer some foam on the top of a newly poured glass, and poor foam leads to a subjective judgment that the beer is of poor quality. The addition of a very low concentration of PGA will provide stable, longer lasting beer foam. A variety of agents are used in the clarification of wine and removal of unwanted coloring—wine fining—but in more difficult cases, it has been found that the addition of sodium alginate can be effective.

The gelling properties of alginate were used in the first production of artificial cherries in 1946. A flavored, colored solution of sodium alginate was allowed to fall, in large drops, into a solution of a calcium salt. Calcium alginate immediately formed as a skin on the outside of the drop and when the drop was allowed to sit in the solution, the calcium gradually penetrated the drop, converting it all into a gel that hardened with further standing. Because the cherry-flavored gels did not melt, they became very popular in bakery products. Fruit substitutes can now be made by automated and continuous processes that are based on similar principles. Either the calcium can be applied externally, as above, or internally. In the latter case, a calcium salt that does not dissolve is added to the fruit puree, together with a weak acid; the weak acid slowly attacks the calcium salt and releases water-soluble calcium that then reacts with the alginate and forms the gel.

Edible dessert jellies can be formed from alginate–calcium mixtures, often promoted as instant jellies or desserts because they are formed simply by mixing the powders with water or milk, no heat being required. Because they do not melt, alginate jellies have a different, firmer mouth feel when compared to gelatin jellies, which can be made to soften and melt at body temperature. Mixtures of calcium salts and sodium alginate can be made to set to a gel at different rates, depending on the rate at which the calcium salt dissolves. Gel formation can also be delayed even after everything is mixed together; this is done using a gel-retarder that reacts with the calcium before the alginate does, so no calcium is available to the alginate until all the retarder is used. In this way, gel formation can be delayed for several minutes if desired, such as when other ingredients need to be added and mixed before the gel starts to set.

Alginate gels are used in restructured or re-formed food products. For example, restructured meats can be made by taking meat pieces, binding them together and shaping them to resemble usual cuts of meat, such as nuggets, roasts, meat loaves, even steaks. The binder can be a powder of sodium alginate, calcium carbonate, lactic acid, and calcium lactate. When mixed with the raw meat, they form a calcium alginate gel that binds the meat pieces together. This is used for meats for human consumption, such as chicken nuggets; it has become especially useful in making loaves of meat for fresh pet food; some abattoir wastes are suitable and cheap ingredients. Up to 1% alginate is used. Similar principles are applied to making shrimp substitutes using alginate, proteins such as soy protein concentrate, and flavors. The mixture is extruded into a calcium chloride bath to form edible fibers which are chopped, coated with sodium alginate, and shaped in a mold. Restructured fish fillets have been made using minced fish and a calcium alginate gel. Onion rings are made from dried onion powder; pimento olive fillings are made using pimento pulp. In 2001, a new line of olives launched in Spain was stuffed with flavored pastes, such as garlic, herbs, hot pepper, lemon, and cheese. Each of these is made with green manzanilla olives and an alginate-based paste containing the appropriate ingredient to provide the flavor.

Calcium alginate films and coatings have been used to help preserve frozen fish. The oils in oily fish such as herring and mackerel can become rancid through oxidation even when quick frozen and stored at low temperatures. If the fish is frozen in a calcium alginate jelly, the fish is protected from the air and rancidity from oxidation is very limited. The jelly thaws with the fish so they are easily separated. If beef cuts are coated with calcium alginate films before freezing, the meat juices released during thaw are reabsorbed into the meat and the coating also helps to protect the meat from bacterial contamination. If desired, the calcium alginate coating can be removed by redissolving it with sodium polyphosphate.

Finally, Table 3.4 (Lupo et al., 2012) exemplifies some applications of microencapsulation with prebiotics and their respective encapsulation techniques.

TABLE 3.4 Applications of Microencapsulation with Prebiotics.

Bacteria	Techniques	Applications
L. acidophilus, B. lactis	Em	Milk, cheese
L. acidophilus, B. bifidum	Ex y em	Kaşar cheese and white cheese
L. plantarum	Em	Yogurt
L. acidophilus, B. lactis	Ex	Fermented milk
L. casei, B. Lactis		Ice cream
L. acidophilus, Bifidobacterium	Em	Frozen desserts
Lactobacillus, L. acidophilus		Yogurt
L. acidophilus	Ex	Vegetable juices
L. reuteri	Ex and Em	Sausages

Note: L = *Lactobacillus*, B = *Bifidobacterium,* Em = emulsion, and Ex = extrusion.

3.4.3 BIOREMEDIATION

Bioremediation is a waste management technique that involves the use of organisms to neutralize or remove pollutants (e.g., petroleum hydrocarbons and toxic metals) from a contaminated site.

Petroleum hydrocarbons are the most common environmental pollutants in the world, and oil spills represent a major threat to terrestrial and marine ecosystems. One of the mechanisms of bioremediation involves the use of biological agents but these may migrate from the source of contamination, to avoid this and thus improve the survival and retention of bioremediation agents at contaminated sites, bacterial cells must be immobilized. This type of resource is widely used for a variety of applications (Bayat et al., 2015).

There are different methods to carry out the immobilization of these agents: adsorption, covalent binding, entrapment, and encapsulation. The different types are schematically exemplified in Figure 3.13.

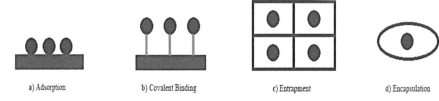

a) Adsorption   b) Covalent Binding   c) Entrapment   d) Encapsulation

FIGURE 3.13   Types of immobilization.

Entrapment method is an irreversible immobilization that is based on the capturing of particles or cells within a support matrix or inside a hollow fiber. In this type of technique, a protective barrier is created around the immobilized microbes that prevents the cells leakage from the polymers into the surrounding medium while allowing mass transfer of nutrients and metabolites. Entrapment is mostly applied to cell immobilization. The advantage of entrapment of cell immobilization method is that it is fast, cheap, and mild conditions are required for the reaction process. The main disadvantages of this technique are costs of immobilization, injury of support material during usage diffusion limitations, deactivation during immobilization and low loading capacity as biocatalysts (Trelles and Rivero, 2013).

Encapsulation is another irreversible technique similar to entrapment. This method can be achieved by enveloping the biological components within various forms of spherical semipermeable membranes with a selectively controlled permeability (Bickerstaff, 1997).

In both, the principle is the same; even the same polymers can be used, but differing in the form. Immobilized particle size to support material pore–size ratio probably is the most important parameter. Taking into account when the pores are too big, the material leaks, which also decreases the loading (Verma et al., 2006).

Alginates are the polymers of choice in most systems of immobilization because they are easy to handle, nontoxic to humans, the environment, and the entrapped microorganisms, legally safe for human use, available in large quantities, and inexpensive. From a physiological perspective, a major advantage of alginate is that immobilized cells do not suffer extreme changes in physicochemical condition during the procedure of immobilization and the gel is transparent and permeable (Buque et al., 2002).

Table 3.5 (Bayat et al., 2015) exemplifies cell immobilization systems for the degradation of different organic compounds.

TABLE 3.5   Some Immobilized Cells for Use in Biodegradation Compounds.

Compounds degraded	Microorganisms
Acrylamide	*Pseudomonas* sp. and *Xanthomonas maltophilia*
Cadmium and zinc	*Pseudomonas fluorescens* G7
Ethylbenzene	*Pseudomonas fluorescens* CS2
Mercury	Nitrogen-fixing bacteria
Naphthalene	*Pseudomonas* sp. strain NGK 1
Pentachlorophenol	*Phanerochaete chrysosporium*
Sodium cyanide and acetonitrile	*Pseudomonas putida*
2,4,6-trinitrotoluene (TNT)	*Arthrobacter* sp.

In some studies, it was demonstrated that the tolerance ability in difficult conditions of immobilized cells was improved mainly due to enhanced modifications of the cell membrane. For example, Kim et al. (2006) examined the effect of co-contaminants (phenol) on the biodegradation of pyridine by free and calcium alginate immobilized *Pseudomonas putida* MK1 (KCTC 12283). They showed that immobilized cells can effectively increase the tolerance to phenol and result in increased degradation of pyridine.

In some cases, microbial metabolism of petroleum hydrocarbons may produce toxic metabolites such as naphthenic acids, which can hamper subsequent biodegradation due to their toxicity that represses microbial metabolism (Lu et al., 2010).

Weir et al. (1995) employed *Pseudomonas aeruginosa* UG14 encapsulated in alginate for the degradation of phenanthrene. They observed that the survival of encapsulated cells was higher after 30 days, whereas free cells endured for 18 days. O'Reilly and Crawford (1989) investigated the degradation of p-cresol by a *Pseudomonas sp.* immobilized in calcium alginate and polyurethane. The results suggested that polyurethane was a better immobilization matrix than calcium alginate owing to its greater mechanical strength and improved oxygen transfer characteristics.

On the other hand, toxic metal pollutants, such as lead, exist widely in industrial wastewater, that is, battery, electroplate, dye, and pigment production (Gautam et al., 2014; Martín-Lara, et al., 2012; Subhashini et al., 2013; Wei et al., 2014). Given the natural physiological toxicity and nonbiodegradability of lead, this material easily accumulates in biological bodies and causes various diseases even at low concentrations (Wu et al., 2013; Zhou et al., 2014; Villa et al., 2014). Common lead processing methods are costly.

In terms of cost and efficiency, adsorption is a promising processing technique for wastewater with low lead concentration (Wu et al., 2011; Gupta et al., 2013; Hadi et al., 2013; Gollavelli et al., 2013).

Researchers have reported that sodium alginate can effectively eliminate heavy metal ions, such as Pb^{2+}, Cu^{2+}, and Cd^{2+} (Lagoa et al., 2009; Bertagnolli et al., 2014; Papageorgiou et al., 2008; Lim et al., 2008). However, sodium alginate is limited by poor stability (Liu et al., 2013), weak water resistance, and serious thermal degradation (Phang et al., 2011). Therefore, sodium alginate requires modification before used to process heavy metal ions in wastewater. Common modifications include oxidation, hydrophobic modification, esterification, and graft copolymerization.

Sodium carboxymethyl cellulose (CMC) is a kind of high-polymer cellulose ether (Pushpamalar et al., 2006; Yaşar et al., 2007) CMC is an anionic high-molecular compound that can produce hydrogels with a 3D cross-linked structure by coordinating with multivalent cations, such as Fe^{3+} and Al^{3+} (Mohamed, 2012).

Based on previous experimental studies (Dewangan et al., 2010, 2011), Huixue et al. (2016) prepared sodium alginate–CMC–Ca–Fe gel beads. The sodium alginate–CMC gel beads improved the performance of a single component, enhanced mechanical strength, and lowered sodium alginate cost. This study provides a novel economical, practical, and easily available heavy metal ion adsorbent.

3.4.4 TEXTILE

Textile materials are excellent media for growing microorganisms, especially those used in hospitals, infant wear, underwear, and sportswear, because of their high surface area of contact for bacteria.

The increasing interest in the personal health and hygiene has created the necessity to improve the antibacterial properties of textiles. For this reason, Li et al. (2017) review the role of alginate in the development of antimicrobial textiles. Antibacterial finishing of textiles has been introduced as a necessary process for various purposes, especially creating a fabric with antimicrobial activities. Currently, the textile industry continues to look for textiles antimicrobial finishing process based on sustainable biopolymers from the viewpoints of environmental friendliness, industrialization, and economic concerns. The availability of free hydroxyl and carboxyl groups of alginate in abundance and its sol-to-gel transformation in the presence of cross-linking cations provide an outstanding candidate to functional finish textiles. At present, techniques used to finish textiles by alginate include nanocomposite coating, ionic cross-linking coating, and layer-by-layer coating.

Zahran et al. (2014) prepared silver nanoparticles (AgNPs)–alginate-composite-coated cotton fabric by the reduction of silver nitrate using alkali hydrolyzed alginate solution. The coated fabrics demonstrated an excellent antibacterial activity against the tested bacteria, *E. coli*, *S. aureus* and *P. aeruginosa*. Although a slight decrease in the antibacterial feature of the cotton fabrics was observed after successive washings, an efficient antibacterial activity still remained on the fabrics.

Bajpai and Sharma (2004) prepared calcium alginate impregnated cotton fabric and loaded with copper nanoparticles (NPs) to impart antimicrobial properties. The fabrics showed an appreciable release of Cu(II) ions, extended over a period of 50 h. The amount of Cu(II) ions released showed a negative dependence on the amount of alginate present within the fabric network and the concentration of cross-linker calcium chloride used. In addition, the fabric showed fair mechanical strength and demonstrated strong biocidal action against *E. coli*.

The abundance of carboxylic groups existing in alginates may provide additional sites for binding of TiO_2 NPs, which makes alginate a potential modifier of textile fiber surfaces. Based on this, Mihailović et al. (2010) used the alginate as a fiber surface modifier to improve the binding efficiency between colloidal TiO_2 NPs and polyester (PES) fabric. Modified PES fabrics exhibited outstanding antibacterial activity and UV protection efficiency even after five washing cycles, indicating the excellent laundering durability (Li et al., 2017).

On the other hand, in textile printing alginates are used as thickeners for the paste containing the dye. These pastes may be applied to the fabric by either screen or roller printing equipment. Alginates became important thickeners with the advent of reactive dyes. These combine chemically with cellulose in the fabric. Many of the usual thickeners, such as starch, react with the reactive dyes, and this leads to lower color yields and sometimes by-products that are not easily washed out. Alginates do not react with the dyes; they easily wash out of the finished textile and are the best thickeners for reactive dyes. The types of alginate required vary from medium-to-high viscosity with older screen printing equipment, to low viscosity if modern, high-speed, roller printing is used. Textile printing accounts for about 50% of the global alginate market.

3.4.5 OTHER USES

The main use for alginate in the "paper industry" is in surface sizing. Alginate added to the normal starch sizing gives a smooth continuous film and a surface with less fluffing. The oil resistance of alginate films gives a size with better oil resistance and enhances greaseproof properties. An improved gloss is obtained with high gloss inks. If papers or boards are to be waxed, alginate in the size will keep the wax mainly at the surface, giving better coating runability on machine coating applications. Alginates are also excellent film formers and improve ink holdout and printability. The alginate also helps to control water loss from the coating suspension into the paper, between the point where the coating is applied and the point where the excess is removed by the trailing blade. The viscosity of the coating suspension must not be allowed to increase by the loss of water into the paper because this leads to uneven removal by the trailing blade and streaking of the coating.

Alginate is also used in starch adhesives for making corrugated boards because it stabilizes the viscosity of the adhesive and allows control of its rate of penetration. One percent sodium alginate, based on the weight of starch used, is usually sufficient.

Alginate can also be modified to become magnetic materials. Garcia et al. (2017) studied magnetic alginate microspheres which are biocompatible due to their alginate matrix, and motion-controllable by applied magnetic fields due to their magnetic character. Therefore, they have the potential of being used as vessels to a broad variety of materials, including drugs and therapeutic agents, facilitating entry to biological systems in a relatively non-invasive manner. Magnetic alginate microspheres respond to magnetic fields forming columnar structures.

ACKNOWLEDGMENTS

The authors acknowledge the financial support from the University of Buenos Aires (UBACyT 20020130100021BA) and CONICET (PIP112–2015–0100443CO). M. N. Pacho and J. E. Tasqué received the doctoral scholarships from CONICET-YTEC. V. E. Manzano and N. B. D´Accorso are research members from CONICET.

SUMMARY

Alginates are hydrocolloids from a family of naturally occurring water-soluble polysaccharides extracted from brown seaweed. It is distributed widely in the cell walls of brown algae, where through binding with water it forms a viscous gum. Thus, alginate is partly responsible for the flexibility of the seaweed. Hydrogels from alginates can be prepared at mild pH and temperature conditions which make them suitable for their use with biomolecules such as proteins and nucleic acids. In this way, alginates hydrogels have been used in biomedical science in applications such as wound healing, drug delivery, in vitro cell culture, and tissue engineering. The use of them is based on its favorable properties, including biocompatibility and ease of gelation. These gels retain structural similarity to the extracellular matrices in tissues and can be manipulated to play several critical roles. In contrast, like other hydrogels, however, alginate gels have very limited mechanical stiffness, and more general physical properties. A continuing challenge is matching the physical properties of alginate gels to the need in a particular application. Consideration of the range of different available cross-linking strategies, using molecules with various chemical structures, molecular weights, and cross-linking functionality will often yield gels suitable for each application. From a chemical point of view, alginates is an unbranched anionic polysaccharide composed of the two monomers, β-D-mannuronate (M) and α-L-guluronate (G), linked $1\rightarrow4$. In this sense, alginates must be regarded as a family of copolymers where the blocks are composed of consecutive G residues, consecutive M residues, and alternating M and G residues. The fact that G and M are C-5 epimers results in a switchover of the monomer chair conformation, giving rise to all four possible glycosidic linkages and at the molecular level. Gelation of alginates is based on the affinity of alginates toward certain ions and the ability to bind these ions selectively and cooperatively. Selective ion binding is strictly linked to the content of guluronate residues (G), or more precisely, the length of the G-blocks. The composition (i.e., M/G ratio), sequence, G-block length, and molecular weight are thus critical factors affecting the physical properties of alginate and its resultant hydrogels. An interesting property of sodium alginate is that it can form ionotropic gels in the presence of multivalent cations (e.g., Ca^{2+}, Zn^{2+}, Ba^{2+}, etc.). Nowadays, the trend is to synthesize the chemical derivatives of alginates in the backbone in order to achieve new properties. For instance, chemical derivatization may tailor in order to improve degradability, the cell surface interactions, tune the anticoagulation properties or the hydrophobic–hydrophilic balance for optimum drug release. In particular, we will center our attention in their chemistry and application of hydrogels of alginates.

KEYWORDS

- **alginate**
- **hydrogels**
- **modified alginates**
- **pharmaceutical applications**

REFERENCES

Agarwal, T.; Narayana, S. N.; Pal, K.; Pramanik, K.; Giri, S.; Banerjee, I. Calcium Alginate-Carboxymethyl Cellulose Beads for Colon-Targeted Drug Delivery. *Int. J. Biol. Macromol.* **2015,** *75,* 409–417.

Agüero, L.; Zaldivar, D.; Pena, L.; Solís, Y.; Ramón, J. A.; Dias, M. L. Preparation and Characterization of pH-Sensitive Microparticles Based on Polyelectrolyte Complexes for Antibiotic Delivery. *Polym. Eng. Sci.* **2015,** *55,* 981–987.

Agüero, L.; Zaldivar-Silva, D.; Peña, L.; Dias, M. L. Alginate Microparticles as Oral Colon Drug Delivery Device, A Review. *Carbohydr. Polym.* **2017,** *168,* 32–43.

Ahmed, E. M. Hydrogel, Preparation, Characterization, and Applications: A Review. *J. Adv. Res.* **2015,** *6,* 105–121.

Akay, S.; Heils, R.; Trieu, H. K.; Smirnova, I.; Yesil-Celiktas, O. An Injectable Alginate-Based Hydrogel for Microfluidic Applications. *Carbohydr. Polym.* **2017,** *161,* 228–234.

Akhta, M. F.; Hanif, M.; Ranjha, N. M. Methods of Synthesis of Hydrogels... A Review. *Saudi Pharm. J.* **2016,** *24,* 554–559.

Alvarez-Lorenzo, C.; Blanco-Fernandez, B.; Puga, A. M.; Concheiro, A. Crosslinked Ionic Polysaccharides for Stimuli-Sensitive Drug Delivery. *Adv. Drug. Delivery Rev.* **2013,** *65,* 1148–1171.

Amer, W.; Abdelouahdi, K.; Ramananarivo, H. R.; Fihri A; Achaby, M. E.; Zahouily, M.; Barakat, A.; Djessas, K.; Clark, J.; Solhy, A. Smart Designing of New Hybrid Materials Based on Brushite-Alginate and Monetite-Alginate Microspheres: Bio-Inspired for Sequential Nucleation and Growth. *Mater. Sci. Eng. C* **2014,** *35,* 341–346.

Arvizu, H. D. L.; Hernández, C.; Rodriguéz-Montesinos, E. Parámetros Que Afectan La Conversión Del Ácido Algínico En Alginato De Sodio. *Cienc. Mar.* **2002,** *28,* 27–36.

Augst, A. D.; Kong, H. J.; Mooney, D. J. Alginate Hydrogels as Biomaterials. *Macromol. Biosci.* **2006,** *6,* 623–633.

Bahram, M.; Mohseni, N.; Moghtader, M. An Introduction to Hydrogels and Some Recent Applications. In *Emerging Concepts in Analysis and Applications of Hydrogels;* Majee,

S. B., Ed.; InTech Open: London, UK, 2016; pp 9–83. DOI: 10.5772/64301. ISBN 978-953-51-2510-5.

Bajpai, S. K.; Sharma, S. Investigation of Swelling/Degradation Behaviour of Alginate Beads Crosslinked with Ca^{2+} and Ba^{2+} Ions. *React. Funct. Polym.* **2004,** *59,* 129–140.

Bansal, D.; Gulbake, A.; Tiwari, J.; Jain, S. K. Development of Liposomes Entrapped in Alginate Beads for the Treatment of Colorectal Cancer. *Int. J. Biol. Macromol.* **2016,** *82,* 687–695.

Bayat, Z.; Hassanshahian, M.; Cappello, S. Immobilization of Microbes for Bioremediation of Crude Oil Polluted Environments: A Mini Review. *Open Microbiol. J.* **2015,** *9,* 48–54.

Bertagnolli, C.; da Silva, M. G.; Guibal, E. Chromium Biosorption Using the Residue of Alginate Extraction from *Sargassum filipendula. Chem. Eng. J.* **2014,** *237,* 362–371.

Bickerstaff, G. F., Jr. *Immobilization of Enzymes and Cells: Methods in Biotechnology;* Humana Press: New Jersey, **1997.**

Braccini, I.; Pérez, S. Molecular Basis of Ca^{2+}-Induced Gelation in Alginates and Pectins: The Egg-Box Model Revisited. *Biomacromolecules* **2001,** *2,* 1089–1096.

Brady, S. A.; Fox, E. K.; Lally, C.; Clarkin, O. M. Optimisation of a Novel Glass-Alginate Hydrogel for the Treatment of Intracranial Aneurysms. *Carbohydr. Polym.* **2017,** *176,* 227–235.

Buque, E. M.; Chin-Joe, I.; Straathof, A. J. J.; et al. Immobilization Affects the Rate and Enantioselectivity of 3-oxo Ester Reduction by Baker's Yeast. *Enzyme Microb. Technol.* **2002,** *31,* 656–664.

Buse, J. B.; DeFronzo, R. A.; Rosenstock, J.; Kim, T.; Burns, C.; Skare, S.; Baron, A.; Fineman, M. The Primary Glucose-Lowering Effect of Metformin Resides in the Gut, Not the Circulation. Results from Short-Term Pharmacokinetic and 12-Week Dose-Ranging Studies. *Diabetes Care* **2016,** *39,* 198–205.

Buwalda, S. J.; Boere, K. W.; Dijkstra, P. J.; Feijen, J.; Vermonden, T.; Hennink, W. E. Hydrogels in a Historical Perspective: from Simple Networks to Smart Materials. *J. Control Release* **2014,** *190,* 254–273.

Caló, E.; Khutoryanskiy, V. V. Biomedical Applications of Hydrogels: A Review of Patents and Commercial Products. *Eur. Polym. J.* **2015,** *65,* 252–267.

Champagne, C. P.; Fustier, P. Microencapsulation for the Improved Delivery of Bioactive Compounds Into Foods. *Curr. Opin. Chem. Biotechnol.* **2007,** *18,* 184–190.

Chan, L. W.; Lee, H. Y.; Heng, P. W. S. Mechanisms of External and Internal Gelation and their Impact on the Functions of Alginate as a Coat and Delivery System. *Carbohydr. Polym.* **2006,** *63,* 176–187.

Chan, E.-S.; Lee, B.-B.; Ravindra, P.; Poncelet, D. Prediction Models for Shape and Size of Ca-Alginate Macrobeads Produced Through Extrusion–Dripping Method. *J. Colloid Interface Sci.* **2009,** *338,* 63–72.

Chirani, N.; Yahia, L. H.; Gritsch, L.; Motta, F. L.; Chirani, S.; Fare, S. History and Applications of Hydrogels. *J. Biomed. Sci.* **2015,** *4,* 2–13.

Chronakis, I. S.; Piculell, L.; Borgstrom, J. Rheology of Kappa-carrageenan in Mixtures of Sodium and Cesium Iodide: Two Types of Gels. *Carbohydr. Polym.* **1996,** *31,* 215–225.

Coleman, R. J.; Lawrie, G.; Lambert, L. K.; Whittaker II, M.; Jack, K. S.; Grøndahl, L. Phosphorylation of Alginate: Synthesis, Characterization, and Evaluation of in Vitro Mineralization Capacity. *Biomacromolecules* **2011,** *12,* 889–897.

Corti, G.; Cirri, M.; Maestrelli, F.; Mennini, N.; Mura, P. Sustained-Release Matrix Tablets of Metformin Hydrochloride in Combination with Triacetyl-ß-Cyclodextrin. *Eur. J. Pharm. Biopharm.* **2008,** *68,* 303–309.

Crow, B. B.; Nelson, K. D. Release of Bovine Serum Albumin from a Hydrogel-Cored Biodegradable Polymer Fiber. *Biopolymers* **2006,** *81,* 419–427.

Das, D.; Pal, S. Modified Biopolymer-Dextrin Based Crosslinked Hydrogels: Application in Controlled Drug Delivery. *RSC Adv.***2015,** *5,* 25014–25050.

Dentini, M.; Rinaldi, G.; Risica, D.; Barbetta, A.; Skjak-Braek, G. Comparative Studies on Solution Characteristics of Mannuronan Epimerized by C-5 Epimerases. *Carbohydr. Polym.* **2005,** *59,* 489–499.

de Vos, P.; Faas, M. M.; Spasojevic, M.; Sikkema, J. Encapsulation for Preservation of Functionality and Targeted Delivery of Bioactive Food Components. *Int. Dairy J.* **2010,** *20,* 292–302.

Dewangan, T.; Tiwari, A.; Bajpai, A. K. Adsorption of Hg(II) Ions Onto Binary Biopolymeric Beads of Carboxymethyl Cellulose and Alginate. *J. Dispersion Sci. Technol.* **2010,** *31*(6), 844–851.

Dewangan, T.; Tiwari, A.; Bajpai, A. K. Removal of Chromium(VI) Ions by Adsorption Onto Binary Biopolymeric Beads of Sodium Alginate and Carboxymethyl Cellulose. *J. Dispersion Sci. Technol.* **2011,** *32*(8), 1075–1082.

Di Colo, G.; Falchi, S.; Zambito, Y. In Vitro Evaluation of a System for pH-Controlled Peroral Delivery of Metformin. *J. Control Release* **2002,** *80,* 119–128.

Draget, K. I.; Skjak Bræk, G; Smidsrød, O. Alginic Acid Gels: the Effect of Alginate Chemical Composition and Molecular Weight. *Carbohydr. Polym.* **1994,** *25,* 31–38.

Draget, K. I.; Skjak-Bræk, G.; Christensen, B. E.; Gaserød, O.; Smidsrød, O. Swelling and Partial Solubilization of Alginic Acid Gel Beads in Acidic Buffer. *Carbohydr. Polym.* **1996,** *29,* 209–215.

Draget, K. I. A. *Handbook of Hydrocolloids;* CRC Press LLC: Cambridge, England, Boca Raton, FL, USA, 2000; pp 379–395.

Drury, J. L.; Boontheekul, T.; Mooney, D. J. Cellular Cross-Linking of Peptide Modified Hydrogels. *J. Biomech. Eng. Trans. ASME* **2005,** *127,* 220–228.

Dunn, C. J.; Peters, D. H. Metformin. A Review of its Pharmacological Properties and Therapeutic Use in Non-Insulin-Dependent Diabetes Mellitus. *Drugs* **1995,** *49,* 721–749.

Dusseault, J.; Tam, S. K.; Ménard, M.; Polizu, S.; Jourdan, G; Yahia, L. H.; Hallé, J. P. Evaluation of Alginate Purification Methods: Effect on Polyphenol, Endotoxin and Protein Contamination. *J. Biomed. Mater. Res. A* **2006,** *76,* 243–251.

Ferreira, N. N.; Ferreira, L. M. B.; Miranda-Gonçalves, V.; Reis, R. M.; Seraphim, T. V.; Borges, J. C.; Baltazar, F.; Gremião, M. P. D. Alginate Hydrogel Improves Anti-Angiogenic Bevacizumab Activity in Cancer Therapy. *Eur. J. Pharm. Biopharm.* **2017,** *119,* 271–282.

Freeman, I.; Kedem, A.; Cohen, S. The Effect of Sulfation of Alginate Hydrogels on the Specific Binding and Controlled Release of Heparin-Binding Proteins. *Biomaterials* **2008,** *29,* 3260–3268.

Fu, S.; Thacker, A.; Sperger, D. M.; Boni, R. L.; Velankar, S.; Munson, E. J.; Block, L. H. Rheological Evaluation of Inter-Grade and Inter-Batch Variability of Sodium Alginate. *AAPS PharmSciTech* **2010,** *11,* 1662–1674.

Fu, S.; Thacker, A.; Sperger, D. M.; Boni, L. R.; Buckner, I. S.; Velankar, S.; Munson, E. J.; Block, L. H. Relevance of Rheological Properties of Sodium Alginate in Solution to Calcium Alginate Gel Properties. *AAPS PharmSciTech* **2011,** *12,* 453–460.

Funami, T.; Fang, Y.; Noda, S.; Ishihara, S.; Nakauma, M.; Draget, K. I.; Nishinari, K.; Phillips, G. O. Rheological Properties of Sodium Alginate in an Aqueous System During Gelation in Relation to Supermolecular Structure and Ca^{2+} Binding. *Food Hydrocolloids* **2009,** *23,* 1746–1756.

Garcia, A. R.; Lacko, C.; Snyder, C.; Bohórquez, A. C.; Schmidt, C. E.; Rinaldi, C. Processing-Size Correlations in the Preparation of Magnetic Alginate. *Colloids Surf. A* **2017**, *529*, 119–127.

Gautam, R. K.; Mudhoo, A.; Lofrano, G.; Chattopadhyaya, M. C. Biomass-Derived Biosorbents for Metal Ions Sequestration: Adsorbent Modification and Activation Methods and Adsorbent Regeneration. *J. Environ. Chem. Eng.* **2014**, *2*, 239–259.

George, M.; Abraham, T. E. Polyionic Hydrocolloids for the Intestinal Delivery of Protein Drugs: Alginate and Chitosan—A Review. *J. Control Release* **2006**, *114*, 1–14.

Gharsallaoui, A.; Roudaut, G.; Chambin, O.; Voilley, A.; Saurel, R, Applications of Spray-drying in Microencapsulation of Food Ingredients: An Overview. *Food Res. Int.* **2007**, *40*, 1107–1121.

Gollavelli, G.; Chang, C.-C.; Ling, Y.-C. Facile Synthesis of Smart Magnetic Graphene for Safe Drinking Water: Heavy Metal Removal and Disinfection Control. *Acs Sustain. Chem. Eng.* **2013**, *1*, 462–472.

Gombotz, W. R.; Wee, S. F. Protein Release from Alginate Matrices. *Adv. Drug Delivery Rev.* **2012**, *64*, 194–205.

González-Rodríguez, M. L.; Holgado, M. A.; Sánchez-Lafuente, C.; Rabasco, A. M.; Fini, A. Alginate/Chitosan Particulate Systems for Sodium Diclofenac Release. *Int. J. Pharm.* **2002**, *232*, 225–234.

Gouin, S. Microencapsulation: Industrial Appraisal of Existing Technologies and Trends. *Trends Food Sci. Technol.* **2004**, *15*, 330–347.

Grant, G. T.; Morris, E. R.; Rees, D. A.; Smith, P. J. C.; Thom, D. Biological Interactions Between Polysaccharides and Divalent Cations: The Egg-Box Model. *FEBS Lett.* **1973**, *32*, 195–198.

Growney Kalaf, E. A.; Flores, R; Bledsoe, J.; Sell, S. A. Characterization of Slow-Gelling Alginate Hydrogels for Intervertebral Disc Tissue-Engineering Applications. *Mater. Sci. Eng. C Mater. Biol. Appl.* **2016**, *63*, 198–210.

Gupta, A. K.; Verma, S. K.; Khan, K; Verma, R. K. Phytoremediation Using Aromatic Plants: A Sustainable Approach for Remediation of Heavy Metals Polluted Sites. *Environ. Sci. Technol.* **2013**, *47*, 10115–10116.

Hadi, P.; Barford, J.; McKay, G. Toxic Heavy Metal Capture Using a Novel Electronic Waste-Based Material—Mechanism, Modeling and Comparison. *Environ. Sci. Technol.* **2013**, *47*, 8248–8255.

Hoffman, A. S. Hydrogels for Biomedical Applications. *Adv. Drug Delivery Rev.* **2012**, *64*, 18–23.

Helgerud, T.; Gåserød, O.; Fjæreide, T.; Andersen, P. O.; Larsen, C. K. A. Alginates. In *Food Stabilizers, Thickeners and Gelling Agents;* Wiley Blackwell: United Kingdom, 2010; pp 50–72.

Hernández, E. M.; López, G. Y. R.; García, P. A. Evaluación De Derivados Carboximetilados Del Alginato De Sodio Como Superabsorbentes. *Revista Cubana De Química* **2005**, *17*(3), 239–240.

Hu, L. D.; Liu, Y.; Tang, X.; Zhang, Q. Preparation and in Vitro/In Vivo Evaluation of Sustained-release Metformin Hydrochloride Pellets. *Eur. J. Pharm. Biopharm.* **2006**, *64*, 185–192.

Huixue, R.; Zhimin, G.; Daoji, W.; Jiahui, J.; Youmin, S.; Congwei, L. Efficient Pb(II) Removal Using Sodium Alginate-Carboxymethyl Cellulose Gel Beads: Preparation, Characterization, and Adsorption Mechanism. *Carbohydr. Polym.* **2016**, *137*, 402–409.

Ikeda, S.; Nishinari, K. "Weak Gel"-Type Rheological Properties of Aqueous Dispersions of Nonaggregated Kappa-Carrageenan Helices. *J. Agric. Food Chem.* **2001,** *49,* 4436–4441.

Kamoun, E. A.; Kenawy, El.-R. S.; Chen, X. A Review on Polymeric Hydrogel Membranes for Wound Dressing Applications: PVA-Based Hydrogel Dressings. *J. Adv. Res.* **2017,** *8,* 217–233.

Kim, D.-W.; Park, J.-B. Development and Pharmaceutical Approach for Sustained-Released Metformin Succinate Tablets. *J. Drug Delivery Sci. Technol.* **2015,** *30,* 90–99.

Kim, M. K.; Singleton, I.; Yin, C. R.; et al. Influence of Phenol on the Biodegradation of Pyridine by Freely Suspended and Immobilized Pseudomonas Putida MK1. *Lett. Appl. Microbiol.* **2006,** *42,* 495–500.

Kuo, C. K.; Ma, P. X. Ionically Crosslinked Alginate Hydrogels as Scaffolds for Tissue Engineering: Part 1. Structure, Gelation Rate and Mechanical Properties. *Biomaterials* **2001,** *22,* 511–521.

Lagoa, R.; Rodrigues, J. R. Kinetic Analysis of Metal Uptake by Dry and Gel Alginate Particles. *Biochem. Eng. J.* **2009,** *46,* 320–326.

Lee, J.; Lee, K. Y. Local and Sustained Vascular Endothelial Growth Factor Delivery for Angiogenesis Using an Injectable System. *Pharm. Res.* **2009,** *26,* 1739–1744.

Lee, K. Y.; Mooney, D. J. Alginate: Properties and Biomedical Applications. *Prog. Polym. Sci.* **2012,** *37,* 106–126.

Lee, K. Y.; Rowley, J. A.; Eiselt, P.; Moy, E. M.; Bouhadir, K. H.; Mooney, D. J. Controlling Mechanical and Swelling Properties of Alginate Hydrogels Independently by Cross-Linker Type and Cross-linking Density. Macromolecules **2000,** *33,* 4291–4294.

Lee, K. Y.; Kong, H. J.; Larson, R. G.; Mooney, D. J. Hydrogel Formation Via Cell Cross-Linking. *Adv. Mater.* **2003,** *15,* 1828–1832.

Leonard, M.; Rastello De Boisseson, M.; Hubert, P.; Dellacherie, E. Production of Microspheres Based on Hydrophobically Associating Alginate Derivatives by Dispersion/Gelation in Aqueous Sodium Chloride Solutions. *J. Biomed. Mater. Res. A* 68A, 335–342 **2004**.

LeRoux, M. A.; Guilak, F.; Setton, L. A. Compressive and Shear Properties of Alginate Gel: Effects of Sodium Ions and Alginate Concentration. *J. Biomed. Mater. Res.* **1999,** *47,* 46–53.

Li, J.; He, J.; Huang, Y. Role of Alginate in Antibacterial Finishing of Textiles. *Int. J. Biol. Macromol.* **2017,** *94,* 466–473.

Li, Y.; Song, J.; Tian, N.; Cai, J.; Huang, M.; Xing, Q.; Wang, Y.; Wu, C.; Hu, H. Improving Oral Bioavailability of Metformin Hydrochloride Using Water-in-Oil Microemulsions and Analysis of Phase Behavior After Dilution. *Int. J. Pharm.* **2014,** *473,* 316–325.

Lim, S.-F.; Zheng, Y.-M.; Zou, S.-W.; Chen, J. P. Characterization of Copper Adsorption Onto an Alginate Encapsulated Magnetic Sorbent by a Combined FT-IR, XPS, and Mathematical Modeling Study. *Environ. Sci. Technol.* **2008,** *42,* 2551–2556.

Liu, Y.; Hu, X.; Wang, H.; Chen, A.; Liu, S.; Guo, Y. Photoreduction of Cr(VI) from Acidic Aqueous Solution Using TiO_2-Impregnated Glutaraldehyde-Crosslinked Alginate Beads and the Effects of Fe(III) Ions. *Chem. Eng. J.* **2013,** *226,* 131–138.

López-Hernández, O. D. Microencapsulación De Sustancias Oleosas Mediante Secado Por Aspersión. *Rev. Cubana Farm.* **2010,** *44,* 381–389.

Lu, M.; Zhang, Z.; Qiao, W. Remediation of Petroleum-contaminated Soil After Composting by Sequential Treatment with Fenton-Like Oxidation and Biodegradation. *Bioresour. Technol.* **2010,** *101,* 2106–2113.

Luna, M. S.; Villegas, A. Instalación de una Planta Productora de Acido Algínico y Derivados en Ensenada, B.C. Ph.D. Dissertation, Facultad de Economía, Universidad Nacional Autónoma de México, **1989,**.

Lupo, P. B.; González, A. C.; Maestro, G. A. Microencapsulación Con Alginato En Alimentos. Técnicas y Aplicaciones. *Rev. Venez. Cienc. y Tecnol. de Aliment.* **2012**, *3,* 130–151.

Maestrelli, F.; Mura, P.; González-Rodríguez, M. L.; Cózar-Bernal, M. J.; Rabasco, A. M.; Di Cesare Mannelli, L.; Ghelardini, C. Calcium Alginate Microspheres Containing Metformin Hydrochloride Niosomes and Chitosomes Aimed for Oral Therapy of Type 2 Diabetes Mellitus. *Int. J. Pharm.* **2017**, *530,* 430–439.

Martín-Lara, M. A.; Blázquez, G.; Ronda, A.; Rodríguez, I. L.; Calero, M. Multiple Biosorption–Desorption Cycles in a Fixed-Bed Column for Pb(II) Removal by Acid-Treated Olive Stone. *J. Ind. Eng. Chem.* **2012**, *18,* 1006–1012.

Martín-Villena, M. J.; Morales-Hernández, M. E.; Gallardo-Lara, V.; Ruíz-Martínez, M. S. Técnicas De Microencapsulación: Una Propuesta Para Microencapsular Probióticos. *ARS Pharm.* **2009**, *50,* 43–50.

McHugh, D. J. Production, Properties and Uses of Alginates. In *Production and Utilization of Products from Commercial Seaweeds: Food and Agriculture Organization of the United Nations;* McHugh, D. J., Ed., FAO: Rome, Italy, 1988; pp 43–91.

Medina, L. H.; Ledo, P. R. M. Alginatos. Propiedades y Uso en la Reducción de Reflujo Gastroesofágico. *Informe Médico,* **2010**, *12* 519–523.

Messaoud, M.; Chadeau, E.; Chaudouët, P.; Oulahal, N.; Langlet, M. Quaternary Ammonium-Based Composite Particles for Antibacterial Finishing of cotton-Based Textiles. *J. Mater. Sci. Technol.* **2014**, *30,* 19–29.

Mihailović, D.; Šaponjić, Z.; Radoičić, M.; Radetić, T.; Jovančić, P.; Nedeljković, J.; Radetić, M. Functionalization of Polyester Fabrics with Alginates and TiO_2 Nanoparticles. *Carbohydr. Polym.* **2010**, *79,* 526–532.

Mofidi, N.; Aghai-Moghadam, M.; Sarbolouki, M. N. Mass Preparation and Characterization of Alginate Microspheres. *Process Biochem.* **2000**, *35,* 885–888.

Mohamed, M. A. Swelling Characteristics and Application of Gamma-Radiation on Irradiated SBR-Carboxymethylcellulose (CMC) Blends. *Arabian J. Chem.* **2012**, *5,* 207–211.

Momoh, M. A.; Adedokun, M. O.; Kenechukwu, F. C.; Ibezim, E. C.; Ugwoke, E. E. Design, Characterization and Evaluation of PEGylated-mucin for Oral Delivery of Metformin Hydrochloride. *Afr. J. Pharm. Pharmacol.* **2013**, *7,* 347–355.

Mørch, Y. A.; Donati, I.; Strand, B. L.; Skjåk-Bræk, G. Effect of Ca2+, Ba2+, and Sr2+ on Alginate Microbeads. *Biomacromolecules* **2006**, *7,* 1471–1480.

Morais, D. S.; Rodrigues, M. A.; Silva, T. I.; Lopes, M. A.; Santos M; Santos, J. D.; Botelho, C. M. Development and Characterization of Novel Alginate-Based Hydrogels as Vehicles for Bone Substitutes. *Carbohydr. Polym.* **2013**, 134–142.

Nayak, A. K.; Pal, D.; Das, S. Calcium Pectinate-Fenugreek Seed Mucilage Mucoadhesive Beads for Controlled Delivery of Metformin HCL. *Carbohydr. Polym.* **2013**, *96,* 349–357.

O'Reilly, K. T.; Crawford, R. L. Kinetics of P-Cresol Degradation by an Immobilized Pseudomonas sp. *Appl. Environ. Microbiol.* **1989**, *55,* 866–870.

Orive, G.; Ponce, S.; Hernández, R. M.; Gascon, A. R.; Igartua, M.; Pedraz, J. L. Biocompatibility of Microcapsules for Cell Immobilization Elaborated with Different Type of Alginates. *Biomaterials* **2002**, *23,* 3825–3831.

Papageorgiou, S. K.; Kouvelos, E. P.; Katsaros, F. K. Calcium Alginate Beads from *Laminaria digitata* for the Removal of Cu^{+2} and Cd^{+2} from Dilute Aqueous Metal Solutions. *Desalination* **2008**, *224,* 293–306.

Page, R. C. L. 42 Insulin, Other Hypoglycemic Drugs, and Glucagon. In *Side Effects of Drugs Annual;* Aronson, J., Ed.; Elsevier; 2011, Vol. 33, pp 889–908.

Parisi, M.; Manzano, V. E.; Flor, S.; Lissarrague, M. H.; Ribba, L.; Lucangioli, S.; D'Accorso, N. B.; Goyanes, S. Polymeric Prosthetic Systems for Site-specific Drug Administration: Physical and Chemical Properties. In *Handbook of Polymers for Pharmaceutical Technologies, Structure and Chemistry, Structure and Chemistry;* Kumar, T. V., Kumari, T. M., Eds.; Wiley: Hoboken, 2015; Vol. 1, 369–412.

Park, H.; Lee, H. J.; An, H.; Lee, K. Y. Alginate Hydrogels Modified with Low Molecular Weight Hyaluronate for Cartilage Regeneration. *Carbohydr. Polym.* **2017,** *162,* 100–107.

Patel, H.; Nagle, A.; Murthy, R. S. Characterization of Calcium Alginate Beads of 5-Fluorouracil for Colon Delivery. *Asian J. Pharm.* **2008,** *2,* 241–245.

Pawar, S. N.; Edgar, K. Alginate Derivatization: A Review of Chemistry, Properties and Applications. *Biomaterials* **2012,** *33,* 3279–3305.

Phang, Y.-N.; Chee, S.-Y.; Lee, C.-O.; Teh, Y.-L. Thermal and Microbial Degradation of Alginate-Based Superabsorbent Polymer. *Polym. Degrad. Stab.* **2011,** *96,* 1653–1661.

Peppas, N. A.; Bures, P.; Leobandung, W.; Ichikawa, H. Hydrogels in Pharmaceutical Formulations. *Eur. J. Pharm. Biopharm.* **2000,** *50,* 27–46.

Pindar, D. F.; Bucke, C. The Biosynthesis of Alginic Acid by Azotobacter Vinelandii. *Biochem. J.* **1975,** *152,* 617–622.

Poncelet, D. Production of Alginate Beads by Emulsification/Internal Gelation. In Bioartificial Organs III: Tissue Sourcing Immunoisolation and Clinical Trials. *Ann. N. Y. Acad. Sci.* **2001,** *944,* 74–82.

Pushpamalar, V.; Langford, S. J.; Ahmad, M.; Lim, Y. Y. Optimization of Reaction Conditions for Preparing Carboxymethyl Cellulose from Sago Waste. *Carbohydr. Polym.* **2006,** *64,* 312–318.

Qin, Y. Alginate Fibres: An Overview of the Production Processes and Applications in Wound Management. *Polym. Int.* **2008,** *57,* 171–180.

Remminghorst, U.; Rehm, B. H. A. Bacterial Alginates: from Biosynthesis to Applications. *Biotechnol. Lett.* **2006,** *28,* 1701–1712.

Rosiak, J. M.; Yoshii, F. Hydrogels and Their Medical Applications. *Nucl. Instrum. Methods Phys. Res. Sect. B* **1999,** *151,* 56–64.

Roy, D.; Cambre, J. N.; Sumerlin, B. S. Future Perspectives and Recent Advances in Stimuli-responsive Materials. *Prog. Polym. Sci.* **2010,** *35,* 278–301.

Sangeetha, K.; Girija, E. K. Tailor Made Alginate Hydrogel for Local Infection Prophylaxis in Orthopedic Applications. *Mater. Sci. Eng. C* **2017,** *78,* 1046–1053.

Scheen, A. J. Clinical Pharmacokinetics of Metformin. *Clin. Pharmacokinet.* **1996,** *30,* 359–371.

Schnaare, R. L.; Block, L. H.; Rohan, L. C. Rheology In *Remington: The Science and Practice of Pharmacy;* 21st ed.; Troy, D., Ed., Wiliams & Wilkins: Philadelphia, 2005; pp 338–357.

Schweiger, R. G. Acetylation of Alginic Acid. II. Reaction of Algin Acetates with Calcium and Other Divalent Ions. *J. Org. Chem.* **1962,** *27,* 1789–1791.

Skjåk-Bræk, G.; Zanetti, F.; Paoletti, S. Effect of Acetylation on Some Solutions and Gelling Properties of Alginates. *Carbohydr. Res.* **1989,** *185,* 131–138.

Smidsrød, O.; Skjak-Bræk, G. Alginate as Immobilization Matrix for Cells. *Trend Biotechnol.* **1990,** *8,* 71–78.

Smidsrød, O.; Glover, R. M.; Whittington, S. G. Relative Extension of Alginates Having Different Chemical Composition. *Carbohydr. Res.* **1973,** *27,* 107–118.

Stokke, B. T.; Smidsrød, O.; Brant, D. A. Predicted Influence of Monomer Sequence Distribution and Acetylation on the Extension of Naturally Occurring Alginates. *Carbohydr. Polym.* **1993,** *22,* 57–66.

Straccia, M. C.; d'Ayala, G. G.; Romano, I.; Oliva, A.; Laurienzo, P. Alginate hydrogels Coated with Chitosan for Wound Dressing. *Mar. Drugs* **2015**, *13,* 2890–2908.

Subhashini, S. S.; Velan, M.; Kaliappan, S. Biosorption of Lead by *Kluyveromyces marxianus* Immobilized in Alginate Beads. *J. Environ. Biol.* **2013**, *34,* 831–835.

Sun, J.; Tan, H. Alginate-Based Biomaterials for Regenerative Medicine Applications. *Materials* **2013**, *6,* 1285–1309.

Trelles, J. A.; Rivero, C. W. Whole Cell Entrapment Techniques. *Methods Mol. Biol.* **2013**, *1051,* 365–374.

Ullah, F.; Othman, M. B. H.; Javed, F.; Ahmad, Z.; Akil, H. M. Classification, Processing and Application of Hydrogels: A Review. *Mater. Sci. Eng. C* **2015**, *57,* 414–433.

Verma, M.; Brar, S. K.; Blais, J. F. Aerobic Biofiltration Processes—advances in Wastewater Treatment. *Pract Period Hazard Toxic Radioact. Waste Manage* **2006**, *10,* 264–276.

Villa, J. E.; Peixoto, R. R.; Cadore, S. Cadmium and Lead in Chocolates Commercialized in Brazil. *J. Agric. Food Chem.* **2014**, *62,* 8759–8763.

Wei, W.; Liu, X.; Sun, P.; Wang II, X.; Hong, M.; Mao, Z. W. Simple Whole-Cell Biodetection and Bioremediation of Heavy Metals Based on an Engineered Lead-Specific Operon. *Environ. Sci. Technol.* **2014**, *48,* 3363–3371.

Weir, S. C.; Dupuis, S. P.; Providenti, M. A. Nutrient-Enhanced Survival of and Phenanthrene Mineralization by Alginate-encapsulated and Free Pseudomonas sp. UG14Lr cells in Creosote-Contaminated Soil Slurries. *Appl. Microbiol. Biotechnol.* **1995**, *43,* 946–951.

Wu, M.-L.; Deng, J.-F.; Lin, K.-P.; Tsai, W.-J. Mercury, and Arsenic Poisoning Due to Topical Use of Traditional Chinese Medicines. *Am. J. Med* **2013**, *126,* 451–454.

Xing, L.; Dawei, C.; Liping, X.; Rongqing, Z. Oral Colon-Specific Drug Delivery for Bee Venom Peptide: Development of a Coated Calcium Alginate Gel Beads-Entrapped Liposome. *J. Control* **2003**, *93,* 293–300.

Yang, J.; Goto, M.; Ise, H.; Cho, C. S.; Akaike, T. Galactosylated Alginate as a Scaffold for Hepatocytes Entrapment. *Biomaterials* **2002**, *23,* 471–479.

Yaşar, F.; Toğrul, H.; Arslan, N. Flow Properties of Cellulose and Carboxymethyl Cellulose from Orange Peel. *J. Food Eng.* **2007**, *81,* 187–199.

Zahran, M. K.; Ahmed, H. B.; El-Rafie, M. H. Surface Modification of Cotton Fabrics for Antibacterial Application by Coating with AgNPs-Alginate Composite. *Carbohydr. Polym.* **2014**, *108,* 145–152.

Zhao, S. P.; Cao, M. J.; Li, H.; Li, L. Y.; Xu, W. L. Synthesis and Characterization of Thermo-Sensitive Semi-IPN Hydrogels Based on Poly(Ethylene Glycol)-Co-Poly(Epsilon-Caprolactone) Macromer, N-isopropylacrylamide, and Sodium Alginate. *Carbohydr. Res.* **2010**, *345,* 425–431.

Zhao, X. H.; Huebsch, N.; Mooney, D. J.; Suo, Z. G. Stress-Relaxation Behavior in Gels with Ionic and Covalent Crosslinks. *J. Appl. Phys.* **2010**, *107,* 1–5.

Zhou, Y.; Fu, S.; Zhang, L.; Levit, M. V. Use of Carboxylated Cellulose Nanofibrils-Filled Magnetic Chitosan Hydrogel Beads as Adsorbents for Pb(II). *Carbohydr Polym.* **2014**, *101,* 75–82.

Zuidam, N. J.; Shimoni, E. Overview of Microencapsulates for Use in Food Products or Processes and Methods to Make Them. In *Encapsulation Technologies for Active Food Ingredients and Food Processing;* Zuidam, N., Nedovic, V., Eds.; Springer: New York, 2010; pp 3–29.

CHAPTER 4

ALGINATE-BASED HYDROGELS: SYNTHESIS, CHARACTERIZATION, AND BIOMEDICAL APPLICATIONS

VANDANA SINGH* and ANGELA SINGH

*Department of Chemistry, University of Allahabad,
Uttar Pradesh 211002, Allahabad, India*

Corresponding author. E-mail: singhvandanasingh@rediffmail.com

4.1 INTRODUCTION

Hydrogels are tridimensional (3D), insoluble, cross-linked, and tissue like network structures of chemically or physically cross-linked hydrophilic polymers. They are capable of taking in and keeping huge quantities of water in their three-dimensional network (Peppas, 1986; Rosiak and Yoshii, 1999; Gehrke, 2000). The hydrogels imbibe and retain a significant amount of water because of their porosity and the presence of many hydrophilic groups on the polymer chains such as $-NH_2$, $-OH$, $-COOH$, $-SO_3H$, and so forth. They resist dissolution in the surrounding medium owing to cross-linking between the polymer chains (Gombotz and Pettit, 1995). They can be derived from natural or synthetic materials by the simple reaction of one or more monomer/polymer/cross-linker units (Langer and Peppas, 1981) and possess a high degree of flexibility. The interaction between polymeric chain networks and water or biological fluids occur through capillary, osmotic, and hydration forces. Hydrogels with characteristic properties such as desired functionality, reversibility, serializability, modifiable chemical properties, biocompatibility, elasticity, the capability to act as a growth medium, and the ability to mimic the extracellular matrix (ECM), have broad uses in biomedical research that spans from drug delivery to regenerative medicine to tissue engineering and are gaining attention due to their ability to encapsulate cells (Augst et al., 2006; Park et al., 1993;

Wichterle and Lim, 1960). In addition, hydrogels can be administered into the body in a noninvasive manner and can fill defects with no limitations on size or shape. Another astonishing feature of hydrogels is their reversible response to different stimuli like pH, temperature, electric field, magnetic field, the ionic strength of the solution, and biological molecules that make them particularly important for a wide range of biomedical applications (Hennink and Van Nostrum, 2002; Slaughter et al., 2009).

Hydrogels based on natural polymers are particularly relevant for drug delivery applications owing to their softness, hydrophilicity, super absorbency, viscoelasticity, biodegradability, biocompatibility, porosity, smoothness, ability to incorporate and release therapeutic agents, and their similarity with ECM (Woerly, 1997). Importantly, hydrogels cause negligible toxicity or tissue damage and do not give inflammatory responses or thrombosis. They can retain a large amount of water or biological fluids and are characterized by a soft rubbery consistency similar to living tissues, and because of this, they have emerged as the ideal materials for drug delivery (Ratner and Hoffman, 1976). Their highly porous structure can easily be tuned by controlling the density of cross-links in the gel matrix and the affinity of the hydrogels for the aqueous environment in which they are swollen. Their porosity also permits loading of drugs into the gel matrix and subsequent drug release at a rate dependent on the diffusion coefficient of the small molecule or macromolecule through the gel network (Harland and Prud'homme, 1992; Ulbrich et al., 1995; Galaev and Mattiasson, 1999).

Alginate (ALG) has several advantages such as high biocompatibility, biodegradability, nontoxicity, non-immunogenicity, chelating ability, and the susceptibility for chemical modification (Tonnesen and Karlsen, 2002; Ertesvag and Valla, 1998; Gombotz and Wee, 1998). It has been tailor-made to suit the requirements of many pharmaceutical and biomedical applications such as implantation of medical devices and artificial organs, tissue engineering, prostheses, ophthalmology, dentistry, bone repair, and drug delivery systems (Lee and Mooney, 2012). ALG is prone to chemical functionalization as it has a number of free hydroxyl and carboxyl groups along its backbone. Its chemical modification can enhance its existing properties (e.g., the strength of its ionic gel can be significantly enhanced by the use of covalent cross-linkers; its hydrophobicity and shelf life can be increased) or new properties can be introduced (such as anticoagulant properties, induction of chemical/biochemical anchors for cell surfaces, and temperature dependent characteristics) (Kong et al., 2003). ALG polymers are known to have hemocompatibility.

The ALG hydrogels possess physiochemical similarity to the native ECM, both compositionally and mechanically, and their high-water content offers them good biocompatibility (Clark and Green, 1936). Biodegradability or dissolution may be designed into hydrogels through enzymatic, hydrolytic, or environmental (e.g., pH, temperature, or electric field) pathways; however, degradation is not always desirable depending on the timescale and location of the drug delivery device (Leonard et al., 2004). Hydrogels are also relatively deformable and can conform to the shape of the surface to which they are applied. In the latter context, the muco- or bioadhesive properties of some hydrogels can be advantageous in immobilizing them at the site of application or in applying them on surfaces that are not horizontal.

4.2 PREPARATION OF ALGINATE HYDROGELS

The strategies of hydrogel fabrication can be divided into two categories such as the non-covalent bonding (physical cross-linking) (Hennink and Nostrum, 2012) and the covalent bonding (chemical cross-linking) (Patil et al., 1997). In chemically cross-linked gels, covalent bonds are present between different polymer chains. In physically cross-linked gels, dissolution is prevented by physical interactions, which exist between the different polymer chains.

4.2.1 PHYSICALLY CROSS-LINKED GELS

4.2.1.1 IONIC CROSS-LINKING

ALGs consist of blocks of similar and alternating residues which have different conformational features and behavior. The block consists of MMMMM, GGGGG, and GMGMGM, and so forth (M stands for mannose and G for glucose residues) (Figure 4.1). ALG hydrogels are crafted by combining an aqueous ALG solution with an ionic cross-linking agent such as divalent cations that is, Ca^{2+}, Sr^{2+}, and Ba^{2+} or trivalent ions (Ştefania et al., 2009) such as Fe^{3+} and $Al.^{3+}$ ALG chelates with divalent cations are formed through ionic interaction and intramolecular bonding between the carboxylic acid groups present mainly at its guluronate blocks (Gaumann et al., 2000). In addition to G-blocks, M and MG blocks also participate by forming weak junctions. Binding studies have revealed that Ca^{2+} is able to bind to G and MG blocks, Ba^{2+} to G and M-blocks, and Sr^{2+} to G-blocks only, while trivalent lanthanide ions (La^{3+}, Pr^{3+}, and Nd^{3+}) show an affinity for both GG and MM segments (De Ramos et al., 1997). The differences in binding affinity are related to the ionic radius, coordination number of the cross-linking ions, and the extent of surrounding water of hydration. The selective binding of divalent metal ions and the corresponding gel increase in the order: MM block<MG block<GG block (Thu et al. 1996).

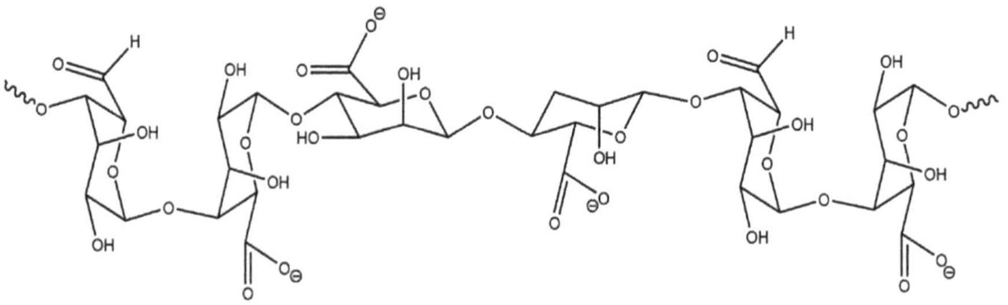

FIGURE 4.1 Possible sequences of L-Guluronic acid (G) and D-Mannuronic acid (M) residues in an alginate (ALG) polymer.

The order of affinity of ALG's for divalent ions decreases in the following order: $Pb^{2+} > Cu^{2+} > Cd^{2+} > Ba^{2+} > Sr^{2+} > Ca^{2+} > Co^{2+}$, Ni^{2+}, $Zn^{2+} > Mn^{2+}$. Ca^{2+} is the most commonly used cation to induce gelation in ALGs because of its nontoxicity (Sutherland, 1991; Badwan et al., 1985). The use of highly toxic cations such as Pb^{2+}, Cu^{2+}, and Cd^{2+} is limited whereas mildly toxic ions such as Sr^{2+} and Ba^{2+} ions have been used in low concentrations for cell immobilization applications. The ionic gel results when divalent cations interact with ALG G-blocks (Fundueanu et al., 1999). The guluronate blocks of one polymer chain form junctions with the guluronate blocks of the adjacent polymer chains through ionic interaction between the guluronic acid groups while the Van der Waal forces between ALG segments result in a three-dimensional gel network. This alignment forms an electronegative cavity consisting of a hydrophilic group that binds the Ca^{2+} through multi coordination using oxygen atoms of the carboxyl groups. This tightly bound polymer configuration results in the formation of a junction zone shaped like an "egg-box," resulting in a gel structure (Figure 4.2). Ca^{2+} and Ba^{2+} bonding with ALG occurs in a planer two-dimensional manner; on the other hand, the trivalent aluminum cation forms a three-dimensional structure with ALG (Gombotz and Wee, 1998; Nokhodchi and Tailor, 2004).

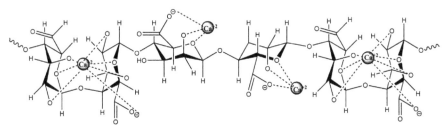

FIGURE 4.2   Ionic interactions between ALG and divalent cations.

Ionic cross-linking of ALG can be further obtained by external or internal gelation and gelation by cooling. The methods differ in the way cross-linking ions are introduced to the ALG polymer (Chan et al., 2006).

External method: In the external method (diffusion controlled), cations diffuse from a higher concentration region to the interior of ALG particle when ALG is extruded drop wise into a cationic solution which instantaneously reacts with the carboxylic groups of guluronic acid residues at the droplet surface. This results in a matrix with a highly cross-linked surface and a less cross-linked interior. At the outermost layer of the hydrogel-cation layer, gelling kinetics is rapid and gel formation is instantaneous. This feature allows ALG to be used in cell or bioactive material where the cell or bioactive species are entrapped in singular ALG gel beads (Figure 4.3).

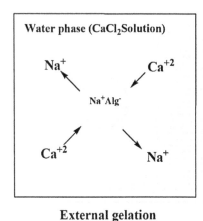

External gelation

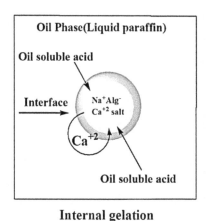

Internal gelation

FIGURE 4.3   Diagram of external gelation and internal gelation.

Internal method: In an internal gelation method (Figure 4.3), the ALG is exposed to the cations in a controlled manner so that a hydrogel having a homogeneous distribution of ALG can be obtained. Inactive forms of calcium salt such as $CaCO_3$ or $CaSO_4$ is added to the ALG solution and the mixture is extruded into the oil. The mixture is then acidified to bring about the release of Ca^{2+} from the insoluble salt to cross-link the ALG. The release of CO_2 from the reaction between the acid and carbonate leads to the formation of abundant cavities within the film. Acidification can be achieved either immediately, by direct addition of a mineral acid such as glacial acetic acid, or in a controlled fashion by slowly hydrolyzing lactone such as D-glucono-δ-lactone.

The ALG gels can also be prepared by the cooling method, for which ALG, calcium salt, and calcium sequestrant are dissolved in a hot medium of 90°C and then allowed to set through cooling. At high-temperature, the high thermal energy of the ALG chains prevents polymeric alignment and their irreversibly destabilize any non-covalent intramolecular bonding between the neighboring chains. Upon cooling at a lower temperature, the reestablishment of the intermolecular bonds between the polymer chains facilitates the formation of an ordered tertiary structure and the resultant homogeneous matrix.

4.2.1.2   HYDROPHOBIC INTERACTION

Hydrophobic bonds are reversible non-covalent interactions, which exist among the nonpolar hydrophobic groups. The motivation for hydrophobic modification of ALGs is to transform the ALG polysaccharide from its predominantly hydrophilic nature to a molecule with amphiphilic or hydro-phobic characteristics (Sinquin and Hubert, 1993). The most straightforward method of stabilizing ALG is to convert its backbone into an amphiphilic polymer by covalent attachment of hydrophobic moieties such as long alkyl chains or aromatic groups (Pawar and Edgar, 2012). The hydrophobic cavities formed could potentially be used as the vehicles for hydrophobic drugs. The hydrophilic portion makes the polymer water-soluble, while the hydrophobic domains tend to aggregate in aqueous solution and form distinct structures with regions rich in hydrophilic and hydrophobic contents. The strength of the association can be tuned by varying degree of substitution (DS) and length/chemical nature of the hydrophobic tails. Hydrophobically modified ALG (HMA), being a derivative of a biocompatible polymer, has a huge potential as a polymeric drug carrier (Kashyap et al., 2005).

The HMA of different DS has been prepared by a simple amide coupling reaction. These amphiphilic polymers form stable gel-like networks in water due to associative hydrophobic interactions. The HMA sol can be further cross-linked with calcium to yield very high modulus hydrogels. The modulus of 2 wt.% HMA gels is of the order of 100 kPa, which is significant for a material with such high-water content. There is a clear evidence of synergy between the two gelation mechanisms; an associative network driven by hydrophobic interaction and the chemical cross-linking (Yang et al., 2011).

The HMA derivatives have been prepared by covalent fixation of dodecyl or octadecyl chains onto the polysaccharide backbone (Leonard et al., 2004). In semi-dilute solution, intermolecular hydrophobic interactions result in the formation of physical hydrogels, the physicochemical properties of which can be controlled through polymer concentration, hydrophobic chain content, and nonthixotropic salts such as sodium chloride. The mechanical properties of these hydrogels can be further reinforced by the addition of calcium chloride. The combination of both calcium bridges and intermolecular hydrophobic interactions decreased the swelling ratio that in turn, decreased the elastic and viscous moduli.

Babak et al. (2000) synthesized new amphiphilic derivatives of sodium ALG (SA) by attaching short polyether chains to the ALG backbone through an amide linkage. α-Amino, ω-benzyloxy tetraoxyethylene $(C_6H_5(OCH_2CH_2)_4NH_2$, (BzlO-TEG-NH$_2$) was used as a coupling reagent in this synthesis. SA was first activated using sodium metaperiodate, which oxidized (20% of the available urinate residues) the two secondary hydroxyl groups to aldehyde groups, which then reacted with BzlO-TEG-NH$_2$ by reductive amination to yield a tetraoxyethylene functionalized amine derivative of ALG (BzlO-TEG-NH-ALG). At the completion of this step, there was a significant drop in the viscosity of the reaction mixture as the molecular weight of ALG decreased due to the extension of chain conformation through ring opening. ALGs containing longer MG block sequences were found to degrade more rapidly than ALGs containing shorter MG blocks. Partial oxidation of ALGs may be advantageous for biomedical applications because they fully degrade in aqueous media.

As the charged (anionic) ALG backbone is decorated with hydrophobic entities, two competing forces emerge – (a) repulsive interactions resulting from the charged carboxylate groups which promote chain extension and (b) attractive interactions resulting from the hydrophobic groups which promote chain collapse. When (b) dominates (a), their cumulative effect leads to the formation of high molecular weight aggregates. For BzlO-TEG-NH-ALG, the electrostatic repulsive forces offset the hydrophobic attractive forces and the formation of high molecular weight derivative is thus prevented.

Yao et al. (2010) developed a new route for the hydrophobic modification of SA. In this modification, butyl methacrylate was grafted onto SA by coupling reaction of poly(butyl methacrylate) with SA. The product matrix showed the prolonged release of bovine serum albumin (BSA) in deionized water and a buffer solution. The release of BSA was faster in the Tris–HCl buffer solution than in deionized water as the release rate depended on the diffusion process and the average pore size of the gel was bigger in the buffer solution (pH = 7.2) than in pure water (pH = 6.8). At high pH value, the carboxyl groups of SA remained in the ionized form and due to the repulsion among the carboxyl groups, the volume and pore size of the hydrogel increased. The release rate was greater in the buffer solution as the diffusion of the protein was easier in the buffer solution.

4.2.1.3   POLYELECTROLYTE COMPLEXATION (PEC)

ALG gels can be prepared by utilizing the electrostatic complex forming ability of ALG. Polycations such as chitosan-poly-L-lysine and albumin have been used for the complexation. In this method, no organic precursors, catalysts, or reactive agents are needed, and thus there was no chance for any cross-reactions with a therapeutic payload (Tsuchida and Abe, 1982). ALG-based polyelectrolyte complex (PEC) network was synthesized by Sarmento et al. (2006), where a low concentration (18 mM) of calcium chloride solution was added to a calculated amount of SA solution under constant stirring. The addition initiated the cross-linking of SA while mechanical stirring prevented bulk gel formation by breaking the pregelled ALG into smaller aggregates. After 60 min, chitosan solution was slowly added into the pregelled ALG solution with constant stirring. The added chitosan formed a PEC with ALG and stabilized the pregelled microgel nucleus into individual sponge-like nanoparticles.

PEC of poly-L-lysine (Donati and Paoletti, 2009) with ALG is reported. In the ALG–albumin system (Zhao et al., 2009), coacervation was less as compared to other polypeptide–polysaccharide systems due to the high viscosity of the albumin–alginic acid complex and its propensity to precipitate. The optimum conditions for maximum coacervate yield were pH 3.9, ionic strength of 1 mM, and 0.15% w/v total polyion concentration. The choice of the cationic molecule for PEC formation is highly dependent upon its charge under physiological conditions because the pH of the hydrogel environment modulates the ionic interactions, and consequently, the properties of PEC hydrogel properties. If electrostatic interactions were sufficiently strong, the physical association between the polymers could be maintained at the physiological pH.

4.2.1.4 HYDROGEN BONDING

Hydrogen bonds (H-bonding) occur between two polar groups, namely hydrogen atom and highly electronegative atom such as nitrogen, oxygen, and fluorine. Though it is relatively weak compared with covalent or ionic bond, concerted H-bonding interactions contribute to the improved bond strength and thus hydrogel formation.

Yuan et al. (2016) reported a poly(vinyl alcohol)-sodium alginate-borax (PVA-SA-borax) hydrogel based on hydrogen bonding. The PVA-SA-borax hydrogels showed complete self-healing behavior in 3 h and demonstrated good barrier properties to hazardous chemicals like sodium cyanide, dichlorvos, and phorate.

4.2.2 CHEMICALLY CROSS-LINKED HYDROGELS

The strength of a physically cross-linked hydrogel is directly related to the chemical properties of the constituent gelators while they have the advantage of forming gels without any chemical modification or the addition of cross-linking entities in vivo. The design flexibility of such hydrogels is limited and it is difficult to manipulate their gelation time, network pore size, chemical functionalization, and degradation time. At the same time, the physically bonded hydrogels have small resident time within the tissue as their dissipation is fast. On the other hand, the covalent cross-linking resists dilution of the hydrogel matrix and also the diffusion of the polymer from the site of administration. Small-molecule cross-linkers have been most often used for designing in situ cross-linked hydrogels (Smidsrød et al., 1973; Zhao et al., 2010).

4.2.2.1 CROSS-LINKING BY CHEMICAL REACTION OF COMPLEMENTARY GROUPS

Water-soluble ALG polysaccharide owes its solubility property to the presence of polar functional groups (mainly OH, COOH). These groups can be utilized for the formation of hydrogels. Covalent linkages between polymer chains can be established by the reaction of functional groups with complementary reactivity, such as an amine-carboxylic acid or an isocyanate-OH reaction, or by Schiff base formation.

4.2.2.1.1 Cross-linking with Aldehydes

Riyajan et al. (2009) used glutaraldehyde cross-linked ALG gel for the encapsulation and controlled release of Neem Azadirachtin-A (Aza-A). Aza-A, an insecticidal tetranortriterpenoid is highly unstable which easily degrades or isomerizes when exposed to light. The degradation of Aza-A could be protected by its microencapsulation within cross-linked ALG gel and its entrapment efficiency was found to be a function of cross-linking time, wherein the efficiency decreased with the increase in time.

The reaction kinetics of ALG gel formation with glutaraldehyde was studied by Chan et al. (2008). An equilibrium swelling model was used to calculate the median pore size of the gel. The reaction rate was zero-order with respect to the ALG concentration, and independent of the ALG M/G composition and sequences. Thus, both M and G were equally reactive towards glutaraldehyde. However, the reaction rate increased upon increasing the ALG molecular weight which reduces the mobility of the chains as now the chains show a better chance to interact with glutaraldehyde. As the temperature was lowered, the rate of network formation slowed down since the acid catalyzed acetalization reactions require high activation energy.

Chan et al. (2009) later reported the synthesis of thermodynamically controlled ALG network gels having pH-responsive properties. Thermodynamic gels were synthesized by allowing the cross-linking reaction to reach the equilibrium.

Even a low concentration of glutaraldehyde is toxic and it may cause cell-growth inhibition, therefore, other alternative cross-linkers have been used, for example, adipic acid dihydrazide (AAD). AAD has been used to cross-link with poly(aldehyde guluronate) of periodate oxidized ALG (Bouhadir et al., 1999). The swelling and degradation of the gels could be controlled by varying the molar ratio of sodium periodates to uronate monosaccharides and a higher number of cross-links could be established by increasing the AAD concentration. An optimum number of intermolecular cross-link junctions were formed when the concentration of AAD was 150 mM. At this concentration, the obtained gel had maximum modulus value. When the hydrogel was prepared in presence of Daunomycin, the drug was loaded onto the polymer matrix through a covalent linkage which was subsequently released on hydrolysis of this linkage in 2 days to 6 weeks time.

Poly(aldehyde guluronate), obtained by periodate oxidation of SA has been transformed into a hydrogel through cross-linking with proteins (such as gelatin) in the presence of low concentrations of sodium tetraborate (borax) (Balakrishnan et al., 2005). These hydrogels were designed for delivery of "Primaquine" and encapsulation of hepatocytes with minimal cytotoxicity. Genipin (a naturally derived chemical from gardenia fruit) has also been found to efficiently cross-link amino-functionalized prepolymers to form hydrogel while exhibiting minimal toxicity to the native tissues (Yun et al., 2015).

In order to improve the biodegradability of ALG, Gao et al. (2009a) performed the oxidation of commercially available high molecular weight ALG with sodium periodate. Oxidized ALG has fully degraded at physiological conditions after 100 h incubation and its molecular weight reduced from 11.2×10^4 to 3.6×10^4 g/mol.

Amine groups interact with aldehyde groups through the formation of imine bonds. Hydrogels prepared by oxidized ALG and acrylamide-modified chitin were able to guide the reconstruction of inorganic biomaterial like hydroxyapatite (HA). The separated pieces of hydrogels with HA could autonomously heal when put together. Furthermore, the lyophilized HA hydrogels retained self-healing property when were rehydrated in water (Ding et al., 2015).

Moe et al. (1991) reported super swelling material which was formed through base catalyzed covalent cross-linking of ALGs with epichlorohydrin. Ca-ALG beads were prepared in water and then subjected to a solvent exchange with 96% ethanol. The cross-linking reaction was performed by suspending the Ca-ALG beads in ethanol containing epichlorohydrin and NaOH. The synthesized beads were able to swell up to 100 times of their dry volume without any mass loss. Volume increases during reswelling of dried beads which remained unaffected by the presence of nonionic solutes such as glucose and glycerol, while the ionic solutes such as NaCl and Na-galacturonate slightly reduced the extent of volume increase. However, the reduction in the degree of swelling (due to the presence of ionic solutes) was significantly lower in magnitude compared to synthetic super swelling materials like cross-linked poly(acrylic acid).

4.2.2.1.2   Cross-linking by Condensation Reactions

Condensation reactions between hydroxyl or amine groups with carboxylic acids or derivatives thereof are frequently applied for the synthesis of polymers such as polyesters and polyamides, respectively. These reactions have also been used for the preparation of hydrogels. Lee et al. (2000) developed covalently cross-linked ALG hydrogels by cross-linking ALG and PEG-diamines using N, N-(3-dimethylaminopropyl)-N-ethyl carbodiimide. The elastic modulus could be controlled by the amount of polyethylene glycol-diamine (PEG-diamine) in the gel and the molecular weight of PEG. The hydrogel properties can be further regulated by multifunctional cross-linking molecules, which provided a wider range and tighter control over degradation rates and mechanical stiffness, as demonstrated by Eiselt et al. (1999). In their work, the hydrogel was formed with either poly(acrylamide-co-hydrazide) as a multifunctional cross-linking molecule or AAD as a bifunctional cross-linking molecule. This multi cross-linking strategy has led to the formation of stronger hydrogels.

Galant et al. (2006) crafted HMA by using 1-ethyl-3-(3-dimethylaminopropyl) carbodiimide hydrochloride as the coupling agent to form amide linkages between amine-containing molecules and the carboxylate moieties on the ALG backbone.

The amide derivative of ALG has been used for the treatment of traumatic disorders of the intervertebral disc (Leone et al., 2008). Na-ALG was first converted to tetrabutylammonium-ALG and then dissolved in DMF. The carboxylic acid groups at ALG were activated by the reaction with 2-Chloro-N-methylpyridinium iodide. A reactive diamine was then used along with triethylamine catalyst to yield the cross-linked ALG. Water uptake and hydration kinetics revealed that the ALG hydrogel swelled up to 250%. The gel was suitable for the injection applications.

Bartley et al. (2003) reported the synthesis of cross-linked ALG hydrogels using water-soluble carbodiimide chemistry. Carboxylic acid groups on the ALG backbone reacted with hydroxyl groups to form a covalently cross-linked matrix.

Bu et al. (2004) reported that the HMA prepared by the Ugi multicomponent condensation reaction, a multicomponent reaction in organic chemistry, involving a ketone or aldehyde, an amine, an isocyanide and a carboxylic acid to form a bis-amide.

4.2.2.1.3 Cross-linking by Polymerization

Preparation of hydrogels, based on grafting involves the polymerization of a monomer on the backbone of a preformed polymer. The main advantage of polymerization is the ease with which a variety of properties can be incorporated into the hydrogel by simply mixing derivatized macromers of choice and subsequently copolymerizing.

Gao et al. (2009b) reported the synthesis of poly[(2-dimethylamino) ethyl methacrylate]-oxidized Na-ALG (PDMAEMA-g-OALG) hydrogel beads by the grafting of poly[(2-dimethylamino) ethyl methacrylate] onto oxidized Na-ALG. This hydrogel was used to study the in vitro controlled release behavior of BSA protein from the hydrogels. The periodate oxidation converted vicinal hydroxyl groups (2-OH and 3-OH at the ALG backbone) to aldehyde groups. These aldehyde groups then reacted with amine terminal of PDMAEMA to form a stable Schiff's base in the form of an imine. Grafting of PDMAEMA chains to the ALG chain allowed a control over the equilibrium swelling ratio of the hydrogels on changing the pH and ionic strength of the media.

Increasing the ionic strength (NaCl concentration) initially increased the swelling ratio due to the disruption of the PECs, and later, it decreased the ratio as the gel network was destroyed by Na-Ca ion exchange.

Kulkarni et al. (2010) prepared electrically responsive ALG-based hydrogels by grafting of acrylamide and subsequently hydrolyzing the amide groups. Similar electro-responsive hydrogels were also synthesized by Yang et al. (2009) by grafting of poly(acrylic acid) onto the ALG backbone. The hydrogels were used as transdermal drug delivery systems for ketoprofen, a model nonsteroidal anti-inflammatory drug. On applying an electrical stimulus across the hydrogel, the positive counterion moved towards the negative electrode, but the negative carboxylate groups remained immobile and consequently, ketoprofen was released from the matrix. Lee et al. (2009) grafted poly(N-isopropylacrylamide) onto the ALG backbone for crafting temperature/and pH-responsive hydrogels.

In recent years, UV-induced polymerization is being utilized for the preparation of hydrogels. In situ photo cross-linking of ALG can be done under physiological conditions in a minimally invasive way using a brief exposure to ultraviolet (UV) light (Jeon et al., 2011). This process occurs under mild conditions and, therefore, can be performed in direct contact with cells. ALG has been modified with 2-aminoethyl methacrylate using carbodiimide chemistry and the methacrylated ALGs were subsequently photo cross-linked on exposure to UV light in the presence of a photoinitiator. Photocross-linkable ALG with controlled degradation and cell adhesive properties has attracted great interest with regard to tissue engineering application, although they are still relatively new and seem to require further studies to assess their effectiveness (Jeon et al., 2009).

4.3 CHARACTERISATION

Circular dichroism (Thom et al., 1982; Morris et al., 1980) which depends on the optical activity of chromophores, provides better understanding of the mechanism of cross-linking and nuclear magnetic resonance spectroscopy (Mammarella and Rubiolo, 2003) provides a quick and nondestructive method to determine the composition and arrangement of ALG uronic acid residues. It also provides the information about the diffusion behavior of the cross-linking cations during the gelation.

Fourier transform infrared spectroscopy is a useful technique for identifying the different functional groups associated in the polymer matrix (Lawrie et al., 2007). It is based on the principle that the basic components of a substance, that is, chemical bonds, usually can be excited and absorb infrared light at frequencies that are typical of the types of the chemical bonds. The resulting IR absorption spectrum represents a fingerprint of the measured sample. This technique is widely used to investigate the structural arrangement in hydrogel by comparison with the starting material.

Scanning electron microscopy is a technique which can be used to provide information about the sample's surface topography, composition, and other properties such as electrical conductivity (Aston et al., 2016). This is a powerful technique, widely used to capture the characteristic "network" structure in hydrogels; while atomic force microscopy provides information about the crystalline homogeneity of the ALG pellets (Zimmermann et al., 2003). It is used for the 3D characterization of the sample as compared to other techniques like electron microscopes, dynamic light scattering, and optical characterization methods.

Gel permeation chromatography coupled online to a multi-angle laser light scattering is a technique which is widely used to determine the molecular distribution and parameters of a polymeric system (Feng et al., 2017).

4.4 BIOMEDICAL APPLICATIONS

4.4.1 PHARMACEUTICAL APPLICATIONS

ALGs are being used as a thickener, gel forming, and stabilizing agent in pharmaceutics where they play a significant role in the controlled release of drugs. Although presently oral dosage formulations of ALGs are more popular in pharmaceutical applications, the use of ALG hydrogels as depots for tissue localized drug delivery is being currently focused.

4.4.1.1   DELIVERY OF DRUGS

Drug delivery systems, capable of releasing the drugs in a controlled manner are very important for health care (Kumar et al., 2001). ALG gels are typically nanoporous and useful as a matrix for cell immobilization, entrapment of bioactive compounds such as low molecular weight drugs, macromolecular drugs including peptide hormones (e.g., insulin, growth hormone), polysaccharides (e.g., heparin), antibiotics, antigens, and enzymes. It is biodegradable and, hence, it degrades and gets absorbed by the body during and/or after drug release without exerting any toxic effects (Tamada and Langer, 1992). Such delivery systems offer numerous advantages as compared to conventional dosage forms such as improved efficacy, reduced toxicity, and improved patient compliance and convenience (Takka et al., 1998). The pore size of the ALG matrix directly affects diffusion and is controlled by various factors. The drug release from the hydrogel may be controlled by several release mechanisms such as diffusion, swelling, chemically controlled, and environmentally-responsive release (Ostberg et al., 1994).

The ionically cross-linked hydrogel consisting of partially oxidized ALG could completely release "Flurbiprofen" within 1.5 h. However, when the drug was incorporated into ALG beads derived from partially oxidized ALG through the combination of ionic and covalent cross-linking (using both calcium ions and AAD), a prolonged release was witnessed because of more intense cross-linking which allowed less swelling (Maiti et al., 2009).

Aslani and Kennedy (1996) investigated the calcium and zinc ALG beads as a sparingly water-soluble drug delivery system using paracetamol as the representative drug and it was observed that the release was fastest in an acidic medium where the complete release was possible in 2 h while the release was slower in water (4–5 h) from Zn ALG beads.

Colinet et al. (2009) prepared ALG grafted with poly(ε-caprolactone) (PCL) hydrogel containing theophylline, a drug with poor water-solubility. The result showed that drug release was completed within 2 h for ALG-graft-PCL/Ca^{2+} as the length of the hydrophobic PCL chains controlled the swelling behavior of the gel beads which slowed the release of theophylline, while for ALG/Ca^{2+} beads, the release was possible in 1 h time.

Zhang et al. (2010) studied the release of theophylline from the carbon nanotube (CNT)-incorporated ALG microspheres. The presence of CNT enhanced the mechanical stability of the gels, whereas the structure and morphology of the microspheres remained unaltered and there was no significant cytotoxicity. Segi et al. (1989) reported an interaction between the anionic carboxyl group of ALGs and the cationic drugs such as propranolol.

The anionic carboxyl groups of ALGs play an important role in determining the loading capacity of cationic drugs, and the total amount of the drug in the beads can be controlled by adjusting the pH of the medium.

The swelling of ALG microspheres was decreased on cross-linking with glutaraldehyde while the loading of the water-soluble drug, (nimesulide) on ion cross-linked hydroxamated alginic acid resulted into prolonged release (Patil and Pokharkar, 2001). The drug release profiles of calcium ALG microspheres loaded with sulfaguanidine were affected by the addition of various copolymers (Heng et al., 2000).

Multiparticulate systems of ALG and chitosan have also been widely exploited in many drug delivery applications. Particulate systems of ALG and chitosan containing triamcinolone were prepared by a complex coacervation/ionotropic gelation method for colonic drug delivery. A higher swelling degree and faster drug release were observed from the particulate systems in a simulated enteric environment (pH 7.5) as compared to a simulated gastric environment (pH 1.2) (Chan et al., 1997; Lucinda-Silva et al., 2010).

Pillay and Fassihi (1999) investigated the release of diclofenac sodium, a sparingly water-soluble drug from cross-linking of SA with calcium ions through ionotropic gelation. There was a negligible drug release at pH 1–4, however, the rate of drug release at pH 6.6 ranged from rapid to slow (i.e., 100% release in 4–10 h) but in a controlled manner.

Magnetic ALG-chitosan beads loaded with albendazole (ABZ) were also prepared for passive targeting to the gastrointestinal tract using physical capture mechanisms (e.g., magnetic field, pH). The beads showed unique pH-dependent swelling behaviors and a continuous release of ABZ (Wang et al., 2010). Amoxicillin loaded chitosan/poly(γ-glutamic acid) nanoparticles have been incorporated into ALG/Ca^{2+} hydrogels for effective treatment of *Helicobacter pylori* infection (Chang et al., 2010).

4.4.1.2   PROTEIN DELIVERY

ALG is an excellent candidate for delivery of protein drugs since proteins can be incorporated into ALG-based formulations under relatively mild conditions due to which their denaturation is avoided; moreover, the gels protect them from degradation until their release. A variety of strategies have been employed to control the rate of protein release from ALG gels. Proteins encapsulated in ALG matrices are released by two mechanisms: (i) diffusion of the protein through the pores of the polymer network, and (ii) degradation of the polymer network (Gombotz and Wee, 2012).

The diffusion of several proteins such as immunoglobulin G, fibrinogen, and insulin has been studied using ALG gels. It was observed that on increasing the concentration of ALG in the beads, the rate of protein diffusion decreased (Tanaka et al., 1984; Chevalier et al., 1987).

Wells et al. (2007) investigated the applicability of ionically cross-linked ALG microspheres as a controlled release system for proteins such as lysozyme and chymotrypsin. The proteins were physically cross-linked with the SA and their release was therefore more sustained.

Gao et al. (2009b) studied the in vitro controlled release of BSA from oxidized SA-graft-poly(2-dimethylamino) ethyl methacrylate hydrogel beads. Tetra-functional acetal-linked and stimuli-responsive gels with adjustable pore sizes have been derived from ALG. The gels were capable of protecting acid-labile proteins (insulin) from denaturation in the gastric environment at pH 1.2, while releasing the loaded protein at near zero-order kinetics at neutral pH. The low encapsulation efficiency and fast release of many proteins from ALG gels were handled by utilizing various cross-linking or encapsulation techniques, and/or by enhancing the mutual interaction between the protein and hydrogel (Chan and Neufeld, 2010).

Insulin-loaded ALG microspheres were crafted by blending ALG with anionic polymers (e.g., cellulose acetate, phthalate, polyphosphate, and dextran sulfate), followed by chitosan-coating in order to protect insulin at gastric pH and achieve its sustained release at intestinal pH (Silva et al., 2006).

ALG microspheres coated with *Bombyx mori* silk fibroin have also been prepared using layer-by-layer deposition technique. The microspheres had a mechanically stable shell, which acted as a diffusion barrier to the encapsulated proteins (Castro et al., 2007).

Lee et al. (2009) prepared an injectable microsphere that served as a depot for proteins/hydrogel combination and enabled the sustained release of BSA. Protein delivery system was formed by the encapsulation of a suspension of poly(d, l-lactide-co-glycolide) (PLGA) microspheres within ALG and then ionic cross-linking was carried out. The author found that the release of protein from this combination delivery system was primarily controlled by the mixing ratio between PLGA microspheres and ALG hydrogels and was totally independent of total BSA content and the size of PLGA microspheres used.

Lee et al. (2009) reported the delivery of heat-shock protein (human immunodeficiency virus) from an injectable microsphere/hydrogel combination system for the treatment of myocardial infarction.

Fluorescein isothiocyanate-labeled bovine serum albumin (FITC-BSA) was incorporated into the three different types of ALG microspheres such as ALG–chitosan system, ALG–CaCl$_2$, and ALG–polylysine. In vitro release studies revealed a large initial burst in all the three cases. After the burst, the release was sustained for 4 days from the ALG–chitosan system which may be due to the strong interaction between the two polymers and a stabilization of the polycation salt by the phosphate ions, while the ALG–CaCl$_2$ and ALG–polylysine systems exhibited a sustained release of FITC-BSA for 6 and 24 h, respectively. The authors attributed the short release time from the ALG–CaCl$_2$ microspheres to the low stability of the chelating junction in a phosphate buffer (> pH 5) (Liu et al., 1997).

4.4.1.3   WOUND HEALING

A wound is a defect or a break in the skin which can result from trauma or medical/physiological conditions. ALG wound management products are more popular than the conventional cotton gauzes as they absorb excess exudate and toxins, keep a good moisture between the wound and the dressing, preserve the wound from external sources of infection, prevent excess heat at the wound, allow good permeability to gases, maintain a physiologically moist microenvironment, and minimize bacterial infection at the wound site (Hooper et al., 2012). They are completely sterile and easy to remove without further trauma to the wound. The sodium ions in wound fluids also slowly convert the cross-linked ALG dressing into a viscous SA liquid, which soothes and protects the wound. A variety of more functional and bioactive ALGs have been studied in a number of wound dressing (Boateng et al., 2008; Queen et al., 2004).

Segal et al. (1991) reported that zinc-containing ALG dressings have a greater potentiating effect on prothrombotic coagulation and platelet activation than calcium. This is due to the role of zinc ions as a cofactor for the coagulation factor XII and the intrinsic pathway of coagulation. ALG fibers cross-linked with zinc ions have also been reported for wound dressings, as zinc ions may have immune modulatory and anti-microbial effects, as well as can enhance keratinocyte migration and increase the levels of endogenous growth factors. Zinc ions aggregate in the vicinity of adenosine diphosphate (ADP) during the wound healing and release ADP from the wound tissues, which in turn activates platelets and facilitate the clotting cascade.

Balakrishnan et al. (2005) reported a hydrogel wound dressing that was prepared from gelatin and oxidized ALG in the presence of borax in small concentration. The composite matrix had the hemostatic effect of gelatin, the wound-healing promoting feature of ALG, and the antiseptic property of borax.

The partially oxidized ALG gels exhibited a sustained release of dibutyryl cyclic adenosine monophosphate, a regulator of human keratinocyte proliferation. It accelerated wound healing, which completed within 10 days in a rat model (Rabbany et al., 2010). Based on the advantages of ALG and Ag nanoparticles, a gel particle was fabricated, resulting in an anti-adhesive and antimicrobial wound dressing. Incorporation of silver into ALG dressings increased antimicrobial activity which plays a key role in determining the process of wound repair and improves the binding affinity for elastase, matrix metalloproteases-2, and pro-inflammatory cytokines. The addition of silver into ALG dressings also enhanced the antioxidant capacity (Agren, 1999).

ALG blend with chitin/chitosan and fucoidan have provided a moist healing environment in rats, with an ease of application and removal (Murakami et al., 2010). The encapsulation of gentamicin in ALG matrices has been carried out for the treatment of osteomyelitis. Implanted ALGs exhibited good biocompatibility with a complete bioabsorption without any sign of rejection or allergic reactions in the neighboring tissues (Sivakumar et al., 2003).

4.4.1.4 CARTILAGE REPAIR AND BONE REGENERATION

ALG-based scaffolds have been widely explored over the past several decades as a vehicle to deliver proteins or cell populations that can direct the regeneration or engineering of various tissues and organs in the body (Lópiz-Morales et al., 2010).

ALG gels have found useful in animal models for the delivery of growth factors, osteoinductive factors, bone-forming cells, or combination of both, that can effectively drive bone regeneration (e.g., bone morphogenetic proteins) as compared to other materials. This is due to their ability to be introduced into the body in a minimally invasive manner, their ability to fill irregularly shaped defects, and the ease of chemical modification with adhesion ligands and controlled release of tissue induction factors. Kolambkar et al. (2011) introduced a hybrid growth factor delivery system that consisted of an electrospun nanofiber mesh tube (for guiding bone regeneration) combined with a peptide-modified ALG hydrogel injected inside the tube. This delivery system resulted in a sustained release of recombinant bone morphogenetic proteins BMP-2 (rhBMP-2). This hybrid technique may be clinically useful for bone regeneration in the case of fracture of nonunions and large bone defects.

Alsberg et al. (2001) used ALG-based devices to transplant cell populations that directly participate in bone formation. The author transplanted primary rat calvarial osteoblasts into mice and found that the arginine-glycine-aspartate (RGD-peptide) ALG gels enhanced in vivo bone formation as compared to control ALG gels.

In addition, co-transplantation of primary chondrocytes and osteoblasts into mice using RGD peptide modified-ALG gels enabled the formation of growth-plate-like structures, which may be potentially used to replace dysfunctional epiphyses (Alsberg et al., 2002).

Barralet et al. (2005) reported degradable and injectable ALG-derived gels, and mixed with rat primary calvarial osteoblasts, and subcutaneously injected into the backs of mice when the mineralized bone tissues were observed after 9 weeks.

The transplantation of stem cells using calcium cross-linked ALG hydrogels has been widely explored in bone tissue engineering. The thickness of Ca-ALG gels was demonstrated to alter the behavior of rat bone marrow cells; however, different geometries did not influence the cell differentiation (Weng et al., 2006)

Calcium cross-linked ALG gels when mixed with bone marrow stromal cells induced the osteoblast pathway in vitro and repaired horizontal alveolar bone defects in dogs (Park et al., 2005). ALG/chitosan gels when entrapped mesenchymal stem cells (MSCs) and bone morphogenetic protein-2 showed potential for trabecular bone formation in mice (Lin and Yeh, 2004). ALG combined with inorganic materials enhanced the bone tissue formation. A separation method has been used for preparing ALG/hydroxyapatite composite scaffolds which exhibited interconnected porous morphology. The composite enhanced the adhesion of osteosarcoma cells. Cell-encapsulating ALG gel beads when introduced into calcium phosphate cement, showed potential for bone tissue engineering under moderate stress-bearing conditions (Weir et al., 2006).

ALG-based injectable hydrogels, solid- and gel-microspheres were found useful for cartilage regeneration. ALG microspheres with human mesenchymal stem cells (MSCs) in hyaluronic acid hydrogels which co-encapsulated transforming growth factor (TGF-β) proved useful for the development of implantable constructs for cartilage repair (Lawson et al., 2004). The Transforming Growth Factor (TGF)-β bioactivity was retained within the scaffold and it promoted chondrogenesis of MSCs when the hydrogels were implanted. Wang et al. (2007) prepared a 3D ALG microsphere scaffold with the help of a microfluidic device. These were effective for chondrocyte culture in vitro. It was shown that the chondrocytes seeded into the ALG microsphere scaffold, survived normally in SCID mice and it regenerated cartilage-like structures after 4 weeks of implantation.

4.5   CONCLUSION

The ALG, being multifunctional is one of most widely studied biopolymer in biomedical and pharmaceutical fields. ALG or its derivative can be easily gelled through cross-linking either through chemical or by physical methods. It has unique physiochemical properties which provide it versatile biological activity. It's swelling property, mucoadhesive nature, and gel-forming ability, gives it a unique place among the starting scaffolds used for the development of advanced drug delivery systems. ALGs have been used in the controlled and targeted release of the drugs and proteins, as a matrix for three-dimensional tissue culture, wound dressings, and cartilage regeneration. The ALG-based nanotherapeutics is of future research interest for the modern therapeutics.

SUMMARY

The polymer hydrogels are the promising vehicles for drug delivery. They provide an easy implementation of the targeted and controlled delivery of drugs to a specific organ. Their use can minimize the unfavorable side effects of classical delivery systems. ALG is an abundant natural polysaccharide that possesses free hydroxyl and carboxyl groups along its backbone and thus is susceptible for chemical modification. ALG-based hydrogels are capable of absorbing huge quantities of water while retaining their structural features. The resemblance of the hydrogels to the living tissue has opened up many opportunities for its biomedical applications, especially for the development of new controlled-released drugs. These have been investigated for delivering therapeutics in a controlled manner to the site of action. ALG-based hydrogels have been designed by using different strategies which are either based on chemical (permanent bonds) or physical cross-linking methods. The chemical methods include radical polymerization, emulsion polymerization, precipitation polymerization, self-assembly, photopolymerization, enzymatic reactions, and covalent cross-linking via linkers such as glutaraldehyde. In contrast, physical cross-linking forms a nonpermanent network with physical interactions such as hydrogen or electrostatic bonds, physical entanglements, and crystal formation. Thus, physically cross-linked hydrogels are formed via ionic interactions using graft copolymers, crystallization, and stereo complex formation. Recent years have witnessed a tremendous growth for ALG-based hydrogels in biomedical areas such as drug delivery, wound healing, and tissue engineering. Due to the increasing interest and great potential of these materials, this chapter is intended to give an overview of the current state-of-the-art technology in producing ALG-based hydrogels and their importance in biomedical applications.

KEYWORDS

- alginate
- hydrogels
- cross-linking
- gels
- biomedical applications

REFERENCES

Agren, M. S. Zinc in Wound Repair. *Arch. Dermatol.* **1999,** *135,* 1273–1274.

Alsberg, E.; Anderson, K. W.; Albeiruti, A.; Franceschi, R. T.; Mooney, D. J. Cell-Interactive Alginate Hydrogels for Bone Tissue Engineering. *J. Dent. Res.* **2001,** *80,* 2025–2029.

Alsberg, E.; Anderson, K. W.; Albeiruti, A.; Rowley, J. A.; Mooney, D. J. Engineering Growing Tissues. *Proc. Natl. Acad. Sci. U. S. A.* **2002,** *99,* 12025–12030.

Aslani, P.; Kennedy, R. A. Effect of Gelation Conditions and Dissolution Media on the Release of Paracetamol from Alginate Gel Beads. *J. Microencapsulation* **1996,** *13,* 601–614.

Aston, R.; Sewell, K.; Klein, T.; Lawrie, G.; Grøndahl, L. Evaluation of the Impact of Freezing Preparation Techniques on the Characterisation of Alginate Hydrogels by Cryo-SEM. *Eur. Polym. J.* **2016,** *82,* 1–15.

Augst, A. D.; Kong, H. J.; Mooney, D. J. Alginate Hydrogels as Biomaterials. *Macromol. Biosci.* **2006,** *6,* 623–33.

Babak, V. G.; Skotnikova, E. A.; Lukina, I. G.; Pelletier, S.; Hubert, P.; Dellacherie, E. Hydrophobically Associating Alginate Derivatives: Surface Tension Properties of Their Mixed Aqueous Solutions with Oppositely Charged Surfactants. *J. Colloid Interface Sci.* **2000,** *225,* 505–510.

Badwan, A. A.; Abumalooh, A.; Sallam, E.; Abukalaf, A.; Jawan, O. A Sustained Release Drug Delivery System Using Calcium Alginate Beads. *Drug Dev. Ind. Pharm.* **1985,** *11,* 239–256.

Balakrishnan, B.; Mohanty, M.; Umashankar, P. R.; Jayakrishnan, A. Evaluation of an in Situ Forming Hydrogel Wound Dressing Based on Oxidized Alginate and Gelatin. *Biomaterials* **2005**, *26,* 6335–6342.

Barralet, J. E.; Wang, L.; Lawson, M.; Triffitt, J. T.; Cooper, P. R.; Shelton, R. M. Comparison of Bone Marrow Cell Growth on 2D and 3D Alginate Hydrogels. *J. Mater. Sci. Mater. Med.* **2005**, *16,* 515–519.

Bartley, J. P.; Johnson, A. R.; Xu, B. J. Preparation and Characterization Of Alginate Hydrogel Membranes Crosslinked Using A Water-Soluble Carbodiimide. *J. Appl. Polym. Sci.* **2003**, *90*, 747–753.

Boateng, J. S.; Matthews, K. H.; Stevens, H. N.; Eccleston, G. M. Wound Healing Dressings and Drug Delivery Systems: A Review. *J. Pharm. Sci.* **2008**, *97*, 2892–2923.

Bouhadir, K.; Hausman, D. S.; Mooney, D. J. Synthesis of Cross-Linked Poly(Aldehyde Guluronate) Hydrogels. *Polymer* **1999**, *40*, 3575–3584.

Bu, H.; Kjoniksen, A. L.; Knudsen, K. D.; Nystrom, B. Rheological and Structural Properties of Aqueous Alginate During Gelation via the Ugi Multicomponent Condensation Reaction. *Biomacromolecules* **2004**, *5,* 1470–1479.

Castro, G. R.; Hu, X.; Kaplan, D. L.; Li, C.; Meinel, L.; Merkle, H.; Wang, X.; Wenk, E. Silk Coatings on PLGA and Alginate Microspheres for Protein Delivery. *Biomaterials* **2007**, *28*, 4161–9.

Chan, A. W.; Neufeld, R. J. Tuneable Semi-Synthetic Network Alginate for Absorptive Encapsulation and Controlled Release of Protein Therapeutics. *Biomaterials* **2010**, *31*, 9040–9047.

Chan, L. W.; Heng, P. W.; Wan, L. S. Effect of Cellulose Derivatives on Alginate Microspheres Prepared by Emulsification. *J. Microencapsulation* **1997**, *14*, 545–555.

Chan, L. W.; Lee, H. Y.; Heng, P. W. S. Mechanisms of External and Internal Gelation and their Impact on the Functions of Alginate as a Coat and Delivery System. *Carbohydr. Polym.* **2006**, 176–187.

Chan, A. W.; Whitney, R. A.; Neufeld, R. J. Kinetic Controlled Synthesis of pH Responsive Network Alginate. *Biomacromolecules* **2008**, *9*, 2536–2545.

Chan, A. W.; Whitney, R. A.; Neufeld, R. J. Semisynthesis of a Controlled Stimuli Responsive Alginate Hydrogel. *Biomacromolecules* **2009**, *10,* 609–616.

Chang, C. H.; Lin, Y. H.; Yeh, C. L.; Chen, Y. C.; Chiou, S. F.; Hsu, Y. M.; Chen, Y. S.; Wang, C. C. Nanoparticles Incorporated in pH-Sensitive Hydrogels as Amoxicillin Delivery for Eradication of Helicobacter Pylori. *Biomacromolecules* **2010**, *11*, 133–142.

Chevalier, P.; Consentino, G. P.; de la Noue, J.; Rakhit, S. Comparative Study on the Diffusion of an IgG from Various Hydrogel Beads. *Biotechnol. Tech.* **1987**, *1*, 201–206

Clark, D. E.; Green, H. C. Alginic Acid and Process of Making Same. U. S. Patent 2,036,922, 1936.

Colinet, I.; Dulong, V.; Mocanu, G.; Picton, L.; Cerf, D. L. New Amphiphilic and pH-Sensitive Hydrogel for Controlled Release of a Model Poorly Water-Soluble Drug. *Eur. J. Pharm. Biopharm.* **2009**, *73,* 345–350.

De Ramos, C. M.; Irwin, A. E.; Nauss, J. L.; Stout, B. E. 13C NMR and Molecular Modeling Studies of Alginic Acid Binding with Alkaline Earth and Lanthanide Metal Ions. *Inorg. Chim. Acta* **1997**, *1,* 69–75.

Ding, F.; Wu, S.; Wang, S.; Xiong, Y.; et al. A Dynamic and Self-Cross-Linked Polysaccharide Hydrogel with Autonomous Self-Healing Ability. *Soft Matter* **2015**, *11,* 3971.

Donati, I.; Paoletti, S. Material Properties of Alginates. In: *Alginates: Biology and Applications;* Rehm, B. H. A., Ed.; Springer-Verlag: Berlin, 2009.

Eiselt, P.; Lee, K. Y.; Mooney, D. J. Rigidity of Two-Component Hydrogels Prepared from Alginate and Poly(Ethylene Glycol)−Diamines. *Macromolecules* **1999**, *32,* 5561–5566.

Ertesvag, H.; Valla, S. Biosynthesis and Applications of Alginates. *Polym. Degrad. Stab.* **1998**, *59,* 85–91.

Feng, L.; Cao, Y.; Xu, D.; Wang, S.; Zhang, J. Molecular Weight Distribution, Rheological Property and Structural Changes of Sodium Alginate Induced by Ultrasound. *Ultrason. Sonochem.* **2017**, *34,* 609–615.

Fundueanu, G.; Nastruzzi, C.; Carpov, A.; Desbrieres, J.; Rinaudo, M. Physicochemical Characterization of Ca-Alginate Microparticles Produced with Different Methods. *Biomaterials* **1999**, *20,* 1427–1435.

Galaev, I. Y.; Mattiasson, B. Smart Polymers and what they could do in Biotechnology and Medicine. *Trends Biotechnol.* **1999**, *17,* 335–340.

Galant, C.; Kjoniksen, A. L.; Nguyen, G. T.; Knudsen, K. D.; Nystrom, B. Altering Associations in Aqueous Solutions of a Hydrophobically Modified Alginate in the Presence of β-Cyclodextrin Monomers. *J. Phys. Chem. B* **2006**, *110,* 190–195.

Gao, C.; Liu, M.; Chen, J.; Zhang, X. Preparation and Controlled Degradation of Oxidized Sodium Alginate Hydrogel. *Polym. Degrad. Stab.* **2009a**, *9,* 1405–1410.

Gao, C.; Liu, M.; Chen, S.; Jin, S.; Chen, J. Preparation of Oxidized Sodium Alginate-Graft-Poly((2-Dimethylamino) Ethyl Methacrylate) Gel Beads and in Vitro Controlled Release Behavior of BSA. *Int. J. Pharm.* **2009b**, *371,* 16–24.

Gaumann, A.; Laudes, M.; Jacob, B.; Pommersheim, R.; Laue, C.; Vogt, W. Effect of Media Composition on Long-Term in Vitro Stability of Barium Alginate and Polyacrylic Acid Multilayer Microcapsules. *Biomaterials* **2000**, *21,* 1911–1917.

Gehrke, S. H. Synthesis and Properties of Hydrogels Used for Drug Delivery. *Drugs Pharm. Sci.* **2000**, *102,* 473–546.

Gombotz, W. R.; Pettit, D. K. Biodegradable Polymers for Protein and Peptide Drug Delivery. *Bioconjugate Chem.* **1995**, *6,* 332–351.

Gombotz, W. R.; Wee, S. Protein Release from Alginate Matrices. *Adv. Drug Delivery Rev.* **1998**, *31,* 267–285.

Gombotz, W. R.; Wee, S. F.; Protein Release from Alginate Matrices. *Adv. Drug Delivery Rev.* **2012**, *64,* 194–205.

Harland, R. S.; Prud'homme, R. K., Eds. *Polyelectrolyte Gels: Properties, Preparation, and Applications;* American Chemical Society: Washington, DC, 1992.

Heng, P. W.; Chan, L. W.; Liew, C. V. Effect of Tabletting Compaction Pressure on Alginate Microspheres. *J. Microencapsulation* **2000**, *17,* 553–564.

Hennink, W. E.; Van Nostrum, C. F. Novel Crosslinking Methods to Design Hydrogels. *Adv. Drug Delivery Rev.* **2002**, *54,* 13.

Hennink, W. E.; Nostrum, C. F. Novel Crosslinking Methods to Design Hydrogels. *Adv. Drug Delivery Rev.* **2012**, *64,* 223–236.

Hooper, S. J.; Percival, S. L.; Hill, K. E.; Thomas, D. W.; Hayes, A. J.; Williams, D. W. The Visualisation and Speed of Kill of Wound Isolates on a Silver Alginate Dressing. *Int. Wound J.* **2012**, *9,* 633–642.

Jeon, O.; Bouhadir, K. H.; Mansour, J. M.; Alsberg, E. Photocrosslinked Alginate Hydrogels with Tunable Biodegradation Rates and Mechanical Properties. *Biomaterials* **2009**, *30,* 2724–2734.

Jeon, O.; Powell, C.; Solorio, L. D.; Krebs, M. D.; Alsberg, E. Affinity-Based Growth Factor Delivery Using Biodegradable, Photo Crosslinked Heparin-Alginate Hydrogels. *J. Controlled Release* **2011**, *154,* 258–266.

Kashyap, N.; Kumar, N.; Kumar, M. N. Hydrogels for Pharmaceutical and Biomedical Applications. *Crit. Rev. Ther. Drug Carrier Syst.* **2005,** *22,* 107–150.

Kolambkar, Y. M.; Dupont, K. M.; et al. An Alginate-Based Hybrid System for Growth Factor Delivery in the Functional Repair of Large Bone Defects. *Biomaterials* **2011,** *32,* 65.

Kong, H. J.; Smith, M. K.; Mooney, D. J. Designing Alginate Hydrogels to Maintain Viability of Immobilized Cells. *Biomaterials* **2003,** *24,* 4023–4029.

Kulkarni, R. V.; Setty, C. M.; Sa, B. Polyacrylamide-g-Alginate-Based Electrically Responsive Hydrogel for Drug Delivery Application: Synthesis, Characterization, and Formulation Development. *J. Appl. Polym. Sci.* **2010,** *115,* 1180–1188.

Kumar, M. N.; Kumar, N. Polymeric Controlled Drug-Delivery Systems: Perspective Issues and Opportunities. *Drug Dev. Ind. Pharm.* **2001,** *27,* 1–30.

Langer, R. S.; Peppas, N. A. Present and Future Applications of Biomaterials in Controlled Drug Delivery Systems. *Biomaterials* **1981,** *2,* 201–214.

Lawrie, G.; Keen, I.; Drew, B.; Rintoul, L.; Fredericks, P.; Grøndahl, L. Interactions Between Alginate and Chitosan Biopolymers Characterized Using FTIR and XPS. *Biomacromolecules* **2007,** *8,* 2533–2541.

Lawson, M. A.; Barralet, J. E.; Wang, L.; Shelton, R. M.; Triffitt, J. T. Adhesion and Growth of Bone Marrow Stromal Cells on Modified Alginate Hydrogels. *Tissue Eng.* **2004,** *10,* 1480–1491.

Lee, K. Y.; Mooney, D. J. Alginate: Properties and Biomedical Applications. *Prog. Polym. Sci.* **2012,** *37,* 106–126.

Lee, J.; Tan, C. Y.; Lee, S. K.; Kim, Y. H.; Lee, K. Y. Controlled Delivery of Heat Shock Protein Using an Injectable Microsphere/Hydrogel Combination System for the Treatment of Myocardial Infarction. *J. Controlled Release* **2009,** *137,* 196–202.

Leonard, M.; De Boisseson, M. R.; Hubert, P.; Dalençon, F.; Dellacherie, E. Hydrophobically Modified Alginate Hydrogels as Protein Carriers with Specific Controlled Release Properties. *J. Controlled Release* **2004,** *98,* 395–405.

Leone, G.; Torricelli, P.; Chiumiento, A.; Facchini, A.; Barbucci, R. Amidic Alginate Hydrogel for Nucleus Pulposus Replacement. *J. Biomed. Mater. Res. A* **2008,** *84,* 391–401.

Lin, H. R.; Yeh, Y. J. Porous Alginate/Hydroxyapatite Composite Scaffolds for Bone Tissue Engineering: Preparation, Characterization, and in Vitro Studies. *J. Biom. Mat. Res. Part B* **2004,** 52–65.

Liu, L. S.; Liu, S. Q.; Ng, S. Y.; Froix, M.; Ohno, T.; Heller, J. Controlled Release of Interleukin-2 for Tumor Immunotherapy Using Alginate/Chitosan Porous Microspheres. *J. Controlled Release* **1997,** *43,* 65–74.

Lópiz-Morales, Y.; Abarrategi, A.; et al. In Vivo Comparison of the Effects of rhBMP-2 and rhBMP-4 in Osteochondral Tissue Regeneration. *Eur. Cells Mater.* **2010,** *20,* 367–378.

Lucinda-Silva, R. M.; Salgado, H. R. N.; Evangelista, R. C. Alginate-Chitosan Systems: in Vitro Controlled Release of Triamcinolone and in Vivo Gastrointestinal Transit. *Carbohydr. Polym.* **2010,** *81,* 260–268.

Maiti, S.; Singha, K.; Ray, S.; Dey, P.; Sa, B. Adipic Acid Dihydrazide Treated Partially Oxidized Alginate Beads for Sustained Oral Delivery of Flurbiprofen. *Pharm. Dev. Technol.* **2009,** *14,* 461–470.

Mammarella, E. J.; Rubiolo, A. C. Cross-Linking Kinetics of Cation Hydrocolloid Gels. *Chem. Eng. J.* **2003,** *94,* 73–77.

Moe, S. T.; Skjåk-Bræk, G.; Smidsrød, O. Covalently Cross-Linked Sodium Alginate Beads. *Food Hydrocolloids* **1991,** *5,* 119–123.

Morris, E. R.; Rees, D. A.; Thom, D. Characterization of Alginate Composition and Block-Structure by Circular Dichroism. *Carbohydr. Res.* **1980**, *81,* 305–314.

Murakami, K.; Aoki, H.; Nakamura, S.; Nakamura, S.; Takikawa, M.; Hanzawa, M.; Kishimoto, S.; Hattori, H. Hydrogel Blends of Chitin/Chitosan, Fucoidan and Alginate as Healing-Impaired Wound Dressings. *Biomaterials* **2010**, *31,* 83–90.

Nokhodchi, A.; Tailor, A. In Situ Cross-Linking of Sodium Alginate with Calcium and Aluminum Ions to Sustain the Release of Theophylline from Polymeric Matrices. *Farmaco* **2004,** *59,* 999–1004.

Ostberg, T.; Lund, E. M.; Graffner, C. Calcium Alginate Matrices for Oral Multiple Unit Administration. IV. Release Characteristics in Different Media. *Int. J. Pharm.* **1994,** *112,* 241–248.

Park, K.; Shalaby, W. S. W.; Park, H., Eds. *Biodegradable Hydrogels for Drug Delivery;* Technomic: Basle, 1993.

Park, D. J.; Choi, B. H.; Zhu, S. J.; Huh, J. Y.; Kim, B. Y.; Lee, S. H. Injectable Bone Using Chitosan Alginate Gel/Mesenchymal Stem Cells/BMP-2 Composites. *J. Craniomaxillofac Surg.* **2005,** *33,* 50–54.

Patil, V.; Pokharkar, V. B. Preparation and Evaluation of Sustained Release Nimesulide Microspheres Prepared from Sodium Alginate. *Indian J. Pharm. Sci.* **2001,** *63,* 15–19.

Patil, N. S.; Li, Y.; Rethwisch, D. G.; Dordick, J. S. Sucrose Diacrylate: A Unique Chemically and Biologically Degradable Crosslinker for Polymeric Hydrogels. *J. Polym. Sci. Part A Polym. Chem.* **1997,** *35,* 2221–2229.

Pawar, S. N.; Edgar, K. J. Alginate Derivatization: A Review of Chemistry, Properties and Applications. *Biomaterials* **2012,** *33,* 3279–3305.

Peppas, N. A., Ed. *Hydrogels in Medicine and Pharmacy;* CRC Press: Boca Raton, FL, 1986; Vol. I, II, III.

Pillay, V.; Fassihi, R. In Vitro Release Modulation from Crosslinked Pellets for Site Specific Drug Delivery to the Gastrointestinal Tract. I. Comparison of pH-Responsive Drug Release and Associated Kinetics. *J. Controlled Release* **1999,** *59,* 229–242.

Queen, D.; Orsted, H.; Sanada, H.; Sussman, G. A. Dressing History. *Int. Wound J.* **2004,** *1,* 59–77.

Rabbany, S. Y.; Pastore, J.; et al. Continuous Delivery of Stromal Cell-Derived Factor-1 from Alginate Scaffolds Accelerates Wound Healing. *Cell Transplant.* **2010,** *19,* 399–408.

Ratner, B. D.; Hoffman, A. S. Synthetic Hydrogels for Biomedical Applications. In *Hydrogels for Medical and Related Applications;* ACS Symposium Series; American Chemical Society: Washington, DC, 1976; Vol. 31, 1–36.

Riyajan, S. A.; Sakdapipanich, J. Development of a Controlled Release Neem Capsule with a Sodium Alginate Matrix, Crosslinked by Glutaraldehyde and Coated with Natural Rubber. *Polym. Bull.* **2009,** *63,* 609–622.

Rosiak, J. M.; Yoshii, F. Hydrogels and their Medical Applications. *Nucl. Instrum. Methods Phys. Res. Sec. B* **1999,** *151,* 56–64.

Sarmento, B.; Ferreira, D.; Veiga, F.; Ribeiro, A. Characterization of Insulin-Loaded Alginate Nanoparticles Produced by Ionotropic Pre-Gelation through DSC and FTIR Studies. *Carbohydr. Polym.* **2006,** *66,* 1–7.

Segal, H. C.; Hunt, B. J.; Gilding, K. The Effects of Alginate and Non-Alginate Wound Dressings on Blood Coagulation and Platelet Activation. *J. Biomater. Appl.* **1991,** *12,* 249–257.

Segi, N.; Yotsuyanagi, T.; Ikeda, K. Interaction of Calcium-Alginate Gel Beads with Propranolol. *Chem. Pharm. Bull.* **1989,** *37,* 3092–3095.

Silva, C. M.; Ribeiro, A. J.; Ferreira, D.; Veiga, F. Insulin Encapsulation in Reinforced Alginate Microspheres Prepared by Internal Gelation. *Eur. J. Pharm. Sci.* **2006,** *29,* 148–159.

Sinquin, A.; Hubert, P.; Dellacherie, E. Amphiphilic Derivatives of Alginate: Evidence for Intra- and Intermolecular Hydrophobic Associations in Aqueous Solution. *Langmuir* **1993,** *9,* 3334–3337.

Sivakumar, M.; Rao, K. P. Preparation, Characterization, and in Vitro Release of Gentamicin from Coralline Hydroxyapatite-Alginate Composite Microspheres. *J. Biomed. Mater. Res.* **2003,** *65,* 222–228.

Slaughter, B. V.; Khurshid, S. S. O.; Fisher, Z.; Peppas, N. A. Hydrogels in Regenerative Medicine. *Adv. Mater.* **2009,** *21,* 3307–3329.

Smidsrød, O.; Glover, R. M.; Whittington, S. G. Relative Extension of Alginates Having Different Chemical Composition. *Carbohydr. Res.* **1973,** *1,* 107–118.

Ştefania, R.; Silvia, V.; Marcel, P.; Cornelia, L. Polysaccharides Based on Micro- and Nanoparticles Obtained by Ionic Gelation and their Applications as Drug Delivery Systems. *Rev. Roum. Chim.* **2009,** *54,* 709–718.

Sutherland, L. W. Alginates. In *Biomaterials: Novel Materials from Biological Sources;* Byron, D., Ed.; Palgrave Macmillan UK, 1991.

Takka, S.; Ocak, O. H.; Acarturk, F. Formulation and Investigation of Nicardipine HCl-Alginate Gel Beads with Factorial Design Based Studies. *Eur. J. Pharm. Sci.* **1998,** *6,* 241–246.

Tamada, J.; Langer, R. The Development of Polyanhydrides for Drug Delivery Applications. J. Biomater. Sci. Polym. Ed. **1992,** *3,* 315–353.

Tanaka, H.; Matsumara, M.; Veliky, I. A. Diffusion Characteristics of Substrates in Ca-Alginate Gel Beads. *Biotechnol. Bioeng.* **1984,** *26,* 53–58.

Thom, D.; Grant, G. T.; Morris, E. R.; Rees, D. A. Characterization of Cation Binding and Gelation of Polyuronates by Circular Dichroism. *Carbohydr. Res.* **1982,** *100,* 29–42.

Thu, B.; Bruheim, P.; Espevik, T.; Smidsrød, O.; Shiong, P. S.; Skjåk-Bræk, G. Alginate Polycation Microcapsules. II. Some Functional Properties. *Biomaterials* **1996,** *17,* 1069–1079.

Tonnesen, H. H.; Karlsen, J. Alginate in Drug Delivery Systems. *Durg Dev. Ind. Pharm.* **2002,** *28,* 621–630.

Tsuchida, E.; Abe, K. Interactions Between Macromolecules in Solution and Inter Macromolecular Complexes. *Adv. Polym. Sci.* **1982,** *45,* 1–119.

Ulbrich, K.; Subr, V.; Podperová, P.; Buresová, M. Synthesis of Novel Hydrolytically Degradable Hydrogels for Controlled Drug Release. *J. Controlled Release* **1995,** *34,* 155–165.

Wang, X.; Wenk, E.; Hu, X.; Castro, G. R.; Meinel, L.; Wang, X.; Li, C.; Merkle, H.; Kaplan, D. L. Silk Coatings on PLGA and Alginate Microspheres for Protein Delivery. *Biomaterials* **2007,** *28,* 4161–4169.

Wang, F. Q.; Li, P.; Zhang, J. P.; Wang, A. Q.; Wei, Q. A Novel pH-Sensitive Magnetic Alginate Chitosan Beads for Albendazole Delivery. *Drug Dev. Ind. Pharm.* **2010,** *36,* 867–877.

Weir, M. D.; Xu, H. H.; Simon, C. G. Strong Calcium Phosphate Cement–Chitosan–Mesh Construct Containing Cell-Encapsulating Hydrogel Beads for Bone Tissue Engineering. *J. Biomed. Mater. Res. Part A* **2006,** *77,* 487–496.

Wells, L. A.; Sheardown, H. Extended Release of High pI Proteins from Alginate Microspheres via a Novel Encapsulation Technique. *Eur. J. Pharm. Biopharm.* **2007,** *65,* 329–335.

Weng, Y.; Wang, M.; Liu, W.; Hu, X.; Chai, G.; Yan, Q.; et al. Repair of Experimental Alveolar Bone Defects by Tissue-Engineered Bone. *Tissue Eng.* **2006,** *12,* 1503–1513.

Wichterle, O.; Lim, D. Hydrophilic Gels for Biological Use. *Nature* **1960,** *185,* 117–118.

Woerly, S. Porous Hydrogels for Neural Tissue Engineering. *Porous Mater. Tissue Eng.* **1997,** *250,* 53–68.

Yang, S.; Liu, G.; Cheng, Y.; Zheng, Y. Electroresponsive Behavior of Sodium Alginate-g-Poly(Acrylic Acid) Hydrogel Under DC Electric Field. *J. Macromol. Sci. Part A* **2009,** *46,* 1078–1082.

Yang, J. S.; Xie, Y. J.; He, W. Research Progress on Chemical Modification of Alginate: A Review. *Carbohydr. Polym.* **2011,** *84,* 33–39.

Yao, B.; Ni, C.; Xiong, C.; Zhu, C.; Huang, B. Hydrophobic Modification of Sodium Alginate and its Application in Drug Controlled Release. *Bioprocess Biosyst. Eng.* **2010,** 33, 457–463.

Yuan, L.; Ren, L.; Tian, X.; Huang, Z.; Xiao, Y.H.; Wei, S.; Wang, Z. Investigation on Polyvinyl-Alcohol-Based Rapidly Gelling Hydrogels for Containment of Hazardous Chemicals. ***RSC Adv.*** **2016,** 6, 71425–71430.

Yun, L.; Chuanjie, Z.; Jinchao, Z.; Yi, G.; Li, C.; Ping, Z. Preparation and Properties of Gelatin/Sodium Alginate (Cross-Linked with Genipin) Interpenetrating Polymeric Network Films. *Acta Mater. Compositae Sin.* **2015,** *32,* 997–1006.

Zhang, X. L.; Hui, Z. Y.; Wan, D. X.; Huang, H. T.; Huang, J.; Yuan, H.; Yu, J. H. Alginate Microsphere Filled with Carbon Nanotube as Drug Carrier. *Int. J. Biol. Macromol.* **2010,** *47,* 389–395.

Zhao, Y.; Li, F.; Carvajal, M. T.; Harris, M. T. Interactions Between Bovine Serum Albumin and Alginate: An Evaluation of Alginate as Protein Carrier. *J. Colloid Interface. Sci.* **2009,** 2, 345–353.

Zhao, X.; Huebsch, N.; Mooney, D. J.; Suo, Z. Stress-Relaxation Behaviour in Gels with Ionic and Covalent Crosslinks. *J. Appl. Phy.* **2010,** *107,* 1–5.

Zimmermann, H.; Hillgartner, M.; Manz, B.; et al. Fabrication of Homogeneously Cross-Linked, Functional Alginate Microcapsules Validated by NMR-, CLSM- and AFM-Imaging. *Biomaterials* **2003,** *24,* 2083–2096.

CHAPTER 5

CHEMICALLY MODIFIED ALGINATES FOR ADVANCED BIOMEDICAL APPLICATIONS

IBRAHIM M. EL-SHERBINY*, MOSTAFA M. ABD AL AZIZ, and ESRAA A. ABDELSALAM

Center for Materials Science, University of Science and Technology (UST), Zewail City of Science and Technology, 6th of October, Giza, Egypt

Corresponding author. E-mail: ielsherbiny@zewailcity.edu.eg

5.1 INTRODUCTION

Alginate, a naturally occurring polysaccharide of the chemical formula $(C_6H_8O_6)_n$, was discovered in the 1880s from British kelp (Panikkar and Brasch, 1996). It is a linear polysaccharide composed of two building units of uronic acids; β-D-mannuronic acid (M) and its C_5 epimer, α-L-guluronic acid (G) linked via (1→4) glycoside bonds. These units are randomly distributed throughout the alginate chain either in MM, GG, or MG manner. Thus, alginate chain contains either homoblocks of GG or MM, or heteroblocks of GM (Figure 5.1). To define the structure of the alginate polymer, important parameters of F_G and N_G are used, where F_G represents the fraction of guluronic acid in the whole polymer, whereas N_G refers to the average number of units of guluronic acid in G-blocks. The ratio G/M could be calculated by ^{1}H NMR.

Alginate is usually extracted from microorganisms whose cell organelles, typically the cell wall, contain an amount of it naturally. Since alginate was discovered by the end of the 19th century, brown algae were the main source of its production. By the 1960s, the production of alginate from bacteria was introduced; however, still, the main source of alginate production is the brown algae such as *Laminaria hyperborea*, *Moroccan Laminaria digitata*,

Sargassum muticum, and *Ascophyllum nodosum*. On the other hand, there are only two genera of bacteria used for alginate production, *Pseudomonas* and *Azotobacter* (McHugh, 1987; Hay et al., 2013). Of note, the G and M monomer sequence in the extracted alginate differs according to the species of algae, its age, the tissues of extraction of the same species, and the time of the year that it is harvested in (Donati et al., 2003). For instance, alginate extracted from the *Laminaria* leaf hyperborean demonstrated lower G content and shorter G-blocks than in that extracted from the stem of the same algal species (Reham, 2009). In addition to the effect of the extraction source, the extraction process can also significantly affect the physicochemical characteristics of the obtained alginate through its effect on the G/M ratio (Hay et al., 2013).

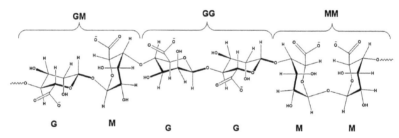

FIGURE 5.1   β-D-mannuronic acid (M) and its C_5 epimer, α-L-guluronic acid (G) monomers distribution throughout alginate chain.

5.2   PHYSICOCHEMICAL PROPERTIES OF ALGINATE

5.2.1   SOLUBILITY

The solubility of alginate in a solvent is determined by the status of its carboxylic group while being in the solvent, the pH as well as the ionic strength. For instance, if the carboxylic group is protonated, the polymer will not be fully soluble in any solvent. Therefore, alginate is water insoluble, but swells in water under normal conditions (McHugh, 1987).

5.2.2   VISCOSITY

Alginate has a thickening effect, which means that a relatively low concentration of it has the ability to increase the overall viscosity of an aqueous solution. On average concentration, alginate solutions have a pseudoplastic behavior where the flow of solutions is more readily as it is pumped or stirred. Of note, the alginate viscosity is affected by its molecular weight, concentration, temperature, pH, and the concentration of calcium ions (McHugh, 1987).

5.2.3 STABILITY

The degree of polymerization (DP) directly affects both the viscosity and stability of a polymer. Therefore, the extent of depolymerization is measured by the loss of viscosity of the polymer upon storage. Alginate of low DP has shown better stability than that of high DP. In addition, the viscosity of alginate is a measure of its stability where the one of low viscosity demonstrates better stability over time than that of high viscosity (McHugh, 1987). Thus, commercial alginates should be stored in the relatively cold condition in order to keep its optimum viscosity (Lee and Mooney, 2012).

5.2.4 DEGRADATION

Alginates are susceptible for three types of degradation—hydrolytic cleavage, enzymatic degradation, and by reducing compounds.

Hydrolytic cleavage: Like all polysaccharides, alginate undergoes hydrolytic cleavage in acidic conditions so commercial alginates should be stored in dry conditions (McHugh, 1987). The mechanism of alginate hydrolysis is illustrated in Figure 5.2.

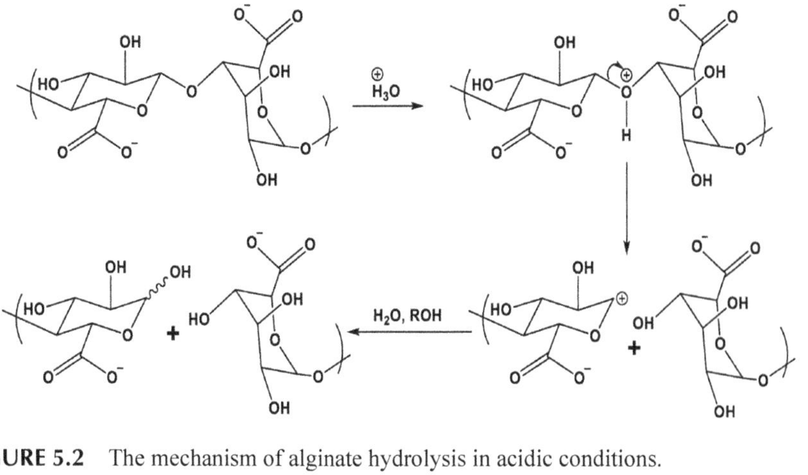

FIGURE 5.2   The mechanism of alginate hydrolysis in acidic conditions.

Enzymatic degradation: It involves a β-elimination reaction by lyase process in strongly alkaline media resulting in unsaturated compounds, followed by the degradation routes shown in Figure 5.3.

Degradation by reducing agent: Not only in basic and acidic pHs but also at neutral media, the alginate is susceptible to degradation but in the presence of a reducing agent such as sodium sulfite, sodium hydrogen sulfide, hydroquinone, ascorbic acid, cysteine, leucomethylene blue, and hydrazine sulfate. In this process, peroxide is formed creating a free radical that causes chain breakdown eventually.

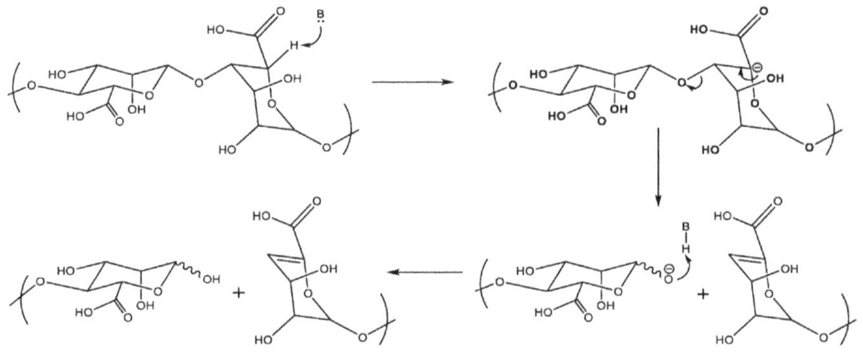

FIGURE 5.3   Alkaline degradation of alginates via β-elimination.

5.3   CHEMICAL MODIFICATION OF ALGINATE

Alginates exhibit fascinating characteristics that make it good candidates for different research areas. In addition, chemical modification of alginates through incorporation of new functions groups further enhances its characteristics and leads to the development of new alginate derivatives of desirable physicochemical and biological properties. It is worth to mention that alginates could be chemically modified at either their hydroxyl groups located at C-2 and C-3, or at the carboxyl group located at C-6. The chemical modification could be done selectively on one of these groups due to the difference in their reactivity (Pawar and Edgar, 2011). Most of the modifications, reported in the literature, aimed at increasing the hydrophobicity of alginates via conjugating hydrophobic moieties to its backbone (Lee and Mooney, 2012). Some other studies reported the modification of alginate in such a way that makes alginates more appropriate for the intended application. For instance, when alginates are desired to be cell interactive, this requires the conjugation of cell-adhesive moiety such as RGD peptide to alginate backbone (Koo et al., 2002). There are three significant factors that should be taken into consideration when selecting the modification approach (as summarized in Figure 5.4):

a) ***Inherent properties:*** As a natural material, alginates' properties vary significantly according to the source from which they were extracted. These changes include, for instance, the ratio of M/G residues and their arrangement along the chain. Thus, it is important to characterize the alginate batches after extraction using advanced techniques.

b) ***Structural reactivity:*** There is a difference in the reactivity between hydroxyl and carboxyl groups of alginates. This difference was not observed between the two types of hydroxyl groups at the alginate backbone, which makes it difficult to modify one of them alone. In addition, there is a difference in the reactivity of the alginate residues, M and G. This difference may control the selective modification of certain residue without the other.

c) ***Type and degree of solubility:*** As the alginate structure implies, it is highly hydrophilic and thus it dissolves readily in water. In addition, it could be also soluble in a mixture of aqueous–organic media. However, the degree of solubility differs according to the nature of the mixture and the used ratio. This range of solubility controls the type of reagents that could be used in modification (Pawar and Edgar, 2012). The following section summarizes the main chemical modifications carried on hydroxyl and carboxyl groups of alginate such as oxidation, amidation, sulfation, and grafting.

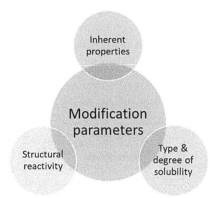

FIGURE 5.4   General parameters that should be considered while performing alginates chemical modification.

5.3.1 CHEMICAL MODIFICATIONS OF THE ALGINATE'S HYDROXYL GROUPS

5.3.1.1 COPOLYMERIZATION

Alginate copolymers have been widely used recently in many applications either through the addition of another polymer (Yang et al., 2016; Zhu and Xin, 2002) or propagation of monomers, such as sodium acrylate, acrylamide, and vinylsulfonic acid onto the alginate hydroxyl groups (Sen et al., 2010; Sand et al., 2010). Figure 5.5 illustrates, for instance, the reaction of alginate copolymerization with sodium acrylate.

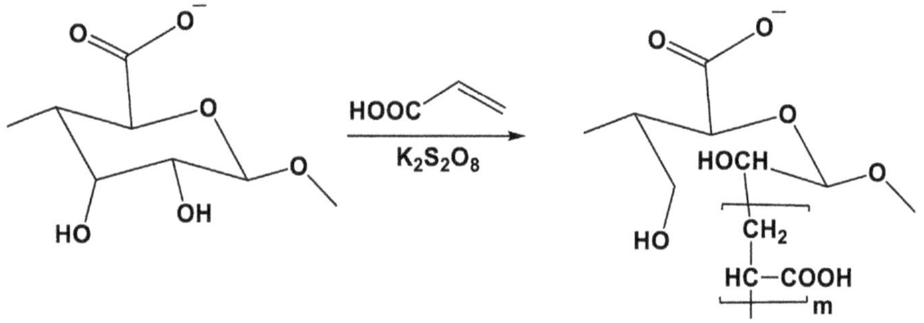

FIGURE 5.5   Copolymerization of sodium acrylate with alginate.

5.3.1.2 SULFATION

Sulfated alginate has been widely used as an anticoagulant for more than 60 years due to the structural resemblance between sulfated alginate and heparin, which provides high blood comparability (Alban et al., 2002; Ronghua et al., 2003). The sulfation reaction of alginate is carried out in the presence of sodium chlorosulfate ($ClSO_3H$) in formamide as shown in Figure 5.6.

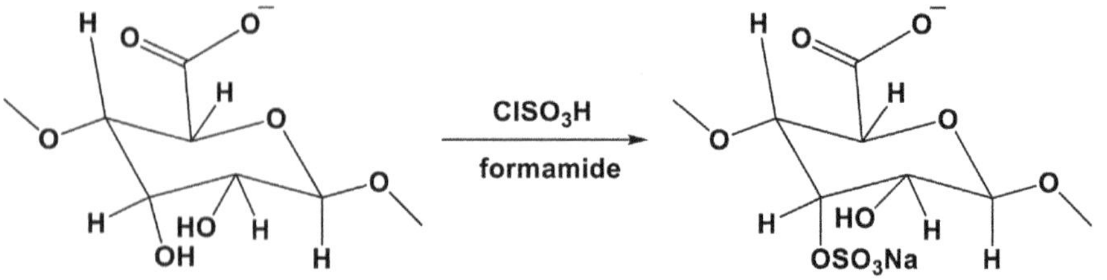

FIGURE 5.6   Sulfation process of sodium alginate using sodium chlorosulfate in formamide.

5.3.1.3   OXIDATION

Oxidized alginate derivatives have more reactive groups and enhanced dero-
gation properties than native alginate. Therefore, the preparation of oxidized
forms of alginate has received much attention in the recent years as it has a
higher potential to be used in various applications, such as drug delivery as
compared to native alginate. The oxidation of alginate has been performed in
the presence of sodium periodate that oxidizes the hydroxyl groups on both
C-3 and C-4 positions in the uronic units as shown in Figure 5.7 (Gomez
et al., 2007). These reactions are carried out in the absence of light in order
to avoid the occurrence of any side reactions. As shown in the figure, the
oxidation reaction leads to the formation of 2,3-dialdehydic alginate via
carbon bond breakage and ring opening. As a result, the oxidized alginate
has a higher degree of rotational freedom along with more active functional
groups (Yang et al., 2011). It was also observed that oxidized alginate has a
lower stiffness and higher biodegradability (Shu-Lan et al., 2005).

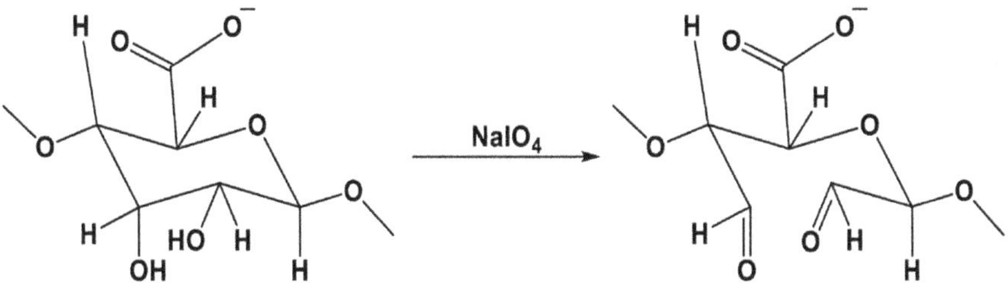

FIGURE 5.7   Oxidation reaction of sodium alginate with the aid of sodium periodate.

5.3.1.4   REDUCTIVE AMINATION OF OXIDIZED ALGINATE

As mentioned above, oxidized alginate has higher reactivity than alginate,
which enables further chemical modifications such as reductive amination.
The reaction is performed by the introduction of alkylamine in the presence
of sodium cyanoborohydride (NaCNBH$_3$) that reduces the imine group in
the pH range of 6–7, as illustrated in Figure 5.8 (Kang et al., 2002; Carré
et al. 1991). The resulting alginamine has amphiphilic characteristics that
increase its potential to be used in many applications, especially biomedical
applications. For instance, amphiphilic alginamine beads were used as a
carrier system for controlled release and delivery of ibuprofen (Zhiyong
et al., 2009). Of note also, the modified alginates, rich in amine groups, could

be used for further modifications such as polymer grafting. For instance, alginate–polyethylene glycol (PEG)-grafted copolymer was synthesized through the addition of monocarboxyl-terminated PEG to alginate, as shown in Figure 5.9. This grafting process provided mixed properties of both alginate and PEG (Laurienzo et al., 2005).

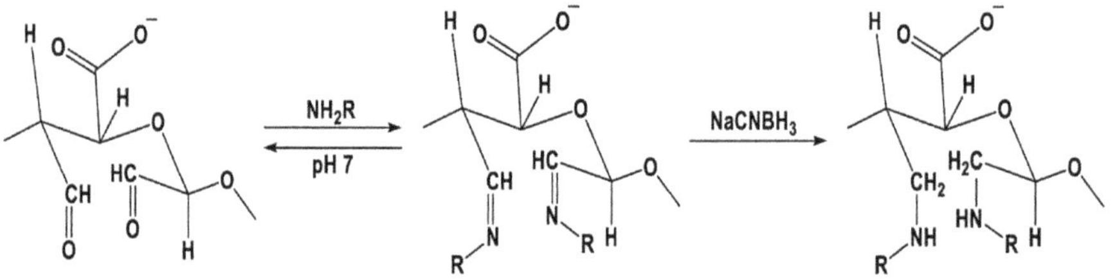

FIGURE 5.8   Reductive amination of oxidized alginate.

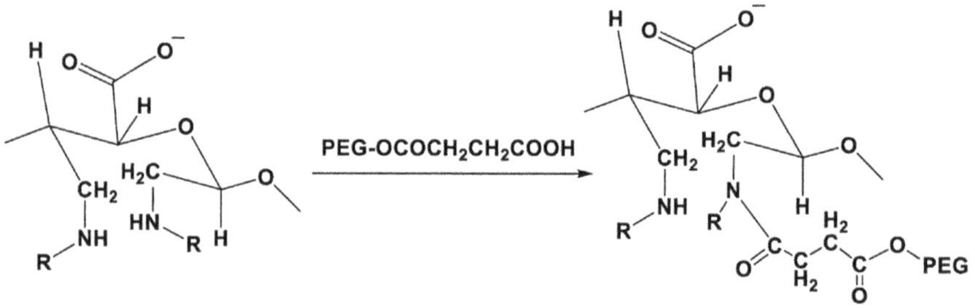

FIGURE 5.9   Preparation of alginate-grafted–PEG copolymer.

5.3.2   CHEMICAL MODIFICATIONS OF THE ALGINATE'S CARBOXYL GROUPS

5.3.2.1   ESTERIFICATION

This type of modification is used particularly to increase the hydrophobicity of alginate through conjugating hydrophobic moieties through ester linkage. The esterification process of alginate is reported to be performed by two major approaches. The first approach involves a direct esterification reaction between an alcohol and the alginate carboxyl group (Yang et al., 2011). The reaction is performed in the presence of a catalyst and an excess of alcohol to guarantee that equilibrium is oriented to product formation (as shown in Figure 5.10). The preparation of many alginate esters has been reported in the literature; however, only one, the propylene glycol ester, has a commercial value to date. It is used mainly as an emulsifier, stabilizer, and as a food additive (Carré et al., 1991).

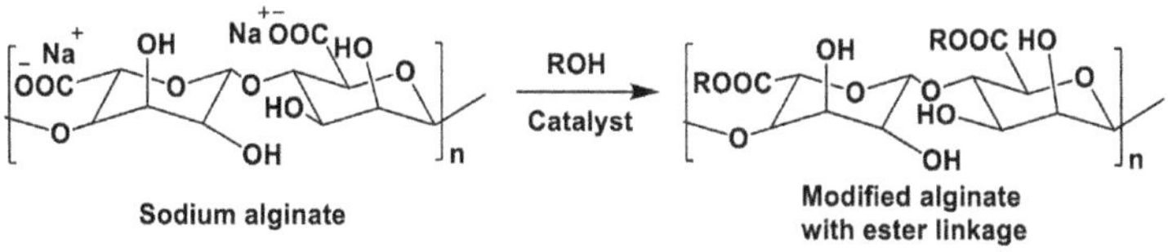

FIGURE 5.10 Direct esterification reaction of sodium alginate in the presence of excess alcohol and catalyst.

Another approach of preparation of alginate esters is through the reaction with alkyl halides (Rastello De Boisseson et al., 2004; Pelletier et al., 2001). The procedure uses alginate in its acidic form, and then a common base, mostly tetrabutylammonium hydroxide (TBA-OH), is added to facilitate the conjugation of alkyl halides. Thereafter, alkyl halide is added to the mixture under stirring for the appropriate time, which leads to conjugation of alkyl moiety to the alginate via ester linkage as illustrated in Figure 5.11.

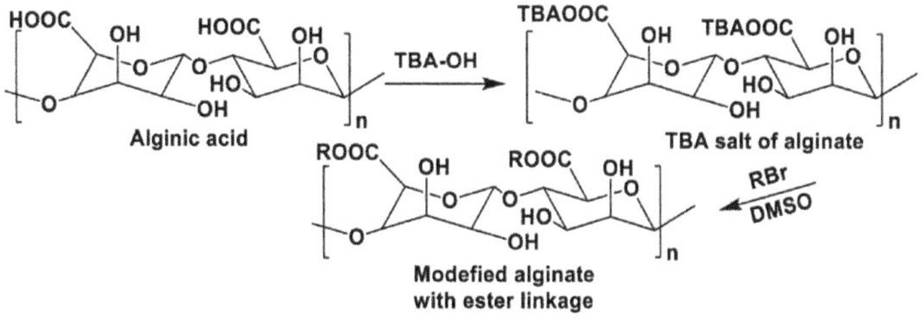

FIGURE 5.11 Esterification process of alginate using alkyl halides.

5.3.2.2   AMIDATION

Typically, amide bonds are formed between a primary or secondary amine, and carboxylate-containing molecules such as alginate. This reaction is performed with the aid of the common water-soluble coupling agent, 1-ethyl-3-(3-dimethylaminopropyl) carbodiimide hydrochloride (EDC-HCl). The reaction begins with the conjugation of EDC-HCl on the alginate carboxyl group. Thereafter, the primary or secondary amine is added to the mixture in order to replace the EDC-HCl, and forming the amide linkage (as shown in Figure 5.12). In order to increase the efficiency of the reaction, N-hydroxysulfosuccinimide (NHS) was reported to be used as a stabilizing agent for EDC intermediates (d'Ayala et al., 2008).

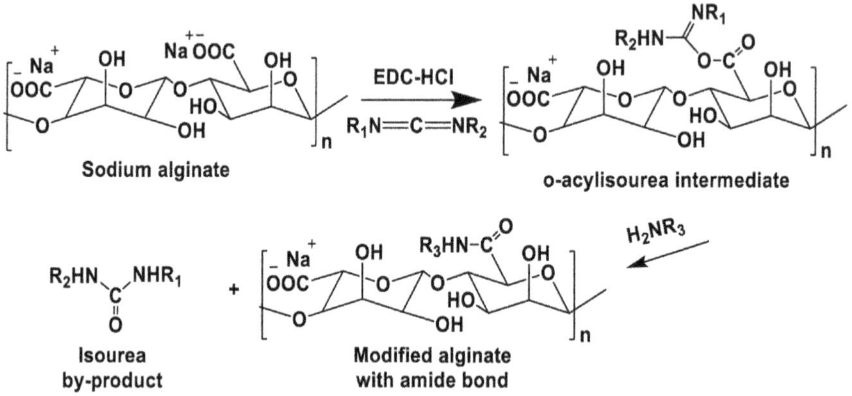

FIGURE 5.12   Amidation of alginate using EDC-HCl.

5.3.2.3   UGI REACTION

Ugi reaction is a common multicomponent organic reaction that is named after the German chemist who reported it, Ivar Karl Ugi. The reaction uses a variety of components: a carboxylic acid, an amine, an isocyanide, and an aldehyde or ketone. All the components are added together with the definite procedure in certain conditions to give a bis-amide (Ugi, 1962). This reaction is used as an approach to increase the hydrophobicity of alginate. Utilizing the presence of carboxyl groups in alginate, the Ugi reaction is performed by gradually adding the rest of components, such as formaldehyde, n-octylamine, and cyclohexyl isocyanide to form a bis-amide alginate that is hydrophobically modified (Bu et al., 2004) (as shown in Figure 5.13).

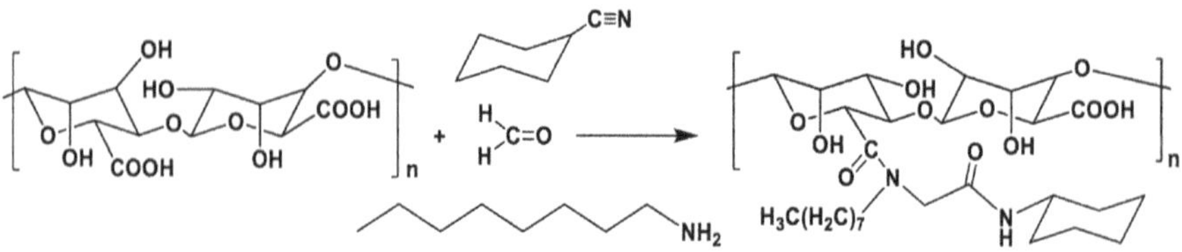

FIGURE 5.13   Modification of alginate using Ugi reaction.

5.4 BIOMEDICAL APPLICATIONS OF ALGINATES AND ITS CHEMICALLY MODIFIED FORMS

5.4.1 WOUND DRESSING

For centuries, open wounds were treated by dressing. The most common type of dressing is gauze due to its low cost and good absorption capability; however, it may cause a second wound while healing (Lee and Mooney, 2012). Thus, new types of dressing have appeared recently such as gels and polymeric sponges. Alginate is a potential candidate, as a highly efficient wound dressing material because of its desirable properties such as tissue compatibility, biodegradability, nontoxicity, and mechanical properties (Sun and Tan, 2013). All these characteristics make it a good resemblant to glycosaminoglycan, an important polysaccharide in the extracellular matrix in human tissues. In addition, alginate is known by its ability to promote epithelialization, the growth of epithelium as a step of wound healing process. In addition, it encourages granulation of tissues through the maintenance of the physiological moist environment for dry wounds (Lee and Mooney, 2012). Moreover, alginate shows a good water absorptivity, optimal water vapor transmission rate, and conformability. On the other hand, it has antiseptic properties (Venkatesan et al., 2015). Therefore, alginate and its chemically modified forms have been commonly used in wound dressing applications either by their own or in a combination with other polymers, such as collagen and chitosan (Kim et al., 2011), or with metals such as silver and zinc (Lee and Mooney, 2012). In many cases, alginate has been chemically modified in order to fit a desired property for wound dressing applications. For instance, oxidized alginate and alginate dialdehyde have been cross-linked with gelatin in the presence of borax forming a hydrogel that showed about 10% enhancement of wound re-epithelialization after 15 days as compared with the control. The modified alginate-based hydrogel dressing demonstrated a high overall healing efficiency along with a quite low water loss noted in the wound. Also, the presence of borax has decreased the probability of microbial growth in the wound (Balakrishnan et al., 2005). This work has been developed further via the addition of cyclic adenosine monophosphate that works as a regulator of proliferation process (Balakrishnan et al., 2006).

5.4.2   TISSUE ENGINEERING

The idea of tissue engineering depends on growing cells on a suitable scaffold in the presence of some protein and growth factor constructing a complete artificial tissue or organ that morphologically and functionally mimics the natural one as a solution to some medical problems, such as tissue loss and organ failure. The features of the used scaffold determine the structure and properties of the final tissue (Sun and Tan, 2013). An ideal scaffold should have some properties such as biocompatibility, controlled biodegradability, porosity, interconnecting pores with appropriate pore size to help in the biointegration and vascularization, three-dimensional, appropriate mechanical properties that mimic the natural ones, as well as appropriate surface chemistry that promotes cell adhesion and proliferation (Martins et al., 2015). Fortunately, alginate fits many of these properties and it was approved as a biopolymer for biomedical applications by the Food and Drug Administration organization; thus, it is widely used in tissue engineering applications.

Degradation of alginate is influenced by the molecular weight of the polymer. Typically, alginate with high molecular weight has a lower degradation rate. The molecular weight can affect not only the degradability but also the stability and the mechanical properties of alginate (Sun and Tan, 2013). Basically, the mechanical properties are also inherently affected by the change in degradation. Of note, the degradation rate of alginate could be controlled by applying chemical modification to it. In general, the degradation rate of alginate is quite slow; thus, Bouhadir et al. hypothesized that the partial oxidation of alginate by periodate may enhance its degradation rates (Bouhadir et al., 2001). The oxidation process, as explained in the modification section, cleaves the carbon–carbon bond of the cis-diol group of the urinate unit that alters the chair conformation of the urinate units into open chains, which provides a free rotation on the glycosidic linkage providing a behavior like acetal group susceptible to hydrolysis. Reported experiments showed that partially oxidized alginate degrades with pH- and temperature-dependent rates. Over the last decade, alginate gels have been used widely in many fields of tissue engineering applications. In order to enhance the properties of the final scaffold, many works tended to chemically modify alginate. In the following section, applications of chemically modified alginate in tissue engineering, such as blood vessels, cartilage, bone, and dental applications are highlighted.

5.4.2.1   SMOOTH MUSCLES AND BLOOD VESSELS

It is quite challenging to recreate an aligned multilayer smooth muscle tissue as the natural ones. Rayatpisheh et al have used the layer-by-layer technique of microchannels to design a homogeneously aligned smooth muscle tissue with an interlayer separation of a mixture of alginate and oxidized alginate hydrogel coated with collagen (Rayatpisheh et al., 2011). That interlayer provided a thicker, three-dimensional tissue in a short time. In a different study, Ruvinov et al. (2011) have used alginate–sulfate gel to encapsulate insulin-like growth factor-1 and hepatocyte growth factor. The study showed the formation of an enhanced mature blood vessel at the infarct site.

5.4.2.2   BONE

Nguyen et al. proposed a composite system based on oxidized alginate, gelatin, and biphasic calcium phosphate for bone regeneration. Within the developed composite, an interaction was attained between the NH_2 groups of gelatin and the CHO groups of oxidized alginate. The scaffold composite system showed enhanced biocompatibility and biodegradability. It was also designed in such a way to have a porous structure along with desirable mechanical properties (Nguyen and Lee, 2012). In some studies, some peptides such as RGD have been bind covalently to alginate-based scaffolds in order to enhance the cell adhesion and homogenous spreading onto the scaffold. For instance, Alsberg et al. have used RGD–alginate to encapsulate pre-osteoblast cells (Alsberg et al., 2001).

5.4.2.3   CARTILAGE

Ghahramanpoor et al. have applied the esterification reaction of octadecyl chains to alginate in order to enhance the alginate overall mechanical and swelling properties in the physiological conditions as well as to render the polymer into more hydrophobic. In addition, the developed hydrogel was reinforced through the addition of calcium chloride, and then used to encapsulate mesenchymal stem cells for cartilage regeneration (Ghahramanpoor et al., 2011). In a different study, Bouhadir et al. have used oxidized alginate hydrogel to encapsulate chondrocytes and introduced it into the dorsal region of mice. After 7 weeks, a white opalescence was observed upon dissection. The investigated oxidized alginate-based hydrogel showed higher degradation rate as compared to native alginate (Bouhadir et al., 2001).

5.4.2.4   DENTAL APPLICATIONS

Moshaverinia et al. have developed an injectable scaffold of oxidized alginate beads to encapsulate periodontal ligament stem cells (PDLSCs) and gingival mesenchymal stem cells (GMSCs). The obtained degradation and swelling properties of the developed oxidized alginate-based injectable scaffold at physiological conditions made it good candidate scaffold of PDLSCs and GMSCs. It showed the capability of directing the differentiation of the stem cells into osteogenic and adipogenic tissues (Moshaverinia et al., 2012).

5.4.3   DRUG DELIVERY

Modified alginates exhibit many prominent properties such as biocompatibility, low toxicity, and gel-forming ability, which are essential for drug delivery applications. This explains why the use of modified alginates in various drug delivery applications is immense (Sun and Tan, 2013). In addition, modified alginates can be prepared in different forms to fit many drug delivery systems. These forms include, for instance, but not limited to, gels, fibers, matrices, nano- and micro-spheres, and membranes of different thicknesses (Jain and Bar-Shalom, 2014). Actually, modified alginates not only can deliver bioactive and pharmaceutical molecules, but they are also capable of delivering bio-cargo such as proteins, cells, and DNA. The type of modification performed on alginates is related to the nature of the cargo need to be delivered. The following section focuses on the applications of some modified alginates in delivering pharmaceutical drugs and biomolecules, particularly proteins.

5.4.3.1   PHARMACEUTICAL DRUGS

Alginates and their derivatives can enhance the pharmacokinetic profile of pharmaceutical drugs. In particular, alginate and its derivatives have the ability to control and sustain the release of encapsulated drugs because of their gelling nature. Besides, they increase the drug concentration in the site of infection, while decreasing its side effects. Moreover, they can encapsulate a variety of drugs (e.g., hydrophobic and hydrophilic ones) according to the type of modification performed. Since the last decade, a lot of research was carried out using alginate and its derivatives in drug delivery applications. For instance, Maiti et al. have prepared beads of partially oxidized sodium alginate for flurbiprofen delivery, a nonsteroidal anti-inflammatory drug. However, the release was so quick that all the drug content was consumed within 90 min. This was attributed to the high rate of diffusion of flurbiprofen molecules from the alginate matrix. To overcome this drawback, the researchers added calcium ions, as ionic cross-linker and adipicdihydrazide as covalent cross-linker. The results showed that the drug release was extended to approximately 8 h depending on the cross-linker ratio. The use of cross-linkers slowed down the swelling behavior of the beads, and thus a decrease in the diffusion rate of the drug (Maiti et al., 2009).

Choudhary et al. managed to chemically modify alginates by conjugating lipophilic moiety (C_8) through amidation reaction (Choudhary et al., 2009). The hydrophobically modified alginate was aimed to deliver the lipophilic drug, sulindac, a nonsteroidal anti-inflammatory drug. In addition, the effect of hydrophobic modification on the drug release profile was studied. The drug release was prolonged in the case of modified alginates compared with pure alginate. Moreover, burst release was not observed in the case of modified alginates unlike the case of alginate. Thus, the hydrophobic modification was confirmed to enhance the release profile of the loaded sulindac drug. In another study, Colinet et al. (2009) managed to prepare amphiphilic alginates by conjugating polycaprolacton (PCL) grafts on the side chains of alginates. This grafting was achieved through esterification reaction with the aid of EDC chemistry. The newly modified amphiphilic alginate was used to deliver a poorly soluble and hydrophobic drug, theophylline. The study focused on the effect of PCL conjugation on the release pattern of theophylline. Release studies showed that PCL conjugation prolonged the release of theophylline to 2 h instead of 1 h in the case of nonconjugated alginates. Colinet et al. suggested that this sustained release is attributed to the emergence of hydrophobic interactions between PCL strands and theophylline which in turn slowed down the swelling behavior of the beads.

5.4.3.2   BIOMOLECULES DELIVERY

Modified alginate matrices can also deliver bioactive molecules, particularly proteins. Basically, proteins are susceptible to denaturation because of the hostile biological environment such as low pH media in the stomach. Thus, alginate matrices are proposed to protect proteins from degradation with the maintenance of their structure and function (Chan and Neufeld, 2010). However, proteins diffuse rapidly from alginates matrices because of their hydrophilicity and the inherent porosity. Thus, certain strategies were used to control the protein release (Lee and Mooney, 2012). One of the significant strategies depends on the chemical modification of alginates via coupling hydrophobic moieties in such a way that increases the loading efficiency and enhances the release profile. In addition, different covalent and ionic cross-linkers were used for further controlling of the protein release. For instance, Yao et al. proposed a new chemical modification on sodium alginate with the aim to increase the loading efficiency and control the release profile through the conjugation to a hydrophobic moiety to control the swelling behavior (Yao et al., 2010). The hydrophobic modification was performed by coupling polybutyl methacrylate onto the sodium alginate backbone through amidation linkage with the aid of EDC chemistry. This new system was used in the delivery of bovine serum albumin (BSA) as a model protein. After chemical modification, the proposed system was incorporated in calcium chloride solution in order to form microspheres. Thereafter, a comparative release study of BSA was conducted between natural sodium alginate and modified alginate microspheres. The results showed prominent enhance-ment in release profile of BSA from the modified alginates microspheres compared to alginate microspheres.

Eldin et al. have prepared L-arginine grafted alginate (Arg-g-Alg) using p-benzoquinone as the activating agent. Thereafter, Arg-g-Alg hydrogels were loaded with BSA as a model protein (Eldin et al., 2015). The purpose of the study was to develop a pH-responsive system that allows a controlled release of BSA in acidic media compared to pure alginate. The results showed that BSA release pattern from pure alginate hydrogel was burst one with only 15% of the protein content was released within 5 h. On the other hand, the release profile from Arg-g-Alg hydrogels was observed to be enhanced at acidic conditions. The study suggested that the enhancement in release profile is attributed to the incorporation of arginine amine groups, which increases the BSA release to 300% of its value in neat alginate.

5.5 CONCLUSION

This chapter has discussed the chemical structure and the extraction sources of alginates. Thereafter, the outstanding physicochemical properties of alginates were elucidated from the applications' perspective. Then, the chapter pointed out the most common chemical modification approaches of alginates, which are performed primarily on both the carboxyl and hydroxyl functional groups. The last part of the chapter had focused on the most advanced biomedical applications of chemically modified alginates. In particular, it covered the up-to-date research performed in the fields of tissue engineering, wound healing and, most importantly, drug delivery applications. In conclusion, it seems obvious that alginate and its chemically modified derivatives are very promising biomaterials for biomedical applications. It is expected that they will have much contribution in the future of drug delivery applications due to their stunning properties.

SUMMARY

Alginate is one of the natural biopolymers that have recently attracted a lot of interest from researchers. It is usually extracted from microorganisms such as brown algae, and basically, it is a linear polysaccharide composed of two building units, β-D-mannuronic acid (M) and α-l-guluronic acid (G)-linked by glycoside bonds. These units are randomly distributed throughout the chain either in MM, GG, or MG manner. Being a natural biopolymer, alginate has many favorable properties such as biocompatibility, biodegradability, and nontoxicity. Besides, alginate characteristics could be further manipulated through facile chemical modification. Therefore, it has been used in a wide range of biomedical applications including tissue engineering, wound dressings, and primarily targeted and sustained drug delivery. There are two main approaches to chemically modify alginate either through its carboxylic or hydroxyl groups. The examples of carboxylic modifications include amidation, esterification, and Ugi reaction. On the other hand, hydroxyl modifications include reductive amination and sulfation. This chapter sheds light on the chemical modification approaches of alginate and the physicochemical characteristics of the modified forms with emphasis on alginate-grafted copolymers. In addition, the second part of this contribution explores the most advanced biomedical applications of alginate and its chemically modified forms, particularly for drug delivery purposes.

KEYWORDS

- **chemical modification**
- **alginate**
- **biomedical**
- **drug delivery**
- **grafting**

REFERENCES

Alban, S.; Schauerte, A.; Franz, G. Anticoagulant Sulfated Polysaccharides: Part I. Synthesis and Structure–Activity Relationships of New Pullulan Sulfates. *Carbohydr. Polym.* **2002,** *47*(3), 267–276. DOI: 10.1016/S0144-8617(01)00178-3.

Alsberg, E.; Anderson, K. W.; Albeiruti, A.; Franceschi, R. T.; Mooney, D. J. Cell-Interactive Alginate Hydrogels for Bone Tissue Engineering. *J. Dent. Res.* **2001,** *80*(11) 2025–2029. DOI: 10.1177/00220345010800111501.

Balakrishnan, B.; Mohanty, M.; Umashankar, P. R.; Jayakrishnan, A. Evaluation of an in Situ Forming Hydrogel Wound Dressing Based on Oxidized Alginate and Gelatin. *Biomaterials* **2005,** *26*(32), 6335–6342. DOI: 10.1016/J.BIOMATERIALS.2005.04.012.

Balakrishnan, B.; Mohanty, M.; Fernandez, A. C.; Mohanan, P. V.; Jayakrishnan, A. Evaluation of the Effect of Incorporation of Dibutyryl Cyclic Adenosine Monophosphate in an in Situ-Forming Hydrogel Wound Dressing Based on Oxidized Alginate and Gelatin. *Biomaterials* **2006,** *27*(8), 1355–1361. DOI: 10.1016/J.BIOMATERIALS.2005.08.021.

Bouhadir, K. H.; Lee, K. Y.; Alsberg, E.; Damm, K. L.; Anderson, K. W.; Mooney, D. J. Degradation of Partially Oxidized Alginate and Its Potential Application for Tissue Engineering. *Biotechnol. Prog.* **2001,** *17*(5), 945–950. DOI: 10.1021/bp010070p.

Bu, H.; Kjøniksen, A.-L.; Kenneth, D. K.; Nyström, B. Rheological and Structural Properties of Aqueous Alginate during Gelation via the Ugi Multicomponent Condensation Reaction. *Biomacromolecules* **2004.** DOI: 10.1021/BM049947+.

Carré, M.-C.; Delestre, C.; Hubert, P.; Dellacherie, E. Covalent Coupling of a Short Polyether on Sodium Alginate: Synthesis and Characterization of the Resulting Amphiphilic Derivative. *Carbohydr. Polym.* **1991,** *16*(4), 367–379. DOI: 10.1016/0144-8617(91)90055-H.

Chan, A. W.; Neufeld, R. J. Tuneable Semi-Synthetic Network Alginate for Absorptive Encapsulation and Controlled Release of Protein Therapeutics. *Biomaterials* **2010,** *31*(34), 9040–9047. DOI: 10.1016/J.BIOMATERIALS.2010.07.111.

Choudhary, S.; Reck, J. M.; Bhatia, S. R. Hydrophobically Modified Alginate for Drug Delivery Systems. In *2009 IEEE 35th Annual Northeast Bioengineering Conference*, 1–2. 2009. IEEE. DOI: 10.1109/NEBC.2009.4967735.

Colinet, I.; Dulong, V.; Mocanu, G.; Picton, L.; Le Cerf, D. New Amphiphilic and pH-Sensitive Hydrogel for Controlled Release of a Model Poorly Water-Soluble Drug. *Eur. J. Pharm. Biopharm.* **2009,** *73*(3), 345–350. DOI: 10.1016/J.EJPB.2009.07.008.

d'Ayala, G. G.; Malinconico, M.; Laurienzo, P. Marine Derived Polysaccharides for Biomedical Applications: Chemical Modification Approaches. *Molecules* **2008**, *13*(9), 2069–2106. DOI: 10.3390/molecules13092069.

Donati, I.; Vetere, A.; Gamini, A.; Skjåk-Bræk, G.; Coslovi, A.; Campa, C.; Paoletti, S. Galactose-Substituted Alginate: Preliminary Characterization and Study of Gelling Properties. *Biomacromolecules* **2003**, 624–631. DOI: 10.1021/BM020114Y.

Eldin, M. S. M.; Kamoun, E. A.; Sofan, M. A.; Elbayomi, S. M. L-Arginine Grafted Alginate Hydrogel Beads: A Novel pH-Sensitive System for Specific Protein Delivery. *Arabian J. Chem.* **2015**, *8*(3), 355–365. DOI: 10.1016/J.ARABJC.2014.01.007.

Ghahramanpoor, M. K.; Hassani Najafabadi, S. A.; Abdouss, M.; Bagheri, F.; Baghaban Eslaminejad, M. A Hydrophobically-Modified Alginate Gel System: Utility in the Repair of Articular Cartilage Defects. *J. Mater. Sci: Mater. Med.* **2011**, *22*(10), 2365–2375. DOI: 10.1007/s10856-011-4396-2.

Gomez, C. G.; Rinaudo, M.; Villar, M. A. Oxidation of Sodium Alginate and Characterization of the Oxidized Derivatives. *Carbohydr. Polym.* **2007**, *67*(3), 296–304. DOI: 10.1016/J.CARBPOL.2006.05.025.

Hay, I. D.; Rehman, Z. U.; Moradali, M. F.; Wang, Y.; Rehm, B. H. A. Microbial Alginate Production, Modification and Its Applications. *Microb. Biotechnol.* **2013**, *6*(6), n/a-n/a. DOI: 10.1111/1751-7915.12076.

Jain, D.; Bar-Shalom, D. Alginate Drug Delivery Systems: Application in Context of Pharmaceutical and Biomedical Research. *Drug Dev. Ind. Pharm.* **2014**, *40*(12), 1576–1584. DOI: 10.3109/03639045.2014.917657.

Kang, H.-A.; Shin, M. S.; Yang, J.-W. Preparation and Characterization of Hydrophobically Modified Alginate. *Polym. Bull.* **2002**, *47*(5), 429–435. DOI: 10.1007/s002890200005.

Kim, G. H.; Ahn, S.; Kim, Y. Y.; Cho, Y.; Chun, W. Coaxial Structured Collagen–Alginate Scaffolds: Fabrication, Physical Properties, and Biomedical Application for Skin Tissue Regeneration. *J. Mater. Chem.* **2011**, *21*(17) 6165. DOI: 10.1039/c0jm03452e.

Koo, L. Y.; Irvine, D. J.; Mayes, A. M.; Lauffenburger, D. A.; Griffith, L. G. Co-Regulation of Cell Adhesion by Nanoscale RGD Organization and Mechanical Stimulus. *J. Cell Sci.* **2002**, 1423–1433. http://jcs.biologists.org/content/joces/115/7/1423.full.pdf.

Laurienzo, P.; Malinconico, M.; Motta, A.; Vicinanza, A. Synthesis and Characterization of a Novel Alginate–Poly(Ethylene Glycol) Graft Copolymer. *Carbohydr. Polym.* **2005**, *62*(3), 274–282. DOI: 10.1016/J.CARBPOL.2005.08.005.

Lee, K. Y.; Mooney, D. J. Alginate: Properties and Biomedical Applications. *Prog. Polym. Sci.* **2012**, *37*(1), 106–126. DOI: 10.1016/J.PROGPOLYMSCI.2011.06.003.

Maiti, S.; Singha, K.; Ray, S.; Dey, P.; Sa, B. Adipic Acid Dihydrazide Treated Partially Oxidized Alginate Beads for Sustained Oral Delivery of Flurbiprofen. *Pharm. Dev. Technol.* **2009**, *14*(5), 461–470. DOI: 10.1080/10837450802712658.

Martins, M.; Barros, A. A. Quraishi, S.; Gurikov, P.; Raman, S. P., Duarte, A. R. C.; Reis, R. L. Preparation of Macroporous Alginate-Based Aerogels for Biomedical Applications. *J. Supercrit. Fluids* **2015**, *106*, 152–159. DOI: 10.1016/J.SUPFLU.2015.05.010.

McHugh, D. J. Production, Properties and Uses of Alginates. In *Production and Utilization of Products from Commercial Seaweeds;* 1987. http://www.fao.org/docrep/x5822e/x5822e04.htm.

Moshaverinia, A.; Chen, C.; Akiyama, K.; Ansari, S.; Xu, X.; Chee, W. W.; Schricker, S. R.; Shi, S. Alginate Hydrogel as a Promising Scaffold for Dental-Derived Stem Cells: An in Vitro Study. *J. Mater. Sci. Mater. Med.* **2012**, *23*(12), 3041–3051. DOI: 10.1007/s10856-012-4759-3.

Nguyen, T.-P.; Lee, B.-T. Fabrication of Oxidized Alginate-Gelatin-BCP Hydrogels and Evaluation of the Microstructure, Material Properties and Biocompatibility for Bone Tissue Regeneration. *J. Biomater. Appl.* **2012,** *27*(3), 311–321. DOI: 10.1177/0885328211404265.

Panikkar, R.; Brasch, D. J. Composition and Block Structure of Alginates from New Zealand Brown Seaweeds. *Carbohydr. Res.* **1996,** *293*(1), 119–132. DOI: 10.1016/0008-6215 (96) 00193-0.

Pawar, S. N.; Edgar, K. J. Chemical Modification of Alginates in Organic Solvent Systems. *Biomacromolecules* **2011,** *12*(11), 4095–4103. DOI: 10.1021/bm201152a.

Pawar, S. N.; Edgar, K. J. Alginate Derivatization: A Review of Chemistry, Properties and Applications. *Biomaterials* **2012,** *33*(11), 3279–3305. DOI: 10.1016/J.BIOMATERIALS. 2012.01.007.

Pelleztier, S.; Hubert, P.; Payan, E.; Marchal, P.; Choplin, L.; Dellacherie, E. Amphiphilic Derivatives of Sodium Alginate and Hyaluronate for Cartilage Repair: Rheological Properties. *J. Biomed. Mater. Res.* **2001,** *54*(1), 102–8. DOI: 10.1002/1097-4636(200101) 54:1<102:AID-JBM12>3.0.CO;2-1.

Rastello De Boisseson, M.; Leonard; M.; Hubert; P.; Marchal; P.; Stequert; A.; Castel; C.; Favre, E.; Dellacherie, E. Physical Alginate Hydrogels Based on Hydrophobic or Dual Hydrophobic/ionic Interactions: Bead Formation, Structure, and Stability. *J. Colloid Interface Sci.* **2004,** *273*(1), 131–139. DOI: 10.1016/J.JCIS.2003.12.064.

Rayatpisheh, S.; Poon, Y. F.; Cao, Y.; Feng, J.; Chan, V.; Chan-Park, M. B. Aligned 3D Human Aortic Smooth Muscle Tissue via Layer by Layer Technique Inside Microchannels with Novel Combination of Collagen and Oxidized Alginate Hydrogel. *J. Biomed. Mater. Res. Part A* **2011,** *98*(2), 235–244. DOI: 10.1002/jbm.a.33085.

Reham, B. *Microbial Production of Biopolymers and Polymer Precursors: Applications and Perspectives*; Horizon Scientific Press. 2009. https://books.google.com.eg/ books?hl=en&lr=&id=Vu9kc0-uSJYC&oi=fnd&pg=PP1&dq=Rehm,+B.H.,+Ed.%3B+M icrobial+production+of+biopolymers+and+polymer+precursors:+applications+and+pers pectives.+Horizon+Scientific+Press,+2009.+&ots=8fHeMA0Ork&sig=sp9x7r7Hc22 6wPY4.

Ronghua, H.; Yumin, D.; Jianhong, Y. Preparation and in Vitro Anticoagulant Activities of Alginate Sulfate and Its Quaterized Derivatives. *Carbohydr. Polym* **2003,** *52*(1), 19–24. DOI: 10.1016/S0144-8617(02)00258-8.

Ruvinov, E.; Leor, J.; Cohen, S. The Promotion of Myocardial Repair by the Sequential Delivery of IGF-1 and HGF from an Injectable Alginate Biomaterial in a Model of Acute Myocardial Infarction. *Biomaterials* **2011,** *32*(2), 565–578. DOI: 10.1016/J. BIOMATERIALS.2010.08.097.

Sand, A.; Yadav, M.; Behari, K. Synthesis and Characterization of Alginate-G-Vinyl Sulfonic Acid with a Potassium Peroxydiphosphate/Thiourea System. *J. Appl. Polym. Sci.* **2010,** *118*(6), 3685–3694. DOI: 10.1002/app.32447.

Sen, G.; Prakash Singh, R.; Pal, S. Microwave-Initiated Synthesis of Polyacrylamide Grafted Sodium Alginate: Synthesis and Characterization. *J. Appl. Polym. Sci.* **2010,** *115*(1), 63–71. DOI: 10.1002/app.30596.

Shu-Lan, H.; Min, Z.; Zhan-Jie, G.; Yu-Ji, Y.; Kang-De, Y. Preparation and Characterization of Partially Oxidized Sodium Alginate. *Chin. J. Appl. Chem.* **2005.** http://en.cnki.com.cn/ Article_en/CJFDTOTAL-YYHX200509020.htm.

Sun, J.; Tan, H. Alginate-Based Biomaterials for Regenerative Medicine Applications. *Materials* **2013,** *6*(4), 1285–1309. DOI: 10.3390/ma6041285.

Ugi, I. The α-Addition of Immonium Ions and Anions to Isonitriles Accompanied by Secondary Reactions. *Angew. Chem. Int. Ed. Engl.* **1962**, *1*(1), 8–21. DOI: 10.1002/anie.196200081.

Venkatesan, J.; Lowe, B.; Anil, S.; Manivasagan, P.; Kheraif, A. A. A.; Kang, K.-H.; Kim, S.-K. Seaweed Polysaccharides and Their Potential Biomedical Applications. *Starch—Stärke* **2015**, *67*(5–6), 381–390. DOI: 10.1002/star.201400127.

Yang, J.-S.; Xie, Y.-J.; He, W. Research Progress on Chemical Modification of Alginate: A Review. *Carbohydr. Polym.* **2011**, *84*(1), 33–39. DOI: 10.1016/J.CARBPOL.2010.11.048.

Yang, J.-S.; Han, S.-Y.; Yang, L.; Zheng, H.-C. Synthesis of Beta-Cyclodextrin-Grafted-Alginate and Its Application for Removing Methylene Blue from Water Solution. *J. Chem. Technol. Biotechnol.* **2016**, *91*(3), 618–623. DOI: 10.1002/jctb.4612.

Yao, B.; Ni, C.; Xiong, C.; Zhu, C.; Huang, B. Hydrophobic Modification of Sodium Alginate and Its Application in Drug Controlled Release. *Bioprocess Biosyst. Eng.* **2010**, *33*(4), 457–463. DOI: 10.1007/s00449-009-0349-2.

Zhiyong, L.; Caihua, N.; Cheng, X.; Qian, L. Preparation and Drug Release of Hydrophobically Modified Alginate. *Chemistry* **2009**. http://en.cnki.com.cn/Article_en/CJFDTOTAL-HXTB 200901020.htm.

Zhu, L. M.; Xin, C. L. Preparation of a Superabsorbent Resistant to Saline Solution by Copolymerization of Acrylic Acid with Sodium Polymannuronate. *Chin. J. Appl. Chem.* **2002**. http://en.cnki.com.cn/Article_en/CJFDTOTAL-YYHX200205010.htm.

CHAPTER 6

BIONANOCOMPOSITES OF ALGINATES, THEIR CHEMISTRY, AND APPLICATIONS

NANCY L. GARCIA[2,3], MARIO CONTÍN[2,4],
CARLOS A. RODRIGUEZ RAMIREZ[2,5], and
NORMA B. D'ACCORSO[1,2,*]

[1]*Universidad de Buenos Aires, Facultad de Ciencias Exactas y Naturales, Departamento de Química Orgánica, Buenos Aires, Argentina*

[2]*CONICET, Universidad de Buenos Aires, Centro de Investigaciones en Hidratos de Carbono (CIHIDECAR), Buenos Aires, Argentina*

[3]*E-mail: nancylis@gmail.com*

[4]*E-mail: mariodc260@hotmail.com*

[5]*E-mail: rodriguezramirez126@gmail.com*

Corresponding author. E-mail: norma@qo.fcen.uba.ar

6.1 INTRODUCTION

Bionanocomposites can be considered as the new emerging group of nano-structured hybrid materials. Bionanocomposites is defined as a mixture of naturally occurring polymer (biopolymer) and inorganic or organic filler materials that have at least one dimension on the nanometer scale (Jawaid et al., 2017). This new class of composites exhibits significant improvements in mechanical, barrier, and thermal properties, and dimensional stability. Furthermore, it also offers benefits such as transparency, low density, better surface properties, good flow properties, and recyclability. Figure 6.1 illustrates the types of composite materials that are classified according to the constituents which determine the structure, properties, functionalities, and applications. To obtain fully renewable and biodegradable nanocomposites, both the polymer matrix and nano reinforcement must be derived from renewable resources (Haafiz et al., 2013).

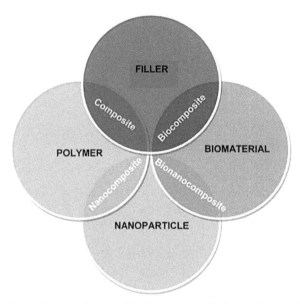

FIGURE 6.1 Types of composite materials that are classified according to the constituents.

Lignin, ALG, and casein members, natural polymers, are a unique class of biomaterials as they can be engineered to meet specific end-use demands that can be selected according to "required" characteristics such as mechanical resistance, permeability, degradability, transparency, and solubility. However, the polymers currently available need to be improved by modifying, in some cases, their properties, especially surface properties. Therefore, for the manufacture of new and improved biocomposites and bionanocomposites (Visakh and Sigrid, 2016), the modification and design of the macromolecules must be carefully adapted to obtain a necessary combination of chemical, mechanical, interfacial, and biological functions.

ALG is one of the functional fibers which possesses many excellent properties. It is made up of ALG acid which is extracted from algae plants in the ocean (Dong et al., 2017). Although alginic acid was initially thought to consist of a uniform polymer of mannuronic acid, the presence of guluronic and mannuronic acid blocks was studied later. More precisely, it consists of $(1\rightarrow4)$-linked β-D-mannuronic acid and α-L-guluronic acid. In alginic acid, both residues exist in the form of a homopolymer block or a heteropolymer block as shown in Figure 6.2. Since ALGs are extracted from certain brown seaweeds, depending on the seaweed source and growing conditions, the ratio of mannuronic acid to guluronic acid can vary in various samples of ALGs. They have the reversible gel-forming ability in the presence of calcium. It has been found that the poly(guluronic acid) blocks can bind calcium ions more effectively than the poly(mannuronic acid) blocks (Visakh and Sigrid, 2016).

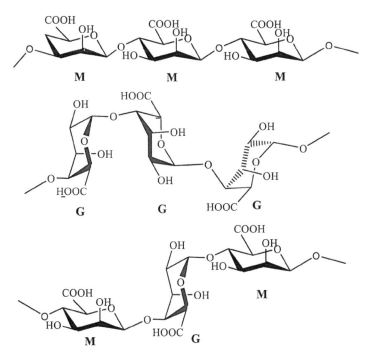

FIGURE 6.2   Repeating D-mannuronic, L-guluronic, and β-D-mannuronic-α-L-guluronic acid blocks in alginic acid (M = β-D-mannuronic acid; G = α-L-guluronic acid).

As this fiber is part of the renewable biomass, it can release to nature by biological decomposition and it will not pollute the environment (Lian et al., 2011). In addition, it possesses many excellent properties, such as high moisture absorption, high oxygen penetration, biocompatibility, biodegradation–absorption, and high ion adsorption (Dong et al., 2017).

These properties of ALG fiber prompt a lot of potential applications in the different fields, for example, in medicinal chemistry as delivery vehicles for drugs and cells, for enzyme entrapment; in the environmental applications as heavy ion scavengers and as adsorption of dye materials. On the other hand, the ALGs have been used as chelators for pulling radioactive toxins, such as iodine-131 and strontium-90, flame-retardant materials, and in recent years, as electromagnetic shielding materials applied in inflexible electronic devices field as a substrate.

Owing to their biocompatible nature, ALGs are well adapted for tissue engineering in biomedicine as medical materials as wound-dressing material (Visakh and Sigrid, 2016). In addition to these applications, they can be used as food additives to provide structures to some food materials, including marine and freshwater products. ALGs can be processed as capsules, beads, and fibers and can be composites with other natural and synthetic polymers or films.

In the field of drug delivery, is reported a new material able to controllably release of olanzapine (OLZ) in the body. To control the dissolution rate, the authors propose a system that incorporates the drug into montmorillonite (MMT) dispersed in a mixture of ALG and xanthan gum biopolymers. It is interesting to note that the OLZ is a thienobenzodiazepine class, which is used in the treatment of schizophrenia and other psychoses. The authors reported that the best results were attained with an incubation time of 24 h, an initial OLZ mass of 300 mg (3.0 mg/mL) and pH 5.8. X-ray diffraction analysis was used to observe the formation of intercalation compounds with different degrees of OLZ incorporation, indicating the possible presence of OLZ through the expansion of the clay mineral structure. The incorporation of the drug in the clay mineral was then confirmed by infrared analysis and quantified through high-performance liquid chromatography–diode-array detector analysis, indicating a maximum incorporation of 47.37 mg of OLZ/100 mg of MMT. In addition to having improved control of the release, the developed material could protect the OLZ when subjected to an oxidative medium, thus presenting a new property for this type of material results of the release test of the MMT–OLZ hybrid were consistent, but the presence of the biopolymers was required to more precisely control the drug release, as well as to improve the bioavailability and to reduce drug insolubility (Oliveira et al., 2017).

Promoting wound healing and assuring the local delivery of the loaded antibiotic, Rădulescu et al. obtained a biocompatible nanostructured composite based on naturally derived biopolymers (chitin and sodium ALG) loaded with commercial antibiotics (either cefuroxime or cefepime) with dual functions (promoting wound healing and assuring the local delivery of the loaded antibiotic). The antimicrobial activity assays revealed a remarkable inhibition of bacterial biofilm development, the best experimental results being obtained for the chitin–sodium ALG composites loaded with the fourth-generation cephalosporin antibiotic cefepime. Therefore, we can conclude that this antibiotic was successfully encapsulated in the polysaccharide composites. This study with a proved biocompatibility and antimicrobial properties seems to be promising for use in the management of wound healing (Rădulescu et al., 2016).

Bionanocomposite beads of halloysite (HAL)/ALG were studied as a medium for drug delivery and adsorption or absorption due to their biocompatibility, renewability, and relatively easy preparation (Chiew et al., 2014). Fourier transform infrared (FTIR) spectroscopy spectra show no chemical interaction between the HAL nanotubes and the ALG polymers. Energy-dispersive X-ray analyzer shows that the HAL nanotubes are embedded within the layers of Ca–ALG hydrogel networks but they are not present in the pores between the matrices. This finding is confirmed by the field emission scanning electron microscopy (FESEM) images which further show that the HAL nanotubes are well dispersed within the ALG matrix. The Young's modulus of the HAL/ALG bionanocomposite beads, determined using uniaxial compression test and Hertz's model, increased by 35% at 100 g/L halloysite nanotube loading compared to that of blank ALG beads. Certainly, it has economic benefits to applications considering the relative cost of HAL nanotubes. However, due to the presence of HAL nanotubes which modified the tortuosity, the HAL/ALG bionanocomposite beads showed slight but noticeable improvements in the resistance to swell-weakening by sodium ions, while incurring only a slight drop in the ease of diffusion by small molecules such as glucose. The enhanced mechanical properties without severely compromising other physicochemical properties make HAL/ALG bionanocomposite a more promising material for a variety of applications including bioprocessing and tissue engineering.

In strategies for bone repair applications, composite scaffolds were prepared by incorporating hydroxyapatite (nHA) and bioactive glass (nBG) into a porous ALG matrix at different particle loads by Valenzuela et al. (2012). nHA and nBG nanoparticles synthesized by the solgel method. The nanoparticles notably accelerate the crystallization process of the apatite phase on the scaffold surfaces. For short immersion times in simulated body fluid (SBF), nBG-based nanocomposites induce more apatite crystallization than nHA-based nanocomposites because of the more reactive nature of the nBG particles. Through a reinforcement effect, HA and BG nanoparticles also improve the mechanical properties and stability of the polymer scaffold matrix in SBF. In addition, in vitro biocompatibility tests show that osteoblast cells are viable and adhere well on the surface of the bionanocomposites.

These results indicate that nHA- and nBG-based bionanocomposites present potential properties for bone repair applications, particularly oriented to accelerate the bone mineralization process.

ALG–bentonite is an improved mixed matrix using natural hydrogels and nanoclays. Green bioprocess using stabilized *Lactobacillus animalis* ATCC 35046 in a bentonite–ALG-based bionanocomposite was developed by Cappa et al. (2016) Scale-up biotransformation to obtain 5-fluorouracil-2-deoxyriboside (floxuridine), a compound extensively used as an antitumor agent, was studied to provide an improved alternative for the synthesis of antitumor compounds. This bioprocess scale-up may be employed in the pharmaceutical industry using a sustainable method.

Another interesting application of bionanocomposites is in the area of eco-friendly insulating materials for construction or in the transport sectors. These nanocomposites are based in starch/ALG bionanocomposite foams reinforced with sepiolite. These foams exhibited good mechanical properties despite their low density with a maximum value of compression modulus. Spectroscopic techniques were applied to assess the interaction mechanism established between the inorganic fibers and the polysaccharide chains, which is established between the hydroxyl groups in the polysaccharide chains and the silanol groups at the external surface of the sepiolite fibers. The textural properties studied by means of mercury intrusion porosimetry, FESEM, and X-ray microtomography revealed a decrease in porosity as the sepiolite content increased. Mechanical properties were also determined for the studied foams, showing an increase in compression moduli from 7.3 MPa in the foam without sepiolite to 29 MPa in foams containing 10% starch, 40% sepiolite, and 50% ALG. Horizontal burning tests were carried out for a preliminary evaluation of the role of the inorganic fibers on the fire resistance properties of the bionanocomposite foams, revealing that bionanocomposite foams with sepiolite content > 25% behave as auto-extinguishable materials. Post-synthesis cross-linking with calcium chloride ($CaCl_2$) was carried out in some of these samples, leading to an increase in the compression modulus up to 40 MPa for the optimal composition. In fact, it was corroborated that porosity of the resulting biofoams can be modulated by varying the content in sepiolite, making possible to tune certain properties like mechanical resistance. These bionanocomposite foams exhibited good mechanical properties despite their low density, with a maximum value of compression modulus of 29 MPa (Darder et al., 2017).

In order to develop new sustainable technologies that can be used as biodegradable mulches in agriculture, a project funded by the European

Commission under the LIFE Environment program, called Biodegradable Coverages for Sustainable Agriculture was initiated. The innovative approach consisted of forming the mulch coating directly in the field by covering the soil with a thin protective geomembrane obtained by spraying water-based solutions of natural polysaccharides, such as sodium ALG (Na–ALG), glucomannan, chitosan, and cellulose (Visakh and Sigrid, 2017). Biocomposites are prepared by sandwiching three layers of unidirectional fibers between four sheets of linear low-density polyethylene and Ca^{2+} ALG. Ratajska and Boryniec (1999) reported results of biodegradation their composites of poly- ethylene filled with Na+ALG studying their morphology. In the film of these composites, was observed the emergence of large-sized holes, which can be seen on the surface and in the cross section of the composites, showing a sponge- like structure. Films filled with cellulose readily degrade in the soil, while films containing sodium ALG biodegrade quite easily in an aqueous medium. An excellent correlation between the results of weight loss and water sorption values was observed in their experiments.

Despite the multiple applications of ALGs, the most interesting can be shown in biomedicine for the reason that the bionanocomposites with nanoparticles of silver and gold will be developed in more detail. Subsequently, a part will be dedicated to the bionanocomposites with ferromagnetic and carbon nanotubes.

6.2 BIONANOCOMPOSITES

6.2.1 *BIONANOCOMPOSITES OF ALGINATE (ALG)–SILVER*

Bionanocomposites are also extensively explored for the utilization in the field of biomedicine such as in drug delivery, bioimaging, chemotherapy, radiation therapy, and tissue engineering (Luo et al., 2012). One of the most commonly used and commercialized are silver nanoparticles because these exhibit versatile characteristics such as conductivity, stability, and catalytic and antimicrobial activities (Li et al., 2010).

Nam et al. (2016) synthesized and characterized ALG/silver bionanocomposites by solutions plasma process. The solution plasma process (SPP) has been proposed as a technique that would synthesize metal nanoparticles and composites of metal–polymer (Takai et al., 2008). SPP involves the sequence of physical and chemical reactions where the water molecules are split into free radicals (H·, OH·, electrons) and solutes (precursors) into ions to nanoparticles during plasma discharge in the solution (Tseng et al., 2011). The process, therefore, could be applied to the synthesis of metal nanoparticles and their simultaneous fabrication into biopolymers (Kim et al., 2014). The biocomposites were synthesized in solutions of $AgNO_3$ and ALG by discharging plasma frequency using a pulsed unipolar power supply and then was analyzed using an ultraviolet (UV)–visible spectrophotometer. The characterization of the ALG/AgNP Bionanocomposites three-dimensional (3D) scaffolds using an FESEM showed that the vast majority of the bionanocomposites had a microporous structure with a smooth surface but a fraction of the nanocompounds showed porous spongy surfaces. For the study of microbiological activity of bionanocomposites, test was performed to observe the growth of various pathogenic bacteria on these bionanocomposites. These nanomaterials exhibited a broad spectrum of microbicidal activity against various pathogens, most effective against Gram-negative bacteria, and then in the case of Gram-positive bacteria, *Candida albicans* and *Aspergillus parasiticus*. They could inhibit the bacterial growth at much lower concentrations than those of other bionanocomposites. The two fungi were quite resistant to the bionanocomposites, resulting that they might be nontoxic to human cells at the concentrations for bactericidal activity and thus safe for medical application. The results suggested that the ALG/AgNP bionanocomposites might have the potential for application as wound-dressing materials (Nam et al., 2016).

Other studies were focusing on the study of microbial activity superabsorbent hydrogel–silver nanocomposite based on polyvinyl alcohol (PVA) and sodium ALG (Na–ALG) (Ghasemzadeh and Ghanaat, 2014). The sodium ALG (Na–ALG) was prepared using free radical polymerization in the presence of acrylamide (AAm). The reactions were conducted under normal atmospheric conditions using ammonium persulfate as an initiator and methylene bisacrylamide as a cross-linking agent. It is important to mention that Ag nanoparticles were synthesized in a green synthesis process (Figure 6.3).

The authors conclude that this methodology allows obtaining highly stable silver nanoparticles using hydrogel networks as nanoreactor. The reduction of silver nitrate is then carried out in situ using sodium borohydride as a reducing agent. Superabsorbent hydrogel–silver nanocomposite based on PVA and sodium ALG (Na–ALG) was prepared using free radical polymerization in the presence of AAm monomer (Figure 6.4) (Ghasemzadeh and Ghanaat, 2014).

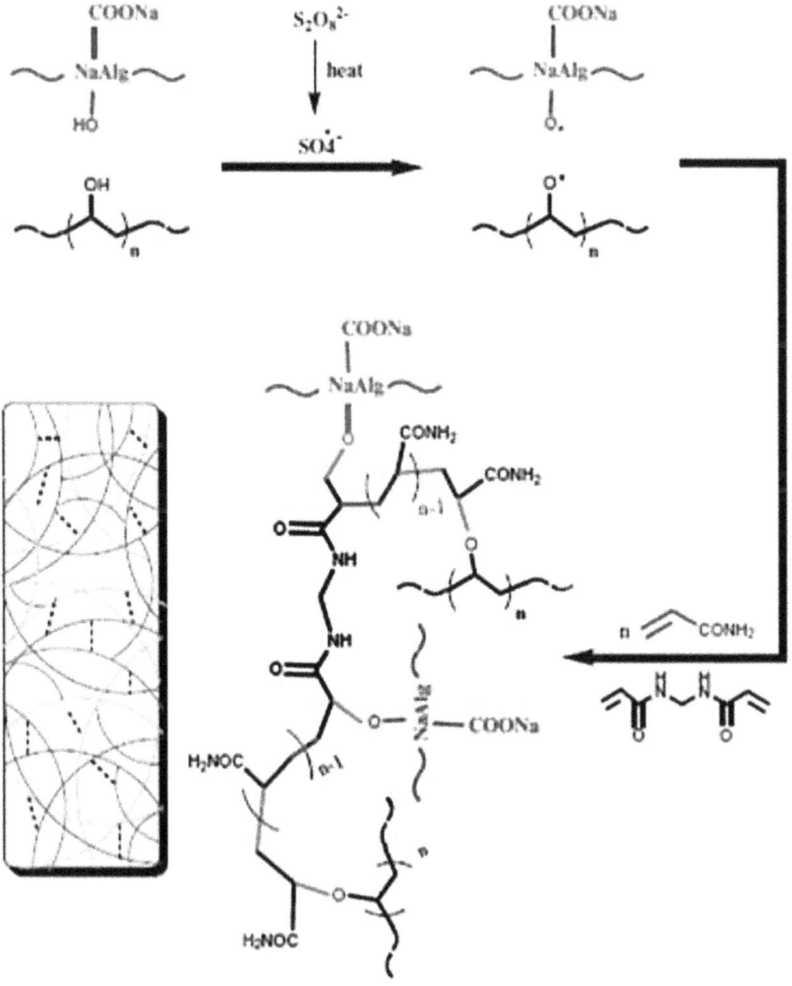

FIGURE 6.3 Proposed mechanistic pathway for the synthesis of (Na–ALG–PVA)-g PAAm hydrogel.

Source: Reprinted from Ghasemzadeh and Ghanaat, 2014 with permission from Universidad de Buenos Aires

The antibacterial activity of the nanocomposite hydrogels was investigated on two model microorganisms, with Gram negative, *Escherichia coli* and Gram positive, *Staphylococcus aureus* cultures in nutrient agar medium. The antibacterial activity is attributed to the difference in cell wall structure between Gram-negative and Gram-positive microorganisms because AgNPs could attach to the bacterial cell wall and alter cell membrane permeability and respiration, causing cell death. It is important to note that smaller AgNPs significantly penetrate bacteria, causing death. The formation of free radicals by AgNPs is also considered to cause cell death. AgNPs bind to membrane proteins, form pits and cause morphological changes, and the binding of AgNPs to membrane surfaces causes leeching of lipopolysaccharides and subsequently loss of structural integrity and impermeability. AgNPs also kill bacteria by damaging DNA by reacting with phosphate groups and other cellular components (Ghasemzadeh and Ghanaat, 2014).

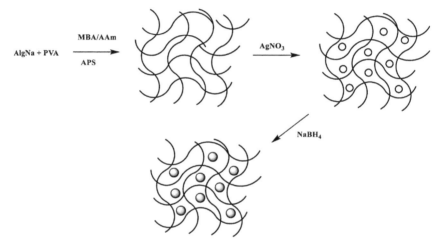

FIGURE 6.4   Schematic representation of the Ag nanoparticles formation in the hydrogel network.

Source: Reprinted from Ghasemzadeh and Ghanaat, 2014 with permission from Universidad de Buenos Aires.

Recent research has focused on the search for new alternatives in the synthetic routes of bionanocomposites of silver–ALG–chitosan (Narayanan and Han, 2017; Bousalem, 2016. Bousalem et al. (2016) synthesized and characterized antibacterial silver–ALG–chitosan bionanocomposite films using UV irradiation at λ=365 nm. The ALG was utilized to inhibit the aggregation of the AgNPs in solution which acts as a multipurpose agent. After performing the microbiological test, the exclusion zone of AgNPs were released out of the discs and adsorbed onto biological molecules inside the bacteria cells (Figure 6.5). This behavior seems to be agreement with the accepted mechanism of silver antimicrobial activity which involves an interaction of silver ions with negatively charged species present within the cytoplasm membrane (Bousalem, 2016).

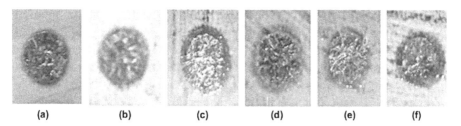

FIGURE 6.5 Comparison of the inhibition zone test of E1 film between: (a) *Escherichia coli*, (b) *Staphylococcus aureus*, (c) *Pseudomonas aeruginosae*, (d) *Citrobacter freundii*, (e) *Bacillus cereus*, and (f) *Acinetobacter baumannii*.

Source: Reprinted from Bousalem, 2016 with permission from Universidad de Buenos Aires.

Other research focused on the study of the silver release from the nano-composites of Ag/ALG hydrogels in the presence of chloride ions (Kostic et al., 2016) and made the comparison between experimental and mathematical data. The AgNPs were stabilized with ALG and produced by electrochemical synthesis using solutions of KNO_3, Na–ALG, and $AgNO_3$. From that research, they could study the different phenomena produced during silver release of the nanocomposite hydrogels in the presence of chloride ions, such as diffusion of AgNPs inside the hydrogel, oxidation/dissolution of AgNP and reaction with chloride ions, and the diffusion of $AgCl_x^{(x-1)}$–ALG hydrogel species. The results implied that transport rates of chloride ions induced higher AgNP oxidation/dissolution rate and higher precipitation of AgCl with lower diffusion coefficient and release of $AgCl_x^{(x-1)}$ species. The results obtained in the present study are highly relevant for the development of silver-containing antimicrobial soft tissue implants and wound dressings based on ALG as a widely used, medically approved biomaterial.

Zvicer et al. (2015) reported the cytotoxicity studies of Ag/ALG where the silver nanoparticles were obtained by electrochemical synthesis and then were aggregated to hydrogels in two-dimensional (2D) monolayer cell cultures and in a 3D explants culture in a biomimetic bioreactor with dynamic compression. On the other hand, the authors noted that the cells in monolayers exhibited moderate cytotoxicity due to their most sensibility in direct contact with the Ag/ALG discs. On the contrary, cartilage explants were not affected by the nanocomposite discs despite the compression. The tests were realized in direct contact of Ag/ALG discs applied in 2D monolayer cultures of bovine calf chondrocytes, while a 3D culture of bovine articular cartilage explants pressed by the discs was established in a biomimetic bioreactor with dynamic compression in the physiological regime. Moderate cytotoxicity was observed in 2D cell cultures as opposed to findings in 3D explants cultures, which were not affected by the Ag/ALG discs despite the compression.

Results reported by Zhao et al. (2017) proved the antibacterial activity and in vitro cytotoxicity evaluation of ALG-AgNP fibers. The cytotoxic effect of the fibers in human cervical cancer (HeLa) cells was assessed by Cell Counting Kit-8 assay and flow cytometry, while the bacterial growth study was performed using a growth kinetic study with *S. aureus* and *E. coli*. Finally, it can be concluded that the treatment showed a high efficiency in the elimination of cells, which makes the ALG AgNP fibers a promising material for biomedical applications.

Montaser et al. (2016) prepared and characterized ALG/silver/nico-tinamide (NIC) nanocomposites for treating diabetic wounds. Nonwoven viscous fabrics were used as a carrier for silver/ALG/nanoparticles composite by impregnating the nonwoven fabrics as per the padding-curing technique. NIC as anti-inflammatory drug was entrapped into Ag-NPS/ALG/nonwoven fabrics. The antibacterial activity of the Ag/ALG/NIC wound-dressing material was evaluated against *E. coli* and *S. aureus*. The wound healing and histological studies were evaluated using burn diabetic rat animals. The result showed that nonwoven viscose fabrics-loaded NIC with outer cross-linking by calcium chloride induced antibacterial resistance as compared with the control sample. It was concluded from the optical observation and histological examinations that fabric-loaded NIC with outer cross-linking provided fast healing character. The insertion of silver nanoparticles in nonwoven viscose fabric for imparting loaded NIC enhanced antibacterial property for a wide range of medical textile applications.

6.2.2 BIONANOCOMPOSITES OF ALG-GOLD

Many efforts have been devoted to the use of macromolecules of biological origin to control the growth of inorganic particles (Sarikaya et al., 2003); thus, in actuality, combining polymeric composites with inorganic materials is a promising modification method of new materials. In recent years, gold nanoparticles (AuNPs) have captured the considerable attention of primitive and modern science due to their size-dependent optical, electrical, and other properties. Moreover, the synthesis of Au/polymer nanocomposite has attracted many researchers since it plays a role as an effective stabilizer, and the characteristic of polymer capping supports the Au nanoparticle (AuNP) functioning (Liu et al., 2006). The excellent optical properties of

AuNP have been widely applied in the colorimetric sensors and biomedical photothermal therapy (Alanazi et al., 2010; Lan and Lin, 2014). In the drug delivery system, such a stable, biocompatible, as well as water-soluble encapsulating agent is highly required (de Folter et al., 2012).

Zhang et al. (2014) established a simple strategy to perform poly (acryl-amide-co-ALG)/gold nanocomposites for the inactivation of bacteria. In the study, the reduction of gold ions by AAm and ALG (AM–SA) occurred before the polymerization and as-obtained gold colloids are stabilized by AM–SA immediately in the absence of commonly used reducing agents and protective reagents (Figure 6.6).

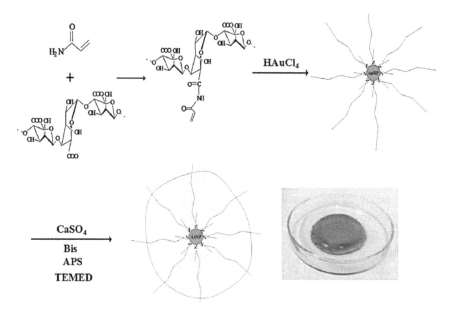

FIGURE 6.6 **(See color insert.)** Schematic illustration of the preparation of the hydrogel/gold nanocomposites.

Source: Reprinted from Zhang, 2014 with permission from Universidad de Buenos Aires.

FTIR spectroscopy and UV–Vis spectroscopy were used to follow up the preparation of the nanobiocomposites. It is important to highlight that the hydrogel/gold nanocomposites showed a non-compromised activity to inhibit the growth of a model bacterium, *E. coli*, also exhibited remarkable stability in the presence of high pHs (Zhang, 2014).

Other research focused on the study in situ of gold colloids growth within ALG films (Jaouen et al., 2010). In this case, gold–ALG bionanocomposite films were prepared by impregnation of ALG films with HAuCl$_4$ followed by reduction with glucose. The process to obtain Au/ALG films consists in three steps: (1) deposition of a pure (i.e., not cross-linked) ALG film, (2) impregnation by aqueous HAuCl$_4$ followed by binding of Au(III) ions by the guluronate units of the polymer, leading to network cross-linking, (3) reduction by glucose to form Au(0) nanoparticles (Figure 6.7).

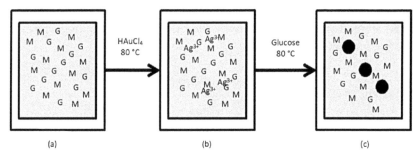

FIGURE 6.7 Schematic description of the Au–alginate (ALG) bionanocomposite film formation: (a) deposition of pure ALG films, (b) impregnation with HAuCl$_4$ leading to cross-linking of the guluronate groups (G) by Au3+, and (c) reduction by glucose leading to colloidal gold formation.

The mannuronate over guluronate ratio (M/G) of the polymer as well as the initial polymer concentration were shown to influence the film thickness, the amount of trapped Au^{3+} ions, and the volume fraction of Au(0) nanoparticles but not the size of these colloids (about 4 nm). The homogeneity of the gold colloid dispersion within the ALG gels was studied by transmission electron microscopy and confirmed by simulation of the surface plasmon resonance spectra using the Maxwell–Garnett model. The calculated spectra also provided fruitful information about the gold colloid/ALG interface. Overall, the whole process is controlled by the balance between the M/G ratio, defining the polymer affinity for Au(III) species, and the solution viscosity, controlling the diffusion phenomena.

On the other hand, Yulizar et al. (2016) used microwave synthesis as an alternative in obtaining thiol-based ligand-modified Au/ALG nanocomposite. This technique helps to complete the reduction of gold precursor. The nanocomposite had lower hydrophilicity compared to that unmodified Au/ALG, as indicated by the decreasing surface tension and increasing contact angle. The hydrophilicity change was influenced by the concentration and type of thiol-based ligand. Using mercaptoundecanoic acid and dodecane thiol simultaneously as thiol-based ligand in Au/ALG, nanocomposites showed a particle-stabilized emulsion o/w (O = chloroform, diesel oil, olive oil/water), namely Pickering emulsion. Emulsification capability increased with increasing nanocomposite concentration. Au/ALG nanocomposite modified was obtained with a facile, simple, and effective route.

6.2.3   *BIONANOCOMPOSITES OF ALG–NANOPARTICLES CELLULOSE*

Actually, the bionanocomposite films developed from biopolymers have gained considerable attention due to their renewability, biodegradability, biocompatibility, low toxicity, and their potential use in the packaging industry (Klemm et al., 2011). In this context, studies based on the use of two biopolymers, such as cellulose and sodium ALG, have received renewed interest. Cellulose, the most ubiquitous biopolymer, has greatly impacted the world and the society in wide areas. The utilization of cellulose as a substrate for understanding and engineering at the atomic and molecular scales is a new ingress in the field of polymer science (Charreau et al., 2013). It is interesting to remark that two novel forms of cellulose, namely cellulose nanofibrils and cellulose nanocrystals were used. These biopolymers exhibit outstanding properties such as low density, low thermal expansion, high aspect ratio, and important mechanical properties, which make them relevant in various applications (Klemm et al., 2011).

The study realized for Huq et al. (2012) developed nanocrystalline cellulose (NCC)-reinforced ALG-based nanocomposite film by solution casting. After incorporating the NCC in ALG matrix, a significant impact on the improvement of physicochemical and thermal properties of ALG-based films was proved, only with 5% w/w of NCC. Similar results were reported when assaying with cellulose nanofibers (Deepa et al., 2016). These nanocomposite films present excellent potential as a new biomaterial for application in food and medicine packaging.

Other investigation reported the study of hybrid injectable hydrogels comprising of ALG, gelatin, and NCC. These materials were formed and processed through adaptation of interpenetrated network of ALG-gelatin, ionic cross-linking of ALG, and supramolecular interaction approach (Wang et al., 2016). The synthesis of hydrogel was carried out using EDC/NHS (1-ethyl-3-(3-dimethylaminopropyl)carbodiimide/N-hydroxy-succinimide) chemistry, zinc ion cross-linking of ALG, and supramolecular interaction with NCC. A schematic of the reactions involved in the synthesis of hydrogel is presented in Figure 6.8.

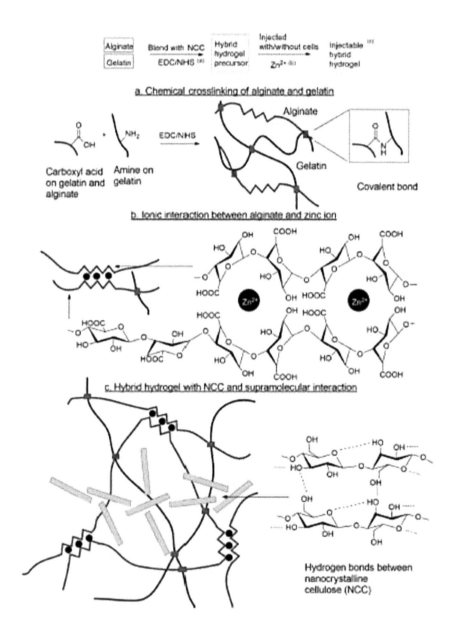

FIGURE 6.8   Schematic of reactions and interactions involved in the synthesis of ALG–gelatin–NCC hydrogels. (a) Chemical cross-linking by EDC/NHS, (b) ionic cross-linking of guluronic acid on ALG, and (c) orientation of NCC by hydrogel bond and hydrophobic interaction.

Source: Reprinted with permission from Wang et al., 2016. © 2016 Elsevier.

Gelatin enabled effective cell adhesion, while ALG and zinc sulfate allowed controllable ionic cross-linking with minimal toxicity and NCC reinforced the mechanical properties. The hybrid hydrogels were characterized by pore diameter and swelling behavior for cell growth and migration. The use of hydrophobic NCC increased crystallinity and stability against degradation. However, hydrophilicity was observed if NCC was used excessively. The constituents of the hybrid hydrogels were biocompatible and had the capability to incorporate osteoblast and bone morphogenetic protein (BMP-2). Homogeneous dispersion of NCC was envisaged to provide guidance to oriented cell growth on the surface or within hydrogels. The studied hybrid hydrogels are potentially cost-effective for delivery of cells and growth factors for the healing of bone defects. Further studies on stem cells differentiation and behavior in vivo are necessary to prove the promising future of the hybrid hydrogels as scaffold materials.

6.2.4 BIONANOCOMPOSITES MAGNETIC NANOPARTICLES MNPS–ALG

Several composites were described where the MNPs were included in an ALG matrix. The most common MNPs are based on magnetite (Fe_3O_4) which can be obtained throw well-known procedures. The most of the syntheses for the nanoparticles of metal oxides belong to one of the following reaction types: (a) hydrolysis, (b) oxidation, and (c) thermal decomposition of the oxygen-rich precursors.

Most of the methods reported for MNPs production are based on the coprecipitation method (a) or a solvothermal method (Hammouda et al., 2015). The first method is based on the addition of a solution of Fe^{2+} and Fe^{3+} in a molar ratio of 1:2 to a solution of high pH to yield Fe_3O_4 according to the reaction of:

$$Fe^{2+} + 2Fe^{3+} + 8OH^- \rightarrow Fe_3O_4 + 4H_2O$$

On the other hand, the former method is based on the thermolysis of an oxygen-rich precursor. A wide number of procedures can be found in the bibliography. A typical procedure consists of the preparation of a solution of $FeCl_3$, sodium acetate, sodium citrate dehydrate ($Na_3Cit \cdot 2H_2O$) and ethylene glycol, transfer to autoclave, and then heat to 200°C for 7 h (Zheng et al. 2014).

Despite the methodology employed, the final product (Fe_3O_4) is recovered by centrifugation or employing a magnet, washed several times with water, and dried.

However, regarding the synthesis of MNPs–ALG, bionanocomposites can be described according to two principal strategies. Fe_3O_4 can be added to a solution of sodium ALG with constant stirring. Then, the above mixture was added dropwise to a solution of a divalent cation for cross-linking to get Fe_3O_4–ALG (Gopalakannan and Viswanathan, 2015) or was prepared in a two-step procedure. First, the ALG beads are prepared by the well-known dripping method. In the second step, the magnetite particles are synthesized in the presence of beads. The dried ALG beads are added to a solution of Fe(III) and Fe(II) ions. Then, the system is kept under mild magnetic stirring at a constant temperature of 60°C for 15 min. Next, ammonium hydroxide solution is added dropwise until pH is raised to 10, while the system was kept at 60°C for another period of 15 min under vigorous stirring for the magnetite formation by coprecipitation. The beads containing the magnetite particles (MNPs) are then washed three times in methanol solution (50% v/v) and dried in the oven at 40°C for 24 h (Kondaveeti et al. 2016).

Many applications that involve ALG–MNPs bionanocomposites can be mentioned. Grumezescu et al. (2014) employed ALG–MNPs composites in the biomedical field, especially on tissue engineering, developing multifunctional porous material with high antimicrobial properties and also a mechanical support for the eukaryotic cells adhesion, exhibiting the advantage of low cytotoxicity in human progenitor cells.

Another important application issue is pollutant removal. Chromium (VI) was deeply studied by many groups. Gopalakannan and Viswanathan (2015) performed Cr^{6+} sorption experiments with Fe_3O_4–ALG-Ce magnetic beads and studied the most significative parameters that influence the adsorption such as pH, contact time, and the presence of other ions. Moreover, the authors proposed two types of kinetic models: reaction-based and diffusion-based models in order to understand Cr(VI) sorption. They concluded that a pseudo-second-order model based on chemisorption is the best option to fit the experimental data.

Above metals, organic compounds were also studied as potential pollutants which were removed by Fe_3O_4–ALG beads. Hammouda et al. (2015) reported the removal of 3-methylindole from aqueous solution. In that case, the authors employed a catalytic property from MNPs, the Fenton reaction that degrades 3-methylindole.

On the other hand, Fe_3O_4 composites are employed in the pharmaceutical research. Chen et al. studied a hyperthermal cancer treatment with Fe_3O_4–ALG bionanocomposites. The magnetic electrospun mats developed, demonstrated a firmly adhesion to the tumor over a prolonged period, killing the tumor directly within an alternating magnetic field. These mats are also made from a biodegradable polymer unlike the larger magnetic electrospun mats that are manufactured using non-biodegradable polymers and organic solvents, causing the problems of elimination after therapy and the suspected biotoxicity associated with the residual solvent (Chen et al., 2016).

Also, in the pharmaceutical field, Seth et al. (2017) evaluated the effect of magnetic retention on the circulation and bioavailability of magnetic beads in the gastrointestinal tract in the presence of an external magnetic field (EMF). The authors developed a composite of iron oxide nanoparticles, a drug (dipeptidyl peptidase-IV inhibitor) and a fluorophore (Alexa Fluor-750) in chitosan–ALG core–shell beads (Figure 6.9). The experiments showed a 2.5-fold increase in drug's bioavailability due to the retention of the magnetic carriers in the presence of an external magnet, which proved the accumulation of these carriers in a specific localization of the intestine.

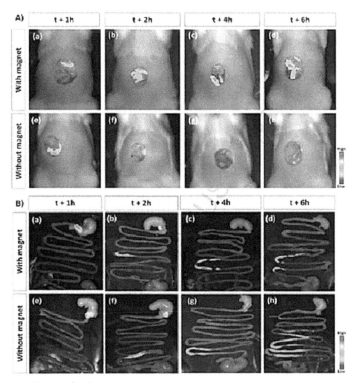

FIGURE 6.9 **(See color insert.)** Fluorescence and bright-field merged images of the beads in the rats intestine (A) under the magnet position, after skin removal and (B) after unfolding the intestine from stomach to caecum at time (a) and (e) 1 h, (b) and (f) 2 h, (c) and (g) 4 h, (d) and (h) 6 h after administration of the beads in the stomach of the rats for animal (a) to (d) with magnet and (e) to (h) without magnet.

Source: Reprinted with permission from Seth, 2017. © 2017 Elsevier.

Dopamine was also integrated into the MNPs–ALG composite. The aim of the work was to enhance dopamine bioavailability. The in vitro release of dopamine from the beads (100 mg) was investigated by immersing them in a buffer solution (pH 7.4), for 26 h in the absence and the presence of static EMF.

As it was observed, the release of dopamine from ALG–MNP increased under EMF. After 26 h, the contents of the released dopamine were 33 and 24% in the presence and the absence of EMF, respectively (Kondaveeti et al. 2016).

6.2.5   GO–ALG

Graphene oxide (GO) is one of the most popular carbon materials. It has a 2D sheet-like carbon structure of graphene and randomly distributed hydroxyl, epoxy, and carboxyl groups on its surface and edges, which makes it easily dispersible in aqueous solutions, enables π–π stacking, hydrogen bonding, cation bonding interactions with adsorbates, large specific surface area, and additional unique physicochemical and excellent mechanical properties. However, its nano-toxicity limits its application in the environment. Fei et al. (2016) developed an ALG gel with encapsulated GO to decrease the nano-toxicity of GO. This fact resulted a decrease in the pore size and improved the pore uniformity. This bionanocomposite was successfully applied to the adsorption of ciprofloxacin.

Go–ALG bionanocomposites were also applied in metal water remediation. Jiao et al (2016) studied GO–ALG composites in the adsorption of Cu^{2+} and Pb^{2+} and concluded from the results of microstructures, mechanical properties, and adsorption capacities and analysis that GO improves ALG beads remarkably and makes GO–ALG a potential candidate in wastewater treatment.

Despite its suspected nano-toxicity, GO was also studied in drug delivery. Fan et al. (2016) loaded doxoribicin onto the surface of GO conjugate via π–π stacking and hydrogen-bonding interaction, which was incorporated into ALG. This bionanocomposite enhances doxorubicin cytotoxicity against HeLa cell with CD44 receptor overexpressed. Fan et al. (2016) and Wang et al. employed 5-fluorouracil as a drug tester to study the in vitro releases from konjac glucomannan/sodium ALG hydrogels. They observed that the burst phenomenon could be avoided at the beginning of release tests and excellent pH sensitivity could be achieved. Nevertheless, the authors do not deny that a lot more systematic exploration is demanded to better understand the in vivo long-term fate and toxicology of graphene (Wang et al., 2014).

6.3 CONCLUSION

Because of the extraordinary mechanical properties of bionanocomposites, much interest lies in mimicking the bone structure such as dental implants and other orthopedic applications as they allow for multilevel integration of material, structural, and biological properties constituted by the polymer and nanofiller combination. The presence of nanosized fillers in bionanocomposites makes them ideally suited for drug delivery as they usually present a torturous diffusion path for encapsulated small molecule/drug, forming an effective barrier and sustained delivery. Furthermore, drug-releasing bionanocomposites are highly suited for wound-dressing applications as they have high water uptake and no cytotoxicity together, high mucoadhesivity, and tear resistance, making them ideal for wound dressing.

However, the use of the ALG matrix, as we have seen, encompasses a very wide variety of applications because ALG is of interest as a potential biopolymer film component due to unique colloidal properties, which includes thickening, stabilizing, suspending, film forming, gel producing, and emulsion stabilizing. The developments of bionanocomposites provide new avenues for fulfilling certain needs of the emerging technologies in matrix formation, tissue regeneration, drug delivery, and wound dressing and will be instrumental in accelerating the evolution of new therapeutics (Rajesh et al., 2018).

SUMMARY

The bionanocomposites are composites materials that contain constituent(s) of biological origin and particles with at least one dimension in the range of 1–100 nm. Choosing an adequate polymer matrix is the key for getting the most salient properties of bionanocomposites related to biocompatibility, biodegradability, and good mechanical properties.

Alginate (ALG) is a preferred biodegradable biomaterial which consists of β-D-mannuronic (M) and α-L-guluronic acid residues used in bionanocomposite formulation, especially in biomedicines such as cell transplantation, regeneration of skin, cartilage, bone, liver, cardiac tissue, wound dressings, and scaffold materials. ALG is a naturally biocompatible polysaccharide with a strong hydrophilic character that maintains a physiologically moist microenvironment, minimizes the bacterial contamination, mild ionotropic gelation, and excellent injectability.

The aim of this chapter is to review the last studies and developments in the field of ALG-based composites, especially in drug delivery by nanoencapsulation and regenerative medicine in the development of bone tissue engineering.

ACKNOWLEDGMENTS

The authors acknowledge the financial support of the University of Buenos Aires (UBACyT 20020130100021BA) and CONICET (PIP112-2015-0100443CO). Marion Contín and Carlos A. Rodriguez Ramirez received a postdoctoral scholarship and doctoral scholarship from CONICET, respectively. Nancy Lis Garcia and N. B. D´Accorso are research members from CONICET.

KEYWORDS

- bionanocomposites
- sepiolite
- nanoencapsulation
- olanzapine
- magnetic nanoparticles

REFERENCES

Alanazi, F. K.; Radwan, A. A.; Alsarra, I. A. Biopharmaceutical Applications of Nanogold. *Saudi Pharm. J.* **2010,** *18,* 179–193.

Bousalem, N.; Benmansour, K.; Cherif, H. Z. Synthesis and Characterization of Antibacterial Silver-Alginate–Chitosan Bionanocomposite Films Using UV Irradiation Method. *Mater. Technol.* **2016,** *32,* 367–377.

Cappa, V. A.; Rivero, C. W.; Sambeth, J. E.; Trelles, J. A. Bioproduction of Floxuridine Using Nanostabilized Biocatalysts. *Chem. Eng. Technol.* **2016,** *39,* 1723–1730.

Charreau, H.; Foresti, M. L.; Vazquez, A. Nanocellulose Patents Trends: A Comprehensive Review on Patents on Cellulose Nanocrystals, Microfibrillated and Bacterial Cellulose. *Recent Pat. Nanotechnol.* **2013,** *7,* 56–80.

Chen, Y. H.; Cheng, C. H.; Chang, W. J.; Lin, Y. C.; Lin, F. H.; Lin, J. C. Studies of Magnetic Alginate-Based Electrospun Matrices Crosslinked with Different Methods for Potential Hyperthermia Treatment. *Mater. Sci. Eng.* **2016,** *62,* 338–349.

Chiew, C. S. C.; Poh, P. E.; Pasbakhsh, P.; Tey, B. T.; Yeoh, H. K.; Chan, E. S. Physicochemical Characterization of Halloysite/Alginate Bionanocomposite Hydrogel. *Appl. Clay Sci.* **2014,** *101,* 444–454.

Darder, M.; Santos Matos, C. R.; Aranda, P.; Figueredo Gouveia, R.; Ruiz-Hitzky, E. Bionanocomposite Foams Based on the Assembly of Starch and Alginate with Sepiolite Fibrous Clay. *Carbohydr. Polym.* **2017,** *157,* 1933–1939.

Deepa, B.; Abraham, E.; Pothan, L.; Cordeiro, N.; Faria, M.; Thomas, S. Biodegradable Nanocomposite Films Based on Sodium Alginate and Cellulose Nanofibrils. *Materials* **2016,** *9,* 50, 2–11.

De Folter, J.; Van Ruijvena, M.; Velikov, K. Oil-Inwater Pickering Emulsions Stabilized by Colloidal Particles from the Water-Insoluble Protein Zein. *Soft Matter* **2012,** *8,* 6807–6815.

Dong, H.; Chen, R.; Mu, Y.; Liu, S.; Zhang, J.; Lin, H. Thermal and Electrical Properties of 3.2 nm Thin Gold Films Coated on Alginate Fiber. ASME. *J. Thermal Sci. Eng. Appl.* **2017,** *10,* 011012-011012-5.

Fan, L.; Ge, H.; Zou, S.; Xiao, Y.; Wen, H.; Li, Y.; Feng, H.; Ni, M. Sodium Alginate Conjugated Graphene Oxide as a New Carrier for Drug Delivery System. *Int. J. Biol. Macromol.* **2016,** *93,* 582–590.

Fei, Y.; Yong, L.; Sheng, H.; Jie, M. Adsorptive Removal of Ciprofloxacin by Sodium Alginate/Graphene Oxide Composite Beads from Aqueous Solution. *J. Colloid Interface Sci.* **2016,** *484,* 196–204.

Ghasemzadeh, H.; Ghanaat, F. Antimicrobial Alginate/PVA Silver Nanocomposite Hydrogel, Synthesis and Characterization. *J. Polym. Res.* **2014,** *21,* 355.

Gopalakannan, V.; Viswanathan, N. Synthesis of Magnetic Alginate Hybrid Beads for Efficient Chromium(VI) Removal. *Int. J. Biol. Macromol.* **2015,** *72,* 862–867.

Grumezescu, A. M.; Holban, A. M.; Andronescu, E.; Mogoşanu, G. D.; Vasilea, B. S.; Chifiriuc, M. C.; Lazar, V.; Andrei, E.; Constantinescu, A.; Maniu, H. Anionic Polymers and 10 nm Fe$_3$O$_4$@UA Wound Dressings Support Human Foetal Stem Cells Normal Development and Exhibit Great Antimicrobial Properties. *Int. J. Pharm.* **2014,** *463,* 46–154.

Haafiz, M. K.; Eichhorn, S. J.; Hassan, A.; Jawaid, M. Isolation and Characterization of Microcrystalline Cellulose from Oil Palm Biomass Residue. *Carbohydr. Polym.* **2013,** *93,* 628–634.

Hammouda, S. B.; Adhoum, N.; Monser, L. Synthesis of Magnetic Alginate Beads Based on Fe$_3$O$_4$ Nanoparticles for the Removal of 3-Methylindole from Aqueous Solution Using Fenton Process. *J. Hazard Mater.* **2015,** *294,* 128–136.

Huq, T.; Salmieria, S.; Khan, A.; Khan, R.; Tien, C.; Riedl, B.; Fraschini, C.; Bouchard, R.; Calderon, J, Kamal, M, Lacroix, M. Nanocrystalline Cellulose (NCC) Reinforced Alginate Based Biodegradable Nanocomposite Film. *Carbohydr. Polym.* **2012,** *90,* 1757–1763.

Jaouen, V.; Brayner, R.; Lantiat, D.; Steunou, N.; Coradin, T. In Situ Growth of Gold Colloids within Alginate Films. *Nanotechnology* **2010,** *21,* 185605.

Jawaid, M.; Salit, M. S.; Alothman, O. Y. *Green Biocomposites: Design and Applications; Green Energy and Technology;* Springer International Publishing: Switzerland, 2017.

Jiao, C.; Xiong, J.; Tao, J.; Xu, S.; Zhang, D.; Lin, H.; Chen, Y. Sodium Alginate/Graphene Oxide Aerogel with Enhancedstrength–Toughness and its Heavy Metal Adsorption Study. *Int. J. Biol. Macromol.* **2016,** *83,* 133–141.

Kim, S.; Lee, S.; Lee, M.; Kim, J. The Synthesis of Pt/Ag Bimetallic Nanoparticles Using a Successive Solution Plasma Process. *J. Nanosci. Nanotechnol.* **2014,** *14*(12), 8925–8929.

Klemm, D.; Kramer, F.; Moritz, S.; Lindstrom, T.; Ankerfors, M.; Gray, D.; Dorris, A. Nanocelluloses: A New Family of Nature-Based Materials. *Angew. Chem. Int. Ed. Engl.* **2011,** *50,* 5438–5466.

Kondaveeti, S.; Cornejo, D. R.; Petri, D. F. S. Alginate/Magnetite Hybrid Beads for Magnetically Stimulated Release of Dopamine. *Colloids Surf. B.* **2016,** *138,* 94–101.

Kostic, D.; Vidovic, S.; Obradovic, B. Silver Release from Nanocomposite Ag/Alginate Hydrogels in the Presence of Chloride Ions: Experimental Result and Mathematical Modeling. *J. Nanopart.* [Online] **2016,** https://link.springer.com/article/10.1007/s11051-016-3384-3 (accessed Oct, 2017).

Lan, Y. J.; Lin, Y. W. A Non-Aggregation Colorimetric Method for Trace Lead(II) Ions Based on the Leaching of Gold Nanorods. *Anal. Methods.* **2014,** *6,* 7234–7242.

Li, W. R.; Xie, X. B.; Shi, Q. S.; Zeng, H. Y.; Ou-Yang, Y. S.; Chen, Y. B. Antibacterial Activity and Mechanism of Silver Nanoparticles on *Escherichia coli. Appl. Microbiol. Biotechnol.* **2010,** *85*(4), 1115–1122.

Lian, Y.; Wu, J. Y.; Zhou, D. P.; Wang, H. M.; Huang, D. W.; Huang, Y. H. Preparation and Properties of Alginate Fibre. *Adv. Mater. Res.* **2011,** *335,* 419–422.

Liu, W.; Yang, X.; Huang, W. Catalytic Properties of Carboxylic Acid Functionalized-Polymer Microsphere-Stabilized Gold Metallic Colloids. *J. Colloid Interface Sci.* **2006,** *304,* 160–165.

Luo, Y.; Wang, C.; Hussein, M.; Qiao, Y.; Ma, L.; An, J.; Su, M. Three-Dimensional Microtissue Assay for High-Throughput Cytotoxicity of Nanoparticles. *Anal. Chem.* **2012,** *84,* 6731–6738.

Montaser, A.; Abdel-Mohsen, A.; Ramadan, M.; Sleem, A.; Sahffie, N.; Jancar, J.; Hebeish, A. Preparation and Characterization of Alginate/Silver/Nicotinamide Nanocomposites for Treating Diabetic Wounds. *Int. J. Biol. Macromol.* **2016,** *92,* 739–747.

Nam, S.; MubarakAli, D.; Kim, J. Characterization of Alginate/Silver Nanobiocomposites Synthesized by Solution Plasma Process and their Antimicrobial Properties. *J. Nanomater.* [Online] **2016,** 4712813. https://www.hindawi.com/journals/jnm/2016/4712813/.

Narayanan, K.; Han, S. Dual-Crosslinked Poly(Vinyl Alcohol)/Sodium Alginate/Silver Nanocomposite Beads—A Promising Antimicrobial Material. *Food Chem.* **2017,** *234,* 103–110.

Oliveira, A. S.; Alcântara, A. C. S.; Pergher, S. B. C. Bionanocomposite Systems Based on Montmorillonite and Biopolymers for the Controlled Release of Olanzapine. *Mater. Sci. Eng. C.* **2017,** *75,* 1250–1258.

Rădulescu, M.; Holban, A. M.; Mogoantă, L.; Bălşeanu, T. A.; Mogoşanu, G. D.; Savu, D.; Popescu, R. C.; Fufă, O.; Grumezescu, A. M.; Bezirtzoglou, E.; Lazar, V.; Chifiriuc, M. C. Fabrication, Characterization, and Evaluation of Bionanocomposites Based on Natural Polymers and Antibiotics for Wound Healing Applications. *Molecules* **2016,** *21,* 761.

Ratajska, M.; Boryniec, S. Biodegradation of Some Natural Polymers in Blends with Polyolefnes. *Polym. Adv. Technol.* **1999,** *10,* 625–633.

Rajesh K. Saini, Anil K., Bajpai, Era Jain. Advances in Bionanocomposites for Biomedical Applications, In *Biodegradable and Biocompatible Polymer Composites;* Navinchandra Gopal Shimpi Ed.; Woodhead Publishing Series in Composites Science and Engineering; Woodhead Publishing: UK, 2018, pp 379–399.

Sarikaya, M.; Tamerler, C.; Jen, A. K.; Schulten, K.; Baneyx, F. Molecular Biomimetics: Nanotechnology Through Biology. *Nat. Mater.* **2003,** *9,* 577–585.

Seth, A.; Lafargue, D.; Poirier, C.; Badier, T.; Delory, N.; Laporte, A.; Delbos, J. M.; Jeannin, V.; Péan, J. M.; Ménager, C. Optimization of Magnetic Retention in the Gastrointestinal Tract: Enhanced Bioavailability of Poorly Permeable Drug. *Eur. J. Pharm. Sci.* **2017,** *100,* 25–35.

Takai, O. Solution Plasma Processing (SPP). *Pure Appl. Chem.* **2008,** *80*(9), 2003–2011.

Tseng, K.; Chen, Y.; Shyue, J. Continuous Synthesis of Colloidal Silver Nanoparticles by Electrochemical Discharge in Aqueous Solutions. *J. Nanopart. Res.* **2011,** *13*(5), 1865–1872.

Valenzuela, F.; Covarrubias, C.; Martínez, C.; Smith, P.; Díaz-Dosque, M.; Yazdani-Pedram, M. Preparation and Bioactive Properties of Novel Bone-Repair Bionanocomposites Based on Hydroxyapatite and Bioactive Glass Nanoparticles. *J. Biomed. Mater. Res.* **2012,** *100*, 1672–1682.

Visakh, P. M.; Sigrid, L. *Polyethylene-Based Biocomposites and Bionanocomposites;* Thermoplastic Bionanocomposites Series; Scrivener Publishing LLC, Wiley: New York, 2016.

Wang, J.; Liu, C.; Shuai, Y.; Cui, X.; Nie, L. Controlled Release of Anticancer Drug Using Graphene Oxide as a Drug-Binding Effector in Konjac Glucomannan/Sodium Alginate Hydrogels. *Colloids Surf. B* **2014,** *113*, 223–229.

Wang, K.; Nune, K.; Misra, R. The Functional Response of Alginate-Gelatin-Nanocrystalline Cellulose Injectable Hydrogels Toward Delivery of Cells and Bioactive Molecules. *Acta Biomater.* **2016,** *36*, 143–151.

Yulizar, Y.; Foliatini; Elita Hafizah, M. A Facile and Effective Technique for the Synthesis of Thiol Modified Au/Alginate Nanocomposite and its Performance in Stabilizing Pickering Emulsion. *Arabian J. Chem.* [Online] **2016,** http://www.sciencedirect.com/science/article/pii/S1878535216300673 (accessed Oct, 2017).

Zhang, Y.; Lou, Z.; Zhang, X.; et al. A Simple Strategy to Fabricate Poly (acrylamide-co-alginate)/Gold Nanocomposites for Inactivation of Bacteria. *Appl. Phys. A* **2014,** *117,* 2009–2018.

Zhao, X.; Li, Q.; Li, X.; Xia, Y.; Wang, B., Zhao, Z. Antibacterial Activity and in Vitro Cytotoxicity Evaluation of Alginate-AgNP Fibers. *Text. Res. J.* **2017,** *87*(11), 1377–1386.

Zheng, J.; Xiao, Y.; Wang, L.; Lin, Z.; Yang, H.; Zhang, L.; Chen, G. Click Synthesis of Glucose-Functionalized Hydrophilic Magnetic Mesoporous Nanoparticles for Highly Selective Enrichment of Glycopeptides and Glycans. *J. Chromatogr. A.* **2014,** *1358,* 29–38.

Zvicer, J.; Samardzic, M.; Miskovic, V.; Obradovie, B. Cytotoxicity Studies of Ag/alginate Nanocomposite Hydrogels in 2D and 3D Cultures. [Online] **2015,** http://ieeexplore.ieee.org/abstract/document/7367664/ (accessed Oct, 2017).

CHAPTER 7

ALGINATE AND ITS APPLICATIONS IN TISSUE ENGINEERING

DILSHAD QURESHI[1], SEEMADRI SUBHADARSHINI[1],
SURAJ KUMAR NAYAK[1], DOMAN KIM[2], PREETAM SARKAR[3],
INDRANIL BANERJEE[1], and KUNAL PAL[1,*]

[1]Department of Biotechnology and Medical Engineering, National Institute of Technology, Rourkela, Odisha 769008, India

[2]Department of International Agricultural Technology, Institute of Green Bio Science and Technology, Seoul National University, Gangwon-do 25354, Republic of Korea

[3]Department of Food Process Engineering, National Institute of Technology, Rourkela, Odisha 769008, India

*Corresponding author. E-mail: kpal.nitrkl@gmail.com

7.1 INTRODUCTION

Evolution has limited the capability of adult humans to regenerate certain tissues in their fully functional form under circumstances of severe trauma and diseases. Researchers have introduced various techniques such as organ transplantation, prosthetics (artificial organs), and surgical operations to tackle the tissue damage problem. Unfortunately, the impediments associated with these techniques like immune rejection of transplants, expensive implants, and long-term surgical problems outweigh their advantages in the medical field (Castells-Sala et al., 2013). The complications associated with the above-specified techniques are circumvented by a new paradigm called "tissue engineering." As the name suggests, tissue engineering (TE) is the application of engineering methodologies in life sciences (Horch, 2012) for developing functional tissues in vitro, which are then easily transplanted in vivo (Sengupta et al., 2014). The tissue constructs are prepared for the cells, which cannot regenerate naturally but have the potential to induce and sustain regeneration under laboratory and natural body conditions (Williams, 2004). This interdisciplinary field is the amalgamation of engineering, medicine, material science, molecular biology, and cell biology. The main objective of this technique is to restore, improve, and maintain the functions of tissues or organs (Horch, 2012), which are damaged and left non-functional by trauma or injuries, birth defects, and diseases like cancer. This old yet still growing field is increasing its scope in the regeneration of all types of body tissues such as nerve, skin, liver, heart, cartilage, bone, and pancreas. Apart from the medical applications, TE has widespread non-therapeutic applications, for example, (i) tissue-engineered constructs serve as in vitro model of an organ to comprehend its physiology, cellular, and molecular processes like apoptosis and carcinogenesis that can help upgrading the medical treatment methods (Nigam and Mahanta, 2014), (ii) the prepared tissue constructs are used in combination with biosensors, to detect the presence of toxic agents, and (iii) for the development of personalized drugs (Hasan, 2017).

The three main pillars of TE are the cells, growth factors (GFs), and scaffolds, which can directly influence the outcome (Gugjoo et al., 2016). Autologous cells are the safest cell source to regenerate own tissues or organs in comparison to allogenic or xenogenic cells (Griffith and Naughton, 2002). Crosstalk between the cells and the cell-matrix is regulated by some set of proteins collectively called as "GFs," which include mitogens, morphogens, and growth-enhancing factors (Lee et al., 2011). In TE, these GFs serve as nature like niche and provide cues for the extracted cells to select a determined lineage and differentiate into an in vitro tissue. Scaffolds are the in vitro counterpart of the extracellular matrix (ECM), present between the varied cells of the tissue under in vivo conditions. They are the custom-tailored three-dimensional (3D) networks, composed of a variety of biomaterials, and provide nature-mimicked porous milieu to the extracted cells for de novo tissue regeneration. Its porous architecture supports cell adhesion in concert with the diffusion of nutrients and controlled release of GFs, thereby enhancing the cell–GF interactions (Castells-Sala et al., 2013). The interactions between the three pillars of TE are the basis of signal transduction through physical, chemical, and mechanical signaling, which guide the scaffold seeded cells to migrate, proliferate, and differentiate (Zhang et Shi al., 2013). The biomaterials from which the scaffolds are fabricated can be categorized as ceramics (e.g., hydroxyapatite [HA] and tri-calcium phosphate), natural polymers (e.g., collagen, proteoglycans, alginate [ALG], and chitosan [CS]), and synthetic polymers (e.g., polystyrene, poly-l-lactic acid [PLLA], polyglycolic acid, and poly-dl-lactic-co-glycolic acid [PLGA])

(O'brien, 2011). Since the engineered tissue, supported by the scaffold, has to be injected or implanted inside the human body, the biomaterials utilized for scaffold fabrication should possess the properties like biocompatibility, biodegradability, biomimetic, non-immunogenicity, non-toxicity (Edgar et al., 2016), and mechanical robustness (Khang, 2017).

The two decades old technique is regularly providing an insight of its infinite possibilities, which are gradually paving the way to cure severe trauma and diseases. But, just like the two sides of the coin, TE also suffers from several real-time complications which pose some risks in its practical applications in the medical field. Contamination of cell sources with viruses, the altered genetic makeup of cells during growth and differentiation, the unknown interaction between cell and scaffold material, and sterility of the prepared tissue construct are the major risks, which limit the translation of TE principles to successful clinical trials (Williams, 2004). To imitate the nature's biological system ex vivo; the cells, the scaffold, and the GFs should be orchestrated. The cell's responsive behavior towards its milieu and GFs can be successfully altered by the type of the biomaterial utilized for the fabrication of the scaffolds since they are in direct contact with each other. Thus, the selection of the biomaterials according to the experiment's demand is a crucial step. Scaffolds, prepared by the naturally occurring polymers such as collagen are prone to enzymatic hydrolysis in the body (Ikada, 2006), have low mechanical strength (O'brien, 2011), and mediate the transfer of pathogens (Zhang et al., 2013). The brittle nature and the inability to sustain the mechanical loading during remodeling restrict the use of ceramic scaffolds in spite of their compatibility with the bone tissue. Synthetic polymers experience rejection by the tissues due to their low biocompatibility, attributed to the presence of monomers (if not purified properly) (O'brien, 2011).

ALG is a linear unbranched polysaccharide of natural origin with characteristics such as biocompatibility, biodegradability, and mild gelation ability (Lee and Mooney, 2012). Interestingly, chemically and physically modified derivatives of ALG rearrange its structure in such a way that new properties, functions, and applications are imparted to it. ALG shows structural resemblance to the glycosaminoglycans (GAGs) of ECM of natural cell system, thereby registering its presence in TE as scaffolds (Bohari et al., 2011). It fulfills the prerequisites of biomaterials, such as their ability to be engineered, compatibility with the tissues in vivo (Cao, 2011), good mechanical properties, and alterable degradation rate in the body to retain the cells for a long time. This chapter concentrates on the use of natural polymer, ALG, as the fabrication material of 3D scaffolds in TE. It covers the brief overview of the fabrication techniques of ALG 3D scaffolds and their applications in various cell-seeded tissue constructs, which are used for the regeneration of different tissues.

7.2 PHYSICAL AND CHEMICAL ASPECTS OF ALGINATE (ALG)

7.2.1 SOURCES OF ALG

The cell wall constituents such as proteins and polysaccharides of the plant, algal, and bacterial cells serve as a structural component. Its main function is to provide rigidity and flexibility in order to communicate with biotic and abiotic environmental stresses around the cells (Popper et al., 2014). "Alginic acid" or its carboxylate salt called "ALG" is a class of natural polysaccharide which is harvested mostly from the cell wall of algal species and some bacterial species (Donati and Paoletti, 2009). *Phaeophyceae* (marine brown algae) was firstly reported as the source of alginic acid, where it was present as an amalgam of its different mono- and divalent salts in the cell wall. It was believed to be a structure-forming compound and was found to account for almost 40% of the algal dry matter (Donati and Paoletti, 2009). Apart from its role as cell wall constituent, ALG contributes as a capsular polysaccharide, biofilms and water reservoir in some other bacterial and algal species (Rehm, 2009). The molecular weight of ALG can vary widely between 50 and 100,000 kDa (Aravamudhan et al., 2014).

7.2.2 CHEMICAL STRUCTURE AND CONFORMATION

The molecular framework of the ALG is depicted as the copolymeric network of anionic uronic sugar monomers, namely, β-D-mannuronic acid (M) and its C-5 epimer α-L-guluronic acid (G) (Rehm, 2009). Interestingly, this unbranched linear polysaccharide is structured with its monomers linked together in a block-wise manner comprising homopolymeric MM and GG blocks with the interspersed heteropolymeric MG blocks (Marković et al., 2016). Mannuronate residues adopt a stable $^4C_1$ chair conformation to avoid steric clashes between the large COOH and other groups present in the ring structure. The hemiacetal mannuronate monomers are linked together by β (1→ 4) glycosidic linkage to form a block of consecutive MM residues (Aravamudhan et al., 2014). The hydroxyl groups of C1 and C4 of the participating M residues in the bond formation notably exhibit equatorial positions (Table 7.1) (De'Nobili et al., 2015). These diequatorial links produce a flat sheetlike pattern in the MM block.

TABLE 7.1 Chemical Structure of Different Components of Alginate (ALG) (Using ChemDraw Trial Version 12.0).

S. No.	Type	Structure
1.	Mannuronate (M)	
2.	Guluronate (G)	
3.	MMM block	
4.	GGG block	
5.	MGM block	

Source: Redrawn from De'Nobili et al. (2015).

Epimerases within the cells perform the C-5 epimerization of mannuronate and convert it to guluronate (Aravamudhan et al., 2014). $^{1}C_{4}$ is the preferred chair conformation of guluronic acid in the ALG and reduces the spatial interference between the groups (Aravamudhan et al., 2014). Guluronate monomers are covalently linked together by α (1→ 4) glycosidic bond, resulting in the formation of a homopolymer G-block. The tacticity of chemical groups around mannuronate and guluronate results in the formation of different molecular conformations. The –OH groups are exclusively present in the axial positions on C1 and C4 of the participating G-residues during G-block formation. The diaxial links between these residues produce the G-block with a rigid helical conformation. This rigidity increases with the gradual increase in the G-content and length of the G-block, which forms stiffer and brittle ALG gels (Andersen et al., 2011). The %G-content present in the polymer is credited to its source and is responsible for assessing the quality of ALG (Aravamudhan et al., 2014).

The alternating arrangement of mannuronate and guluronate (GM + MG) in equal or unequal proportion frames the third component (apart from G- and M-blocks), which influence the ALG's macroscopic and microscopic properties. Unlike M- and G-blocks, this diad component comprises either GM or MG as the repeating unit and acquires a certain fraction of the polysaccharide (Draget et al., 2005). The monomers of the repeating unit consist of alternate equatorial-axial or axial-equatorial (1→ 4) linked glycosidic bonds for GM or MG, respectively. Apart from the above-specified four diad (i.e., GG, MM, MG, and GM) blocks, the monomers are also found to be arranged in mixed proportion (Andersen et al., 2011). On assigning the degree of stiffness, these three blocks arrange themselves in the order of GG > MM > MG due to their characteristic bonding pattern (Harding et al., 2017).

The source, the constitutional profile, and the distribution of the aforesaid blocks are the prime features, which determine the microstructural and the behavioral properties of ALG (Dominguez, 2013). The monomeric profile determines the location and the function of ALG in the various algal and bacterial species. Till date, species of algae such as *Laminaria hyperborea,* *Macrocystis pyrifera,* and *Laminaria digitata* are the prominent reservoir of ALG (Rehm, 2009). Subtle differences exist between the functional profile of ALG in bacteria and algae. Several genera of bacteria such as *Azotobacter* and *Pseudomonas* confirm the presence of ALG as their extracellular polymeric material. *Pseudomonas aeruginosa*, an opportunistic pathogen, is found to secrete notable amounts of ALG in its slime layer while infecting cystic fibrosis patients and dormant cysts of *Azotobacter* was found to have stiffer ALG (Hay et al., 2013).

7.3 ALG-BASED SCAFFOLD ARCHITECTURES FOR TISSUE ENGINEERING (TE)

Exploiting the structural properties of ALG, synthesis of different kinds of scaffold architectures has been proposed. A general overview of the different techniques for synthesizing scaffolds using ALG has been described in this section.

7.3.1 ALG HYDROGEL

Hydrogel is a formulation, which is prepared by a cross-linked polymer and stores a large amount of water. The polymer chains contain a large number of hydrophilic functional groups (Ahmed, 2015). The void spaces within the polymer provide porosity to the hydrogel network. The presence of these spaces supports diffusion of nutrients, GFs, and cells, rendering the hydrogels as an important candidate to synthesize scaffold architectures for TE applications (Sun and Tan, 2013). The hydrated polymer architecture resembles the microenvironment of the cell's ECM and hence allows the spatial distribution, proliferation, and differentiation of the seeded cells (Sun and Tan, 2013). The type, size, and molecular weight of the polymer used, the type of cross-linkers and their concentration, and the fabrication technique used to produce the desired 3D structure are important considerations for the synthesis of scaffolds. By varying these properties, the mechanical strength and the degradation rate of the hydrogels can easily be tailored (Nakanishi, 2015). Interestingly, ALG fulfills the requirements of a polymer to be used as scaffold biomaterial due to its hydrophilic behavior, biocompatible nature, and matrix-like microstructure. Cross-linking of the polymer strands is achieved either by physical or chemical method. ALG is a polyanionic polymer. Owing to the presence of carboxylic groups, ALG shows an affinity towards polyvalent cations, resulting in the formation of hydrogels (Gwon et al., 2015). ALG gels can be prepared by a list of methods such as:

7.3.1.1 IONIC CROSS-LINKING

Owing to its polyanionic nature, ALG shows an affinity towards monovalent and divalent ions. The associated salts alter the solubility of the cross-linked polymer matrix in water. The sodium, potassium, and ammonium salts of

ALG are water-soluble in nature (Guiraldo et al., 2014). After exchanging these monovalent ions with divalent ions, a distinct change occurs in the ALG structural and macroscopic properties. Due to its monomeric profile, ALG exhibits varied affinity towards divalent cations in the decreasing order of Pb > Cu > Cd > Ba > Sr > Ca > Co, Ni, Zn > Mn (da Silva et al., 2017). Calcium is the most common divalent ion used to prepare ALG hydrogels. Calcium chloride ($CaCl_2$) solution is often used as a cross-linker solution (Lee and Mooney, 2012). Unlike the nonspecific electrostatic interactions responsible for the monovalent ion binding, Ca^{2+} binds to the ALG with a specific chelation process with specified coordinate bonds. This coordinate bonding is mainly dependent on the G-block distribution in the ALG structure (Montanucci et al., 2015). The requirement of correct arrangement of COOH groups within a specified distance for chelation of Ca^{2+} ions is mainly fulfilled by G-blocks of ALG polymer (Montanucci et al., 2015). The two adjacent G-blocks of different ALG polymer strands get interconnected with a centrally coordinated Ca^{2+}, forming "eggbox" junction zones of gelation (Bowman et al., 2016). This results in the cross-linking of the ALG polymer strands leading to the formation of an ordered hydrogel. Polyguluronate blocks dominate the cross-linking capacity, but, researches indicate that mannuronate residues (in MM and MG blocks) also contribute to the chelation of ions with weak junction zones (Rinaudo, 2014; da Silva et al., 2017). Ma et al. (2015) reported the formation of thermostable cross-linked ALG gels utilizing lanthanide ions (europium ions [Eu^{3+}] or terbium ions [Tb^{3+}]) due to their high coordination numbers (Ma and Wang, 2015).

Cross-linking between the ALG polymeric chains by the divalent ions can be achieved by two broadly categorized processes, namely, "external gelation or diffusion method" and "internal gelation or internal setting" (Pawar and Edgar, 2012; Kaklamani et al., 2014). As the name suggests, the diffusion method employs the diffusion of Ca^{2+} ions in the polymeric architecture of ALG solution and initiates the interchain bonding (Pawar and Edgar, 2012). This method involves the incorporation of sodium ALG in the calcium chloride ($CaCl_2$) solution reservoir in a dropwise fashion, which gives rise to ALG hydrogel bead (Figure 7.1).

Internal gelation is achieved by incorporating inactive cross-linking agents such as $CaCO_3$, $CaSO_4$, and so forth in the ALG solution, which starts solubilizing when the solution approaches an acidic pH with the help of glucono-δ-lactone or acetic acid. Lower pH triggers slow release of Ca^{2+} ions in the ALG solution with the subsequent initiation of the internal gelation (Figure 7.2) (Cao, 2011).

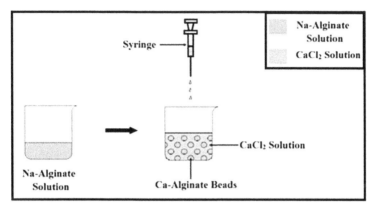

FIGURE 7.1   External gelation process.

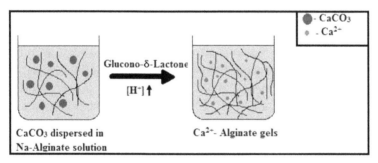

FIGURE 7.2   Internal gelation process.

7.3.1.2   COVALENT CROSS-LINKING

According to the application, appropriate changes in the polymer properties are desirable. ALG, owing to the presence of –COOH or –OH groups, allows early tailoring of the architecture by tuning its physical, chemical, and mechanical properties. Covalent cross-linking replaces the plastic behavior of the ALG gels under stress conditions to an elastic one (Lee and Mooney, 2012). Different chemical modification approaches of the functional groups of ALG have been investigated to date. Oxidation, reductive amination, sulfonation, copolymerization, and cyclodextrin linkage are the methods to modify –OH groups, while –COOH groups are modified by esterification and amidation (Yang et al., 2011). In the presence of oxidants like periodate, oxidation of –OH group occurs and results in the cleavage of the C2–C3 bond of the sugar rings, dialdehyde formation, and depolymerization of ALG

(Marinho Carvalho Bjørge, 2016). High degradation rate and low stiffness evolve as the properties of the oxidized ALG (Kalaf and Sell, 2016).

The open ring structure is prone to other chemical modifications such as "reductive amination." Alkyl amine reacts with the open ring to form a Schiff base (Marinho Carvalho Bjørge, 2016), following treatment with a reducing agent such as $NaBH_3CN$ (Yang et al., 2011). This reaction endows ALG with properties such as low surface tension and adsorbent for heavy metals (Kalaf and Sell, 2016).

Sulfating agents such as SO_3/complexes, sulfuric acid-carbodiimide, and chlorosulfonic acid-formamide are responsible for the esterified sulfation of –OH groups present on the uronic acid monomers of ALG (Mhanna et al., 2017). This modification increases the overall negative charge on the ALG polymer, which closely mimic the abundant GAG, heparin (HN). It increases its biocompatibility in blood and anticoagulant, antioxidant, and anti-inflammatory nature (Kalaf and Sell, 2016; Kerschenmeyer et al., 2017).

The conversion of uronic acids of ALG into amides is achieved by carbodiimide chemistry, in which 1-ethyl-(dimethylaminopropyl) carbodiimide along with a co-reactant, N-hydroxysulfosuccinimide couple –COOH groups of the ALG polymers with the compounds which contain primary or secondary amines (d'Ayala et al., 2008). Carboxylic acid groups esterified with long alkyl chains impart hydrophobic and amphiphilic nature to ALG (Kalaf and Sell, 2016). Murdzheva and Denev (2016) investigated the effect of ultrasound frequency and power on the speed of esterification reaction between ALG–COOH groups and varied alcohols. The research reported that ultrasound-assisted alginic acid esterification proceeded approximately 10 times faster than the conventional esterification reaction, performed under normal conditions (Figure 7.3) (Murdzheva and Denev, 2016).

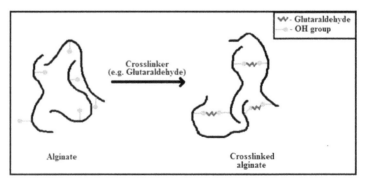

FIGURE 7.3   Chemical cross-linking of alginate (ALG) with cross-linker, for example, glutaraldehyde.

7.3.1.3 THERMAL GELATION

Thermal gelation is a process in which solution phase of a polymer is converted to hydrogel under the stimulus of varying temperature. The threshold phase transition temperature below which polymer prevails in sol form is referred to as "lower critical solution temperature" (LCST) (Klouda, 2015). ALG thermosensitive hydrogelation can be achieved by grafting some polymers, such as *N*-isopropylacrylamide (NiPAAM) polymers, poly(ethylene oxide)–*b*-poly(propylene oxide)–*b*-poly(ethylene oxide) (PEO–PPO–PEO), and polyethylene glycol (PEG)-biodegradable polyester copolymers on ALG. Poly(N-isopropylacrylamide) (PNIPAM) is the most widely and commonly utilized thermosensitive polymer with an LCST near to the physiological temperature (32°C) of the body (Lee and Mooney, 2012). The interpenetrating network formed by the graft copolymerization of ALG polymer by PNIPAM hydrogel has been studied. This interpenetration evolves with the high mechanical strength of PNIPAM thermosensitive hydrogel and viscoelastic gel formation of ALG (Figure 7.4) (Lee and Mooney, 2012).

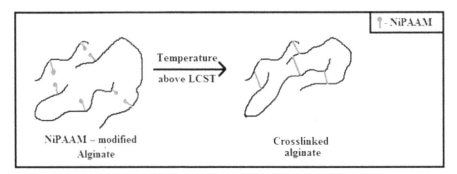

FIGURE 7.4 Thermal gelation of ALG.

7.3.1.4 CELL CROSS-LINKING

Cells which we deliver to regenerate the tissues can also work as cross-linkers for the formation of ALG hydrogels. Since ALG lack cell-interactive functional groups, it is normally tailored by chemically coupling short peptides, composed of arginine–glycine–aspartate (RGD) sequence applying carbodiimide chemistry. Incorporating and dispersing cells in the modified ALG solution initiate hydrogel 3D network formation through specific ligand–receptor interaction between cells and RGD sequences of different

ALG strands even in the absence of the cross-linkers (Figure 7.5) (Sun and Tan, 2013).

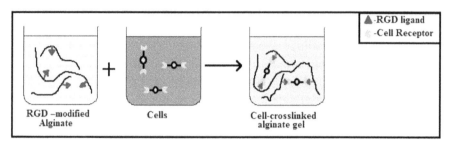

FIGURE 7.5   Cell cross-linking of ALG.

7.3.1.5   FREE RADICAL POLYMERIZATION

ALG strands can be intertwined with each other to produce a porous gel-like structure by employing a common technique of free-radical polymerization. Grafting of ALG with polymerizable groups and induction of covalent cross-linking among them by the free radicals generated from the UV-irradiated initiators is the normal free-radical polymerization approach. However, acknowledging the cytotoxic nature of the photo-initiators, new regimes of cross-linking, compatible with the body, have been developed (Sun and Tan, 2013). Temperature-induced gelation of ALG, grafted with photo cross-linkable groups such as glacidyl methacrylate (GMA), for injectable scaffolds have been studied. Cross-linking of ALG–GMA macromonomers was achieved by free radicals produced by cytocompatible initiator molecules such as ammonium persulfate and N,N,N′,N′-tetramethylethylenediamine (Wang et al., 2015).

Nowadays, radiation-induced chemical cross-linking between the modified ALG strands circumvent the requirement of initiators. Elsayed et al. (2016) prepared photo-cross-linkable styryl-pyridine-modified ALG (ASP-ALG), which was casted into a membrane. Exposure of the ASP-ALG to the UV-radiation induced cycloaddition addition reaction between the photoactive ASP groups. This ultimately resulted in the joining of the ALG strands in an interconnected 3D structure. XRD, SEM, FTIR, UV–visible spectra, swelling behavior, and biodegradability analyses of the prepared photo-cross-linked hydrogel revealed its promising applications in drug delivery (Figure 7.6) (Elsayed et al., 2016).

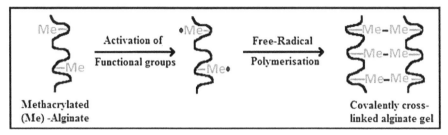

FIGURE 7.6 Free-radical polymerization of ALG.

7.3.2 MICROPARTICLES

In vivo delivery of substances such as cells, proteins, GFs, and small drug molecules in their biologically active form is a critical issue as they are highly prone to the environmental degradation at the injected site. Enzymatic and physical factors limit their active life, release profile and dosage before or after they reach the site of action by degrading and denaturing them. The current approach to terminate the above-specified problems is the fabrication of delivery systems of micrometer dimension. The process of encapsulation of the delivery materials within a coating of polymeric material and having the size range of micrometers is termed as "microencapsulation." The product obtained from this process is called as "microparticle" whose diameter ranges between 1 and 1000 μm (Comolli and Clark, 2014). These microparticles are used as carriers for the delivery of cells, proteins, GFs, and drugs with several advantages such as: (i) encapsulation provides a boundary to the delivery material to protect it through the transfer process (to its action site), (ii) reduced action of enzymes and environmental factors at the site of action to maintain its therapeutic efficacy, and (iii) prolonged and sustained release of the delivered material.

Microparticles are broadly categorized as "microspheres" and "microcapsules." Microspheres are so called due to their spherical morphology in which the active ingredient is present either as fully dissolved or as dispersion. Microcapsules are the formulations in which the active ingredient is present in more discrete domains known as "core" with a coating of hydrogel matrix around it as the "shell" (Figure 7.7) (Muhaimin, 2013).

ALG microspheres are generally prepared by an external gelation method in which the ALG sol is already mixed with the material to be encapsulated and is dropped in the isotonic $CaCl_2$ solution in dropwise fashion through a needle (Paques et al., 2014). Production of ALG hydrogel spheres encapsulating *Ganoderma lucidum* spores (GLSs) employing elec-trospraying technique has been reported. The aqueous sol containing GLS/ALG is extruded through a stainless steel needle and induced to convert into fine highly charged aerosol droplets by electric charge applied to the needle. The droplet size covers a wide range of micrometers and then added to the $CaCl_2$ solution to form uniform-sized hydrogel beads (Zhao et al., 2016). Water-in-oil emulsion solvent diffusion method with post Ca^{2+} cross-linking has been reported to prepare ALG gel spheres. The aqueous solution containing ALG and hydrophilic "Blue Dextran" is added to an oil phase, composed of ethyl acetate, drop-by-drop under continuous stirring. ALG microspheres collected by centrifugation were then incubated in the $CaCl_2$ bath for post-cross-linking, recollected, and freeze-dried (Figure 7.8) (Baimark and Srisuwan, 2014).

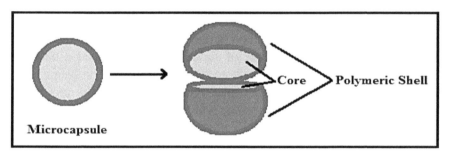

FIGURE 7.7   Structure of microcapsule.

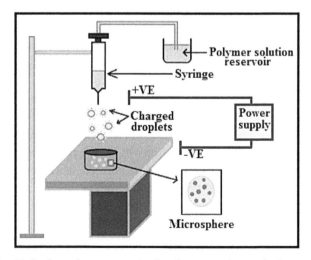

FIGURE 7.8   ALG microsphere preparation by electrospraying method.

Encapsulation of *Bifidobacterium* BB-12 in the microcapsular morphology of ALG hydrogel by emulsification/internal gelation technique has been reported. ALG aqueous solution containing $CaCO_3$ and freeze-dried cells was dispersed in the rapeseed oil phase under magnetic stirring in the presence of emulsifier (Tween 80) and glacial acetic acid. Prepared capsules were separated, processed to remove the oil phase, and subsequently freeze-dried (Holkem et al., 2016).

Adherence of cells and mutual interaction are the prerequisites of scaffold material to be used for cell encapsulation. ALG, regardless of its resemblance with the ECM, profoundly lacks the property to support cell–matrix interactions and cell-adhesion. RGD–ALG has been reported to encapsulate cells with higher adhesivity and maintain interactive microenvironment. Encapsulation of genetically modified mesenchymal stem cells (MSCs) used to release erythropoietin from RGD–ALG microcapsules prepared by electrostatic drop generator has been previously reported (Garate et al., 2015).

7.3.3   POROUS SCAFFOLDS LIKE SPONGES, FOAMS, AND FIBERS

In TE applications, micro-architecture of the prepared scaffolds should provide a 3D network which closely simulates the in vivo niche of the cells. The porosity of the scaffold reinforces the diffusion process of nutrients and oxygen, structural support for the attachment of the cells, and signal transduction, which stimulates the correct differentiation of the cells (Chen et al., 2015). Acknowledging gelling properties of ALG, its development as porous scaffolds in a variety of forms such as sponges, fibers, and foams has been reported.

7.3.3.1   SPONGES

ALG has been fabricated into interconnected porous structures called as sponges, which has found its application as scaffolds. Freeze-drying is the most frequently applied technique for converting ALG solution into sponge. Principally, the process covers three stages: (i) cross-linking of ALG solution to form a hydrogel, (ii) freezing of the hydrogel, and (iii) lyophilization (Song et al., 2015). The concentration of the ALG, G/M ratio, initial concentration of the ALG solution, and the type and the concentration of the cross-linker used have a significant effect on the microstructural properties such as pore size and pore number of the sponges (Shapiro and Cohen, 1997).

7.3.3.2 FOAMS

Macroporous architecture such as foam is formed when the polymer strands are arranged as porous interconnecting channel network. Foams have potential advantages over normal hydrogels, which include: (i) support for anchorage-dependent cell lines, (ii) boost nutrient transport, and (iii) avert necrotic center formation (Dhandayuthapani et al., 2011). ALG-based foams are now attaining attention as artificial ECM in vitro so as to maintain an interface with the biological system in vivo for TE applications. One of the most common methods of ALG-based foam preparation is carried out in the following steps: (i) preparation of ALG solution containing foaming agents (to stabilize wet foam), ion source (to initiate gelation), and plasticizers, (ii) continuous aeration of the viscous ALG sol with high-shear mixing, and (iii) air-drying of the hydrated foam to remove the aqueous fraction, thereby leaving behind porous interconnected 3D structure (Figure 7.9) (Andersen, 2013; Iannace and Park, 2015).

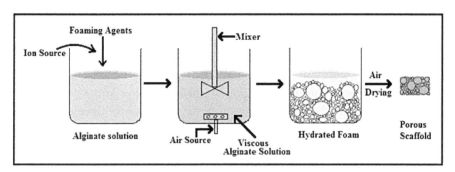

FIGURE 7.9   ALG foam preparation.

7.3.3.3 FIBERS

Fabricating ALG hydrogel as nanofibers have paved a new way to imitate extracellular matrices at nanoscale environment with high surface-to-volume ratio and highly ordered structure. Its role as a carrier and supporting architecture for cells in TE has gained importance due to their capability to support the morphogenesis of the cells along a particular pattern (Liu et al., 2014).

Over the period of years, electrospinning has become evident as the methodology to fashion ALG solution into finely tunable ultrathin nanofiber mats (Sridhar et al., 2015). ALG is woven into nanofiber mats through electrospinning which works on the principle of applying a high voltage around the spinneret during the extrusion of the polymeric solution. High voltage charges heat the solution droplet to such an extent that decreases the surface tension of the solution. This phenomenon causes instability and lengthening of the droplet in the form of fibers. The fibers can be post-cross-linked by incubating in the aqueous $CaCl_2$ bath (Zhao et al., 2015; Xue et al., 2017).

7.4 FABRICATION OF SCAFFOLDS

Cells are not present as a secluded entity in the tissues. They interact with the adjacent cells and surrounding matrix, which governs their behavioral response according to the biological, physicochemical, and mechanical cues. Scaffolds serve as ECM analog for the seeding of the cells in vitro and maintaining a sustained niche like microenvironment until these cells construct their own ECM in vivo before scaffold degradation. Therefore, porosity, pore structure, and interconnectivity of the polymeric scaffold are the critical issues for optimizing mechanical strength, stiffness, cell attachment, survival, proliferation, and migration (Annabi et al., 2010). These variables can be narrowed for various scaffold architectures according to our requirements with the advent of scaffold fabrication techniques.

7.4.1 ELECTROSPINNING

Electrospinning is a technique which transforms the aqueous or melted solution of polymer into long threaded fibers. The dimension of the polymer fibers ranges in between nano- to micrometers by applying an electrostatic field. The polymeric solution is filled in a syringe (or polymer solution reservoir) and is subsequently extruded out through a thin needle, called as "spinneret." It serves as one of the electrodes in the setup. The fibers are collected onto a second electrode, "collector." The extruded drop of the solution starts accumulating same surface charges as that of the spinneret. The spherical shape of the drops starts destabilizing when a high electric voltage is applied between the two electrodes, spinneret and collector. At the very point when the generated charge exceeds the surface tension, the drop reforms itself into an elongated and stretched Taylor cone. A jet of polymer, in a spiral trajectory with a much-reduced diameter, starts ejecting from the cone towards the collector with continuous solvent evaporation. The fibers are collected as electrospun fiber mats. Ultrathin fibers, fabricated using this technique, have a high porosity which aid in the nutrient supply to the cells, formation of interconnected mesh architecture, and high surface area-to-volume ratios. This provides an ordered surface for cell attachment (Figure 7.10).

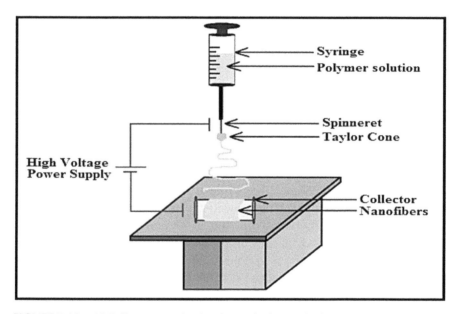

FIGURE 7.10   ALG fiber preparation by elecrospinning method.

The rate of flow of the polymeric solution from the spinneret, the concentration of the polymer solution, and the interspace between the two electrodes are some of the factors that regulate the diameter of the electrospun fibers (Loh and Choong, 2013). A reduction in the fiber diameter gradually increases the crystalline structure of the polymer matrix, with a subsequent increment in the tensile strength, tensile modulus, and shear modulus. It provides the scaffold enough mechanical strength to tune cell growth by overcoming cell cytoskeleton forces (Dahlin et al., 2011).

Due to the polyanionic nature of the ALG backbone, electrostatic repulsion between the chains limits its capability to be woven in electrospunned fibers. Repulsive forces can be overcome by blending ALG with other polymers (Kyzioł et al., 2017). Hu et al. (2015) reported the preparation of nanofibers of sodium ALG, by blending it with PEO, an uncharged synthetic polymer. It interacts with ALG chains through hydrogen bonding and masks the repulsive forces to successfully create crystalline nanofibers (Hu et al., 2015). Kusumastuti et al. (2016) optimized the process parameters, such as composition, concentration, and conductivity of polymeric solutions, to fabricate uniform electrospun nanofibers of CS–ALG with polyvinyl alcohol. The conducted research resulted in the formation of fibers having diameters in the range of 200–400 nm (Kusumastuti et al., 2016).

Considering the low capacity of the ALG hydrogels to allow adherence of the seeded cells, Wongkanya et al. (2017) reported the formation of nanofiber mats of soy protein modified ALG. Electrospinning of an aqueous solution of sodium ALG blended with a copolymer PEO, soy protein isolated (SPI), and antibacterial drug (vancomycin) was used to prepare nanosize fibers. The antibacterial and the biocompatibility studies reported that drug-loaded sodium ALG (SA)/PEO/SPI fibers were able to release the drug in its active form. The mats were biocompatible and noncytotoxic. This study reported that SA/PEO/SPI electrospun fibers can be a suitable candidate for biomedical applications (Wongkanya et al., 2017).

7.4.2   FREEZE-DRYING

This very technique exploits the differences in the temperatures of sublimation of organic or aqueous solvents and the polymers whose fabrication into a 3D structure is the target. Scaffolds are normally fabricated by preparing a solution of polymers in aqueous or organic solvents which is subsequently resuspended in a water phase. After loading the emulsion into a mold, freezing at around (−70 to −80°C) temperature results in the solvent crystallization. Frozen samples are then placed under vacuum, which generates enough heat to sublimate the solvent crystals without entering into a liquid phase. This leaves behind a porous interconnected structure of the polymer (Garg et al., 2012; Lu et al., 2013). Morphology of the scaffolds, such as pore size and porosity, prepared by freeze-drying can be varied with the alteration in the instrumental parameters (e.g., freezing rate and freezing temperature) and solution parameters (e.g., molecular weight, concentration of the polymer, and the viscosity of the formulation). Solovieva et al. (2017) designed a series of freeze-dried ALG–fibrinogen (FG) composite scaffolds for engineering of skin tissues severely damaged by burns and trauma. The novel procedure for scaffold preparation follows the order: (i) mixing of ALG and FG solutions in different proportions, (ii) conversion of FG to fibrin, anti-fibrinolysis, and gelation were achieved with thrombin, ε-aminocapronic acid, and $CaCl_2$, respectively, and (iii) the prepared gels were subsequently frozen and dried under vacuum to obtain intact porous structure, possessing an average pore size from about 60 to 300 μm. Biocompatibility of the scaffolds was confirmed with the adhesion, survival, proliferation, and differentiation of four different skin cell lines, while their re-vascularization capability was studied by mouse aortic ring sprouting model (Figure 7.11) (Solovieva et al., 2017).

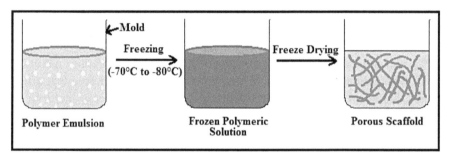

FIGURE 7.11   Porous scaffold preparation by freeze-drying technique.

7.4.3   RAPID PROTOTYPING

Among the plethora of scaffold fabrication techniques, rapid prototyping also known as "solid free-form fabrication (SFF)" or "additive manufacturing process" is gaining importance in the current day world. The name signifies rapid fabrication of finely tuned 3D porous architectures, models, or prototypes directly from computer files in the form of "computer-aided design" (Yagnik, 2014) or from scanned images of computed tomography, and magnetic resonance imaging. The scaffold materials are deposited on one above the other in an additive approach. Conventional techniques have limited microstructure variability owing to the restricted shapes of porogens and 3D molds, while SFF provides more freedom for the fabrication of more ordered and complex internal structure of the scaffolds for homogeneous cell seeding (Chia and Wu, 2015). Various techniques come under this technique such as 3D printing, stereolithography, selective laser sintering (SLS), and fused deposition modeling (FDM) with their own advantages and limitations (Wang et al., 2015).

7.4.3.1 THREE-DIMENSIONAL PRINTING

This technique allows the creation of ECM identical scaffolds with controlled 3D contour for in vivo implantation. Unlike the conventional scaffold preparation techniques which are subtractive in nature, it is an additive process. A 3D printing employs extrusion of binding material or binder through a computerized nozzle in a manner already programmed according to an electronic blueprint. The printhead selectively deposits the binder solution on powdered polymer layered on the computerized platform (Chia and Wu, 2015). Synchronization of the platform and the nozzle assembles the polymer in a 2D form in layer-by-layer fashion, ultimately constructing a physical 3D form of a scaffold. Scaffold fabrication with this technique offers some advantages such as: (i) controlled pore size, structure, and porosity, and (ii) ability to form complex frameworks (Do et al., 2018). On account of the various properties of polyuronide ALG, such as rapid gelation kinetics in the cationic environment, shear thinning rheological behavior, controllable viscosity by modulating its molecular weight and concentration, and its use as "bioinks" in 3D bioprinters, it has been promoted (Axpe and Oyen, 2016). To improve its mechanical properties, ALG is normally amended through chemical processes or by developing its composites with other polymers (Axpe and Oyen, 2016). Microfluidic channels are an effective approach to increase the viability of the encapsulated cells by providing nutrient flow to them. Zhang et al. (2013) reported the successful direct bioprinting of vessel-like tubular microfluidic channels with ALG and CS hydrogels which were found to support cell viability through their effective media exchange capability (Zhang et al., 2013). Wang et al. (2015) demonstrated 3D printing of an anti-inflammatory composite scaffold, amalgamating the feature of a stable hydrogel formation of ALG, osteoconductive ability of hydroxyapatite particles (nHAp), and anti-inflammatory nature of atsttrin protein. The in vivo and in vitro analysis concluded that the scaffold was non-cytotoxic and it maintained a controlled release profile of atsttrin, which in turn, promoted bone defect regeneration with tumor necrosis factor (TNF)/tumor necrosis factor receptor (TNFR) signaling involvement (Wang et al., 2015). Pan et al. (2016) reported the 3D bioplotter-mediated scaffold preparation from the ALG/gelatin composite. Mechanical robustness, water absorption capacity, and degradation rate of the composite scaffolds were optimized by post-cross-linking its components, that is, ALG and gelatin, with $CaCl_2$ and glutaraldehyde, respectively (Figure 7.12) (Pan et al., 2016).

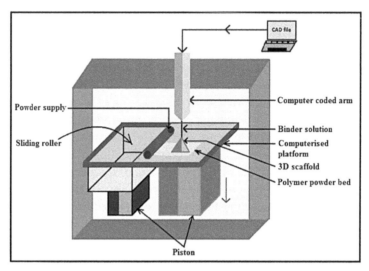

FIGURE 7.12   Three-dimensional (3D) scaffold fabrication by 3D printing approach.

The authors have not reported the fabrication of ALG scaffold by other rapid prototyping methods such as stereolithography, SLS, and FDM.

7.4.4   GAS FOAMING

Use of toxic organic solvents, nonhomogeneous pore size and porosity, and poor interconnected geometry are some of the major limitations of the conventional porous scaffold fabrication techniques (Elamparithi and Moorthy, 2017). To circumvent these drawbacks, gas foaming technique, which exploits the solubility nature of gases in the polymeric solutions to synthesize porous scaffolds, has been proposed (Daskalaki, 2009). In this technique, gases delivered at low/high pressures or its release through chemical reaction starts nucleation and growth of gas bubbles throughout the dispersion medium. When the pressure drops, the preformed bubbles frame the porous cavities in the polymer with good interconnectivity (Dehghani and Annabi, 2011). Various factors such as solubility of a gas in the polymer, nucleation and growth rate of bubbles, and diffusion rate of the gas molecules at the site of nucleation govern the overall porosity and pore structure of the prepared scaffold (Tomlins, 2015). Ceccaldi et al. (2017) proposed the fabrication of macroporous ALG-based foam scaffold by gas foaming technique for the 3D culture of MSCs. Foaming of the ALG solution with the gas forming agent, that is, sodium carbonate, followed by freezing and lyophilization resulted in ALG-based foam. The formed foams were subsequently seeded with MSCs. The research also proposed that varying of the type and the concentration of the surfactant, it is possible to tailor the porosity and the pore structure of the scaffold (Ceccaldi et al., 2017).

7.4.5 THERMALLY INDUCED PHASE SEPARATION (TIPS)

Fabrication of scaffolds with high interconnected and varied range of pore architecture has been widely explored by the technique called "thermally induced phase separation (TIPS)." It is based on the alteration of the temperature of the polymer-diluent system in order to alter their miscibility with each other (Conoscenti et al., 2017). The general series of events comprising TIPS technique include: (i) preparation of polymer-diluent homogenous solution at elevated temperatures, (ii) casting of the solution into the desired mold followed by controlled removal of thermal energy, which induces phase separation, thereby dividing the system into a polymer-rich and a polymer-lean phases, (iii) polymer starts crystallizing in the polymer-rich phase, while amorphous polymer containing diluent (polymer-lean phase) is subsequently extracted by solvent extraction (Lloyd et al., 1990; Martínez-Pérez et al., 2011), and (iv) evaporation of the extractant which leads to the formation of a microporous scaffold architecture (Ishigami et al., 2014). The scaffold morphology, shape, and pore size can be controlled by modulating the process parameters, such as type and concentration of polymer, solvent composition, (Akbarzadeh and Yousefi, 2014), phase separation conditions, and crystallization kinetics (Lloyd et al., 1990; Martínez-Pérez et al., 2011). Zhang et al. (2015) reported the preparation of silk fibroin (SF)/SA composite nanofibrous scaffolds through TIPS method. The authors could achieve pore diameter in the range of 50–500 nm and >85% porosity. Nanofibrous SF/SA scaffolds showed good cytocompatibility with MG63 cells (Figure 7.13) (Zhang et al., 2015).

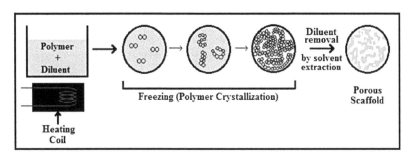

FIGURE 7.13 Microporous scaffold fabrication by thermally induced phase separation.

7.5 APPLICATIONS OF ALG SCAFFOLDS IN TE

ALG is widely used for the preparation of the scaffolds in various TE applications like bone and cartilage regeneration, cell encapsulation, drug and GF delivery, and so forth. This can be accounted to its unique properties like biocompatibility, biodegradability, and porous microstructure that are quite advantageous for TE application. Below is a list of ongoing ALG scaffold applications in various TE fields over a span of last 5 years (Table 7.2).

7.5.1 BONE TE

Bone repair and reconstruction is a much-talked-about issue and is a major concern in the healthcare industry. Where the conventional clinical practices fail, TE has emerged as a promising alternative. Bone TE deals with methods and practices involved in fabrication of constructs that resemble the physical, chemical, and biological properties of natural bone tissue. Sharma et al. (2016) fabricated nano-biocomposite scaffolds using CS, gelatin, ALG, and HA that showed improved biocompatibility and enhanced osteoblast proliferation. Wang et al. (2016) developed self-setting iPSMSC–ALG–calcium phosphate paste for bone TE, which showed success in cranial bone reconstruction in vivo (Wang et al., 2016). Venkatesan et al. (2014) made a comparative study between CS and ALG (CS-ALG) scaffold and CS–ALG biocomposite scaffold blended with fucoidan (CS-ALG-fucoidan). The scaffolds were prepared by freeze-drying method. They suggested that CS–ALG–fucoidan scaffolds as a promising blend for bone TE applications (Venkatesan et al., 2014). Sajesh et al. (2013) incorporated polypyrrole–ALG (PPy-ALG) blend with CS to develop a conducting polypyrrole-based scaffold using lyophilization method for bone TE (Sajesh et al., 2013). Marsich et al. (2013) developed nanocomposite scaffolds of ALG–HA. The addition of silver nanoparticles endowed antibacterial properties to the scaffolds. The scaffolds were prepared by internal gelation-cum-freeze-drying method. The scaffolds promoted osteoblast proliferation (Marsich et al., 2013).

7.5.2 CARTILAGE TE

Articular cartilage defects and injuries are prevalent and very common in old age people. This leads to numerous health problems because the

TABLE 7.2 Recent Applications of ALG in Different Types of Tissue Engineering.

Application domain	Composition	Purpose	Reference
Bone tissue engineering (TE)	Peptide incorporated 3D porous ALG Scaffold	Bone-forming peptide 1 (BFP-1) combined with ALG formed peptide-incorporated PAS (p-PAS) for bone repair.	(Luo et al., 2016)
	Hap-coated chitosan (CS)–ALG PEC porous scaffold	CS–ALG polyelectrolyte complex 3D porous hybrid scaffold supported attachment and proliferation of MG63 osteosarcoma cells in vitro.	(Patil et al., 2017)
	ALG/cockle shell powder nanocomposite bone scaffold	The scaffold facilitated osteoblast growth, proliferation, and viability.	(Ahmed et al., 2017)
	ALG–CS–gelatin composite 3D scaffold incorporating bacterial cellulose nanocrystals	The scaffold showed excellent biocompatibility, cytocompatibility, and stability and facilitated the proliferation, attachment, and differentiation of osteoblastic MC3T3-E1 cells.	(Yan et al., 2017)
Cartilage TE	Polycaprolactone (PCL) and chondrocyte cell-encapsulated ALG hydrogel	Improved type II collagen fibril formation and cartilage tissue in the PCL–ALG gel (+TGFβ) hybrid scaffold	(Kundu et al., 2015)
	Nanocellulose–ALG bioink	3D bioprinting of human chondrocytes	(Markstedt et al., 2015)
	Poly(l-glutamic acid) and ALG hydrogel	The study showed rapid in vivo gel formation, injectability, cell growth, mechanical stability, and ectopic cartilage formation.	(Yan et al., 2014)
	Self-cross-linked oxidized ALG/gelatin hydrogel	The study showed self-cross-linked oxidized ALG/gelatin hydrogel as an effective cell-attracting, injectable adhesive matrix for the formation of neo-cartilage in the osteoarthritis treatment and management.	(Balakrishnan et al., 2014)
Drug and growth factor (GF) delivery	Calcium phosphate cement with ALG	Biological proteins like lysozyme and bovine serum albumin were loaded onto and effectively released from the scaffold.	(Lee et al., 2011)

TABLE 7.2 (Continued)

Application domain	Composition	Purpose	Reference
	Spray-dried ALG microparticles in collagen–hydroxyapatite scaffolds	Sustained release of vascular endothelial GF in rat calvarial defect model in vivo that enhanced bone regeneration and improved vessel formation.	(Quinlan et al., 2017)
	CS–ALG scaffold	Sustained GF delivery and bioactivity with TGF-β1 release aiding in homogeneous matrix deposition and chondrogenesis.	(Reed and Wu, 2017)
	ALG and DNA scaffold	Suitable delivery system for diabetic wound healing tested in mouse models of diabetes mellitus.	(Tellechea et al., 2015)
	ALG-based hybrid scaffold/nanofiber mesh	Sustained GF release and controlled delivery of recombinant bone morphogenetic protein-2 for bone and cartilage tissue repair	(Kolambkar et al., 2011)
Cardiac TE	ALG and hyaluronic acid hydrogels	Therapeutic heart muscle reconstruction by in situ cross-linking of hydrogel that improved its functionality and mechanical properties apt for a myocardial tissue.	(Dahlmann et al., 2013)
	ALG	Treatment of myocardial infarction	(Ruvinov and Cohen, 2016)
	ALG scaffold with immobilized RGD peptide	Contributed to better preservation of regenerated tissue in the culture media and formation of functional cardiac muscle tissue.	(Shachar et al., 2011)
	Gold nanoparticle-decellularized ALG matrix hybrids	For the treatment of myocardial infarction. The hybrid scaffold patches were found better than pristine patches with superior functions like faster calcium transients, lower excitation thresholds, and stronger contraction force.	(Shevach et al., 2014)

TABLE 7.2 *(Continued)*

Application domain	Composition	Purpose	Reference
	Electrospun sodium ALG/polyethylene oxide core-shell nanofibers scaffolds	High potential for cardiac TE as it promoted fibroblast cell proliferation and attachment.	(Ma et al., 2012)
Skin TE	Hybrid ALG-Collagen Biopolymer	Tissue substitutes and 3D in vitro models by laser-assisted bioprinting technique for skin TE.	(Koch et al., 2012)
	Aligned poly(lactic acid)–CS nanofibers	Novel parallel blade collector method was used to fabricate electrospun PLA-CS nanofibers for skin TE	(Shalumon et al., 2012)
	Bilayer scaffold of CS/PCL nanofibrous mat and PLLA microporous disk	Bilayer scaffolds lead to a great increase in cell proliferation. The bilayer scaffold microenvironment closely resembled that present during the initial phase of wound healing, the native extracellular matrix.	(Lou et al., 2014)
	N-acetylglucosamine modified ALG sponges as scaffolds	Tested with HaCaT and HUVEC cells and found that it was noncytotoxic and promoted IL-10 and TNF-alpha levels at a small rate which is helpful for skin TE.	(Demirbilek et al., 2017)
	Injectable bioactive akermanite/ALG composite hydrogels	Designing multifunctional bioactive biomaterials for wound healing and in situ skin TE with enhanced cell proliferation and re-epithelialization.	(Han et al., 2017)

tissue has poor self-healing capability. TE provides certain solutions to this problem by designing methods and strategies to repair and regenerate the damaged and defective cartilage tissue. Focaroli et al. (2016) prepared a functional scaffold using calcium–cobalt ALG microbeads for cartilage tissue regeneration. This scaffold helped direct differentiation of the human adipose-derived mesenchymal stem cells into cartilage-producing chondrocyte (Focaroli et al., 2016). Yan et al. (2014) used ALG and poly(L-glutamic acid) (PLGA/Alg) to design a self-cross-linking in situ injectable hydrogel for cartilage TE and pharmaceutical delivery. Ectopic cartilage formation, cell in growth, and mechanical stability of the scaffold were tested and found to be suitable for the above purpose (Yan et al., 2014). Park and Lee (2014) designed oxidized ALG/hyaluronate hydrogels that are biodegradable for cartilage tissue regeneration. This was done by partially oxidizing ALG by using sodium periodate. The in vivo testing was done in mice by injecting primary chondrocytes. Further, the expression of chondrogenic marker genes and secretion of sulfated glycosaminoglycans were observed. They concluded that the dAl/HA hydrogel was found suitable for cartilage TE purpose (Park and Lee, 2014).

7.5.3 DRUG AND GROWTH FACTOR DELIVERY

Delivery of drug and GFs is essential in the maintenance of tissue homeostasis and internal regularization. Yan et al. (2016) designed a biodegradable and injectable ALG-based composite gel scaffold integrated with gelatin microspheres and HAp. The gel scaffold effectively released tetracycline hydrochloride in a controlled way (Yan et al., 2016). Quinlan et al. (2015) developed a collagen–hydroxyapatite scaffold integrated with PLGA microparticles and bioactive rhBMP-2 with high encapsulation efficiency. Pro-osteogenic factor (rhBMP-2) was found to be delivered in an effective way (Quinlan et al., 2015). Miao et al. (2014) performed a comparative study on ALG, ALG-graft-polyethylene glycol-S-S-arginine-glycine-aspartic acid, and ALG-graft-polyethylene glycol microspheres for intracellular GF delivery. The results demonstrated that the intracellular delivery of vascular endothelial growth factor A and the internalization of ALG-based microspheres supports drug delivery and intracrine mechanism to enhance osteogenic differentiation and to control the fate of human MSCs (Miao et al., 2014).

7.5.4 CARDIAC TE

With the increase in the cardiac diseases and unavailability of donors, various new theories and scientific methods have come up for cardiac disease treatment. Thankam and Muthu (2015) devised a hybrid ALG–polyester comacromer-based hydrogel for cardiac TE with both biologically and physiologically favored characteristics. Poly(mannitol fumarate-co-sebacate) and ALG were copolymerized to synthesize the hybrid scaffold. The biological performance of the prepared scaffolds, such as cell cycle proliferation and long-term cell viability, was greatly influenced. The authors found the scaffolds to be suitable for cardiac TE (Thankam and Muthu, 2015). Fleischer et al. (2017) described various platforms and scaffold designing techniques for cardiac TE. The layer-by-layer assembly 3D printing technique and bionic TE are prominent areas of research these days (Fleischer et al., 2017).

7.5.5 SKIN TE

Skin TE is a promising alternative to classical severe skin damage treatments like grafting, which is limited by the availability of autogenic skin. Sarkar et al. (2013) fabricated a CS–collagen–ALG scaffold with micro- and nanofibrous structure for skin TE applications. Before testing on animals, the scaffold was tested ex vivo in a human skin equivalent wound model that showed wound re-epithelization and keratinocyte migration, two very important characteristics for skin TE. HaCat keratinocytes and 3T3 fibroblasts were used for experimentation to test the cytocompatibility of the scaffolds (Sarkar et al., 2013). Chandika et al. (2015) fabricated an integrated scaffold using fish collagen/ALG/chitooligosaccharides that provided improved biological, physical, and chemical characteristics that are suitable for skin TE (Chandika et al., 2015). Shi et al. (2017) for the purpose of skin TE fabricated sodium ALG/gelatin composite scaffold by extrusion free-forming, a 3D printing technique that could be used as dermal substitutes in case of severe skin injuries, thus establishing a promising novel therapeutic strategy (Shi et al. 2017). Han et al. (2017) designed a bioactive injectable composite hydrogel that was composed of akermanite/ALG for skin TE. The interaction between biopolymer and bioactive bioceramic lead to the regeneration of damaged skin tissue (Han et al., 2017). Koh et al. (2016) conducted a study to test the fracture toughness of several fiber–hydrogel composites like hydrated, dehydrated, and ALG small intestinal submucosa (SIS) of cattle for skin TE. They found the SIS–ALG composite scaffold to have a similar toughness as that of natural skin (Koh et al., 2016).

7.6 CONCLUSION

ALG has traveled the path from a seaweed polysaccharide to the prescribed biomaterial for the treatment of patients in the medical industry due to its easily persuasive material properties. Chemical and physical modifications, blending with other polymers, and grafting of ligands of ALG impart astounding alterations to its physical, chemical, and mechanical aspects. Due to its ECM-like features, ALG-based scaffolds are nowadays framed in different architectures like hydrogels, sponges, foams, aerogels, fibers, and microparticles by finely tuning its properties. Plethora of techniques such as electrospinning, particulate leaching, freeze-drying, gas foaming, 3D printing, and TIPS have made possible ALG 3D scaffolds to be fashioned in a controlled manner. In different areas of TE, ALG is registering its presence as injectable scaffolds, delivery vehicle of therapeutics like drugs and cells, and regenerative environment builder for the repair process of bone, cartilage, heart, and skin.

SUMMARY

Cells, GFs, and scaffolds play the role of the fundamental units of "TE." As the scaffolds directly embrace the cells and the GFs, the type of material preferred for its fabrication should be selected accordingly. This chapter discusses the application of a natural polysaccharide, namely, ALG as the biomaterial for constructing scaffolds by virtue of its biodegradable, biocompatible, and modifiable properties. Along with the morphology of the ALG-based scaffolds, their fabrication techniques have also been outlined. Recent advancements in the applications of ALG from repair and regeneration of bone, skin, cartilage, and heart to potential cell and drug delivery vehicles have been proposed.

ACKNOWLEDGMENT

The authors would like to acknowledge the funds accredited from the project (INT/Korea/P-37), sanctioned by the Department of Science and Technology, Government of India.

KEYWORDS

- **alginate**
- **scaffolds**
- **tissue engineering**
- **biocompatible**

REFERENCES

Ahmed, E. M. Hydrogel: Preparation, Characterization, and Applications: A Review. *J. Adv. Res.* **2015,** *6*(2), 105–121.

Akbarzadeh, R.; Yousefi, A. M. Effects of Processing Parameters in Thermally Induced Phase Separation Technique on Porous Architecture of Scaffolds for Bone Tissue Engineering. *J. Biomed. Mater. Res. B Appl. Biomater.* **2014,** *102*(6), 1304–1315.

Andersen, T. Alginate Foams as Biomaterials. Ph.D. Dissertation, Norges Teknisk-Naturvitenskapelige Universitet, 2013.

Andersen, T.; Strand, B. L.; Formo, K.; Alsberg, E.; Christensen, B. E. Alginates As Biomaterials In Tissue Engineering. In *Carbohydrate Chemistry Chemical Biological Approaches;* Rauter, A. P., Lindhorst, T. K., Queneau, Y., André, I., Aubry, J.-M., Augé, J., Ballet, C., Barberot, C., Beau, J.-M., Benvegnu, T., Eds.; Royal Society of Chemistry: UK, 2011; Vol. 37, pp 227–258.

Annabi, N.; Nichol, J. W.; Zhong, X.; Ji, C.; Koshy, S.; Khademhosseini, A.; Dehghani, F. Controlling the Porosity and Microarchitecture of Hydrogels for Tissue Engineering. *Tissue Eng. Part B* **2010,** *16*(4), 371–383.

Aravamudhan, A.; Ramos, D. M.; Nada, A. A.; Kumbar, S. G. Natural Polymers: Polysaccharides and Their Derivatives for Biomedical Applications. In *Natural and Synthetic Biomedical Polymers;* Elsevier, 2014; pp 67–89.

Axpe, E.; Oyen, M. L. Applications of Alginate-Based Bioinks in 3d Bioprinting. *Int. J. Mol. Sci.* **2016,** *17*(12), 1976.

Baimark, Y.; Srisuwan, Y. Preparation of Alginate Microspheres by Water-in-Oil Emulsion Method for Drug Delivery: Effect of Ca^{2+} Post-Cross-Linking. *Adv. Powder Technol.* **2014,** *25*(5), 1541–1546.

Balakrishnan, B.; Joshi, N.; Jayakrishnan, A.; Banerjee, R. Self-Crosslinked Oxidized Alginate/Gelatin Hydrogel as Injectable, Adhesive Biomimetic Scaffolds for Cartilage Regeneration. *Acta Biomater.* **2014,** *10*(8), 3650–3663.

Bohari, S. P.; Hukins, D. W.; Grover, L. M. Effect of Calcium Alginate Concentration on Viability and Proliferation of Encapsulated Fibroblasts. *Biomed. Mater. Eng.* **2011,** *21*(3), 159–170.

Bowman, K. A.; Aarstad, O. A.; Nakamura, M.; Stokke, B. T.; Skjåk-Bræk, G.; Round, A. N. Single Molecule Investigation of the Onset and Minimum Size of the Calcium-Mediated Junction Zone in Alginate. *Carbohydr. Polym.* **2016,** *148,* 52–60.

Cao, N. Fabrication of Alginate Hydrogel Scaffolds and Cell Viability in Calcium-Crosslinked Alginate Hydrogel. Graduation Thesis, University of Saskatchewan Saskatoon, 2011.

Castells-Sala, C.; Alemany-Ribes, M.; Fernández-Muiños, T.; Recha-Sancho, L.; López-Chicón, P.; Aloy-Reverté, C.; Caballero-Camino, J.; Márquez-Gil, A.; Semino, C. E. Current Applications of Tissue Engineering in Biomedicine. *J. Biochips Tissue Chips.* **2013**, (S2), 1.

Ceccaldi, C.; Bushkalova, R.; Cussac, D.; Duployer, B.; Tenailleau, C.; Bourin, P.; Parini, A.; Sallerin, B.; Girod Fullana, D. Elaboration and Evaluation of Alginate Foam Scaffolds for Soft Tissue Engineering. *Int. J. Pharm.* **2017**, *524*(1), 433–442.

Chandika, P.; Ko, S.-C.; Oh, G.-W.; Heo, S.-Y.; Nguyen, V.-T.; Jeon, Y.-J.; Lee, B.; Jang, C. H.; Kim, G.; Park, W. S.; et al. Fish Collagen/Alginate/Chitooligosaccharides Integrated Scaffold for Skin Tissue Regeneration Application. *Int. J. Biol. Macromol.* **2015**, *81*, 504–513.

Chen, C.-Y.; Ke, C.-J.; Yen, K.-C.; Hsieh, H.-C.; Sun, J.-S.; Lin, F.-H. 3d Porous Calcium-Alginate Scaffolds Cell Culture System Improved Human Osteoblast Cell Clusters for Cell Therapy. *Theranostics* **2015**, *5*(6), 643.

Chia, H. N.; Wu, B. M. Recent Advances in 3d Printing of Biomaterials. *J. Biol. Eng.* **2015**, *9*(1), 4.

Comolli, N. K.; Clark, C. E. Polymeric Microparticles. In *Engineering Polymer Systems for Improved Drug Delivery;* John Wiley & Sons, 2014; pp 85–116.

Conoscenti, G.; Carrubba, V. L.; Brucato, V. A Versatile Technique to Produce Porous Polymeric Scaffolds: The Thermally Induced Phase Separation (Tips) Method. *Arch. Chem. Res.* **2017**, *1*(2), 1–3.

d'Ayala, G. G.; Malinconico, M.; Laurienzo, P. Marine Derived Polysaccharides for Biomedical Applications: Chemical Modification Approaches. *Molecules* **2008**, *13*(9), 2069–2106.

da Silva, T. L.; Vidart, J. M. M.; da Silva, M. G. C.; Gimenes, M. L.; Vieira, M. G. A. Alginate and Sericin: Environmental and Pharmaceutical Applications. In *Biological Activities and Application of Marine Polysaccharides;* InTechOpen, 2017; pp 57–85.

Dahlin, R. L.; Kasper, F. K.; Mikos, A. G. Polymeric Nanofibers in Tissue Engineering. *Tissue Eng. Part B* **2011**, *17*(5), 349–364.

Dahlmann, J.; Krause, A.; Möller, L.; Kensah, G.; Möwes, M.; Diekmann, A.; Martin, U.; Kirschning, A.; Gruh, I.; Dräger, G. Fully Defined in Situ Cross-Linkable Alginate and Hyaluronic Acid Hydrogels for Myocardial Tissue Engineering. *Biomaterials* **2013**, *34*(4), 940–951.

Daskalaki, A. *Dental Computing and Applications: Advanced Techniques for Clinical Dentistry;* Medical Information Science Reference: Hershey, New York, 2009.

De'Nobili, M. D.; Curto, L. M.; Delfino, J. M.; Pérez, C. D.; Bernhardt, D.; Gerschenson, L. N.; Fissore, E. N.; Rojas, A. M. Alginate Utility in Edible and Non-Edible Film Development and the Influence of its Macromolecular Structure in the Antioxidant Activity of a Pharmaceutical/Food Interface.In *Alginic acid: Chemical structure, uses, and health benefits; NOVA*, 2015; pp 119–169.

Dehghani, F.; Annabi, N. Engineering Porous Scaffolds Using Gas-Based Techniques. *Curr. Opin. Biotechnol.* **2011**, *22*(5), 661–666.

Demirbilek, M.; Türkoğlu, N.; Aktürk, S. N-Acetylglucoseamine Modified Alginate Sponges as Scaffolds for Skin Tissue Engineering. *Turkish J. Biol.* **2017**, *41*(5), 796–807.

Dhandayuthapani, B.; Yoshida, Y.; Maekawa, T.; Kumar, D. S. Polymeric Scaffolds in Tissue Engineering Application: A Review. *Int. J. Polym. Sci.* **2011**, *2011*, 1–19.

Do, A.-V.; Smith, R.; Acri, T. M.; Geary, S. M.; Salem, A. K. 3d Printing Technologies for 3d Scaffold Engineering. In *Functional 3d Tissue Engineering Scaffolds;* Deng, Y. and Kuiper, J., Eds., Elsevier, 2018; pp 203–234.

Dominguez, H. *Functional Ingredients from Algae for Foods and Nutraceuticals;* Woodhead Publishing Limited: Cambridge, UK, 2013.

Donati, I.; Paoletti, S. Material Properties of Alginates. In *Alginates: Biology and Applications;* Rehm, B. H., Eds., Springer, Berlin: Heidelberg, Germany 2009; pp 1–53.

Draget, K. I.; Smidsrød, O.; Skjåk-Bræk, G. Alginates from Algae. In *Biopolymers Online;* Wiley-VCH Verlach GmbH: Weinheim, Germany, 2005; Vol. 1, pp 1–30.

Edgar, L.; McNamara, K.; Wong, T.; Tamburrini, R.; Katari, R.; Orlando, G. Heterogeneity of Scaffold Biomaterials in Tissue Engineering. *Materials* **2016**, *9*(5), 332.

Elamparithi, D.; Moorthy, V. On Various Porous Scaffold Fabrication Methods. *Mapana J. Sci.* **2017**, *16*(4), 47–52.

Elsayed, N. H.; Monier, M.; Alatawi, R. A. Synthesis and Characterization of Photo-Crosslinkable 4-Styryl-Pyridine Modified Alginate. *Carbohydr. Polym.* **2016**, *145,* 121–131.

Fleischer, S.; Feiner, R.; Dvir, T. Cutting-Edge Platforms in Cardiac Tissue Engineering. *Curr. Opin. Biotechnol.* **2017**, *47,* 23–29.

Focaroli, S.; Teti, G.; Salvatore, V.; Orienti, I.; Falconi, M. Calcium/Cobalt Alginate Beads as Functional Scaffolds for Cartilage Tissue Engineering. *Stem Cells Int.* **2016**, *2016,* 1–12.

Garate, A.; Ciriza, J.; Casado, J. G.; Blazquez, R.; Pedraz, J. L.; Orive, G.; Hernandez, R. M. Assessment of the Behavior of Mesenchymal Stem Cells Immobilized in Biomimetic Alginate Microcapsules. *Mol. Pharm.* **2015**, *12*(11), 3953–3962.

Garg, T.; Singh, O.; Arora, S.; Murthy, R. Scaffold: A Novel Carrier for Cell and Drug Delivery. *Crit. Rev. Ther. Drug Carrier Syst.* **2012**, *29*(1), 1–63.

Griffith, L. G.; Naughton, G. Tissue Engineering–Current Challenges and Expanding Opportunities. *Science* **2002**, *295*(5557), 1009–1014.

Gugjoo, M.; Amarpal; Sharma, G.; Aithal, H.; Kinjavdekar, P. Cartilage Tissue Engineering: Role of Mesenchymal Stem Cells Along with Growth Factors and Scaffolds. *Indian J. Med. Res.* **2016**, *144*(3), 339.

Guiraldo, R. D.; Berger, S. B.; Consani, R. L. X.; Consani, S.; de Carvalho, R. V.; Lopes, M. B.; Meneghel, L. L.; da Silva, F. B.; Sinhoreti, M. A. C. Characterization of Morphology and Composition of Inorganic Fillers in Dental Alginates. *BioMed. Res. Int.* **2014**, *2014,* 1–6.

Gwon, S. H.; Yoon, J.; Seok, H. K.; Oh, K. H.; Sun, J.-Y. Gelation Dynamics of Ionically Crosslinked Alginate Gel With Various Cations. *Macromol. Res.* **2015**, *23*(12), 1112–1116.

Han, Y.; Li, Y.; Zeng, Q.; Li, H.; Peng, J.; Xu, Y.; Chang, J. Injectable Bioactive Akermanite/Alginate Composite Hydrogels for in Situ Skin Tissue Engineering. *J. Mater. Chem. B* **2017**, *5*(18), 3315–3326.

Harding, S. E.; Tombs, M. P.; Adams, G. G.; Paulsen, B. S.; Inngjerdingen, K. T.; Barsett, H. *An Introduction to Polysaccharide Biotechnology;* CRC Press: Boca Raton, FL, 2017.

Hasan, A. *Tissue Engineering for Artificial Organs: Regenerative Medicine, Smart Diagnostics and Personalized Medicine;* John Wiley & Sons, Verlag GmbH & Co. KGaA: Weinheim, Germany, 2017.

Hay, I. D.; Rehman, Z. U.; Moradali, M. F.; Wang, Y.; Rehm, B. H. Microbial Alginate Production, Modification and its Applications. *Microb. Biotechnol.* **2013**, *6*(6), 637–650.

Holkem, A. T.; Raddatz, G. C.; Nunes, G. L.; Cichoski, A. J.; Jacob-Lopes, E.; Grosso, C. R. F.; de Menezes, C. R. Development and Characterization of Alginate Microcapsules Containing *Bifidobacterium* BB-12 Produced by Emulsification/Internal Gelation Followed by Freeze Drying. *LWT-Food Sci. Technol.* **2016**, *71,* 302–308.

Horch, R. New Developments and Trends in Tissue Engineering: An Update. *J. Tissue Sci. Eng.* **2012,** *3*(2), 1–6.

Hu, C.; Gong, R.; Zhou, F. Electrospun Sodium Alginate/Polyethylene Oxide Fibers and Nanocoated Yarns. *Int. J. Polym. Sci.* **2015,** *2015,* 1–12.

Iannace, S.; Park, C. B. *Biofoams: Science and Applications of Bio-Based Cellular and Porous Materials;* CRC Press: Boca Raton, FL, 2015.

Ikada, Y. Challenges in Tissue Engineering. *J. R. Soc. Interface* **2006,** *3*(10), 589–601.

Ishigami, T.; Nii, Y.; Ohmukai, Y.; Rajabzadeh, S.; Matsuyama, H. Solidification Behavior of Polymer Solution During Membrane Preparation by Thermally Induced Phase Separation. *Membranes* **2014,** *4*(1), 113–122.

Kaklamani, G.; Cheneler, D.; Grover, L. M.; Adams, M. J.; Bowen, J. Mechanical Properties of Alginate Hydrogels Manufactured Using External Gelation. *J. Mech. Behav. Biomed. Mater.* **2014,** *36,* 135–142.

Kalaf, E.; Sell, S. Inscribing the Blank Slate: The Growing Role of Modified Alginates in Tissue Engineering. *Adv. Tissue Eng. Regener. Med. Open Access* **2016,** *1*(2), 32–33. DOI: 10.15406/atroa.2016.01.00006.

Kerschenmeyer, A.; Arlov, Ø.; Malheiro, V.; Steinwachs, M.; Rottmar, M.; Maniura-Weber, K.; Palazzolo, G.; Zenobi-Wong, M. Anti-Oxidant and Immune-Modulatory Properties of Sulfated Alginate Derivatives on Human Chondrocytes and Macrophages. *Biomater. Sci.* **2017,** *5*(9), 1756–1765.

Khang, G. *Handbook of Intelligent Scaffolds for Tissue Engineering and Regenerative Medicine;* Pan Stanford Publishing Pte. Ltd.: Singapore 2017.

Klouda, L. Thermoresponsive Hydrogels in Biomedical Applications: A Seven-Year Update. *Eur. J. Pharm. Biopharm.* **2015,** *97,* 338–349.

Koch, L.; Deiwick, A.; Schlie, S.; Michael, S.; Gruene, M.; Coger, V.; Zychlinski, D.; Schambach, A.; Reimers, K.; Vogt, P. M. Skin Tissue Generation by Laser Cell Printing. *Biotechnol. Bioeng.* **2012,** *109*(7), 1855–1863.

Koh, C. T.; bin Kamarudin, A. D. Z.; Khoo, W.; Binti Mohamed, N. S. In *Fiber-Hydrogel Composites for Skin Tissue Engineering.* Biomedical Engineering and Sciences (IECBES), 2016 IEEE EMBS Conference, IEEE, 2016; 627–630.

Kolambkar, Y. M.; Dupont, K. M.; Boerckel, J. D.; Huebsch, N.; Mooney, D. J.; Hutmacher, D. W.; Guldberg, R. E. An Alginate-Based Hybrid System for Growth Factor Delivery in the Functional Repair of Large Bone Defects. *Biomaterials* **2011,** *32*(1), 65–74.

Kundu, J.; Shim, J. H.; Jang, J.; Kim, S. W.; Cho, D. W. An Additive Manufacturing-Based PCL–Alginate–Chondrocyte Bioprinted Scaffold for Cartilage Tissue Engineering. *J. Tissue Eng. Regener. Med.* **2015,** *9*(11), 1286–1297.

Kusumastuti, Y.; Putri, N. R. E.; Dary, A. R. Electrospinning Optimization and Characterization of Chitosan/Alginate/Polyvinyl Alcohol Nanofibers. In *AIP Conference Proceedings*, AIP Publishing, 2016; 150007.

Kyzioł, A.; Michna, J.; Moreno, I.; Gamez, E.; Irusta, S. Preparation and Characterization of Electrospun Alginate Nanofibers Loaded with Ciprofloxacin Hydrochloride. *Eur. Polym. J.* **2017,** *96,* 350–360.

Lee, K. Y.; Mooney, D. J. Alginate: Properties and Biomedical Applications. *Prog. Polym. Sci.* **2012,** *37*(1), 106–126.

Lee, G.-S.; Park, J.-H.; Shin, U. S.; Kim, H.-W. Direct Deposited Porous Scaffolds of Calcium Phosphate Cement with Alginate for Drug Delivery and Bone Tissue Engineering. *Acta Biomater.* **2011a,** *7*(8), 3178–3186.

Lee, K.; Silva, E. A.; Mooney, D. J. Growth Factor Delivery-Based Tissue Engineering: General Approaches and a Review of Recent Developments. *J. R. Soc. Interface* **2011b,** *8*(55), 153–170.

Liu, L.; Jiang, L.; Xu, G.; Ma, C.; Yang, X.; Yao, J. Potential of Alginate Fibers Incorporated with Drug-Loaded Nanocapsules as Drug Delivery Systems. *J. Mater. Chem. B* **2014,** *2*(43), 7596–7604.

Lloyd, D. R.; Kinzer, K. E.; Tseng, H. Microporous Membrane Formation via Thermally Induced Phase Separation. I. Solid-Liquid Phase Separation. *J. Membr. Sci.* **1990,** *52*(3), 239–261.

Loh, Q. L.; Choong, C. Three-Dimensional Scaffolds for Tissue Engineering Applications: Role of Porosity and Pore Size. *Tissue Eng. Part B: Rev.* **2013,** *19*(6), 485–502.

Lou, T.; Leung, M.; Wang, X.; Chang, J. Y.; Tsao, C. T.; Sham, J. G.; Edmondson, D.; Zhang, M. Bi-Layer Scaffold of Chitosan/PCL-Nanofibrous Mat and PLLA-Microporous Disc for Skin Tissue Engineering. *J. Biomed. Nanotechnol.* **2014,** *10*(6), 1105–1113.

Lu, T.; Li, Y.; Chen, T. Techniques for Fabrication and Construction of Three-Dimensional Scaffolds for Tissue Engineering. *Int. J. Nanomed.* **2013,** *8,* 337.

Luo, Z.; Yang, Y.; Deng, Y.; Sun, Y.; Yang, H.; Wei, S. Peptide-Incorporated 3d Porous Alginate Scaffolds with Enhanced Osteogenesis for Bone Tissue Engineering. *Colloids Surf. B* **2016,** *143,* 243–251.

Ma, G.; Fang, D.; Liu, Y.; Zhu, X.; Nie, J. Electrospun Sodium Alginate/Poly(Ethylene Oxide) Core–Shell Nanofibers Scaffolds Potential for Tissue Engineering Applications. *Carbohydr. Polym.* **2012,** *87*(1), 737–743.

Ma, Q.; Wang, Q. Lanthanide Induced Formation of Novel Luminescent Alginate Hydrogels and Detection Features. *Carbohydr. Polym.* **2015,** *133,* 19–23.

Marinho Carvalho Bjørge, I. Degradation of Calcium Gels of Alginate and Periodate Oxidised Alginate. Ph.D. Dissertation. NTNU, 2016.

Marković, D.; Zarubica, A.; Stojković, N.; Vasić, M.; Cakić, M.; Nikolić, G. Alginates and Similar Exopolysaccharides in Biomedical Application and Pharmacy: Controled Delivery of Drugs. *Adv. Technol.* **2016,** *5*(1), 39–52.

Markstedt, K.; Mantas, A.; Tournier, I.; Martínez Ávila, H.; Hägg, D.; Gatenholm, P. 3d Bioprinting Human Chondrocytes with Nanocellulose–Alginate Bioink for Cartilage Tissue Engineering Applications. *Biomacromolecules* **2015,** *16*(5), 1489–1496.

Marsich, E.; Bellomo, F.; Turco, G.; Travan, A.; Donati, I.; Paoletti, S. Nano-Composite Scaffolds for Bone Tissue Engineering Containing Silver Nanoparticles: Preparation, Characterization and Biological Properties. *J. Mater. Sci. Mater. Med.* **2013,** *24*(7), 1799–1807.

Martínez-Pérez, C. A.; Olivas-Armendariz, I.; Castro-Carmona, J. S.; García-Casillas, P. E. Scaffolds for Tissue Engineering via Thermally Induced Phase Separation. In *Advances in Regenerative Medicine;* InTech Open, 2011; pp 275–294.

Mhanna, R.; Becher, J.; Schnabelrauch, M.; Reis, R. L.; Pashkuleva, I. Sulfated Alginate as a Mimic of Sulfated Glycosaminoglycans: Binding of Growth Factors and Effect on Stem Cell Behavior. *Adv. Biosyst.* **2017,** *1*(7), 1–7.

Miao, T.; Rao, K. S.; Spees, J. L.; Oldinski, R. A. Osteogenic Differentiation of Human Mesenchymal Stem Cells Through Alginate-Graft-Poly(Ethylene Glycol) Microsphere-Mediated Intracellular Growth Factor Delivery. *J. Controlled Release* **2014,** *192,* 57–66.

Montanucci, P.; Terenzi, S.; Santi, C.; Pennoni, I.; Bini, V.; Pescara, T.; Basta, G.; Calafiore, R. Insights in Behavior of Variably Formulated Alginate-Based Microcapsules for Cell Transplantation. *BioMed. Res. Int.* **2015,** *2015,* 1–11.

Muhaimin. Study of Microparticle Preparation by the Solvent Evaporation Method Using Focused Beam Reflectance Measurement (FBRM). Ph.D. Dissertation, Freie Universität, 2013.

Murdzheva, D.; Denev, P. Chemical Modification of Alginic Acid by Ultrasonic Irradiation. *Acta Sci. Nat.* **2016,** *3*(1), 13–18.

Nakanishi, Y. *Hydrated Materials: Applications in Biomedicine and the Environment;* CRC Press: Boca Raton, FL, 2015.

Nigam, R.; Mahanta, B. An Overview of Various Biomimetic Scaffolds: Challenges and Applications in Tissue Engineering. *J. Tissue Sci. Eng.* **2014,** *5*(2), 1.

O'brien, F. J. Biomaterials and Scaffolds for Tissue Engineering. *Mater. Today* **2011,** *14*(3), 88–95.

Pan, T.; Song, W.; Cao, X.; Wang, Y. 3d Bioplotting of Gelatin/Alginate Scaffolds for Tissue Engineering: Influence of Crosslinking Degree and Pore Architecture on Physicochemical Properties. *J. Mater. Sci. Technol.* **2016,** *32*(9), 889–900.

Paques, J. P.; van der Linden, E.; van Rijn, C. J.; Sagis, L. M. Preparation Methods of Alginate Nanoparticles. *Adv. Colloid Interface Sci.* **2014,** *209,* 163–171.

Park, H.; Lee, K. Y. Cartilage Regeneration Using Biodegradable Oxidized Alginate/ Hyaluronate Hydrogels. *J. Biomed. Mater. Res. Part A* **2014,** *102*(12), 4519–4525.

Patil, T.; Saha, S.; Biswas, A. In *Preparation and Characterization of HAp Coated Chitosan-Alginate PEC Porous Scaffold for Bone Tissue Engineering.* Macromolecular Symposia, Wiley Online Library, 2017.

Pawar, S. N.; Edgar, K. J. Alginate Derivatization: A Review of Chemistry, Properties and Applications. *Biomaterials* **2012,** *33*(11), 3279–3305.

Popper, Z. A.; Ralet, M.-C.; Domozych, D. S. Plant and Algal Cell Walls: Diversity and Functionality. *Ann. Bot. (London)* **2014,** *114*(6), 1043–1048.

Quinlan, E.; López-Noriega, A.; Thompson, E.; Kelly, H. M.; Cryan, S. A.; O'brien, F. J. Development of Collagen–Hydroxyapatite Scaffolds Incorporating PLGA and Alginate Microparticles for the Controlled Delivery of rhBMP-2 for Bone Tissue Engineering. *J. Controlled Release* **2015,** *198,* 71–79.

Quinlan, E.; López-Noriega, A.; Thompson, E. M.; Hibbitts, A.; Cryan, S. A.; O'Brien, F. J. Controlled Release of Vascular Endothelial Growth Factor from Spray-Dried Alginate Microparticles in Collagen–Hydroxyapatite Scaffolds for Promoting Vascularization and Bone Repair. *J. Tissue Eng. Regener. Med.* **2017,** *11*(4), 1097–1109.

Reed, S.; Wu, B. M. Biological and Mechanical Characterization of Chitosan-Alginate Scaffolds for Growth Factor Delivery and Chondrogenesis. *J. Biomed. Mater. Res. B Appl. Biomater.* **2017,** *105*(2), 272–282.

Rehm, B. H. *Alginates: Biology and Applications;* Springer, Verlag Berlin: Heidelberg, Germany 2009.

Rinaudo, M. Biomateriales basados en un polisacárido natural: El alginato. *TIP Revista especializada en ciencias químico-biológicas* **2014,** *17*(1), 92–96.

Ruvinov, E.; Cohen, S. Alginate Biomaterial for the Treatment of Myocardial Infarction: Progress, Translational Strategies, and Clinical Outlook: From Ocean Algae to Patient Bedside. *Adv. Drug Delivery Rev.* **2016,** *96,* 54–76.

Sajesh, K.; Jayakumar, R.; Nair, S. V.; Chennazhi, K. Biocompatible Conducting Chitosan/ Polypyrrole–Alginate Composite Scaffold for Bone Tissue Engineering. *Int. J. Biol. Macromol.* **2013,** *62,* 465–471.

Sarkar, S. D.; Farrugia, B. L.; Dargaville, T. R.; Dhara, S. Chitosan–Collagen Scaffolds with Nano/Microfibrous Architecture for Skin Tissue Engineering. *J. Biomed. Mater. Res. Part A* **2013,** *101*(12), 3482–3492.

Sengupta, D.; Waldman, S. D.; Li, S. From in Vitro to in Situ Tissue Engineering. *Ann. Biomed. Eng.* **2014,** *42*(7), 1537–1545.

Shachar, M.; Tsur-Gang, O.; Dvir, T.; Leor, J.; Cohen, S. The Effect of Immobilized RGD Peptide in Alginate Scaffolds on Cardiac Tissue Engineering. *Acta Biomater.* **2011,** *7*(1), 152–162.

Shalumon, K.; Sathish, D.; Nair, S.; Chennazhi, K.; Tamura, H.; Jayakumar, R. Fabrication of Aligned Poly(Lactic Acid)-Chitosan Nanofibers by Novel Parallel Blade Collector Method for Skin Tissue Engineering. *J. Biomed. Nanotechnol.* **2012,** *8*(3), 405–416.

Shapiro, L.; Cohen, S. Novel Alginate Sponges for Cell Culture and Transplantation. *Biomaterials* **1997,** *18*(8), 583–590.

Sharma, C.; Dinda, A. K.; Potdar, P. D.; Chou, C.-F.; Mishra, N. C. Fabrication and Characterization of Novel Nano-Biocomposite Scaffold of Chitosan–Gelatin–Alginate–Hydroxyapatite for Bone Tissue Engineering. *Mater. Sci. Eng. C* **2016,** *64,* 416–427.

Shevach, M.; Fleischer, S.; Shapira, A.; Dvir, T. Gold Nanoparticle-Decellularized Matrix Hybrids for Cardiac Tissue Engineering. *Nano Lett.* **2014,** *14*(10), 5792–5796.

Shi, L.; Xiong, L.; Hu, Y.; Li, W.; Chen, Z.; Liu, K.; Zhang, X. Three-Dimensional Printing Alginate/Gelatin Scaffolds as Dermal Substitutes for Skin Tissue Engineering. *Polym. Eng. Sci.* **2017,** *0,* 1–9.

Solovieva, E. V.; Fedotov, A. Y.; Mamonov, V. E.; Komlev, V. S.; Panteleyev, A. A. Fibrinogen-Modified Sodium Alginate as a Scaffold Material for Skin Tissue Engineering. *Biomed. Mater.* **2017,** *13,* 1–27.

Song, J. E.; Kim, A. R.; Lee, C. J.; Tripathy, N.; Yoon, K. H.; Lee, D.; Khang, G. Effects of Purified Alginate Sponge on the Regeneration of Chondrocytes: In Vitro and in Vivo. *J. Biomater. Sci. Polym. Ed.* **2015,** *26*(3), 181–195.

Sridhar, R.; Lakshminarayanan, R.; Madhaiyan, K.; Barathi, V. A.; Lim, K. H.; Ramakrishna, S. Electrosprayed Nanoparticles and Electrospun Nanofibers Based on Natural Materials: Applications in Tissue Regeneration, Drug Delivery and Pharmaceuticals. *Chem. Soc. Rev.* **2015,** *44*(3), 790–814.

Sun, J.; Tan, H. Alginate-Based Biomaterials for Regenerative Medicine Applications. *Materials* **2013,** *6*(4), 1285–1309.

Tellechea, A.; Silva, E. A.; Min, J.; Leal, E. C.; Auster M. E.; Pradhan-Nabzdyk, L.; Shih, W.; Mooney, D. J.; Veves, A. Alginate and DNA Gels are Suitable Delivery Systems for Diabetic Wound Healing. *Int. J. Lower Extremity Wounds* **2015,** *14*(2), 146–153.

Thankam, F. G.; Muthu, J. Alginate–Polyester Comacromer Based Hydrogels as Physio-chemically and Biologically Favorable Entities for Cardiac Tissue Engineering. *J. Colloid Interface Sci.* **2015,** *457,* 52–61.

Tomlins, P. *Characterisation and Design of Tissue Scaffolds;* Woodhead Publishing: Cambridge, UK, 2015.

Venkatesan, J.; Bhatnagar, I.; Kim, S.-K. Chitosan-Alginate Biocomposite Containing Fucoidan for Bone Tissue Engineering. *Mari. Drugs* **2014,** *12*(1), 300–316.

Wang, X.; Hao, T.; Qu, J.; Wang, C.; Chen, H. Synthesis of Thermal Polymerizable Alginate-GMA Hydrogel for Cell Encapsulation. *J. Nanomater.* **2015a,** *2015,* 5.

Wang, Q.; Xia, Q.; Wu, Y.; Zhang, X.; Wen, F.; Chen, X.; Zhang, S.; Heng, B. C.; He, Y.; Ouyang, H. W. 3d-Printed Atsttrin-Incorporated Alginate/Hydroxyapatite Scaffold Promotes Bone Defect Regeneration with TNF/TNFR Signaling Involvement. *Adv. Healthcare Mater.* **2015b,** *4*(11), 1701–1708.

Wang, P.; Song, Y.; Weir, M. D.; Sun, J.; Zhao, L.; Simon, C. G.; Xu, H. H. A Self-Setting iPSMSC-Alginate-Calcium Phosphate Paste for Bone Tissue Engineering. *Dent. Mater.* **2016,** *32*(2), 252–263.

Williams, D. Benefit and Risk in Tissue Engineering. *Mater. Today* **2004,** *7*(5), 24–29.

Wongkanya, R.; Chuysinuan, P.; Pengsuk, C.; Nooeaid P. Electrospinning of Alginate/Soy Protein Isolated Nanofibers and their Release Characteristics for Biomedical Applications. *J. Sci. Adv. Mater. Devices* **2017,** *2,* 309–316.

Xue, J.; Xie, J.; Liu, W.; Xia, Y. Electrospun Nanofibers: New Concepts, Materials, and Applications. *Acc. Chem. Res.* **2017,** *50*(8), 1976–1987.

Yagnik, D. In *Fused Deposition Modeling – A Rapid Prototyping Technique for Product Cycle Time Reduction Cost Effectively in Aerospace Applications.* International Conference on Advances in Engineering and Technology (ICAET); 2014; pp 62–68.

Yan, S.; Wang, T.; Feng, L.; Zhu, J.; Zhang, K.; Chen, X.; Cui, L.; Yin, J. Injectable in Situ Self-Cross-Linking Hydrogels Based on Poly(l-Glutamic Acid) and Alginate for Cartilage Tissue Engineering. *Biomacromolecules* **2014,** *15*(12), 4495–4508.

Yan, J.; Miao, Y.; Tan, H.; Zhou, T.; Ling, Z.; Chen, Y.; Xing, X.; Hu, X. Injectable Alginate/ Hydroxyapatite Gel Scaffold Combined with Gelatin Microspheres for Drug Delivery and Bone Tissue Engineering. *Mater. Sci. Eng. C* **2016,** *63,* 274–284.

Yan, H.; Chen, X.; Feng, M.; Shi, Z.; Zhang, D.; Lin, Q. Layer-by-Layer Assembly of 3d Alginate-Chitosan-Gelatin Composite Scaffold Incorporating Bacterial Cellulose Nanocrystals for Bone Tissue Engineering. *Mater. Lett.* **2017,** *209,* 492–496.

Yang, J.-S.; Xie, Y.-J.; He, W. Research Progress on Chemical Modification of Alginate: A Review. *Carbohydr. Polym.* **2011,** *84*(1), 33–39.

Zhang, Y.; Yu, Y.; Ozbolat, I. T. Direct Bioprinting of Vessel-Like Tubular Microfluidic Channels. *J. Nanotechnol. Eng. Med.* **2013a,** *4*(2), 0210011–0210017.

Zhang, Z.; Gupte, M. J.; Ma, P. X. Biomaterials and Stem Cells for Tissue Engineering. *Expert Opin. Biol. Ther.* **2013b,** *13*(4), 527–540.

Zhang, H.; Liu, X.; Yang, M.; Zhu, L. Silk Fibroin/Sodium Alginate Composite Nano-Fibrous Scaffold Prepared Through Thermally Induced Phase-Separation (Tips) Method for Biomedical Applications. *Mater. Sci. Eng. C* **2015,** *55,* 8–13.

Zhao, X.; Li, Q.; Ma, X.; Xiong, Z.; Quan, F.; Xia, Y. Alginate Fibers Embedded with Silver Nanoparticles as Efficient Catalysts for Reduction of 4-Nitrophenol. *RSC Adv.* **2015,** *5*(61), 49534–49540.

Zhao, D.; Li, J.-S.; Suen, W.; Chang, M.-W.; Huang, J. Preparation and Characterization of Ganoderma Lucidum Spores-Loaded Alginate Microspheres by Electrospraying. *Mater. Sci. Eng. C* **2016,** *62,* 835–842.

CHAPTER 8

ALGINATE-BASED SCAFFOLDS IN BONE TISSUE ENGINEERING APPLICATIONS

S. VIJI CHANDRAN, V. SANJAY, and N. SELVAMURUGAN*

Department of Biotechnology, School of Bioengineering, SRM Institute of Science and Technology, Kattankulathur 603203, Tamil Nadu, India

Corresponding author. E-mail: selvamn2@yahoo.com; selvamurugan.n@ktr.srmuniv.ac.in

8.1 INTRODUCTION: BONE TISSUE ENGINEERING (BTE)

Trauma, injury, or disease can often cause tissue damage which might result in considerable morbidity which in turn increases the need for enhanced and more reliable strategies for bone regeneration. Though bone possesses the property of regeneration and remodeling, clinical assistance is required for bone repair. The current clinical practices involve utilization of bone grafting and transplantation methods. Autologous and transplantations are the most traditional methods, and each method has its advantages and disadvantages. This is where the evolution of bone tissue engineering (BTE) and regenerative medicine come into play. BTE is an interdisciplinary field which bridges different scientific fields of interest. It involves utilization of cells, biomaterials, and appropriate growth factors to assist tissue regeneration, thereby proving to be a potent alternative to autografts and allografts. In general, BTE involves the culturing of mesenchymal stem cells (MSCs), which are subsequently seeded on to the 3D scaffold matrix, thereby directed towards regeneration of bone via osteoinductive signals (Fig 8.1) (Wang et al., 2006; Binulal et al., 2010; Sahithi et al., 2010; Swetha et al., 2010; Saranya et al., 2011; Tripathi et al., 2012; Sowjanya et al., 2013; Kumar et al., 2014; Dhivya et al., 2015b; Saravanan et al., 2016a; LogithKumar et al., 2016;

Marolt et al., 2010; Balagangadharan et al., 2017). MSCs are simultaneously involved in the regeneration of tissue by their indirect contribution
via secretion of soluble factors and modulation of inflammatory responses.
Osteoinductive cytokines, which are present in the bone matrix along with
growth factors such as transforming growth factor-beta (TGF-β), platelet-
derived growth factor, vascular endothelial growth factor (VEGF), fibroblast
growth factor, or insulin-like growth factor, produce a profile of chemotaxis
which induce the differentiation of MSCs towards osteoblasts (Venkatesan
et al., 2015). Bone regeneration also involves the activation of intracellular
signaling pathways such as TGF-β, bone morphogenetic protein (BMP),
Ca^{2+}, Wnt, and other regulators such as microRNAs in MSCs (Moorthi et al.,
2013; Vimalraj et al., 2014; Sriram et al., 2015; Vimalraj et al., 2016; Leena
et al., 2017; Rao et al., 2017).

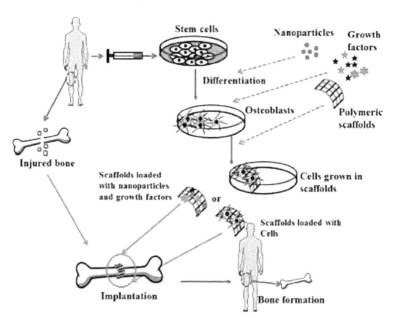

FIGURE 8.1   (See color insert.) Bone tissue engineering involves the use of cells and
biomaterials or a combination of cells loaded onto biodegradable scaffolds to treat critical-
sized bone defects. Mesenchymal stem cells isolated from the patient donor are differentiated
into osteoblasts in vitro prior to its loading into scaffolds. The cell-free construct is also used
along with bioactive molecules and nanoparticles for enhancing bone formation.

Source: Reprinted with permission from Saravanan et al., 2016b. © 2016 Elsevier.

Bone constructs obtained via tissue engineering potentially have the
ability to mimic extracellular matrix (ECM), aid in the formation of new

bone, and provide structural integrity (Saravanan et al., 2016b; Balag-angadharan et al., 2017). Osteoconductivity, osteoinductivity, osteogenicity, and biodegradability are some of the vital properties that scaffolds need to possess to facilitate the adhesion, survival, and migration of osteogenic cells (Saravanan et al., 2016b). The appropriate architecture of scaffolds with interconnecting porous tissues is often essential for enhanced cell penetration, new tissue formation, nutrient transportation, and neovascularization. Scaffolds can be prepared using two or more materials and that scaffold fabrication initiates a synergistic effect which improves its mechanical strength and also facilitates cell adhesion, proliferation, and differentiation (Dhandayuthapani et al., 2011; Saravanan et al., 2016b; Sharma et al., 2016; Saravanan et al., 2017; Wei et al., 2017). A number of materials such as polymers and ceramics have been widely used in BTE. Polymers are categorized as natural or synthetic based on their origin. Chitosan (CS), alginate (ALG), gelatin (GEL), and collagen (COL) are some of the commonly used natural polymers in BTE (Serra et al., 2015; Kuttappan et al., 2016; Yan et al., 2016). Synthetic polymers such as poly(L-lactic acid) (PLLA), polycaprolactone (PCL), and poly(lactic-co-glycolic acid) (PLGA) have been used extensively (Van Bael et al., 2013; Yazdimamaghani et al., 2015; Nie et al., 2015; Shao et al., 2016; Mao et al., 2017; Fernandes et al., 2017). These polymers along with ceramics or metal ions are blended and made as biocomposite scaffolds, thereby improving their physiochemical and biological properties (Chen et al., 2014; Cuozzo et al., 2014; Cordero-Arias et al., 2015a; Mao et al., 2017; Kanasan et al., 2017). There are certain salient features that biomaterials need to possess for them to be fabricated into the efficient scaffolds and used in BTE applications (Howk et al., 2006; Lin et al., 2007; Kim et al., 2014; Wu et al., 2014; Ribeiro et al., 2015; Gómez et al., 2016; Lie et al., 2017).

1) It is essential that the scaffolds are biocompatible and nontoxic with a sufficient amount of surface area.
2) The mechanical strength of the scaffolds must be just as good as that of a cortical bone.
3) Promotion of cell proliferation and cell migration is essential.
4) Osteoblast and osteoclast differentiation must occur in a balanced manner.
5) Biomaterials used to fabricate the scaffolds must be inexpensive.

ALG, CS, and GEL are the most preferred natural polymers for scaffold fabrication due to their availability, easy handling, and low cost. There is growing evidence indicating that ALG has a great potential for its application in BTE. ALG, as an anionic polymer, is combined and modified with other materials into many forms such as hydrogels, aerogels, 3D scaffolds, fibers, sponges, microspheres, microcapsules, and foams. The highly hydrophilic and porous nature of this polymer provides a matrix for bone tissue regeneration. ALG is a linear unbranched polymer which contains β-(1,4)-linked D-mannuronic acid (M) and α-(1,4)-linked L-guluronic acid (G) residues. The composition of the blocks involves the presence of consecutive G residues (GGGGGG), consecutive M residues (MMMMMM), and alternating M and G residues (GMGMGM). They are anionic, biocompatible, and biodegradable polymers which are hydrophilic (Lee and Mooney, 2012). The structure of ALG resembles glycosaminoglycan, which apparently is one of the major components of ECM in human tissue (Chae et al., 2013). ALG undergoes many exchanges when cross-linked in the presence of divalent ions. These exchanges usually occur between sodium ions and the divalent ions during the gelation of the ALG solution. When sodium ion from glucuronic acid exchanges with divalent cations, a structure referred to as "egg box" is created due to its subsequent cross-linking, which in turn paves the way to the possibility of incorporation or entrapment of desired substances. Divalent cations bind to blocks of α-L-glucuronic acid in such a manner that it enables the association with more than 20 monomers. Dimerization of each chain of ALG may occur to create links with other chains, resulting in a constructed framework of gel (Luo et al., 2015). This ability of ALG to form gels is one of the most important reasons for it to be used as an entrapping matrix for biological molecules such as proteins, drugs, cell, and so forth (Cardoso et al., 2014a; Cuozzo et al., 2014). ALG as a biomaterial is easily be formulated into a variety of soft gels, fibers, foams, nanoparticles, and multilayers at certain physiological conditions, thereby ensuring the preservation of cell viability and function (Valente et al., 2012; Morais et al., 2013; Cunniffe et al., 2015; Wongkanya et al., 2017).

Low mechanical strength and poor control over the micro-internal architecture due to excessive hydrophilicity are the main limitations of ALG and its use in hard tissue engineering. Unfortunately, ALG on its own showed reduced cell attachment in vitro due to its hydrophilicity, negative charge, as well as poor osteoconductivity. To address these limitations, ALG is being used in combination with other biomaterials to produce biocomposite scaffolds which would make use of both the biological advantages of ALG and greater mechanical strength of the reinforcement added (Lee and Mooney, 2012; Chae et al., 2013; Sarker et al., 2014; Kim and Kim, 2015). When ALG was used in combination with other materials, a synergistic effect was noticed with enhanced mechanical strength along with increased cell attachment, proliferation, and differentiation (Rajesh and Ravichandran, 2015; Venkatesan et al., 2015; Lee et al., 2016; Sharma et al., 2016).

ALG is combined with natural polymers like silk, CS, GEL, or ceramics, such as tricalcium phosphate (TCP) and hydroxyapatite (HAp) to improve its mechanical properties (Sharma et al., 2016). The molecular weight (MW) of ALG has the potential to alter the rate of degradation and mechanical properties of ALG-based biomaterials. Higher MW contributes towards the decrease in the number of reactive positions available for hydrolysis degradation. This further helps in slowing down the degradation rate. Additionally, degradation also directly influences the mechanical properties which bring about structural changes both at molecular and macroscopic levels (Sun and Tan, 2013). ALG is one of the leading suitors for 3D bioprinting due to its easy and customizable gelation process and natural hydrogel structure which is very similar to native ECM. Printability of the system is not affected by cell culture media or cell suspension. The hydrogel matrix encapsulated with cell increases the possibility of potential for tissue healing and reduces the difficulties such as nonuniform cell infiltration and tissue regeneration caused by as post-fabrication seeding processes (Axpe and Oyen, 2016; He et al., 2016; Wu et al., 2016; Shang et al., 2017).

The mechanical properties of ALG are improved by blending it with an inorganic material, especially HAp. Inorganic materials when encapsulated in bioresorbable polymers can alter the polymer degradation behavior by influencing the pH of the nearby solution and thereby preventing the autocatalytic effect of the acidic groups which result due to hydrolysis of polymer chains. HAp's inability to stimulate osteogenetic process and the uncontrollability of the burst release of the loaded drugs are the disadvantages of using it all alone. To solve these issues, the fabrication of Hap-incorporated ALG–biocomposite scaffolds has come into existence, which possessed better biomechanical and bioactive properties. Moreover, the incorporation of HAp could potentially prolong the drug release (Li et al., 2016).

8.2   ALGINATE (ALG)–INORGANIC BIOCOMPOSITES IN BTE

8.2.1   ALG–CALCIUM PHOSPHATE

Calcium phosphate (CaP) has been extensively studied in BTE due to its being close to the mineral phase of bone which contributes towards their ability to promote bone regeneration to a great extent (Venkatesan et al.,

2015). CaP, in general, has proved to be an excellent prospective to be used as a drug-eluting stent. TCP, another well-renowned form of CaP, possesses sublime properties such as biocompatibility, good bioactivity, and thermodynamic stability. Its ability to get easily attached to the natural bone surface, be gradually absorbed, and get replaced by actual bone itself makes it a promising biomaterial. TCP, when compared to HAp, has much better solubility and is resorbed swiftly in vivo which concludes it an obvious choice to be chosen ahead of apatites for the fabrication of completely biodegradable and reliable biocomposites. But, TCP, unfortunately, is brittle due to which it is necessary to use it in combination with other biopolymers (Yamamoto and Tabata et al., 2008).

Polymers and bioceramics blended together showed the development of osteochondral tissue scaffolds, thereby successfully overcoming poor mechanical integrity of the biopolymer and brittle nature of bioceramics (Yamamoto and Tabata, 2008). Additionally, they also promoted the adhesion of growth factors and adsorption of proteins onto their surfaces which led to the promotion of osteoblast adhesion, thereby rendering CaP to become osteoconductive which in turn made it suitable for repairing bone defects and injury. TCP–ALG scaffolds fabricated using powder printing technique which is a two-step method that first involves the printing of inorganic matrix followed by the subsequent integration of the ALG phase by vacuum infiltration and analyzed for its applicability in BTE. ALG, in the presence of divalent cations, such as calcium ions (Ca^{2+}) gets cross-linked easily and is clearly preferred over other biopolymers. Apart from this, in vitro studies suggested ALG used in combination with ceramics promoted osteoblastic cell attachment, proliferation, and osteogenic activity on the whole in a broader perspective (Castilho et al., 2015). Calcium phosphate cements (CPCs), variants of CaP, have emerged into prominence due to their possessing excellent cell and tissue compatibility. Their ability to self-set makes them very potent injectable materials which require minimally invasive surgery, and moreover, they possibly can carry incorporated therapeutic molecules within the particular formulation. However, CPCs have one noteworthy limitation wherein its degradation rate is slower than that of the rate of bone formation (Qiao et al., 2013). The application of CPC-based materials in BTE requires them to be able to form 3D scaffolds along with biopolymers as they enhance cell proliferation and cell–material composite construction. ALG here proved to be the right candidate to be combined with CPCs, and scaffolds were fabricated which were, in particular, a fibrous network formulated by the direct deposition of composite suspension under a Ca^{2+}-containing solution. This deposited suspension quickly solidified, thereby yielding a gelled network. The porous scaffolds were hard enough and were considered to be cell compatible as shown by their cell attachment efficiency on 7 and 14 days, making them potent enough to be put to use in BTE (Figure 8.2). Moreover, these scaffolds are considered to be load bearing and an efficient drug delivery vehicle. Histological studies done after 6 weeks post-surgery on critical-sized calvarial defect further confirmed the potential for bone formation and biocompatibility of the scaffolds (Fig 8.3) (Lee et al., 2011).

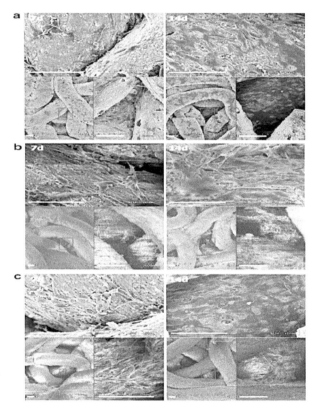

FIGURE 8.2   Cell morphology observed on calcium phosphate cement/alginate (ALG) scaffolds with different level of porosity during 7- and 14-day culture. (a) Low porosity; (b) medium porosity; (c) high porosity. Cells on day 7 adhered well to the underlying fibrous stems, showing a highly elongated cell shape with many filopodia. By day 14, the cells had proliferated, were in contact with each other, and covered the surface of stems almost completely. This cell growth and morphology were similarly observed for all porous scaffolds. Moreover, many cells were found inside the scaffold (deep in the pore channels), particularly in the samples with high porosity. Bar scale 50 µm.

Source: Reprinted with permission from Lee et al., 2011. © 2011 Elsevier.

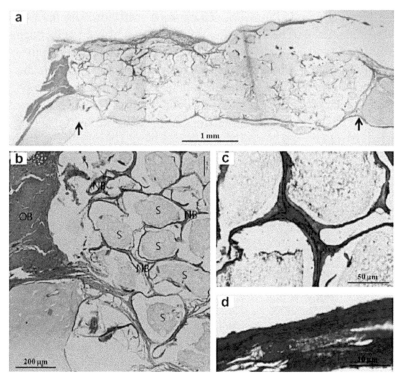

FIGURE 8.3   Histological staining of the tissues generated by the scaffold with high porosity at 6 weeks post-operation: (a, b) hematoxylin and eosin stain; (c, d) Masson's trichrome (MT) stain at different magnifications. Arrows indicate defect margins (a). OB, old bone; NB, new bone; S, scaffold (b). Connective bone tissue filled the pore channel of the scaffold throughout the defect region (a), and newly formed tissue lined the fiber stems of the scaffold (b). Pale or dark blue areas stained with MT demonstrate the formation of bony tissue, the major bone extracellular matrix.

Source: Reprinted with permission from Lee et al., 2011. © 2011 Elsevier.

Lipson and collaborators built an open-source 3D printer known as Fab@ Home which is one of the newest of its kinds used for the manufacture of 3D scaffolds. Beta-tricalcium phosphate (β-TCP)/ALG scaffolds were produced using this technique and they showed a high degree of control, including pore size optimization (Malone and Lipson, 2007; Diogo et al., 2014). Additionally, this system is comparatively easier to assemble, and it promotes the fabrication of structures in a quick manner with high reproducibility without compromising the uniformity of the biological scaffolds. Cells seeded onto the 3D porous β-TCP and ALG scaffolds facilitated the controlled BMP-2 growth factor release in vitro, and further enhanced osteogenesis in vivo

(Florczyk et al., 2012). ALG with HAp prepared using the phase separation method enhanced the attachment of osteosarcoma cells (Lin and Yeh, 2004; Turco et al., 2009). Different types of scaffolds produced using ALG and HAp are being investigated to assess the extent until which they could mimic natural bone functions (Chae et al., 2013; Luo et al., 2016; Cai et al., 2016; Jo et al., 2017). ALG combined with HAp improved its compressive strength, cell adhesion, and proliferation, and these scaffolds showed pore size ranging around 150 μm and porosity well over 82%. (Venkatesan et al., 2015). Rat osteoblastic cells (UMR106), seeded in the ALG/HAp biocomposite scaffolds, showed better cell attachment compared to that of the pure ALG scaffolds (Lin and Yeh, 2004). In vivo studies have also been performed using HAp/ALG scaffolds in the calvarial region of rats wherein new bone formation was observed. This might be due to the ability of ALG molecules to form highly anionic complexes and their capability of adsorbing important factors recognized by integrins present in osteoblasts (De Paulo et al., 2009; Nazarpak et al., 2012). A promising core–shell design of ALG along with α-TCP was prepared for controlled delivery of protein in situ (Perez and Kim, 2013). Core–shell-structured fibrous scaffolds were fabricated using a uniquely designed concentric nozzle (inner 17G and outer 23G) to which ALG/α-TCP was fed into both outer and inner syringe, and this syringe was clubbed with an injection pump connected via a microtube (Perez and Kim, 2013).

Protein cytochrome C (cytC) was used as a model protein to study its release from ALG scaffolds, and the results showed a burst effect due to the applied cross-linking conditions. The release pattern was found to be more sustained when α-TCP was mixed with ALG (Perez and Kim et al., 2013). In another study, human umbilical cord MSCs were encapsulated in microbeads produced by combining ALG hydrogel and CaP. There was no change in cell viability in the hydrogel and the mechanical properties drastically improved (Venkatesan et al., 2015). An injectable calcium silicate–sodium ALG hybrid variety of hydrogel was designed by Han et al in 2013, which made use of a novel material composition design. An eye-catching feature of these scaffolds was that the gelling time could be controlled varying from the 30 s to 10 m by bringing about some alterations to the amount of D-gluconic acid δ-lactone (GDL). The pore size ranged between 50 and 200 μm in the interconnected porous structure. These scaffolds also proved to possess properties such as good viability and proliferation which in turn led to higher levels of alkaline phosphatase (ALP) expression and subsequently angiogenesis (Han et al., 2013). In another work, ALG hydrogel beads were used to encapsulate CaP/CS containing mouse pre-osteoblasts (MC3T3-E1), and they showed good elastic strength (Venkatesan et al., 2015).

8.2.2   ALG-HYDROXYAPATITE

Hydroxyapatite (HAp) is a natural component of bone which forms the mineral phase imparting mechanical strength and osteoconductivity. HAp-based scaffolds have higher cell attachment capacity due to their surface roughness and protein adsorption ability. Sintered HAp is brittle, thus limiting its applicability in tissue engineering. Combining with natural biodegradable polymers such as ALG forms a composite of organic (ALG) and inorganic (HAp) phases mimicking natural bone. This also enhances mechanical strength and induces partial elasticity to the composites ideal for tissue engineering applications (Kamalaldin et al., 2016).

ALG has less potential for offering cell attachment on its surface due to its hydrophilic nature and negative charge. Addition of COL and HAp to ALG suspension increased their osteoconductivity, osteoblast cell attachment, and proliferation (Cardoso et al., 2014a). In situ polymerization of hydrogels is advantageous over already lyophilized scaffolds. HAp in the form of granules used for bone defects can migrate to other regions reducing its efficiency, and HAp blocks used are not able to fill the complete defective areas which are major disadvantages for tissue engineering applications. Hence, hydrogel made by combining HAp with ALG showed an efficient alternative to overcome these difficulties (Borhan et al., 2016). ALG/COL/HAp scaffolds were prepared either by addition of HAp and COL lyophilized powder to ALG solution or by nucleation of apatite crystals on to COL fibers by incubating them in simulated body fluid (Bendtsen and Wei, 2015). Addition of GEL to ALG/HAp improved the crystallinity of hydrogel by providing Ca binding sites on the carboxylic groups of GEL (Sangeetha et al., 2013). Modified ALG such as oxidized had better reactivity than native ALG, and it was achieved by reacting ALG with sodium periodate (Sarker et al., 2015). The presence of HAp granules in oxidized ALG/GEL/CaP hydrogel amplified bone regeneration by improving osseointegration and osteoconductivity. Reinforcing materials to ALG/HAp composites also showed enhancement of mechanical strength and osteogenic differentiation potential of the scaffolds (Rajesh and Ravichandran et al., 2015).

Growth factors such as BMPs, VEGF, and so forth have been incorporated into scaffolds for increased osteogenesis, angiogenesis, and vascular permeability (Quinlan et al., 2015). Recombinant bone morphogenetic protein 2 was encapsulated in HAp granules due to their high adsorption ability, and they were further combined with oxidized ALG to form biocomposites for bone regeneration (Cai et al., 2016). VEGF encapsulated in ALG microparticles showed an encapsulation efficiency of 49%. The sustained release profile of VEGF enhanced its bioactivity (Quinlan et al., 2015).

Due to swelling, ALG/HAp scaffolds tend to lose their mechanical integrity. An effective way to overcome this problem was the addition of synthetic hydrophobic polymers such as PCL or PLLA to inner pore wall of the scaffolds. This can be achieved via one-step or two-step process. One-step process to form scaffolds was achieved by templating scaffolds on oil-in-water high internal phase emulsion (Hu et al., 2017). These synthetic polymers also acted as drug carriers and provided sustained and prolonged release of drug from the scaffolds. Bovine serum albumin (BSA) was incorporated into such scaffolds by dissolving it along with ALG solution before combining the water and oil phase (Hu et al., 2016). Increased concentration of PCL increased the mechanical strength of the scaffolds along with a prolonged and sustained release of BSA.

Personalized tissue substitutes are the latest advancement in the field of tissue engineering which is achieved using 3D printing. Direct mixing of ALG with HAp lacks homogeneity in particle distribution which in turn limits their bioactivity. The 3D plotting of ALG solution mixed with 500 mM Na_2HPO_4 and later cross-linking with $CaCl_2$ produced the mineralized core-shelled structure of scaffolds with homogeneous distribution of HAp particles. Such scaffolds showed higher ALP activity compared to ALG alone. The ALG/HAp scaffolds also exhibited sustained delivery of BSA for a time period of 25 days (Luo et al., 2015). Addition of polyvinyl alcohol (PVA) to ALG/HAp solution increased the viscosity of the solution, thereby supported its printability, while ALG and HAp provided biocompatibility and ability for cell encapsulation. About 95.6% average cell viability in 3D bioprinted ALG/HAp/polyvinyl pyrrolidone scaffolds has been reported which was significantly higher than 60.1% in scaffolds made from ALG solution (Bendtsen et al., 2017). HAp nanowires were also used for improving the mechanical strength of hydrogels. HAp nanowires were synthesized by the dropwise addition of $CaCl_2$, NaOH, and Na_2HPO_4 solution to a mixture of oleic acid, water, and methanol. The product obtained was dried at 180°C for 24 h and washed with deionized water, ethanol, and cyclohexane. These HAp nanowires were mixed with ALG to produce ALG/HAp nanowire hydrogels with $CaCl_2$ cross-linking, and the results showed that these nanowires increased in their compressive strength, elasticity, and tensile strength suitable for bone tissue repair (Jiang et al., 2017).

ALG microspheres are widely used for drug delivery applications but they have various limitations such as uncontrolled release kinetics and low drug entrapment efficiency (Lee and Mooney, 2012; Venkatesan et al., 2015). Incorporation of HAp into ALG improved mechanical and bioactive properties of the composites. HAp resorption is less, thus restricting the formation of new bone tissue. Substitution of one of the phosphate groups with a carbonate group is used to overcome this limitation (Valiense et al., 2016). HAp substituted with strontium (Sr) and incorporated into ALG microspheres (Sr/HAp/ALG) showed a better drug (vancomycin)-loading efficiency and slow release kinetics compared to both ALG and Sr/HAp microspheres. The release of Sr ions improved bone tissue formation (Li et al., 2016). Sr is an important metal during early stages of bone development. It can enhance osteogenesis as well as inhibit osteoclast formation (Dhivya et al., 2015a; Valiense et al., 2016). Similarly, a sustained release of atsttrin (progranulin) was observed from ALG/nHAp scaffolds prepared via pneumatic bioprinting system with vertical pores in which size of the strand was controlled by speed of deposition and pressure of extrusion. Atsttrin inhibited the effect of TNF-α, enhanced gene expression of various osteoblast markers such as COL1A, osteocalcin (OCN), and osteopontin (OPN), and improved bone healing in rat calvarial models (Wang et al., 2015). ALG/HAp/GEL microspheres containing tetracyclin enhanced their bioactivity by a controlled release of drug and increased osteoblast proliferation efficiency (Yan et al., 2016). Ascorbic acid or vitamin C, a component required for osteogenesis, incorporated into ALG/HAp scaffolds showed a sustained release of the ascorbic acid which improved its bioavailability for a longer time period with target specificity (Ilie et al., 2016).

ALG-containing COL/HAp biocomposite scaffolds showed better mechanical strength along with biological activity. These types of biocomposites had higher cell viability, enhanced cell proliferation, and upregulation of hyaline cartilage marker gene expression which suggested the suitability of these biocomposites for osteochondral tissue regeneration (Zheng et al., 2014). Addition of graphene oxide into ALG/HAp composites enhanced their compressive strength (Xiong et al., 2015). The polymeric coating on metal implants increased its bioactivity. For example, the incorporation of a polymeric material such as ALG to TiO2 and HAp increased their mechanical stiffness, enhanced cell attachment, and proliferation (Naik et al., 2016). Incorporation of HAp in ALG-based biomaterials showed their enhancement of mechanical properties, cell attachment, and osteoblastic differentiation potential. In vivo results identified an increase in bone growth on ALG/nHAp scaffolds compared to ALG scaffolds alone (Wang et al., 2016). Due to a controlled delivery of growth factors from scaffolds, bone regeneration enhanced. In one such study, BMP2 was loaded into CS/ALG/HAp scaffolds and their potential for bone regeneration was determined. BMP2 showed a sustained release for a time period of 21 days which was essential for bone regeneration (He et al., 2014). Alizarin red staining and ALP activity were done to determine differentiation potential of the scaffolds at the cellular level. The mRNA expression of COL1A, OCN, and OPN was analyzed for determining the same at the molecular level. Both results showed that incorporation of BMP2 enhanced the differentiation potential of the scaffolds as shown in Figure 8.4. Further, in vivo studies were carried out on critical-sized rat calvarial defect by treating with CS/ALG/HAp/BMP2 and the results showed an enhanced bone regeneration with respect to both bone mineral density and area of new bone formation (Fig 8.5), confirming its bone regeneration potential (He et al., 2014). Fibroin, a natural biopolymer from silkworms, was added to ALG/HAp solution to prepare biocomposite particles which had an enhanced calvarial bone healing effect in vivo (Jo et al., 2017).

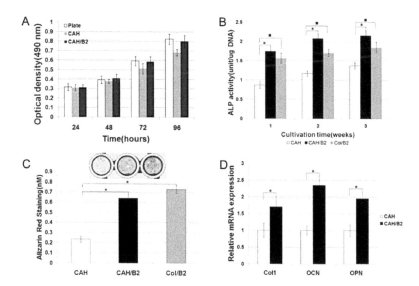

FIGURE 8.4 Biocompatibility and effects of chitosan (CS)/HAp/ALG/bone morphogenetic protein 2 (BMP2) on osteoblast differentiation. (A) MTS assay of MSCs cultured with CAH and CAH/B2 scaffolds. The cells were also cultured in plates as a control. Data represent the mean+SD of n=5 samples. No statistically significant differences were seen between groups. (B) Effects of CAH/B2 on in vitro alkaline phosphatase (ALP) activity. ALP activity in the CAH/B2 group was higher than that in the CAH group. One-way analyses of variance suggest that there are significant differences among three groups. The significant post hoc test results are identified by symbol *. N=5. P<0.001: CAH versus CAH/B2. (C) The level of calcium deposition in 3-week cultures was evaluated by AR-S. The values indicated are means±SD, (n=5) p<0.005 as compared with deposition in the CAH group. (D) qRT-PCR analysis of osteoblast marker genes, showing that MSCs cultured on a CAH/B2 scaffold exhibited increased collagen I, OCN, and OPN gene expression. Data represent the mean+SD of n=5 samples. P<0.05.

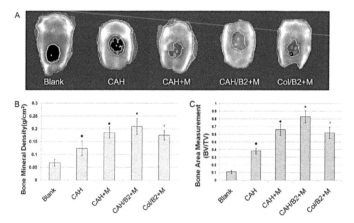

FIGURE 8.5 CS/HAp/ALG/BMP2 scaffolds enhance bone regeneration in the rat critical-sized calvarial defect model. (A) Image of calvarial bone from the Lunar PIXImus system, 12 weeks after surgery. The areas of bone regeneration were labeled in different colors. A black area circled with a blue line (*) is a low-density area. The dark gray area between inside blue line and inside yellow line (#) is an area of thin bone, the area between two yellow lines (Δ) is considered an area of normal bone density, and the density in this area is close to that of normal bone tissue. (B) Quantitative analysis of bone density. N = 6, * p < 0.05: CAH/B2 + M versus four other groups. • p < 0.05: CAH + M versus CAH or blank. ♦ p < 0.05: CAH versus blank. (C) Quantitative analysis of bone area in the implanted region showed a significantly larger bone area within the CAH/B2 + M group when compared with the other four groups. BV, bone area in the implant; TV, total implant area. N=6, * p < 0.05: CAH/B2 + M versus four other groups. • p < 0.05: CAH + M versus CAH or blank. ♦ p < 0.05: CAH versus blank.

Reprinted from He et al., 2014. https://creativecommons.org/licenses/by/4.0/

In consideration of ALG clearance by renal system in vivo, ALG should be less than 50 kDa in size, since human body lacks enzymes which can disintegrate ALG. Treatments such as gamma irradiation and partial oxidation along with thermal treatments are given to ensure the size of ALG used. Among these techniques, gamma irradiation is the most powerful strategy which causes rapid loss of material integrity, whereas partial oxidation is less destructive. Repeated cycles of thermal treatment using autoclaving can reduce MW in mild and controlled manner without affecting composite integrity (Cardoso et al., 2014b).

8.2.3 ALG–SILICA

Silica (Si) (silicon dioxide, SiO_2) has the excellent properties such as enhancement in biomineralization, mechanical stiffness, cell proliferation, and differentiation, which makes it an ideal choice for tissue engineering applications (Pattnaik et al., 2011; Sowjanya et al., 2013; Kumar et al., 2014; Moorthi et al., 2014; Ajita et al., 2015; Sainitya et al., 2015; Saravanan et al., 2015; Saravanan et al., 2016a). The presence of silicate showed an anabolic effect on osteogenic potential and inhibitory action on osteoclastogenesis, which were essential for bone regeneration application (Beck et al., 2012; Schröder et al., 2012; Schloßmacher et al., 2013; Müller et al., 2015; Qiu et al., 2013). Introduction of tricalcium silicate to ALG hydrogels improved their handling properties due to in situ hydrogel formation. The ionic extracts from the hydrogels also enhanced cell proliferation (Xu et al., 2018). ALG with mesoporous Si nanoparticles (MSN) was used for targeted drug delivery applications. It was synthesized using air dynamical atomization technique. Briefly, ALG solution containing MSN was loaded into a syringe and extruded out using a syringe pump along with air flow into $CaCl_2$ solution dropwise. Due to cross-linking of ALG, MSN-encapsulated ALG beads were produced. For the preparation of drug-loaded ALG beads, a model drug was mixed in required concentration to MSN/ALG solution for 24 h before loading into the syringe for extrusion. Experimental results showed that by controlling instrumental parameters such as flow rate of solution, nozzle diameter, stirring speed of cross-linker solution, distance of syringe from cross-linker solution, and pressure, different composites suitable for various applications were synthesized. Particles with 20 μm in size showed sustained release, excellent biocompatibility, and target specificity (Liao et al., 2014). In calcium silicate, Sr was substituted and combined with ALG to improve osteoblast proliferation and inhibit osteoclastogenesis for enhancement of bone tissue repair (Qiu et al., 2017). The 3D bioplotting was utilized for fabrication of composites containing Si and ALG. Addition of COL to this biocomposite increased the interaction of scaffolds with cells. There was an improved cell proliferation of pre-osteoblasts along with increased gene expression of osteoblast differentiation markers such as COL, OCN, and BMP2 in the ALG/COL scaffolds containing Si, which suggested the potential nature of these scaffolds for BTE applications (Lee et al., 2014).

8.2.4 ALG–BIOGLASS

Bioactive glass (BG) is a form of inorganic biomaterial containing ions such as Si, Ca, P, and so forth in it. These ions have shown their stimulatory effect on the proliferation and osteoblast differentiation (Au et al., 2010; Wu et al.,

2011; Moorthi et al., 2014; Ajita et al., 2015; Mo et al., 2016; Gong et al., 2017). Ca and Si ions adjust the chemical environment to regulate cell cycle phase. Bioglass 45S5 has been shown to possess osteostimulatory effects suitable for BTE. Nanosized BG (nBG) showed higher biological activity regarding proliferation and differentiation compared to micron-sized BG. The 13-93 BG is a modified form of BG 45S5 with higher content of SiO_2, making it mechanically stronger (Luo et al., 2017). BG in the form of powder is not sufficient for tissue engineering applications. These, when formed into scaffolds, provided mechanical strength to the implants, and injectability of these materials increased by combining it with water-soluble polymers such as ALG. nBG composites with ALG and HAc were tested for their stability, osteogenesis, and cytotoxicity. Results showed that nBG/ALG composites were more mechanically stable than nBG/HAc scaffolds. Biocomposites with nBG/ALG/HAc showed a higher release of Si ions into the medium, thus having higher osteogenic effects (Sohrabi et al., 2014). Addition of BG to ALG enhanced the degree of cross-linking due to the presence of Ca ions in BG, thereby increasing the mechanical strength (Sarker et al., 2016). In another study, BG was synthesized from the tetraethyl orthosilicate, calcium nitrate tetrahydrate, and triethyl phosphate and used to fabricate BG/ALG scaffolds using the 3D printing method. The result showed that scaffolds had enhanced the effect on osteogeneis (Zhao et al., 2016). The 3D printing was useful to fabricate the biocomposites containing BG with controlled pore size and scaffold architecture (Luo et al., 2017). The 3D printed scaffolds containing ALG/13-93 BG were fabricated and analyzed for their bone regeneration potential. The scaffolds showed the compressive strength of 10–16 MPa and moduli of 40–80 MPa which were similar to cancellous bone. The release of Mg and Si ions from scaffolds enhanced MSC differentiation towards osteoblast, suggesting their potential application in BTE applications (Luo et al., 2017).

ALG/CS was codoped with octacalcium phosphate (OCP)/nBG and fabricated into membranes using layer-by-layer method for bone regeneration applications. There was enhanced cell adhesion and proliferation of human bone marrow stromal cells in the ALG/CS membranes with OCP/nBG compared to ALG/CS membranes alone (Xu et al., 2016). Alginate dialdehyde/GEL hydrogel containing BG showed better cell attachment due to the presence of GEL. BG affected in controlled degradation and release of GEL due to the increased covalent cross-linking (Rottensteiner et al., 2014; Sarker et al., 2016). A similar composition was fabricated as a biocomposite hydrogel using 3D bioplotting and constructs were obtained with the grid-like structure. They showed a sustained release of model drug and proved to be a feasible technique for cell encapsulation due to the milder conditions (Leite et al., 2016).

Both direct and alternating currents are used for electrophoretic deposition of BG/ALG onto stainless steel implants. Among these two techniques, alternating current deposition showed higher corrosion resistance and adhesion strength. Various biological entities were immobilized on to surfaces using an alternating current method which made it superior to direct current electrophoretic deposition (Chen et al., 2013). Addition of PVA to BG/ALG increased adhesion of the coating to the substrate (Chen et al., 2014). BG/ALG hydrogels have the potential to be used as cell carriers for bone regeneration. Incorporation of BG into ALG regulated the microstructure of biocomposites to aid controlled release of encapsulated growth factors and peptides (Zeng et al., 2014). Risk of infection is another major challenge in the success of implants. Zinc oxide nanoparticles (ZnO) have the antibacterial activity (Tripathi et al., 2012; Swetha et al., 2012; Niranjan et al., 2013; Dhivya et al., 2015a; Dhivya et al., 2015b) and inclusion of ZnO in the BG/ALG composites showed a possible solution for this infection problem (Cordero-Arias et al., 2015a). TiO_2 also has antibacterial properties, and thus, it is used instead of ZnO in BG/ALG biocomposites for producing a coating on the surface of stainless steel implants for reduction of infection risks. This electrophoretic coating also provided corrosion protection to implants along with enhanced osteogenesis effects (Cordero-Arias et al., 2015b).

8.2.5 OTHERS

Materials such as oyster shell powder (OSP), cockle shell powder, and halloysite nanotubes (HNTs) are used along with ALG to form scaffolds for tissue engineering applications. Oyster shell is a waste product in mariculture. It is rich in $CaCO_3$ and can be utilized after processing as an alternative to inorganic phosphates in biocomposites for bone regeneration. Oyster shell also has slow resorption rate, good biocompatibility, and osteogenic potential. The scaffolds with ALG/hydroxypropyl trimethyl ammonium chloride chitosan (HACC)/OSP had better their physicochemical properties, antimicrobial activity, and mineralization effects. Addition of OSP in ALG/HACC scaffolds increased their protein adsorption and biomineralization activities. The scaffolds also showed biocompatibility to cells (Chen et al., 2016). Cockleshell powder comprises more than 95% $CaCO_3$ and has similarities with coral exoskeletons. $CaCO_3$ present in cockleshell powder is in the form of aragonite which is a denser form of $CaCO_3$, making it promising candidate in material engineering, and it can also be easily converted into nanoparticles to increase the surface area. Addition of cockle shell powder to ALG scaffolds showed enhanced osteoblast cell attachment and growth (Bharathy et al., 2014; Ahmad et al., 2017).

Carbon nanotubes (CNTs) act as effective cross-linkers for ALG hydrogels. Single-walled CNTs increase compressive strength and modulus of ALG struts. HNTs are one-dimensional particles with unique tubular microstructure. When compared to other nanoparticles, nanotubes have better biocompatibility, higher dispersion, hydrophilicity, entrapment of drugs, and low cost. HNTs were incorporated into ALG for sustained drug release. They increased the thermal stability of the composites, and increased concentration of HNTs in ALG increased a number of cells attached to the scaffolds (Liu et al., 2015). They also enhanced cell proliferation of mouse pre-osteoblasts (MC3T3-E1), proving their potential to be used for bone regeneration applications (Huang et al., 2017).

8.3   FABRICATION METHODS OF SCAFFOLDS

In BTE applications, ALG is prepared along with other materials as 3D biocomposites in various structures including scaffolds, electrospun fibers, hydrogels, microspheres, and so forth. Scaffolds are 3D structures fabricated using the techniques such as lyophilization/freeze-drying, solvent/porogen leaching, and additive manufacturing (AM; 3D printing, powder printing, fused deposition modeling, etc.). They are mainly used for bone defects at the load-bearing site due to their mechanical properties. Scaffolds used in larger bone defects or at the load-bearing sites should be tested for their compressive strength before use, and they should have the compressive strength similar to natural bone. Scaffolds fabricated by lyophilization can have isotropic or anisotropic pore structures (Kolewe et al., 2013; Porrelli et al., 2015). Electrospun fibers are majorly used in nonload-bearing sites. Nanofibers provide a larger surface area for cell attachment and spreading. Electrospun fibers can also entrap drugs in it, and the studies showed that release profile of drugs from fibers is more controlled than other forms such as scaffolds, hydrogels, and microspheres (Song et al., 2013; Weng and Xie, 2015; Yao et al., 2016; Tang et al., 2016; Balagangadharan et al., 2017). Hydrogels are ideal for bone regeneration due to their injectability and noninvasive nature along with efficient drug delivery (Sotome et al., 2004; Luginbuehl et al., 2005; Chung et al., 2007; Kretlow et al., 2007; Bhattarai et al., 2010; Lee et al., 2011). Reconstruction of osseous defects using prefabricated implants has many disadvantages such as fibrous encapsulation due to the presence of voids. Hydrogels can accommodate cells and growth factors inside them for tissue regeneration process. They are prepared using various solgel polymerization techniques such as ionic cross-linking, covalent cross-linking, photopolymerization, and so forth (Lu et al., 2003; Cardoso et al., 2014a; Lai and He, 2016; Barthes et al., 2017; Yang et al., 2017). Microspheres act as the matrix for cell entrapment and drug delivery during tissue regeneration process. Drug loading in ALG microspheres was carried out using emulsion solvent evaporation technique (Li et al., 2016). The following section explains the fabrication methods for preparation of the scaffolds including ALG as one of the biomaterials used in BTE.

8.3.1 LYOPHILIZATION

Lyophilization/freeze-drying is a commonly used in scaffold fabrication technique in which the solution containing materials for scaffolds is freeze-dried at −40°C in a vacuum. Pore size can be controlled by stepwise reduction of temperature in the lyophilizer. ALG and inorganic phosphate materials can be prepared separately and then mixed thoroughly using stirrers or ultrasonicator for uniform dispersion of the mixture and then freeze-dried at −45°C. Initial freezing of the solution helps in the freezing of water molecules and followed by reduction of surrounding pressure sublimes the frozen molecules to get converted from solid to liquid phase. The regions occupied by the water molecules form pores in the final scaffolds thus formed. Thus, scaffolds can have interconnected pore structure which enhances water uptake, nutrient exchange, and waste removal from the scaffolds more efficiently during the process of bone regeneration (Kim et al., 2015; Chen et al., 2016; Leena et al., 2017).

8.3.2 ELECTROSPINNING

Electrospinning is a more reliable technique to obtain fibers at nano- and microscales. Rapid evaporation of solvent occurs during electrospinning process, resulting in the formation of nonwoven mesh with 3D interconnected pores having high surface area structurally mimicking ECM (Jeong et al., 2010; Bonino et al., 2011; Saquing et al., 2013; Balagangadharan et al., 2017). Nanofibers are more suitable for cell attachment and migration, diffusion of oxygen, high drug-loading capacity, and vascularization due to their unique topography. ALG at higher concentrations becomes viscous, and thus, it may not be suitable for electrospinning. In such cases, ALG can be mixed with polyethylene oxide copolymer for fabrication of nanofibers (Saquing et al., 2013; Venkatesan et al., 2015). Inorganic phosphates are also mixed along with ALG solution for electrospinning process of biocomposite fibers. Nanoparticles tend to flocculate during the process of electrospinning, resulting in an uneven distribution of inorganic phosphates on the ALG mesh. In such situation, in situ synthesis of HAp crystals had been performed where uniform distribution of nanocrystals was obtained on the matrices (Chae et al., 2013).

8.3.3 ELECTROPHORETIC DEPOSITION

Bioinert metallic implants are used in load-bearing site bone defects. These implants have the porous structure which allows vascular as well as bone tissue ingrowths. Making these metallic implants by mimicking natural bone characteristics can enhance bone formation. Coating with inorganic phosphates had an effect on the enhancement of osseointegration in vivo (Kollath et al., 2016). Biomimetic is a widely used technique for coating with inorganic phosphates. It was carried out as follows: the experimental setup consisted a glass beaker inside which a concentric circle of the diameter larger than the metallic implant made of stainless steel foil was placed as demonstrated in Figure 8.6A. The metallic implant was connected with either positive or negative electrode, whereas the stainless steel foil acted as the counter electrode. The prepared CaP/ALG solution was filled in the glass beaker, and an electric potential was applied. A slight turbulence was given by stirring at a low speed to ensure uniform deposition on to the surface. Electrophoretic deposition is mediated by different solvents such as acetone, acetylacetone, water, water/ethanol mixture, and so forth. Figure 8.6B indicated the deposition of CAp/ALG on implants (Kollath et al., 2016). A similar procedure was done on stainless steel for deposition of ALG/TiO2 or ALG/BG biocomposite mixture onto it. Coated substrates were air-dried before use (Cordero-Arias et al., 2014).

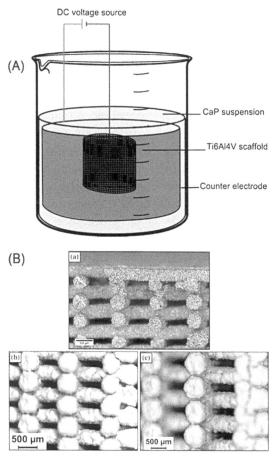

FIGURE 8.6 (A) Schematic representation of electrophoretic deposition(B) Optical micrographs of uncoated a and HA–Alg-coated sample before(b) and after (c) sintering step (Kollath, V.O.; Chen, Q.; Mullens, S.; Luyten, J.; Traina, K.; Boccaccini, A.R. and Cloots, R. Electrophoretic deposition of hydroxyapatite and hydroxyapatite–alginate on rapid prototyped 3D Ti6Al4V scaffolds. *Journal of Materials Science.* 2016, *51*(5), 2338-2346. With Permission)

8.3.4 ADDITIVE MANUFACTURING

Scaffold architecture is an important parameter for implantable biomaterials. Among the various techniques available, AM technique has superior control over scaffold architecture. 3D powder printing, 3D plotting, fused deposition modeling, and so forth are the various AM techniques currently available which can be used to make personalized tissue constructs. A patient's computed tomography scan or magnetic resonance imaging is used to construct repaired computer-aided design model of tissue/organ within 24 h. The model is then converted into stereolithography file in 3D printer software. This determines the filling path in XY direction scanning movement, forming the 3D structured scaffolds (Xu et al., 2015). These techniques are more suitable for scaffolds containing ceramics. Powder printing technology is based on combining different powder composition using a binder material such as phosphoric acid, and unreacted powder is then removed after drying the scaffolds by immersing it in an acidic solution. In this technique, the selection of binder material limits the application of powder printing for materials with multiple layers containing different composition. A 3D plotting is done in a layer-by-layer fashion of starting materials (polymer/mineral components) by simple inkjet processing at room temperature which makes it suitable for applications involving thermosensitive materials and incorporation of growth factors or live cells. Size of the strands can be adjusted using the speed of deposition and pressure of extrusion yielding structures with regular vertically connected pores to get a uniform deposition of inorganic ceramics throughout the scaffolds (Wang et al., 2015). Fused deposition modeling is similar to 3D plotting but using higher temperatures in which polymers melted and extruded to form layer-by-layer model of scaffolds (Kumar et al., 2016).

8.3.5 SOLVENT CASTING EVAPORATION

This method is used for fabrication of composite films. In this technique, the components are dissolved in solvents (usually water), stirred thoroughly with or without cross-linker and poured onto casting chambers. After solvent evaporation is completed, the films are incubated with cross-linker solution for overnight and then washed several times to adjust the pH to 7.0 and dried at 37°C. This technique was used for fabrication of GEL/ALG/HAc/bone ash biocomposite films with EDC as cross-linker and results showed that films possessed high mechanical strength and sustained drug release (Alemdar, 2016; Xu et al., 2016).

8.3.6 FOAMING METHOD

It is one of the economic scaffold fabrication techniques available in which polymer foam is produced upon agitation of the polymer solution and thereby cross-linking/solidifying the polymer foam. ALG/GEL mixture, when agitated in the presence of NaHCO3, produced foam to which glutaraldehyde was added as a cross-linker. This polymer foam was slowly added to CS solution containing HAp, resulting in the formation of scaffold beads. These beads were then washed to remove any excess glutaraldehyde present and immersed in glycine solution to block any free aldehyde group present in the scaffolds (Sharma et al., 2016).

8.3.7   EXTRUSION FREE-FORMING

It is a rapid prototyping technique used to make scaffolds with the tailored porous structure for BTE applications. The key parameters for extrusion free-forming are sintering conditions, slurry properties, and printing. Sodium ALG solution containing inorganic components dispersed uniformly was used as the slurry for the process. The scaffolds were then fabricated using the microsyringe extrusion free-forming system. Thus, the prepared scaffolds were cross-linked by incubating them in calcium chloride solution for 24 h. ALG/HAp scaffolds sintered at relatively lower temperatures showed interconnected pores with a rougher surface containing microparticles (Zhou et al., 2015).

8.3.8   SOLGEL POLYMERIZATION

Solgel polymerization is a commonly used technique for the preparation of hydrogels which can be injected directly into defect sites for bone and cartilage regeneration. ALG hydrogel containing inorganic compounds was prepared by mixing and stirring along with $CaCO_3$ which acted as a cross-linker. Glucono-d-lactone (GDL) was then added which controlled the release of Ca^{2+} from $CaCO_3$ (Yan et al., 2016). Solgel polymerization is also used for the production of microspheres. Microspheres encapsulated with a drug provided a sustained and prolonged release of the drug, thus increased its bioavailability (Wang et al., 2016).

8.3.9   ICE-SEGREGATION-INDUCED SELF-ASSEMBLY

This method is used to introduce anisotropy in the scaffolds. It was achieved by immersing the samples in liquid nitrogen or on dry ice at a controlled speed. By controlling the freezing velocity, the solvent composition, the concentration of particles, and the morphology of pores were modulated. These structures had an effect on the promotion of osteoblast growth due to their anisotropic pores for cell colonization (Porrelli et al., 2015).

8.4 CONCLUSION

ALG is a promising material for BTE applications owing to its low cost and excellent biocompatibility. Even though ALG lacks mechanical strength, stable ALG biocomposites were prepared using cross-linkers and other biomaterials. ALG along with other biomaterials in the form of various 3D structures by a number of fabrication methods showed enhanced cell proliferation and osteoblast differentiation. Their encapsulation with cells/bioactive growth factors promoted bone tissue regeneration by a sustained and prolonged release of bioactive growth factors. The emerging techniques such as 3D printing for personalized tissue constructs using ALG-containing biocomposites would possibly be the best alternatives for autografts and metallic implants in the field of BTE.

SUMMARY

BTE encompasses the principles of bone biology and engineering disciplines to augment bone loss through the use of temporary matrices called scaffolds. ALG is an anionic polymer having promising potential for its applications in BTE since it can easily be modified in many forms such as hydrogels, aerogels, 3D scaffolds, fibers, sponges, microspheres, microcapsules, and foams. The highly hydrophilic and porous nature of this polymer can provide a matrix for bone tissue regeneration. ALG appears to have reduced risk of immune rejection, along with low toxicity and relatively small cost which make it suitable for BTE applications. However, ALG lacks mechanical strength, and hence, ALG was blended with inorganic materials (mainly hydroxyapatite, β-TCP, silica, and bioglass) or carbon nanotubes as biocomposite scaffolds and they showed enhanced mechanical properties. Encapsulation of these biocomposite scaffolds with stem cells, osteoblasts, or growth factors increased their bioactivity by a controlled delivery of growth factors. Thus, this chapter summarizes recent developments in synthesis and formation of ALG-based scaffolds with inorganic compounds and their applications in the field of BTE.

ACKNOWLEDGMENT

This work was in part supported by the SRM University.

KEYWORDS

- **bone**
- **alginate**
- **tissue engineering**
- **scaffolds**
- **drug delivery**

REFERENCES

Ahmad, N.; Bharatham, H. B.; Hamid, Z. A.; Zulkipli, N. Z. Cytotoxicity and Oxidative Stress Evaluation of Alginate/Cockle Shell Powder Nanobiocomposite Bone Scaffold on Osteoblast. *Jurnal Sains Kesihatan Malaysia (Malays. J. Health Sci.)*. **2017,** *15*(1), 97–103.

Ajita, J.; Saravanan, S. Selvamurugan, N. Effect of Size of Bioactive Glass Nanoparticles on Mesenchymal Stem Cell Proliferation for Dental and Orthopedic Applications. *Mater. Sci. Eng. C* **2015,** *53,* 142–149.

Alemdar, N. Fabrication of A Novel Bone Ash-Reinforced Gelatin/Alginate/Hyaluronic Acid Composite Film for Controlled Drug Delivery. *Carbohydr. Polym.* **2016,** *151,* 1019–1026.

Andrades, J. A.; Narváez-Ledesma, L.; Cerón-Torres, L.; Cruz-Amaya, A. P.; López-Guillén, D.; Mesa-Almagro, M. L.; Moreno-Moreno, J. A. Bone Engineering: a Matter of Cells, Growth Factors and Biomaterials. In *Regenerative Medicine and Tissue Engineering;* 2013; InTech, pp 615–641. DOI: 10.5772/56389

Au, A. Y.; Au, R. Y.; Demko, J. L.; McLaughlin, R. M.; Eves, B. E.; Frondoza, C. G. Consil Bioactive Glass Particles Enhance Osteoblast Proliferation and Selectively Modulate Cell Signaling Pathways in Vitro. *J. Biomed. Mater. Res. Part A* **2010,** *94*(2), 380–388.

Axpe, E.; Oyen, M. L. Applications of Alginate-Based Bioinks in 3D Bioprinting. *Int. J. Mol. Sci.* **2016,** *17*(12), 1976.

Balagangadharan, K.; Dhivya, S.; Selvamurugan, N. Chitosan Based Nanofibers in Bone Tissue Engineering. *Int. J. Biol. Macromol.* **2017,** *104,* 1372–1382.

Barthes, J.; Mutschler, A.; Dollinger, C.; Gaudinat, G.; Lavalle, P.; Le Houerou, V.; McGuinness, G. B.; Vrana, N. E. Establishing Contact Between Cell-Laden Hydrogels and Metallic Implants with a Biomimetic Adhesive for Cell Therapy Supported Implants. *Biomed. Mater*. **2017,** *13*(1), 015015.

Beck, G. R., Jr.; Ha, S. W.; Camalier, C. E.; Yamaguchi, M.; Li, Y.; Lee, J. K.; Weitzmann, M. N. Bioactive Silica-Based Nanoparticles Stimulate Bone-Forming Osteoblasts, Suppress

Bone-Resorbing Osteoclasts, and Enhance Bone Mineral Density in Vivo. *Nanomed. Nanotechnol. Biol. Med.* **2012**, *8*(6), 793–803.

Bendtsen, S. T.; Wei, M. Synthesis and Characterization of a Novel Injectable Alginate–Collagen–Hydroxyapatite Hydrogel for Bone Tissue Regeneration. *J. Mater. Chem. B* **2015**, *3*(15), 3081–3090.

Bendtsen, S. T.; Quinnell, S. P.; Wei, M. Development of a Novel Alginate-Polyvinyl Alcohol-Hydroxyapatite Hydrogel for 3D Bioprinting Bone Tissue Engineered Scaffolds. *J. Biomed. Mater. Res. Part A* **2017**, *105*(5), 1457–1468.

Bharatham, B.H.; Bakar, A.; Zuki, M.; Perimal, E.K.; Yusof, L.M.; Hamid, M. Development and Characterization of Novel Porous 3D Alginate-Cockle Shell Powder Nanobiocomposite Bone Scaffold. *Biomed. Res. Int.* 2014, *2014*, Article ID 146723.

Bhattarai, N.; Gunn, J.; Zhang, M. Chitosan-Based Hydrogels for Controlled, Localized Drug Delivery. *Adv. Drug Delivery Rev.* **2010**, *62*(1), 83–99.

Binulal, N. S.; Deepthy, M.; Selvamurugan, N.; Shalumon, K. T.; Suja, S.; Mony, U.; Jayakumar, R.; Nair, S. V. Role of Nanofibrous Poly (Caprolactone) Scaffolds in Human Mesenchymal Stem Cell Attachment and Spreading for in Vitro Bone Tissue Engineering—Response to Osteogenic Regulators. *Tissue Eng. Part A.* **2010**, *16*(2), 393–404.

Bonino, C. A.; Krebs, M. D.; Saquing, C. D.; Jeong, S. I.; Shearer, K. L.; Alsberg, E.; Khan, S. A. Electrospinning Alginate-Based Nanofibers: from Blends to Crosslinked Low Molecular Weight Alginate-Only Systems. *Carbohydr. Polym.* **2011**, *85*(1), 111-119.

Borhan, S.; Hesaraki, S.; Nezafati, N. Synthesis and Rheological Evaluations of Novel Injectable Sodium Alginate/ Chitosan-Nanostructured Hydroxyapatite Composite Bone Pastes. *J. Aust. Ceram. Soc.* **2016**, *52*(2), 120–127.

Cai, Y.; Yu, J.; Kundu, S. C.; Yao, J. Multifunctional Nano-Hydroxyapatite and Alginate/ Gelatin Based Sticky Gel Composites for Potential Bone Regeneration. *Mater. Chem. Phys.* **2016**, *181*, 227–233.

Calasans-Maia, M. D.; Alves, A. T. N. N.; Resende, R. F. D. B.; Louro, R. S.; Sartoretto, S. C.; Granjeiro, J. M.; Alves, G. G. Cytocompatibility and Biocompatibility of Nanostructured Carbonated Hydroxyapatite Spheres for Bone Repair. *J. Appl. Oral Sci.* **2015**, *23*(6), 599–608.

Cardoso, D. A.; Ulset, A. S.; Bender, J.; Jansen, J. A.; Christensen, B. E.; Leeuwenburgh, S. C. Effects of Physical and Chemical Treatments on the Molecular Weight and Degradation of Alginate–Hydroxyapatite Composites. *Macromol. Biosci.* **2014a**, *14*(6), 872–880.

Cardoso, D. A.; Van Den Beucken, J. J. J. P.; Both, L. L. H.; Bender, J.; Jansen, J. A.; Leeuwenburgh, S. C. G. Gelation and Biocompatibility of Injectable Alginate–Calcium Phosphate Gels for Bone Regeneration. *J. Biomed. Mater. Res. Part A* **2014b**, *102*(3), 808–817.

Castilho, M.; Rodrigues, J.; Pires, I.; Gouveia, B.; Pereira, M.; Moseke, C.; Groll, J.; Ewald, A.; Vorndran, E. Fabrication of Individual Alginate-TCP Scaffolds for Bone Tissue Engineering by Means of Powder Printing. *Biofabrication* **2015**, *7*(1), 015004.

Chae, T.; Yang, H.; Leung, V.; Ko, F.; Troczynski, T. Novel Biomimetic Hydroxyapatite/ Alginate Nanocomposite Fibrous Scaffolds for Bone Tissue Regeneration. *J. Mater. Sci. Mater. Med.* **2013**, *24*(8), 1885–1894.

Yamamoto, M.; Tabata, Y. A. Tissue Engineering Scaffolds from Bioactive Glass and Composite Materials. In *Topics Tissue Engineering;* Chen, Q., Roether, J. A., Boccaccini, Eds., 2008; Vol.4, pp 1–27.

Chen, Q.; Cordero-Arias, L.; Roether, J. A.; Cabanas-Polo, S.; Virtanen, S.; Boccaccini, A. R. Alginate/Bioglass® Composite Coatings on Stainless Steel Deposited by Direct Current and Alternating Current Electrophoretic Deposition. *Surf. Coat. Technol.* **2013**, *233*, 49–56.

Chen, Q.; Cabanas-Polo, S.; Goudouri, O. M. Boccaccini, A. R. Electrophoretic Co-Deposition of Polyvinyl Alcohol (PVA) Reinforced Alginate–Bioglass® Composite Coating On Stainless Steel: Mechanical Properties And In-Vitro Bioactivity Assessment. *Mater. Sci. Eng. C* **2014**, *40*, 55–64.

Chen, C. Y.; Ke, C. J.; Yen, K. C.; Hsieh, H. C.; Sun, J. S.; Lin, F. H. 3D Porous Calcium-Alginate Scaffolds Cell Culture System Improved Human Osteoblast Cell Clusters for Cell Therapy. *Theranostics* **2015**, *5*(6), 643.

Chen, T.-Y.; Huang, H.-C.; Cao, J.-L.; Xin, Y.-J.; Luo, W.-F. Ao, N.-J. Preparation and Characterization of Alginate/HACC/Oyster Shell Powder Biocomposite Scaffolds for Potential Bone Tissue Engineering Applications. *RSC Adv.* **2016**, *6*(42), 35577–35588.

Chung, H. J.; Park, T. G. Surface Engineered and Drug Releasing Pre-Fabricated Scaffolds for Tissue Engineering. *Adv. Drug Delivery Rev.* **2007**, *59*(4), 249–262.

Coathup, M. J.; Edwards, T. C.; Samizadeh, S.; Lo, W. J.; Blunn, G. W. The Effect of an Alginate Carrier on Bone Formation in a Hydroxyapatite Scaffold. *J. Biomed. Mater. Res. Part B Appl. Biomater.* **2016**, *104*(7), 1328–1335.

Cordero-Arias, L.; Cabanas-Polo, S.; Gilabert, J.; Goudouri, O. M.; Sanchez, E.; Virtanen, S.; Boccaccini, A. R. Electrophoretic Deposition of Nanostructured TiO_2/Alginate and TiO_2-Bioactive Glass/Alginate Composite Coatings on Stainless Steel. *Adv. Appl. Ceram.* **2014**, *113*(1), 42–49.

Cordero-Arias, L.; Cabanas-Polo, S.; Goudouri, O. M.; Misra, S. K.; Gilabert, J.; Valsami-Jones, E.; Sanchez, E.; Virtanen, S.; Boccaccini, A. R. Electrophoretic Deposition of ZnO/Alginate and ZnO-Bioactive Glass/Alginate Composite Coatings for Antimicrobial Applications. *Mater. Sci. Eng. C* **2015a**, *55*, 137–144.

Cordero-Arias, L.; Cabanas-Polo, S.; Virtanen, S.; Boccaccini, A. R. Electrophoretic Deposition of Nanostructured Titania-Bioactive Glass/Alginate Coatings on Stainless Steel. *Key Eng. Mater.* **2015b**, *654*, 159–164.

Cunniffe, G. M.; Vinardell, T.; Thompson, E. M.; Daly, A. C.; Matsiko, A.; O'Brien, F. J.; Kelly, D. J. Chondrogenically Primed Mesenchymal Stem Cell-Seeded Alginate Hydrogels Promote Early Bone Formation in Critically Sized Defects. *Eur. Polym. J.* **2015**, *72*, 464–472.

Cuozzo, R. C., da Rocha Leão, M. H. M., de Andrade Gobbo, L., da Rocha, D. N., Ayad, N. M. E., Trindade, W., Costa, A. M.; da Silva, M. H. P. Zinc Alginate–Hydroxyapatite Composite Microspheres for Bone Repair. *Ceram. Int.* **2014**, *40*(7), 11369–11375.

De Paula, F. L.; Barreto, I. C.; Rocha-Leão, M. H.; Borojevic, R.; Rossi, A. M.; Rosa, F. P.; Farina, M. Hydroxyapatite-Alginate Biocomposite Promotes Bone Mineralization in Different Length Scales in Vivo. *Front. Mater. Sci. China.* **2009**, *3*(2), 145–153.

Dhandayuthapani, B.; Yoshida, Y.; Maekawa, T.; Kumar, D. S. Polymeric Scaffolds in Tissue Engineering Application: a Review. *Int. J. Polym. Sci.* **2011**, *2011*, 1–19.

Dhivya, S.; Ajita, J.; Selvamurugan, N. Metallic Nanomaterials for Bone Tissue Engineering. *J. Biomed. Nanotechnol.* **2015a**, *11*(10), 1675–1700.

Dhivya, S.; Saravanan, S.; Sastry, T. P.; Selvamurugan, N. Nanohydroxyapatite-Reinforced Chitosan Composite Hydrogel for Bone Tissue Repair in Vitro and in Vivo. *J. Nanobio-technol.* **2015b**, *13*(1), 40.

Diogo, G. S.; Gaspar, V. M.; Serra, I. R.; Fradique, R.; Correia, I. J. Manufacture of β-TCP/Alginate Scaffolds Through a Fab@Home Model for Application in Bone Tissue Engineering. *Biofabrication* **2014**, *6*(2), 025001.

Dittrich, R.; Tomandl, G.; Despang, F.; Bernhardt, A.; Hanke, Th.; Pompe, W.; Gelinsky, M. Scaffolds for Hard Tissue Engineering by Ionotropic Gelation of Alginate–Influence of Selected Preparation Parameters. *J. Am. Ceram. Soc.* **2007**, *90*(6), 1703–1708.

Fernandes, J. S.; Reis, R. L.; Pires, R. A. Wetspun Poly-L-(lactic acid)-Borosilicate Bioactive Glass Scaffolds for Guided Bone Regeneration. *Mater. Sci. Eng C* **2017**, *71*, 252–259.

Florczyk, S. J.; Leung, M.; Jana, S.; Li, Z.; Bhattarai, N.; Huang, J. I.; Hopper, R. A.; Zhang, M. Enhanced Bone Tissue Formation by Alginate Gel-Assisted Cell Seeding in Porous Ceramic Scaffolds and Sustained Release of Growth factor. *J. Biomed. Mater. Res. Part A* **2012**, *100*(12), 3408–3415.

Gomez, C. G.; Lambrecht, M. V. P.; Lozano, J. E.; Rinaudo, M.; Villar, M. A. Influence of the Extraction–Purification Conditions on Final Properties of Alginates Obtained from Brown Algae (*Macrocystis pyrifera*). *Int. J. Biol. Macromol.* **2009**, *44*(4), 365–371.

Gómez, S.; Vlad, M. D.; López, J.; Fernández, E. Design and Properties of 3D Scaffolds for Bone Tissue Engineering. *Acta Biomater.* **2016**, *42*, 341–350.

Gong, W.; Dong, Y.; Wang, S.; Gao, X.; Chen, X. A Novel Nano-sized Bioactive Glass Stimulates Osteogenesis via the MAPK Pathway. *RSC Adv.* **2017**, *7*(23), 13760–13767.

Han, Y.; Zeng, Q.; Li, H.; Chang, J. The Calcium Silicate/Alginate Composite: Preparation and Evaluation of its Behavior as Bioactive Injectable Hydrogels. *Acta Biomater.* **2013**, *9*(11), 9107–9117.

He, X.; Liu, Y.; Yuan, X.; Lu, L. Enhanced Healing of Rat Calvarial Defects with MSCs Loaded on BMP-2 Releasing Chitosan/Alginate/Hydroxyapatite Scaffolds. *PloS One.* **2014**, *9*(8), e104061.

He, Y.; Yang, F.; Zhao, H.; Gao, Q.; Xia, B.; Fu, J. Research on the Printability of Hydrogels in 3D Bioprinting. *Sci. Rep.* **2016**, *6*, 29977.

Howk, D.; Chu, T. M. Design Variables for Mechanical Properties of Bone Tissue Scaffolds. *Biomed. Sci. Instrum.* **2006**, *42*, 278–283.

Hu, Y.; Ma, S.; Yang, Z.; Zhou, W.; Du, Z.; Huang, J.; Yi, H.; Wang, C. Facile Fabrication of Poly (L-Lactic Acid) Microsphere-Incorporated Calcium Alginate/Hydroxyapatite Porous Scaffolds Based on Pickering Emulsion Templates. *Colloids Surf. B* **2016**, *140*, 382–391.

Hu, Y.; Han, W.; Chen, Y.; Zou, R.; Ouyang, Y.; Zhou, W.; Yang, Z.; Wang, C. One-Pot Fabrication of Poly (ε-Caprolactone)-Incorporated Bovine Serum Albumin/Calcium Alginate/Hydroxyapatite Nanocomposite Scaffolds by High Internal Phase Emulsion Templates. *Macromol. Mater. Eng.* **2017**, *302*(4), 1600367.

Huang, B.; Liu, M.; Long, Z.; Shen, Y.; Zhou, C. Effects of Halloysite Nanotubes on Physical Properties and Cytocompatibility of Alginate Composite Hydrogels. *Mater. Sci. Eng C* **2017**, *70*, 303–310.

Ilie, A.; Ghiţulică, C.; Andronescu, E.; Cucuruz, A.; Ficai, A. New Composite Materials Based on Alginate and Hydroxyapatite as Potential Carriers for Ascorbic Acid. *Int. J. Pharm.* **2016**, *510*(2), 501–507.

Jeong, S. I.; Krebs, M. D.; Bonino, C. A.; Khan, S. A.; Alsberg, E. Electrospun Alginate Nanofibers with Controlled Cell Adhesion for Tissue Engineering. *Macromol. Biosci.* **2010**, *10*(8), 934–943.

Jiang, Y. Y.; Zhu, Y. J.; Li, H.; Zhang, Y. G.; Shen, Y. Q.; Sun, T. W.; Chen, F. Preparation and Enhanced Mechanical Properties of Hybrid Hydrogels Comprising Ultralong Hydroxyapatite Nanowires And Sodium Alginate. *J. Colloid Interface Sci.* **2017**, *497*, 266–275.

Jo, Y. Y.; Kim, S. G.; Kwon, K. J.; Kweon, H.; Chae, W. S.; Yang, W. G.; Lee, E. Y.; Seok, H. Silk Fibroin-Alginate-Hydroxyapatite Composite Particles in Bone Tissue Engineering Applications in Vivo. *Int. J. Mol. Sci.* **2017**, *18*(4), E858.

Kamalaldin, N.A.; Yahya, B.H.; Nurazreena, A. Cell Evaluation on Alginate/Hydroxyapatite Block for Biomedical Application. *Procedia Chem.* **2016**, *19*, 297–303.

Kanasan, N.; Adzila, S.; AzimahMustaffa, N.; Gurubaran, P. The Effect of Sodium Alginate on the Properties of Hydroxyapatite. *Procedia Eng.* **2017,** *184*, 442–448.

Kim, J.; Bae, W. G.; Lim, K. T.; Jang, K. J.; Oh, S.; Jang, K. J.; Jeon, N. L.; Suh, K. Y.; Chung, J. H. Density of Nanopatterned Surfaces for Designing Bone Tissue Engineering Scaffolds. *Mater. Lett.* **2014,** *130*, 227–231.

Kim, Y. B.; Kim, G. H. PCL/Alginate Composite Scaffolds for Hard Tissue Engineering: Fabrication, Characterization, and Cellular Activities. *ACS Comb. Sci.* **2015,** *17*(2), 87–99.

Kim, H. L.; Jung, G. Y.; Yoon, J. H.; Han, J. S.; Park, Y. J.; Kim, D. G.; Zhang, M. Kim, D. J. Preparation and Characterization of Nano-Sized Hydroxyapatite/Alginate/Chitosan Composite Scaffolds for Bone Tissue Engineering. *Mater. Sci. Eng. C* **2015,** *54*, 20–25.

Kolewe, M. E.; Park, H.; Gray, C.; Ye, X.; Langer, R.; Freed, L. E. 3D Structural Patterns in Scalable, Elastomeric Scaffolds Guide Engineered Tissue Architecture. *Adv. Mater.* **2013,** *25*(32), 4459-4465.

Kollath, V. O.; Chen, Q.; Mullens, S.; Luyten, J.; Traina, K.; Boccaccini, A. R.; Cloots, R. Electrophoretic Deposition of Hydroxyapatite and Hydroxyapatite–Alginate on Rapid Prototyped 3D Ti6Al4V Scaffolds. *J. Mater. Sci.* **2016,** *51*(5), 2338–2346.

Kretlow, J. D.; Klouda, L.; Mikos, A. G. Injectable Matrices and Scaffolds for Drug Delivery in Tissue Engineering. *Adv. Drug Delivery Rev.* **2007,** *59*(4), 263–273.

Kumar, J. P.; Lakshmi, L.; Jyothsna, V.; Balaji, D. R.; Saravanan, S.; Moorthi, A.; Selvamurugan, N. Synthesis and Characterization of Diopside Particles and their Suitability Along with Chitosan Matrix for Bone Tissue Engineering in Vitro and in Vivo. *J. Biomed. Nanotechnol.* **2014,** *10*(6), 970–981.

Kumar, A.; Akkineni, A. R.; Basu, B.; Gelinsky, M. Three-Dimensional Plotted Hydroxyapatite Scaffolds with Predefined Architecture: Comparison of Stabilization by Alginate Cross-Linking Versus Sintering. *J. Biomater. Appl.* **2016,** *30*(8), 1168–1181.

Kuttappan, S.; Mathew, D.; Nair, M. B. Biomimetic Composite Scaffolds Containing Bioceramics and Collagen/Gelatin for Bone Tissue Engineering – a Mini Review. *Int. J. Biol. Macromol.* **2016,** *93*, 1390–1401.

Lai, W. F.; He, Z. D. Design and Fabrication of Hydrogel-Based Nanoparticulate Systems for in Vivo Drug Delivery. *J. Controlled Release.* **2016,** *243*, 269–282.

Lee, K. Y.; Mooney, D. J. Alginate: Properties and Biomedical Applications. *Prog. Polym. Sci.* **2012,** *37*(1), 106–126.

Lee, G. S.; Park, J. H.; Shin, U. S.; Kim, H. W. Direct Deposited Porous Scaffolds of Calcium Phosphate Cement with Alginate for Drug Delivery and Bone Tissue Engineering. *Acta Biomaterialia* **2011,** *7*(8), 3178–3186.

Lee, H.; Kim, Y.; Kim, S.; Kim, G. Mineralized Biomimetic Collagen/Alginate/Silica Composite Scaffolds Fabricated by a Low-Temperature Bio-Plotting Process for Hard Tissue Regeneration: Fabrication, Characterisation and in Vitro Cellular Activities. *J. Mater. Chem. B* **2014,** *2*(35), 5785–5798.

Lee, J. Y.; Chung, J.; Chung, W. J.; Kim, G. Fabrication and in Vitro Biocompatibilities of Fibrous Biocomposites Consisting of PCL and M13 Bacteriophage-Conjugated Alginate for Bone Tissue Engineering. *J. Mater. Chem. B* **2016,** *4*(4), 656–665.

Leena, R. S.; Vairamani, M.; Selvamurugan, N. Alginate/Gelatin Scaffolds Incorporated with Silibinin-Loaded Chitosan Nanoparticles for Bone Formation in Vitro. *Colloids Surf. B* **2017,** *158*, 308–318.

Lei, Y.; Xu, Z.; Ke, Q.; Yin, W.; Chen, Y.; Zhang, C.; Guo, Y. Strontium Hydroxyapatite/ Chitosan Nanohybrid Scaffolds with Enhanced Osteoinductivity for Bone Tissue Engineering. *Mater. Sci. Eng. C* **2017,** *72*, 134–142.

Leite, Á. J.; Sarker, B.; Zehnder, T.; Silva, R.; Mano, J. F.; Boccaccini, A. R. Bioplotting of a Bioactive Alginate Dialdehyde-Gelatin Composite Hydrogel Containing Bioactive Glass Nanoparticles. *Biofabrication* **2016**, *8*(3), 035005.

Lewandowska-Łańcucka, J.; Mystek, K.; Mignon, A.; Van Vlierberghe, S.; Łatkiewicz, A.; Nowakowska, M. Alginate- and Gelatin-Based Bioactive Photocross-Linkable Hybrid Materials for Bone Tissue Engineering. *Carbohydr. Polym.* **2017**, *157*, 1714–1722.

Li, H.; Jiang, F.; Ye, S.; Wu, Y.; Zhu, K.; Wang, D. Bioactive Apatite Incorporated Alginate Microspheres with Sustained Drug-Delivery for Bone Regeneration Application. *Mater. Sci. Eng. C* **2016**, *62*, 779–786.

Liao, Y. T.; Wu, K. C.-W.; Yu, J. Synthesis of Mesoporous Silica Nanoparticle-Encapsulated Alginate Microparticles for Sustained Release and Targeting Therapy. *J. Biomed. Mater. Res. Part B* **2014**, *102*(2), 293–302.

Lin, H. R.; Yeh, Y. J. Porous Alginate/Hydroxyapatite Composite Scaffolds for Bone Tissue Engineering: Preparation, Characterization, and in Vitro Studies. *J. Biomed. Mater. Res. Part B* **2004**, *71*(1), 52–65.

Lin, L.; Tong, A.; Zhang, H.; Hu, Q.; Fang, M. In The Mechanical Properties of Bone Tissue Engineering Scaffold Fabricating via Selective Laser Sintering. In *International Conference on Life System Modeling and Simulation,* Springer: Berlin, Heidelberg, 2007; pp 146–152.

Linh, N. T.; Paul, K.; Kim, B.; Lee, B. T. Augmenting in Vitro Osteogenesis of a Glycine-Arginine-Glycine-Aspartic-Conjugated Oxidized Alginate-Gelatin-Biphasic Calcium Phosphate Hydrogel Composite and In Vivo Bone Biogenesis Through Stem Cell Delivery. *J. Biomater. Appl.* **2016**, *31*(5), 661–673.

Liu, M.; Dai, L.; Shi, H.; Xiong, S.; Zhou, C. In Vitro Evaluation of Alginate/Halloysite Nanotube Composite Scaffolds for Tissue Engineering. *Mater. Sci. Eng. C* **2015**, *49*, 700–712.

LogithKumar, R.; Keshav Narayan, A.; Dhivya, S.; Chawla, A.; Saravanan, S.; Selvamurugan, N. A Review of Chitosan and its Derivatives in Bone Tissue Engineering. *Carbohydr. Polym.* **2016**, *151*, 172–188.

Lu, L.; Liu, X.; Qian, L.; Tong, Z. Sol–Gel Transition in Aqueous Alginate Solutions Induced by Cupric Cations Observed with Viscoelasticity. *Polym. J.* **2003**, *35*(10), 804–809.

Luginbuehl, V.; Wenk, E.; Koch, A.; Gander, B.; Merkle, H. P.; Meinel, L. Insulin-like Growth Factor I–Releasing Alginate-Tricalcium Phosphate Composites for Bone Regeneration. *Pharm. Res.* **2005**, *22*(6), 940–950.

Luo, Y.; Lode, A.; Sonntag, F.; Nies, B.; Gelinsky, M. Well-Ordered Biphasic Calcium Phosphate–Alginate Scaffolds Fabricated by Multi-Channel 3D Plotting Under Mild Conditions. *J. Mater. Chem. B* **2013**, *1*(33), 4088–4098.

Luo, Y.; Lode, A.; Wu, C.; Chang, J.; Gelinsky, M. Alginate/Nanohydroxyapatite Scaffolds with Designed Core/Shell Structures Fabricated by 3D Plotting and in Situ Mineralization for Bone Tissue Engineering. *ACS Appl. Mater. Interfaces* **2015**, *7*(12), 6541–6549.

Luo, G.; Ma, Y.; Cui, X.; Jiang, L.; Wu, M.; Hu, Y.; Luo, Y.; Pan, H.; Ruan, C. 13–93 Bioactive Glass/Alginate Composite Scaffolds 3D Printed Under Mild Conditions for Bone Regeneration. *RSC Adv.* **2017a**, *7*(20), 11880–11889.

Luo, H.; Zuo, G.; Xiong, G.; Li, C.; Wu, C.; Wan, Y. Porous Nanoplate-Like Hydroxyapatite–Sodium Alginate Nanocomposite Scaffolds for Potential Bone Tissue Engineering. *Mater. Technol.* **2017b**, *32*(2), 78–84.

Malone, E.; Lipson, H. Fab@Home: The Personal Desktop Fabricator Kit. *Rapid Prototyping J.* **2007**, *13*(4), 245–255.

Mao, D.; Li, Q.; Bai, N.; Dong, H.; Li, D. Porous Stable Poly (Lactic Acid)/Ethyl Cellulose/ Hydroxyapatite Composite Scaffolds Prepared by a Combined Method for Bone Regeneration. *Carbohydr. Polym.* **2017,** 180, 104–111.

Marolt, D.; Knezevic, M.; Vunjak-Novakovic, G. Bone Tissue Engineering with Human Stem Cells. *Stem Cell Res. Ther.* **2010,** *1*(2), 10.

Mo, X.; Wei, Y.; Zhang, X.; Cai, Q.; Shen, Y.; Dai, X.; Meng, S.; Liu, X.; Liu, Y.; Hu, Z.; Deng, X. Enhanced Stem Cell Osteogenic Differentiation by Bioactive Glass Functionalized Graphene Oxide Substrates. *J. Nanomater.* **2016,** *2016,* 5613980.

Moorthi, A.; Vimalraj, S.; Avani, C.; He, Z.; Partridge, N. C.; Selvamurugan, N. Expression of MicroRNA-30c and its Target Genes in Human Osteoblastic cells by Nano-Bioglass Ceramic-Treatment. *Int. J. Bio. Macromol.* **2013,** *56*, 181–185.

Moorthi, A.; Parihar, P. R.; Saravanan, S.; Vairamani, M.; Selvamurugan, N. Effects of Silica and Calcium Levels in Nanobioglass Ceramic Particles on Osteoblast Proliferation. *Mater. Sci. Eng. C* **2014,** *43*, 458–464.

Morais, D. S.; Rodrigues, M. A.; Silva, T. I.; Lopes, M. A.; Santos, M.; Santos, J. D.; Botelho, C. M. Development And Characterization of Novel Alginate-Based Hydrogels as Vehicles for Bone Substitutes. *Carbohydr. Polym.* **2013,** *95*(1), 134–142.

Müller, W. E.; Schröder, H. C.; Feng, Q.; Schlossmacher, U.; Link, T.; Wang, X. Development of a Morphogenetically Active Scaffold for Three-Dimensional Growth of Bone Cells: Biosilica-Alginate Hydrogel for SaOS-2 Cell Cultivation. *J. Tissue Eng. Regener. Med.* **2015,** *9*(11), E39-50.

Naik, K.; Chandran, V. G.; Rajashekaran, R.; Waigaonkar, S.; Kowshik, M. Mechanical Properties, Biological Behaviour and Drug Release Capability of Nano TiO2-HAp-Alginate Composite Scaffolds for Potential Application as Bone Implant Material. *J. Biomater. Appl.* **2016,** *31*(3), 387–399.

Nazarpak, M. H.; Pourasgari, F.; Aghajamali, M.; Sarbolouki, M. Preparation and Evaluation of Porous Alginate/ Hydroxyapatite Composite Scaffold Coated with a Biodegradable Triblock Copolymer. *Asian Biomed.* **2012,** *6*(5), 753–758.

Nie, L.; Chen, D.; Fu, J.; Yang, S.; Hou, R.; Suo, J. Macroporous Biphasic Calcium Phosphate Scaffolds Reinforced by Poly-L-Lactic Acid/Hydroxyapatite Nanocomposite Coatings for Bone Regeneration. *Biochem. Eng. J.* **2015,** *98*, 29–37.

Niranjan, R.; Koushik, C.; Saravanan, S.; Moorthi, A.; Vairamani, M.; Selvamurugan, N. A Novel Injectable Temperature-Sensitive Zinc Doped Chitosan/β-Glycerophosphate Hydrogel for Bone Tissue Engineering. *Int. J. Biol. Macromol.* **2013,** *54*, 24–29.

Pattnaik, S.; Nethala, S.; Tripathi, A.; Saravanan, S.; Moorthi, A.; Selvamurugan, N. Chitosan Scaffolds Containing Silicon Dioxide and Zirconia Nano Particles for Bone Tissue Engineering. *Int. J. Biol. Macromol.* **2011,** *49*(5), 1167–1172.

Perez, R. A.; Kim, H.-W. Core–Shell Designed Scaffolds of Alginate/Alpha-Tricalcium Phosphate for the Loading and Delivery of Biological Proteins. *J. Biomed. Mater. Res. Part A* **2013,** *101A*(4), 1103–1112.

Porrelli, D.; Travan, A.; Turco, G.; Marsich, E.; Borgogna, M.; Paoletti, S.; Donati, I. Alginate–Hydroxyapatite Bone Scaffolds with Isotropic or Anisotropic Pore Structure: Material Properties and Biological Behavior. *Macromol. Mater. Eng.* **2015,** *300*(10), 989–1000.

Qiao, P.; Wang, J.; Xie, Q.; Li, F.; Dong, L.; Xu, T. Injectable Calcium Phosphate-Alginate-Chitosan Microencapsulated MC3T3-E1 Cell Paste for Bone Tissue Engineering in Vivo. *Mater. Sci. Eng. C* **2013,** *33*(8), 4633–4639.

Qiu, Z.-Y.; Noh, I.-S.; Zhang, S.-M. Silicate-Doped Hydroxyapatite and its Promotive Effect on Bone Mineralization. *Front. Mater. Sci.* **2013,** *7*(1), 40–50.

Qiu, M.; Chen, D.; Shen, C.; Shen, J.; Zhao, H.; He, Y. Preparation of in Situ Forming and Injectable Alginate/Mesoporous Sr-Containing Calcium Silicate Composite Cement for Bone Repair. *RSC Adv.* **2017,** *7*(38), 23671–23679.

Quinlan, E.; López-Noriega, A.; Thompson, E.; Kelly, H. M.; Cryan, S. A.; O'brien, F. J. Development of Collagen–Hydroxyapatite Scaffolds Incorporating PLGA and Alginate Microparticles for the Controlled Delivery of rhBMP-2 for Bone Tissue Engineering. *J. Controlled Release* **2015,** *198,* 71-79.

Quinlan, E.; López-Noriega, A.; Thompson, E. M.; Hibbitts, A.; Cryan, S. A.; O'Brien, F. J. Controlled Release of Vascular Endothelial Growth Factor from Spray-Dried Alginate Microparticles in Collagen-Hydroxyapatite Scaffolds for Promoting Vascularization and Bone Repair. *J. Tissue Eng. Regener. Med.* **2017,** *11*(4), 1097–1109.

Rafienia, M.; Saberi, A.; Poorazizi, E. A Novel Fabrication of PVA/Alginate-Bioglass Electrospun for Biomedical Engineering Application. *Nanomed. J.* **2017,** *4*(3), 152–163.

Rajesh, R.; Ravichandran, Y. D. Development of a New Carbon Nanotube–Alginate–Hydroxyapatite Tricomponent Composite Scaffold for Application in Bone Tissue Engineering. *Int. J. Nanomed.* **2015,** *10*(Suppl 1), 7.

Rao, S. H.; Harini, B.; Shadamarshan, R. P. K.; Balagangadharan, K.; Selvamurugan, N. Natural and Synthetic Polymers/Bioceramics/Bioactive Compounds-mediated Cell Signaling in Bone Tissue Engineering. *Int. J. Biol. Macromol.* **2017,** *110,* 88–96.

Ribeiro, M.; de Moraes, M. A.; Beppu, M. M.; Garcia, M. P.; Fernandes, M. H.; Monteiro, F. J.; Ferraz, M. P. Development of Silk Fibroin/Nanohydroxyapatite Composite Hydrogels for Bone Tissue Engineering. *Eur. Polym. J.* **2015,** *67,* 66–77.

Rottensteiner, U.; Sarker, B.; Heusinger, D.; Dafinova, D.; Rath, S. N.; Beier, J. P.; Kneser, U.; Horch, R. E.; Detsch, R.; Boccaccini, A. R.; Arkudas, A. In Vitro and In Vivo Biocompatibility of Alginate Dialdehyde/Gelatin Hydrogels with and without Nanoscaled Bioactive Glass for Bone Tissue Engineering Applications. *Materials* **2014,** *7*(3), 1957–1974.

Sahithi, K.; Swetha, M.; Ramasamy, K.; Srinivasan, N.; Selvamurugan, N. Polymeric Composites Containing Carbon Nanotubes for Bone Tissue Engineering. *Int. J. Biol. Macromol.* **2010,** *46*(3), 281–283.

Sainitya, R.; Sriram, M.; Kalyanaraman, V.; Dhivya, S.; Saravanan, S.; Vairamani, M.; Sastry, T. P. and Selvamurugan, N. Scaffolds Containing Chitosan/Carboxymethyl Cellulose/ Mesoporous Wollastonite for Bone Tissue Engineering. *Int. J. Biol. Macromol.* **2015,** *80,* 481–488.

Sangeetha, K.; Thamizhavel, A.; Girija, E. K. Effect of Gelatin on the in Situ Formation of Alginate/Hydroxyapatite Nanocomposite. *Mater. Lett.* **2013,** *91,* 27–30.

Saranya, N.; Saravanan, S.; Moorthi, A.; Ramyakrishna, B.; Selvamurugan, N. Enhanced Osteoblast Adhesion on Polymeric Nano-Scaffolds for Bone Tissue Engineering. *J. Biomed. Nanotechnol.* **2011,** *7*(2), 238–244.

Saravanan, S.; Vimalraj, S.; Vairamani, M.; Selvamurugan, N. Role of Mesoporous Wollastonite (Calcium Silicate) in Mesenchymal Stem Cell Proliferation and Osteoblast Differentiation: a Cellular and Molecular Study. *J. Biomed. Nanotechnol.* **2015,** *11*(7), 1124–1138.

Saravanan, S.; Selvamurugan, N. Bioactive Mesoporous Wollastonite Particles for one Tissue Engineering. *J. Tissue Eng.* **2016a,** *7,* 2041731416680319.

Saravanan, S.; Leena, R. S.; Selvamurugan, N. Chitosan Based Biocomposite Scaffolds for Bone Tissue Engineering. *Int. J. Biol. Macromol.* **2016b,** *93,* 1354–1365.

Saravanan, S.; Chawla, A.; Vairamani, M.; Sastry, T. P.; Subramanian, K. S.; Selvamurugan, N. Scaffolds Containing Chitosan, Gelatin and Graphene Oxide for Bone Tissue Regeneration in Vitro and in Vivo. *Int. J. Biol. Macromol.* **2017,** *104*(Pt B), 1975–1985.

Sarker, B.; Singh, R.; Silva, R.; Roether, J. A.; Kaschta, J.; Detsch, R.; Schubert, D. W.; Cicha, I.; Boccaccini, A. R. Evaluation of Fibroblasts Adhesion and Proliferation on Alginate-Gelatin Crosslinked Hydrogel. *PLoS One.* **2014,** *9*(9), e107952.

Sarker, A.; Amirian, J.; Min, Y. K.; Lee, B. T. HAp Granules Encapsulated Oxidized Alginate–Gelatin–Biphasic Calcium Phosphate Hydrogel for Bone Regeneration. *Int. J. Biol. Macromol.* **2015,** *81,* 898–911.

Sarker, B.; Li, W.; Zheng, K.; Detsch, R.; Boccaccini, A. R. Designing Porous Bone Tissue Engineering Scaffolds with Enhanced Mechanical Properties from Composite Hydrogels Composed of Modified Alginate, Gelatin, and Bioactive Glass. *ACS Biomater. Sci. Eng.* **2016,** *2*(12), 2240–2254.

Saquing, C. D.; Tang, C.; Monian, B.; Bonino, C. A.; Manasco, J. L.; Alsberg, E.; Khan, S. A. Alginate–polyethylene Oxide Blend Nanofibers and the Role of the Carrier Polymer in Electrospinning. *Ind. Eng. Chem. Res.* **2013,** *52*(26), 8692–8704.

Schloßmacher, U.; Schröder, H. C.; Wang, X.; Feng, Q.; Diehl-Seifert, B.; Neumann, S.; Trautwein, A.; Müller, W. E. G. Alginate/Silica Composite Hydrogel as a Potential Morphogenetically Active Scaffold for Three-Dimensional Tissue Engineering. *RSC Adv.* **2013,** *3*(28), 11185–11194.

Schröder, H. C.; Wang, X. H.; Wiens, M.; Diehl-Seifert, B.; Kropf, K.; Schloßmacher, U.; Müller, W. E. G. Silicate Modulates the Cross-Talk between Osteoblasts (SaOS-2) and Osteoclasts (RAW 264.7 cells): Inhibition of Osteoclast Growth and Differentiation. *J. Cell. Biochem.* **2012,** *113*(10), 3197–3206.

Serra, I. R.; Fradique, R.; Vallejo, M. C. S.; Correia, T. R.; Miguel, S. P.; Correia, I. J. Production and Characterization of Chitosan/Gelatin/B-TCP Scaffolds for Improved Bone Tissue Regeneration. *Mater. Sci. Eng. C* **2015,** *55,* 592–604.

Shang, W.; Liu, Y.; Wan, W.; Hu, C.; Liu, Z.; Wong, C. T.; Fukuda, T.; Shen, Y. Hybrid 3D Printing and Electrodeposition Approach for Controllable 3D Alginate Hydrogel Formation. *Biofabrication* **2017,** *9*(2), 025032.

Shao, W.; He, J.; Sang, F.; Wang, Q.; Chen, L.; Cui, S.; Ding, B. Enhanced Bone Formation in Electrospun Poly (L-lactic-co-glycolic acid)–Tussah Silk Fibroin Ultrafine Nanofiber Scaffolds Incorporated with Graphene Oxide. *Mater. Sci. Eng. C* **2016,** *62,* 823–834.

Sharma, C.; Dinda, A. K.; Potdar, P. D.; Chou, C. F.; Mishra, N. C. Fabrication and Characterization of Novel Nano-Biocomposite Scaffold of Chitosan-Gelatin-Alginate-Hydroxyapatite for Bone Tissue Engineering. *Mater. Sci. Eng. C* **2016,** *64,* 416–427.

Silva, R.; Bulut, B.; Roether, J. A.; Kaschta, J.; Schubert, D. W.; Boccaccini, A. R. Sonochemical Processing and Characterization of Composite Materials Based on Soy Protein and Alginate Containing Micron-Sized Bioactive Glass Particles. *J. Mol. Struct.* **2014,** *1073,* 87–96.

Sohrabi, M.; Hesaraki, S.; Kazemzadeh, A. The Influence of Polymeric Component of Bioactive Glass-Based Nanocomposite Paste on its Rheological Behaviors and in Vitro Responses: Hyaluronic Acid Versus Sodium Alginate. *J. Biomed. Mater. Res. Part B* **2014,** *102*(3), 561–573.

Song, W.; Yu, X.; Markel, D. C.; Shi, T.; Ren, W. Coaxial PCL/PVA Electrospun Nanofibers: Osseointegration Enhancer and Controlled Drug Release Device. *Biofabrication* **2013,** *5*(3), 035006.

Sotome, S.; Uemura, T.; Kikuchi, M.; Chen, J.; Itoh, S.; Tanaka, J.; Tateishi, T.; Shinomiya, K. Synthesis and in Vivo Evaluation of a Novel Hydroxyapatite/Collagen–Alginate as a Bone Filler and a Drug Delivery Carrier of Bone Morphogenetic Protein. *Mater. Sci. Eng. C* **2004,** *24*(3), 341–347.

Soundarya, S. P.; Sanjay, V.; Menon, A. H.; Dhivya, S.; Selvamurugan, N. Effects of Flavonoids Incorporated Biological Macromolecules Based Scaffolds in Bone Tissue Engineering. *Int. J. Biol. Macromol.* **2017,** *110,* 74–87.

Sowjanya, J. A.; Singh, J.; Mohita, T.; Sarvanan, S.; Moorthi, A.; Srinivasan, N.; Selvamurugan, N. Biocomposite Scaffolds Containing Chitosan/Alginate/Nano-Silica for Bone Tissue Engineering. *Colloids Surf B* **2013,** *109,* 294–300.

Sriram, M.; Sainitya, R.; Kalyanaraman, V.; Dhivya, S. and Selvamurugan, N. Biomaterials Mediated MicroRNA Delivery for Bone Tissue Engineering. *Int. J. Biol. Macromol.* **2015,** *74,* 404–412.

Sun, J.; Tan, H. Alginate-Based Biomaterials for Regenerative Medicine Applications. *Materials* **2013,** *6*(4), 1285–1309.

Swetha, M.; Sahithi, K.; Moorthi, A.; Srinivasan, N.; Ramasamy, K.; Selvamurugan, N. Biocomposites Containing Natural Polymers and Hydroxyapatite for Bone Tissue Engineering. *Int. J. Biol. Macromol.* **2010,** *47*(1), 1–4.

Swetha, M.; Sahithi, K.; Moorthi, A.; Saranya, N.; Saravanan, S.; Ramasamy, K.; Srinivasan, N.; Selvamurugan, N. Synthesis, Characterization, and Antimicrobial Activity of Nano-Hydroxyapatite-Zinc for Bone Tissue Engineering Applications. *J. Nanosci. Nanotechnol.* **2012,** *12*(1), 167–172.

Tang, S.; Zhao, Z.; Chen, G.; Su, Y.; Lu, L.; Li, B.; Liang, D.; Jin, R. Fabrication of Ampicillin/Starch/Polymer Composite Nanofibers with Controlled Drug Release Properties by Electrospinning. *J. Sol-Gel Sci. Technol.* **2016,** *77*(3), 594–603.

Torres, A. L.; Gaspar, V. M.; Serra, I. R.; Diogo, G. S.; Fradique, R.; Silva, A. P.; Correia, I. J. Bioactive Polymeric-Ceramic Hybrid 3D Scaffold for Application in Bone Tissue Regeneration. *Mater. Sci. Eng. C* **2013,** *33*(7), 4460–4469.

Tripathi, A.; Saravanan, S.; Pattnaik, S.; Moorthi, A.; Partridge, N. C.; Selvamurugan, N. Bio-Composite Scaffolds Containing Chitosan/Nano-Hydroxyapatite/Nano-Copper-Zinc for Bone Tissue Engineering. *Int. J. Biol. Macromol.* **2012,** *50*(1), 294–299.

Turco, G.; Marsich, E.; Bellomo, F.; Semeraro, S.; Donati, I.; Brun, F.; Grandolfo, M.; Accardo, A.; Paoletti, S. Alginate/Hydroxyapatite Biocomposite for Bone Ingrowth: a Trabecular Structure with High and Isotropic Connectivity. *Biomacromolecules* **2009,** *10*(6), 1575–1583.

Valente, J. F. A.; Valente, T. A. M.; Alves, P.; Ferreira, P.; Silva, A.; Correia, I. J. Alginate Based Scaffolds for Bone Tissue Engineering. *Mater. Sci. Eng. C* **2012,** *32*(8), 2596–2603.

Valiense, H.; Barreto, M.; Resende, R. F.; Alves, A. T.; Rossi, A. M.; Mavropoulos, E.; Granjeiro, J. M.; Calasans-Maia, M. D. In vitro and in Vivo Evaluation of Strontium-Containing Nanostructured Carbonated Hydroxyapatite/Sodium Alginate for Sinus Lift in Rabbits. *J. Biomed. Mater. Res. Part B* **2016,** *104*(2), 274–282.

Van Bael, S.; Desmet, T.; Chai, Y. C.; Pyka, G.; Dubruel, P.; Kruth, J. P.; Schrooten, J. In Vitro Cell-Biological Performance and Structural Characterization of Selective Laser Sintered and Plasma Surface Functionalized Polycaprolactone Scaffolds for Bone Regeneration. *Mater. Sci. Eng. C* **2013,** *33*(6), 3404–3412.

Venkatesan, J.; Bhatnagar, I.; Manivasagan, P.; Kang, K. H.; Kim, S. K. Alginate Composites for Bone Tissue Engineering: a Review. *Int. J. Biol. Macromol.* **2015,** *72,* 269–281.

Vimalraj, S.; Selvamurugan, N. MicroRNAs Expression and their Regulatory Networks during Mesenchymal Stem Cells Differentiation Toward Osteoblasts. *Int. J. Biol. Macromol.* **2014,** *66,* 194–202.

Vimalraj, S.; Saravanan, S.; Vairamani, M.; Gopalakrishnan, C.; Sastry, T. P.; Selvamurugan, N. A Combinatorial Effect of Carboxymethyl Cellulose Based Scaffold and MicroRNA-15b on Osteoblast Differentiation. *Int. J. Biol. Macromol.* **2016,** *93,* 1457–1464.

Wang, Y.; Kim, H. J.; Vunjak-Novakovic, G.; Kaplan, D. L. Stem Cell-Based Tissue Engineering with Silk Biomaterials. *Biomaterials* **2006,** *27*(36), 6064–6082.

Wang, Q.; Xia, Q.; Wu, Y.; Zhang, X.; Wen, F.; Chen, X.; Zhang, S.; Heng, B. C.; He, Y.; Ouyang, H. W. 3D-Printed Atsttrin-Incorporated Alginate/Hydroxyapatite Scaffold Promotes Bone Defect Regeneration with TNF/TNFR Signaling Involvement. *Adv. Healthcare Mater.* **2015,** *4*(11), 1701–1708.

Wang, M. O.; Bracaglia, L.; Thompson, J. A.; Fisher, J. P. Hydroxyapatite-Doped Alginate Beads as Scaffolds for the Osteoblastic Differentiation of Mesenchymal Stem Cells. *J. Biomed. Mater. Res. Part A* **2016,** *104*(9), 2325–2333.

Wei, M.; Li, S.; Le, W. Nanomaterials Modulate Stem Cell Differentiation: Biological Interaction and Underlying Mechanisms. *J. Nanobiotechnol.* **2017,** *15*(1), 75.

Weng, L.; Xie, J. Smart Electrospun Nanofibers for Controlled Drug Release: Recent Advances and New Perspectives. *Curr. Pharm. Design.* **2015,** *21*(15), 1944–1959.

Wongkanya, R.; Chuysinuan, P.; Pengsuk, C.; Techasakul, S.; Lirdprapamongkol, K.; Svasti, J.; Nooeaid, P. Electrospinning of Alginate/Soy Protein Isolated Nanofibers and their Release Characteristics for Biomedical Applications. *J. Sci. Adv. Mater. Devices.* **2017,** *2*(3), 309–316.

Wu, C.; Miron, R.; Sculean, A.; Kaskel, S.; Doert, T.; Schulze, R.; Zhang, Y. Proliferation, Differentiation and Gene Expression of Osteoblasts in Boron-Containing Associated with Dexamethasone Deliver from Mesoporous Bioactive Glass Scaffolds. *Biomaterials* **2011,** *32*(29), 7068–7078.

Wu, S.; Liu, X.; Yeung, K. W.; Liu, C.; Yang, X. Biomimetic Porous Scaffolds for Bone Tissue Engineering. *Mater. Sci. Eng. R Rep.* **2014,** *80,* 1–36.

Wu, Z.; Su, X.; Xu, Y.; Kong, B.; Sun, W.; Mi, S. Bioprinting Three-Dimensional Cell-Laden Tissue Constructs with Controllable Degradation. *Sci. Rep.* **2016,** *6,* 24474.

Xiong, G.; Luo, H.; Zuo, G.; Ren, K. Wan, Y. Novel Porous Graphene Oxide and Hydroxyapatite Nanosheets-Reinforced Sodium Alginate Hybrid Nanocomposites for Medical Applications. *Mater. Charact.* **2015,** *107,* 419–425.

Xu, Y.; Zhou, J.; Sun, W.; Li, D.; Dang, L. Preparation Process Analysis and Performance Research on Hydroxyapatite/Sodium Alginate Composite Bone Scaffold. *Mater. Res. Innovations* **2015,** *19*(sup8), S8–365.

Xu, S.; Chen, X.; Yang, X.; Zhang, L.; Yang, G.; Shao, H.; He, Y.; Gou, Z. Preparation and in Vitro Biological Evaluation of Octacalcium Phosphate/Bioactive Glass-Chitosan/ Alginate Composite Membranes Potential for Bone Guided Regeneration. *J. Nanosci. Nanotechnol.* **2016,** *16*(6), 5577–5585.

Xu, C.; Wang, X.; Zhou, J.; Huan, Z.; Chang, J. Bioactive Tricalcium Silicate/Alginate Composite Bone Cements with Enhanced Physicochemical Properties. *J. Biomed. Res. Part B: Appl. Biomater.* **2018,** *106*(1), 237–244.

Yan, J.; Miao, Y.; Tan, H.; Zhou, T.; Ling, Z.; Chen, Y.; Xing, X.; Hu, X. Injectable Alginate/ Hydroxyapatite Gel Scaffold Combined with Gelatin Microspheres for Drug Delivery and Bone Tissue Engineering. *Mater. Sci. Eng. C* **2016,** *63,* 274–284.

Yang, J.; Zhang, Y. S.; Yue, K.; Khademhosseini, A. Cell-Laden Hydrogels for Osteochondral and Cartilage Tissue Engineering. *Acta Biomater.* **2017,** *57,* 1–25.

Yao, J.; Zhang, S.; Li, W.; Du, Z.; Li, Y. In Vitro Drug Controlled-Release Behavior of an Electrospun Modified Poly(lactic Acid)/Bacitracin Drug Delivery System. *RSC Adv.* **2016,** *6*(1), 515–521.

Yazdimamaghani, M.; Razavi, M.; Vashaee, D.; Tayebi, L. Surface Modification of Biodegradable Porous Mg Bone Scaffold using Polycaprolactone/Bioactive Glass Composite. *Mater. Sci. Eng. C* **2015,** *49,* 436–444.

Yu, C. C.; Chang, J. J.; Lee, Y. H.; Lin, Y. C.; Wu, M. H.; Yang, M. C.; Chien, C. T. Electrospun Scaffolds Composing of Alginate, Chitosan, Collagen and Hydroxyapatite for Applying in Bone Tissue Engineering. *Mater. Lett.* **2013,** *93,* 133–136.

Zeng, Q.; Han, Y.; Li, H.; Chang, J. Bioglass/Alginate Composite Hydrogel Beads as Cell Carriers for Bone Regeneration. *J. Biomed. Mater. Res. Part B* **2014,** *102*(1), 42–51.

Zhao, F.; Zhang, W.; Fu, X.; Xie, W.; Chen, X. Fabrication and Characterization of Bioactive Glass/Alginate Composite Scaffolds by a Self-Crosslinking Processing for Bone Regeneration. *RSC Adv.* **2016,** *6*(94), 91201–91208.

Zheng, L.; Jiang, X.; Chen, X.; Fan, H.; Zhang, X. Evaluation of Novel in Situ Synthesized Nano-Hydroxyapatite/Collagen/Alginate Hydrogels for Osteochondral Tissue Engineering. *Biomed. Mater.* **2014,** *9*(6), 065004.

Zhou, K.; Zhang, X.; Chen, Z.; Shi, L.; Li, W. Preparation and Characterization of Hydroxyapatite–Sodium Alginate Scaffolds by Extrusion Freeforming. *Ceram. Int.* **2015,** *41*(10), 14029–14034.

ALGINATE PROPERTIES, PHARMACEUTICAL AND TISSUE ENGINEERING APPLICATIONS

K. S. JOSHY[1], SNIGDHA S[1], and SABU THOMAS[1,2,*]

[1]*International and Inter University Centre for Nanoscience and Nanotechnology, Mahatma Gandhi University, Kottayam, Kerala 686560, India*

[2]*School of Chemical Sciences, Mahatma Gandhi University, Kottayam, Kerala 686560 India*

Corresponding author. E-mail: sabuthomas@mgu.ac.in

9.1 INTRODUCTION

Traditionally, the biomaterials were designed to be inert and separated from the biological systems in the host. Naturally derived materials such as wood have been used as prosthetics since ancient times to replace lost tissues as a result of disease or trauma (Martinsen et al., 1989; Szekalska et al., 2016). The recent developments clearly define any biomaterial as an agent that can provide an interface with biological systems and this can be used to repair, modify, or replace any tissue or organ in the body (Lee et al., 2012). The applications of biomaterials are increasing day by day. The recent trends in biomaterials design are aimed at stimulating the function and structure extracellular matrices of the target body tissues in order to incorporate the biomaterials in the host system in a conducive and controlled manner. Materials derived from nature have been garnering the vast amount of attention due to their in-built biocompatibility.

Regenerative medicine brings together tissue engineering and drug delivery and it combines multidisciplinary aspects and fundamentals of materials engineering, polymer technology, and life sciences to effectively engineer excellent scaffolding material for tissues and organs that are very similar to the native tissues and organs. Alginate (ALG) is a natural anionic polymer typically extracted from brown seaweed. It has been extensively studied and applied in various biomedical practices as a result of its outstanding biocompatibility, nontoxicity, low cost, and the ability to form gel when divalent cations such as Ca^{2+} are added (Smidsrod and Skjåk Bræk, 1990). ALG hydrogels are usually prepared by using cross-linking methods, which can be altered accordingly to suit biological tissue matrices. This allows for various combinations and permutations in creating scaffolds and drug delivery vectors which are in great demand in regenerative medicine, tissue engineering, and drug delivery. ALG wound dressings provide a physiologically complacent moist microenvironment and minimize bacterial infection at the wound area, thereby facilitating wound healing. Therapeutics ranging from small chemical drugs to macromolecular proteins can be encapsulated and released from ALG gels in a controlled manner. This controlled release can be engineered by varying the type, amount, and methods of cross-linking. Moreover, the ALG gels can be administrated in a minimally invasive manner, parenterally or intravenously. ALG gels are therefore promising candidates for cell transplantation and pharmaceutical applications (Clark and Green, 1936; Rinaudo, 2008).

9.2 ALGINATE (ALG) PRODUCTION

The raw material for ALG production is the brown algae (Phaeophyceae) which grow abundantly in the ocean all over the world. Commercially available ALG is extracted from Phaeophyceae such as *Laminaria hyperborea, Laminaria digitata, Laminaria japonica, Ascophyllum nodosum*, and *Macrocystis pyrifera* (Qin, 2008); these are selected, dried, and pulverized to be used in ALG production. The pulverized seaweed is then treated with metal cations such as calcium, which results in the conversion of alginic acid in the brown algae to an insoluble ALG gel. When the seaweed is again rinsed with acidic water, it results in the swelling of the weed. This swollen seaweed is then treated with aqueous alkali solutions, usually with NaOH to produce water-soluble sodium ALG (Remminghorst and Rehm, 2006). The extract thus obtained is filtered, and allowed to react with either sodium or calcium chloride until ALG is precipitated. The treatment of this ALG salt with dilute HCl yields alginic acid, which after further purification and conversion, yields water-soluble sodium ALG powder (Kuo and Ma, 2001). Various algae have been investigated for ALG production and different plants yield a different amount of ALG powder. The ALG contents of 22–30% for *A. nodosum* and 25–44% for *L. digitata* have been reported (Sachan et al., 2009).

Bacterial biosynthesis has been reported to yield ALG with more pronounced chemical and physical properties when compared to their seaweed-derived counterparts. ALG of bacterial origin are usually produced by *Azotobacter* and *Pseudomonas* spp. The pathway of ALG is represented in Figure 9.1 (Remminghorst and Rehm, 2006). Advancements in metabolic regulation of pathways involved in ALG biosynthesis in bacteria and the possibility of easy modification of bacterial systems may facilitate faster and controlled production of ALG for a large number of applications in the biomedical field.

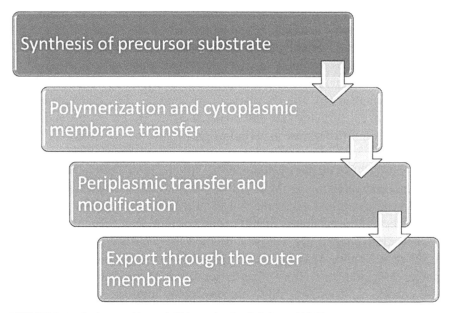

FIGURE 9.1   Pathway of bacterial biosynthesis of alginate (ALG).

9.3   CHEMICAL PROPERTIES

ALG are linear polymers of biological origin made up of 1,4-linked-D-mannuronic acid (M) and 1,4-L-guluronic acid (G) residues, arranged in homogenous (poly-G, poly-M) or heterogenous (MG) blocklike patterns (Hillberg et al., 2013). The biological and physical properties of ALG in aqueous media are dependent on the M/G ratio (obtained by proton nuclear magnetic resonance) and also on the distribution of M and G units along the polymer chain. Commercial ALG may differ in composition and the sequence of G- and M-blocks based on the source material. The distribution pattern of M-block and G-block are responsible for their physicochemical properties such as viscosity, solgel transition, and water-uptake ability. On raising the G-block content or molecular weight, more stronger or brittle ALG gels may be synthesized.

Commercial ALG are exclusively processed from algal sources although alternative production by microbial fermentation has been recently explored in order to provide ALG with more defined physicochemical properties (Draget et al., 1994).

Commercially available ALG possess a high degree of physicochemical heterogeneity which influences their quality and determines potential applicability. ALG are commercially available in various grades of molecular weight, composition, and distribution pattern of M-block and G-block. The molecular weight of commercial ALG varies between 33,000 and 400,000 g/mol. Alginic acid is insoluble in water and organic solvents, whereas ALG monovalent salts and ALG esters are water soluble and form stable, viscous solutions (Brault et al.). The 1% w/v aqueous solution of sodium alginate has a dynamic viscosity, that is, 20–400 mPa·s at 20°C. ALG solubility is limited by the solvent pH (a decrease in pH below pKa 3.38–3.65 may lead to polymer precipitation), ionic strength, and the content of "gelling ions" (Shimokawa et al., 1996). ALG with more heterogeneous structure (MG-blocks) are soluble at low pH compared to poly-M or poly-G ALG molecules, which precipitate under these conditions (Boontheekul et al., 2005). Apart from molecular weight, the gelling capability of ALG solutions may vary depending on their concentration, solvent pH, temperature, and the presence of divalent ions (Maiti et al., 2009). ALG has the unique ability of solgel transition, which enables easy transition from diverse semisolid to solid structures under mild conditions. Therefore, ALG are commonly used as viscosity-altering agents, thickeners, and as suspension and emulsion stabilizers in food and pharmaceutical industry. Among various ALG, sodium alginate is the most widely investigated one in the biomedical and allied fields. ALG is a gold mine for biomedical field because of its biocompatibility, biodegradability, nonantigenicity, and chelating ability (Wiegand et al., 2009). The chelating ability enables the preparation of pH-responsive hydrogels which can effectively interact with cationic polyelectrolytes and proteoglycans. ALG can be chelated with divalent cations under ambient conditions. Thus, efficient and practical drug delivery vehicles for various therapeutics can be obtained by altering and making use of simple electrostatic interactions. Purified ALG also find widespread industrial uses especially due to their ability to form hydrogels, beads, fibers, or films (Cao et al., 2007).

9.4 ALG IN BIOMEDICAL APPLICATIONS

ALG are extensively exploited in the biomedical and allied industries due to their multitudinous advantages. In the biomedical realm, ALG are used for controlled drug release, cells encapsulation, scaffolds for tissue engineering, or to prepare molds in dentistry (in the presence of slow-release calcium salt). Pharmaceutical industries make use of purified ALG as thickener, stabilizer in solution and dispersion of solid substances. ALG could play a significant role in controlled release of drug and other products. Oral administration is the most frequently used form in pharmaceutics; it is encouraging to note that ALG hydrogels are also being used as repositories for localized drug/probiotic delivery as well.

ALG can be easily modified chemically or by physical cross-linking to improve physicochemical properties and/or biological activity. ALG cross-linking can be achieved by ionic cross-linking, covalent cross-linking, cell cross-linking, phase transition (thermal gelation), "click" reaction, and free radical polymerization. An alteration of the M- to G-block proportion or an enrichment of polymer backbone in M-, G-, or MG-blocks is being practiced; this can be achieved by enzymatic epimerization using mannuronan C-5 epimerases. This enzyme, isolated from the soil bacterium *Azotobacter vinelandii* and expressed in *Escherichia coli*, converts mannuronic acid residues into guluronic acid residues in the polymer backbone without breaking the glycosidic bond. Oligosaccharides have also been isolated from ALG backbone and these contain polymer fragments with three to ten simple monosaccharides. There are two methods commonly employed for the ALG oligosaccharides preparation: enzymatic depolymerization and acid hydrolysis.

The common chemical modification of ALG hydroxyl groups includes oxidation, sulfation, graft copolymerization, acetylation, and phosphorylation. Modification of the carboxyl groups may be achieved by esterification and amidation. ALG solubility can be changed by modification of hydroxyl groups (in positions C-2 and C-3) or the carboxyl groups (in C-6 position) through covalent attachment of long alkyl chains or aromatic groups to the polymer backbone. Increasing ALG hydrophobicity provides decreasing polymer dissolution and erosion. Additionally, there are many studies, which include production of ALG derivatives by grafting with different substances such as polyacrylamide, methacrylate, galactose, lectin, sulfate, cysteine, cyclodextrins, propylene glycol, and dodecylamine (Gu et al., 2004; Zhao et al., 2006; Wong et al., 2011; Chang, 1998).

9.4.1   APPLICATIONS IN DRUG DELIVERY

Various reports indicate that low-molecular-weight drug delivery using ALG gels have been extensively studied. It has been observed that a primary or secondary bond between the drug and ALG can help regulate the drug release kinetics. ALG gels typically have pores that are nanometric in size (~5 nm); this could lead to rapid diffusion of small molecules through the gel. For example, in a study dealing with flurbiprofen, the release of drug from partially oxidized and ionically cross-linked ALG gels was almost completed in 1.5 h. However, when the drug was introduced into ALG beads of partially oxidized ALG using a combination of ionic and covalent cross-linking, an increased number of cross-links and consequently reduced swelling was observed. The controlled and localized delivery of antineoplastic agents has also been achieved using partially oxidized ALG gels. Microspheres have been extensively exploited to deliver cells, growth factors, proteins, genes, and other drugs in tissue engineering (Serra et al., 2011; Kong et al., 2003; Man et al., 2012; Yu et al., 2010). The microencapsulation technique can provide a protective shell for various bioactive compounds such as live cells, cytokines, and small proteins. Biodegradable micro- and nanoparticles made up of polymers such as poly(lactic acid), poly(lactide-co-glycolide) (PLGA), chitosan, and gelatin, are being extensively used as drug carriers (Freiberg and Zhu, 2004; Chen and Subirade, 2006; Liu et al., 2012; Huang et al., 2012). ALG effortlessly form gel and solid-microspheres which can be suitably engineered and applied as delivery systems. Typically, ALG gel-spheres are prepared in aqueous media through ionic cross-linking, and they are used for encapsulation of various cells, trophic factors, and proteins (Yao et al., 2012; Li et al., 2011; Meli et al., 2012). ALG solid-spheres can be fabricated by emulsion-solvent evaporation techniques, which are usually used to encapsulate drugs. ALG-based gel microspheres and solid-microspheres exhibit excellent biocompatibility. Although many synthetic microspheres have been studied as delivery systems for various bioactive therapeutics, their activities may be denatured and wasted due to extreme conditions involved in the preparation, especially if organic solvents are used (Sugaya et al., 2012). The organic solvents in combination with high shear stresses can have adverse effects on the bioactivity and structure of encapsulated substances. In general, if encapsulated under these conditions, the growth factors/therapeutics can be efficiently transported to a target site where it can be released in a sustained dosage form. ALG solutions tend to rapidly form hydrogels under mild conditions when exposed to divalent cations. ALG gel-spheres, which are ionically cross-linked in the presence of Ca^{2+}, have been used widely for the controlled delivery of cells and growth factors (Liu et al., 2011; Sun and Tan, 2013; Lee et al., 2000; Zhao et al., 2011). It has been found that microspheres/nanoparticles are rapidly cleared from circulation by the mononuclear phagocyte system (MPS) following intravenous injection. The MPS is involved in the uptake of such particles include macrophages of the liver, the spleen, and circulating monocytes that are primarily involved in uptake of such particles. The higher the hydrophobicity, the faster is their uptake from circulation. This can be controlled by varying the size of the particle and its surface properties (Petka et al., 1998; MacKay et al., 2009). Therefore, it is desirable to have ALG microspheres and nanoparticles that are hydrophilic with an electronegative surface in order to prevent their uptake. Usually, drugs are loaded in ALG microspheres by emulsion solvent evaporation technique where the drugs are mixed with the ALG solution evenly, followed by emulsification under sonication. The mixture is then being added dropwise into an organic emulsion under continuous stirring. The carriers based on ALG can protect drugs from degradation, thereby improving plasma halftime and ensuring transport and release of drugs at the appropriate site. In addition, the ALG solid-microspheres can also be employed as cell microcarriers, which is essentially an injectable cell scaffold for tissue engineering. ALG-based hollow microcapsules have a great potential application as drug delivery vehicle, biosensors, and micro-reactors (Sculean et al., 2001). Hollow microcapsules are typically synthesized by the layer-by-layer technique, where a sequential assembly of negatively and positively charged polyelectrolytes is carried out. These drug-carrying microcapsules have been studied thoroughly with regard to their property to control loading and release of the drug. Biopolymer microcapsules have been fabricated by using sacrificial colloid particles as core and depositing chitosan/ALG polymers alternately onto these decomposable core particles, followed by core removal. This process resulted in the production of hollow microcapsules that were biocompatible and possessed electrostatic interaction. The properties of ALG/chitosan microcapsules could be fine-tuned by varying the parameters involved in coating around the sacrificial template. Another study revealed that the addition of PEG to the ALG-based microcapsules led to protection against an acidic environment. Recently, a three-dimensional (3D) high-throughput screening assay for drug screening and diagnostic devices was developed using tissue engineering approach. A 3D ALG hydrogel platform was used for microarray systems and surface micro-patterning (Huang et al., 2011). The gelation solution was selectively trapped in areas that were hydrophilic by a dipping process. These ALG gel-patterns were then used to selectively capture cells with different adhesion properties. The results of the study indicated that the 3D platform provided near in vivo conditions that allowed cells to reach their natural phenotypes. The upregulation of several enzymes and growth factor was observed in these 3D microarray cultures. ALG have been used extensively in drug delivery applications but ALG-based delivery systems for functional genetic materials such as DNAs or siRNAs are more promising and have not been reported so far. In such applications, ALG modified to be cationic could be used to enhance the efficiency of DNA or siRNA transfection to target cells. Simultaneous or sequential delivery of multiple drugs can be achieved using ALG-based gels. The release kinetics of the drugs incorporated in ALG matrix will be dependent on chemical structure of and mode of incorporation of the drugs. For example, methotrexate, which does not interact with ALG, was rapidly released by diffusion, whereas doxorubicin which covalently attaches to the ALG moieties was released upon the chemical hydrolysis of the cross-linker. Mitoxantrone, which ionically complexed with ALG, could only be released after the gel was dissociated. Amphiphilic gel beads could be prepared in order to modulate the release of hydrophobic drugs. The advancement of recombinant DNA technology has led to the development of various protein-based drugs and ALG can act as an excellent carrier for protein drugs as these can be incorporated under mild conditions into delivery systems. These mild conditions of drug carrier synthesis minimize the denaturation of the proteins, and the gels matrix can also protect the drugs from the harsh physiological environment. Many strategies have been used to modulate the release rate of proteins from ALG gels. The release rate of proteins is generally fast due to porosity and hydrophilic nature of the ALG gels. Some proteins such as vascular endothelial growth factor (VEGF) or basic fibroblast growth factor, which are heparin-binding growth factors, exhibit reversible binding to ALG gels which can lead to a sustained and localized release (Ali and Mooney, 2008). Thus, the release of proteins in such cases can be engineered by altering the degradation of the gels (e.g., by using partially oxidized ALG). This will enable the release of protein to be partially dependent on the degradation rate of the gels. The controlled release of angiogenic molecules from ALG gels have been investigated especially as they are not heparin binding. ALG microspheres were found to effectively encapsulate proteins with high pI such as lysozyme and chymotrypsin; these proteins seem to physically cross-link with the sodium alginate gel, thereby facilitating their sustained release. Amino group-terminated poly((2-dimethylamino)ethyl methacrylate) was made to react with oxidized ALG, in the absence of a catalyst, to obtain an ALG derivative. This was dropped into an aqueous $CaCl_2$ solution to obtain particles for parenteral delivery of proteins (Hashimoto et al., 2002). ALG has also been used as a building block to synthesize tetrafunctional acetal-linked polymer network to prepare stimuli-responsive gels with adjustable pore sizes. The gels-protected proteins such as insulin from the harsh acidic conditions in the stomach and the proteins were released in neutral pH. ALG gels are disadvantageous due to their low encapsulation efficiency and burst release profiles. These can be overcome by using various cross-linking or encapsulation techniques, and/or by enhancing protein–hydrogel interactions. For example, ALG microspheres that encapsulated insulin was prepared by blending ALG with anionic polymers and this was followed by coating with chitosan to guard insulin from acidic conditions of the gastric environment and also to promote its release at intestinal pH. *Bombyx mori* silk fibroin has also been used as a coating for ALG microspheres, which provided mechanical stability in the form of strong shells and also as a diffusion barrier to the encapsulated therapeutics. Protein-entrapped microspheres embedded in ALG hydrogels can also facilitate sustained protein release. Bovine serum albumin (BSA), a model protein was encapsulated in poly(d,l-lactide-co-glycolide) (PLGA) microspheres and the microspheres were dispersed in ALG prior to ionic cross-linking. A homogeneous dispersion of the polymeric microspheres was observed by scanning electron microscope, and it was also noted that the release of BSA from this system was controlled primarily by the mixing ratio between PLGA microspheres and ALG hydrogels. However, it was also found that the release rates were independent of total BSA content and the dimensions of PLGA microspheres. Another study indicated that the release behavior of TAT-HSP27 was also regulated by varying the ratio between microspheres and gels. ALG gels which release proteins are being exploited for engineering of tissue and regenerative medicine (Vacharathit et al., 2011).

9.4.2 TISSUE ENGINEERING APPLICATIONS OF ALG

Poor healing has been a limiting factor in the treatment of bone injuries. ALG gels have a great scope in bone healing and repair as they can be used to deliver osteo-inductive factors, osteoclasts, or a combination of both. ALG gels can be introduced anywhere in the body through minimally invasive procedures, which makes them attractive for application in bone and cartilage repair. They have the added capacity to fill irregular defects, controlled release of factors, and the ease of chemical modification. However, these gels are not mechanically robust, which could create problems in the initial stages of regeneration if fixations are not used. ALG gels inherent ability to not degrade under physiological conditions, which highlights the necessity to engineer their degradation so that they do not interfere with the regeneration process. ALG gels for the delivery of growth factors have proved to be successful in animal models.

9.4.2.1   CARTILAGE REPAIR

The tissue-engineered cartilage is in high demand and has great clinical significance. One of the leading causes of disability is the traumatic and degenerative lesions of the articular cartilage. Injectable therapies are preferred for cartilage repair as it allows the implant to be maintained within the defect and it also allows weight-bearing due to the stiffness and strength rendered by the gels. The ALG hydrogel can be easily engineered to be similar to the articular cartilage and also to match its mechanical properties to that of the native tissue. ALG-based solid and gel-like injectable hydrogels have been reported in cartilage regeneration. The use of stem cells in cartilage regeneration is very attractive due to the invasive and destructive processes required to obtain primary chondrocytes from tissues. Encapsulation in ALG can regulate differentiation of stem cells, and in particular, chondrogenesis may be enhanced. It has been demonstrated that chondrogenic lineage of adult stem cells could be regulated through the introduction of soluble factors and biophysical cues in 3D cell culture systems (Guilak et al., 2009). In addition, it has been hypothesized that chondrogenesis of stem cells relates to the morphology of the encapsulated cells (i.e., round cell shape), and ALG gels promote a rounded morphology that may promote the cellular differentiation process.

9.4.2.2   BONE REGENERATION

Bone regeneration has always been a major challenge in the field of reconstructive surgery. There could be several reasons for loss of bone tissue, such as trauma or surgical removal. In situ osteogenesis could prove to be a desirable system for repair of bone tissue. Stem cells seeded into an injectable scaffold could be induced to differentiate, thereby leading to bone tissue formation. Numerous studies involving injectable ALG-based scaffolds for bone regeneration have been reported so far. ALG, therefore, could be an excellent candidate for generating tissue in gels for inducing osteogenesis as well as angiogenesis. A chemically modified ALG has been extensively used to promote periodontal regeneration.

9.4.2.3   *MUSCLE, NERVE, PANCREAS, AND LIVER*

ALG gels are being used extensively for the regeneration and engineering of numerous tissues such as skeletal muscle, nerve, pancreas, and liver. Skeletal muscle regeneration methods make use of replacement, trophic factor delivery, or a combination of both strategies. ALG gels can have great potential in such areas. ALG gels were used for the combined delivery of VEGF and insulin-like growth factor-1 and this was found to induce both angiogenesis and myogenesis. The targeted and sustained delivery of the trophic factors induced a significant amount of muscle regeneration and functional muscle formation. ALG gels were also found to exhibit the sustained delivery of hepatocyte growth factor and fibroblast growth factor-2 which resulted in long-term survival and migration of primary myoblasts into damaged muscle tissue in vivo. This resulted in repopulation of host muscle tissues with increased regeneration of muscle fibers at the wound location.

ALG gels have been extensively used in the repair and restoration of the central and peripheral nerve systems as well. Highly anisotropic capillary gels, based on ALG, when introduced into acute cervical spinal cord lesions in adult rats, were easily integrated into the spinal cord parenchyma without serious inflammatory responses and promoted axonal regrowth. A 50-mm gap in cat's sciatic nerves was bridged using ALG gel that was covalently cross-linked with ethylenediamine. Similarly, the outgrowth of regenerating axons and astrocyte was observed when ALG gels were applied at the stump of transected spinal cords in young rats. These gels have also been used as glue to repair gaps of the peripheral nerve that were impossible to be sutured. ALG gels have also found great potential in the field of cell-based neural therapies; mouse-derived neural stem cells retained their ability for multilineage differentiation when they were cultured in calcium ALG beads (Dashtdar et al., 2011).

Tissue engineering has a great potential to help replace hepatic tissues of damaged or failing liver. Hepatocytes encapsulated in ALG gels could be used for developing an artificial liver as these gels can be easily tailored to suit various needs and can also be cryopreserved. ALG gels were engineered in order to possess interconnected pore network which efficiently harbored hepatocytes and maintained hepatocellular functions. One of the earliest uses of ALG gels in tissue engineering involved the introduction of encapsulated pancreatic islet grafts to cure Type I diabetes. In this study, the gel provided protection for the foreign hepatocytes from the host immune system, thereby circumventing the use of immunosuppressive drugs. This approach has been successful in effectively treating Type I diabetes in animal models without the need for immunosuppressant therapy. Such pancreatic islet-encapsulated ALG beads usually have a coating made up of poly(amino acids), such as poly-L-lysine, that tend to maintain a fluid core structure while decreasing the outer pore size. ALG composition and purity can be varied in order to effectively reduce the transplant volume of encapsulated islet cells. However, the mechanical and chemical instability of ALG beads is matter of major concern that affects the long-term preservation of the transplanted islets in vivo. These instabilities have brought on various investigations where different poly(amino acids) has been examined as coating materials. Various micro-fabrication techniques have also been explored (Tuan et al. 2002).

9.5 CONCLUSIONS AND FUTURE PERSPECTIVES

ALG have proved to be excellent biomaterials that have immense potential for almost every biomedical application. The ALG is particularly impressive owing to its biocompatibility, gentle gelation conditions, facile chemical modification, and lack of immunogenicity, which aid in preparation of tailor-made ALG derivative for personalized treatment. ALG has been proved to be safe for clinical uses as a wound-dressing material and also as a therapeutic component. However, ALG hydrogels are limited due to their inferior mechanical and a few other physical performances. To overcome these limitations, different cross-linking strategies can be applied. These strategies could involve the use of molecules with different chemical composition, molecular weights, and cross-linking ability. Covalent cross-linking reactions could adversely affect the cells that are to be encapsulated; this calls for the choice of appropriate and biologically safe chemical reagents. Thorough clearance of unreacted reagents and by-products is also to be carried out strictly for such applications. Hopefully, the near future holds great scope for the use of ALG-based materials used in medicine. Although ALG gels play a passive role in wound-healing applications, it is very likely that the dressings of the future will offer a more active role for this efficient biopolymer. ALG dressings can be effectively used to deliver one or more bioactive materials that aid wound healing/tissue repair. Such gels have proved to be effective in sustaining concentrations of various factors, such as proteins, over long periods of time in localized areas. Dynamic control over precise delivery of drugs can help in improving the safety and efficacy of the drugs used. Through appropriate engineering of components, precise control can be gained over delivery of single/multiple drugs and/or sustained/sequential release of these components to the external environment. On-demand release of drugs from ALG gels can also be achieved by engineering responsiveness to various stimuli such as mechanical signals and magnetic fields. Tissue engineering approaches will greatly benefit from the introduction of cell–matrix interaction features. Further explorations of the fundamental properties of ALG and development of state-of-the-art features such as cell and tissue-interactive hydrogels would greatly benefit the biomedical science and engineering fields. New ALG polymers and their functional derivatives could be potentially exploited by using genetic engineering techniques to control bacterial synthesis of this biopolymer. The ability to engineer such variants will help in creating tailor-made treatments available for tissue/organ loss. New variants of ALG possessing precisely controlled chemical and physical properties could help revolutionize the future of tissue engineering and regenerative medicine.

SUMMARY

Alginate, a natural polysaccharide of algal origin is being used widely in various biomedical applications. Its popularity is primarily due to its superior biocompatibility and biodegradability. The ease of processability of this biomaterial makes it attractive in applications such as drug delivery, wound healing, and three-dimensional scaffolds such as hydrogels, capsules, foams, and fibers. The ALG hydrogels closely resemble the extracellular matrices found in tissues, thereby acting as excellent scaffolding materials. This chapter covers the general characteristics of ALG and recent developments in the use and applications of ALG and its derivatives in the biomedical sector.

KEYWORDS

- alginate hydrogels
- drug delivery
- microcapsules
- vascular endothelial growth factor
- nanoparticles

REFERENCES

Ali, O. A.; Mooney, D. J. Sustained GM-CSF and PEI Condensed pDNA Presentation Increases the Level and Duration of Gene Expression in Dendritic Cells. *J. Controlled Release* **2008,** *132*(3), 273–278.

Boontheekul, T.; et al. Controlling Alginate Gel Degradation Utilizing Partial Oxidation and Bimodal Molecular Weight Distribution. *Biomaterials* **2005,** *26*(15), 2455–2465.

Brault, D.; Heyraud, A; Lognone, V; Roussel, M. Methods for Obtaining Oligomannuronates and Guluronates, Products Obtained and Use Thereof. May 26, 2003.

Cao, L.; et al. Spatiotemporal Control over Growth Factor Signaling for Therapeutic Neovascularization. *Adv. Drug Delivery Rev.* **2007,** *59*(13), 1340–1350.

Chang, T. M. Pharmaceutical and Therapeutic Applications of Artificial Cells Including Microencapsulation. *Eur. J. Pharma. Biopharm.* **1998,** *45*(1), 3–8.

Chen, L.; Subirade, M. Alginate–Whey Protein Granular Microspheres as Oral Delivery Vehicles for Bioactive Compounds. *Biomaterials* **2006,** *27*(26), 4646–4654.

Clark, D. E.; Green, H. C. Alginic Acid and Process of Making Same. U.S. Patent 2,036,922, April 7, 1936.

Dashtdar, H.; et al. A Preliminary Study Comparing the Use of Allogenic Chondrogenic Pre Differentiated and Undifferentiated Mesenchymal Stem Cells for the Repair of Full Thickness Articular Cartilage Defects in Rabbits. *J. Orthop. Res.* **2011,** *29*(9), 1336–1342.

Draget, K. I.; et al. Alginic Acid Gels: The Effect of Alginate Chemical Composition and Molecular Weight. *Carbohydr. Polym.* **1994,** *25*(1), 31–38.

Freiberg, S.; Zhu, X. X. Polymer Microspheres for Controlled Drug Release. *Int. J. Pharm.* **2004,** *282*(1–2), 1–18.

Gu, F.; et al. Sustained Delivery of Vascular Endothelial Growth Factor with Alginate Beads. *J. Controlled Release* **2004,** *96*(3), 463–472.

Guilak, F.; et al. Control of Stem Cell Fate by Physical Interactions with the Extracellular Matrix. *Cell Stem Cell* **2009,** *5*(1), 17–26.

Hashimoto, T.; et al. Peripheral Nerve Regeneration Through Alginate Gel: Analysis of Early Outgrowth and Late Increase in Diameter of Regenerating Axons. *Exp. Brain Res.* **2002,** *146*(3), 356–368.

Hillberg, A. L.; et al. Improving Alginate-Poly-L-Ornithine-Alginate Capsule Biocompatibility through Genipin Crosslinking. *J. Biomed. Mater. Res. Part B* **2013,** *101*(2), 258–268.

Huang, S. H.; Hsueh, H. J.; Jiang, Y. L. Light-Addressable Electrodeposition of Cell-Encapsulated Alginate Hydrogels for a Cellular Microarray Using a digital Micromirror Device. *Biomicrofluidics* **2011,** *5,* 34109–3410910.

Huang, X.; et al. Microenvironment of Alginate-Based Microcapsules for Cell Culture and Tissue Engineering. *J. Biosci. Bioeng.* **2012,** *114*(1), 1–8.

Kong, H. J.; et al. Designing Alginate Hydrogels to Maintain Viability of Immobilized Cells. *Biomaterials* **2003,** *24*(22), 4023–4029.

Kuo, C. K.; Ma, P. X. Ionically Crosslinked Alginate Hydrogels as Scaffolds for Tissue Engineering: Part 1. Structure, Gelation Rate and Mechanical Properties. *Biomaterials* **2001,** *22*(6), 511–521.

Lee, K. Y.; et al. Controlled Growth Factor Release from Synthetic Extracellular Matrices. *Nature* **2000,** *408*(6815), 998.

Lee, K. Y.; et al. Alginate: Properties and Biomedical Applications. *Prog. Polym. Sci.* **2012,** *37*(1), 106–126.

Li, H.; et al. Hydrogel Droplet Microarrays with Trapped Antibody-Functionalized Beads for Multiplexed Protein Analysis. *Lab Chip* **2011,** *11*(3), 528–534.

Liu, X.; Ma, L.; Mao, Z.; Gao, C. Chitosan-Based Biomaterials for Tissue Repair and Regeneration. In *Chitosan for Biomaterials II;* Rangasamy, J., Prabaharan, M., Muzzarelli, R. A. A., Eds., Springer Berlin: Heidelberg, 2011; pp 81–127.

Liu, J.; et al. Fast-Degradable Microbeads Encapsulating Human Umbilical Cord Stem Cells in Alginate for Muscle Tissue Engineering. *Tissue Eng. Part A* **2012,** *18*(21–22), 2303–2314.

MacKay, J. A.; et al. Self-Assembling Chimeric Polypeptide–Doxorubicin Conjugate Nanoparticles that Abolish Tumours After a Single Injection. *Nat. Mater.* **2009,** *8*(12), 993.

Maiti, S.; et al. Adipic Acid Dihydrazide Treated Partially Oxidized Alginate Beads for Sustained Oral Delivery of Flurbiprofen. *Pharm. Dev. Technol.* **2009,** *14*(5), 461–470.

Man, Y.; et al. Angiogenic and Osteogenic Potential of Platelet-Rich Plasma and Adipose-Derived Stem Cell Laden Alginate Microspheres. *Biomaterials* **2012,** *33*(34), 8802–8811.

Martinsen, A. G.; et al. Alginate as Immobilization Material: I. Correlation Between Chemical and Physical Properties of Alginate Gel Beads. *Biotechnol. Bioeng.* **1989,** *33*(1), 79–89.

Meli, L.; et al. Influence of a Three-Dimensional, Microarray Environment on Human Cell Culture in Drug Screening Systems. *Biomaterials* **2012,** *33*(35), 9087–9096.

Petka, W. A.; et al. Reversible Hydrogels from Self-Assembling Artificial Proteins. *Science* **1998,** *281*(5375), 389–392.

Qin, Y. Alginate Fibres: An Overview of the Production Processes and Applications in Wound Management. *Polym. Int.* **2008,** *57*(2), 171–180.

Remminghorst, U.; Rehm, B. H. Bacterial Alginates: From Biosynthesis to Applications. *Biotechnol Lett.* **2006,** *28*(21), 1701–1712.

Rinaudo, M. Main Properties and Current Applications of Some Polysaccharides as Biomaterials. *Polym. Int.* **2008,** *57*(3), 397–430.

Sachan, N. K.; et al. Sodium Alginate: The Wonder Polymer for Controlled Drug Delivery. *J. Pharm. Res.* **2009,** *2*(8), 1191–1199.

Sculean, A.; et al. Effect of an Enamel Matrix Protein Derivative (Emdogain®) on ex Vivo Dental Plaque Vitality. *J. Clin. Periodontol.* **2001,** *28*(11), 1074–1078.

Serra, M.; et al. Microencapsulation Technology: A Powerful Tool for Integrating Expansion and Cryopreservation of Human Embryonic Stem Cells. *PLoS One* **2011,** *6.* DOI: 10.1371/journal.pone.0023212.

Shimokawa, T.; et al. Preparation of Two Series of Oligo-Guluronic Acids from Sodium Alginate by Acid Hydrolysis and Enzymatic Degradation. *Biosci. Biotechnol. Biochem.* **1996,** *60*(9), 1532–1534.

Smidsrod, O.; Skjåk Bræk, G. Alginate as Immobilization Matrix for Cells. *Trends Biotechnol.* **1990,** *8,* 71–78.

Sugaya, S.; et al. Micropatterning of Hydrogels on Locally Hydrophilized Regions on PDMS by Stepwise Solution Dipping and in Situ Gelation. *Langmuir* **2012,** *28*(39), 14073–14080.

Sun, J. Tan, H. Alginate-Based Biomaterials for Regenerative Medicine Applications. *Materials* **2013,** *6*(4), 1285–1309.

Szekalska, M.; et al. Alginate: Current Use and Future Perspectives in Pharmaceutical and Biomedical Applications. *Int. J. Polym. Sci.* **2016,** *2016,* 7697031.

Tuan, R. S.; et al. Adult Mesenchymal Stem Cells and Cell-Based Tissue Engineering. *Arthritis Res Ther* **2002,** *5*(1), 32.

Vacharathit, V.; et al. Viability and Functionality of Cells Delivered from Peptide Conjugated Scaffolds. *Biomaterials* **2011,** *32,* 3721–3728.

Wiegand, C.; et al. Comparative in Vitro Study on Cytotoxicity, Antimicrobial Activity, and Binding Capacity for Pathophysiological Factors in Chronic Wounds of Alginate and Silver-Containing Alginate. *Wound Repair Regener.* **2009,** *17*(4), 511–521.

Wong, Y. Y.; et al. Degradation of PEG and non-PEG Alginate-Chitosan Microcapsules in Different pH Environments. *Polym. Degrad. Stab.* **2011,** *96,* 2189–2197.

Yao, R.; et al. Alginate and Alginate/Gelatin Microspheres for Human Adipose-Derived Stem Cell Encapsulation and Differentiation. *Biofabrication* **2012,** *4*(2), 025007.

Yu, J.; et al. The Use of Human Mesenchymal Stem Cells Encapsulated in RGD Modified Alginate Microspheres in the Repair of Myocardial Infarction in the Rat. *Biomaterials* **2010,** *31*(27), 7012–7020.

Zhao, Q.; et al. Assembly of Multilayer Microcapsules on CaCO$_3$ Particles from Biocompatible Polysaccharides. *J. Biomater. Sci. Polym. Ed.* **2006,** *17*(9), 997–1014.

Zhao, X.; et al. Active Scaffolds for On-Demand Drug and Cell Delivery. *Proc. Natl. Acad. Sci.* **2011,** *108*(1), 67–72.

CHAPTER 10

ALGINATE: DRUG DELIVERY AND APPLICATION

GAUTAM SINGHVI*, RAPALLI VAMSHI KRISHNA,
KOWTHAVARAPU V. KRISHNA, and SUNIL KUMAR DUBEY

*Department of Pharmacy, Birla Institute of Technology and Science
(BITS), Vidyavihar, Pilani, Rajasthan 333031, India*

Corresponding author. E-mail: singhvigautam@gmail.com

10.1 INTRODUCTION

Alginates (ALGs) are naturally occurring anionic unbranched polysac-charide processed from seaweeds (brown algae) and bacterial strains (Szekalska et al., 2016). ALG is most widely used in biomedical, pharma-ceutical, food industries, tissue engineering, and cosmetic application due to its biocompatibility, low toxicity, and inexpensive in availability (Lee and Mooney, 2012). ALGs are widely used in drug delivery as a matrix system for entrapment of drug/cell due to several unique properties. ALGs are inert, with good dissolution, biodegradable properties in physiological conditions and have high gel porosity for macromolecules diffusion through the matrix (Gombotz and Wee, 2012). ALG exhibits mucoad-hesive property with mucin. Carboxyl groups of ALG form hydrogen bonding on interaction with mucin and exhibit pH-dependent mucoadhe-sive property. Commonly used ALGs in food, pharmaceutical industry is alginic acid, sodium ALG, ammonium ALG, calcium ALG and propylene glycol ALG (Szekalska et al., 2016; Haugstad et al., 2015). ALGs are used in combination with water-insoluble materials such as clay (Montmoril-lonite) to improve the drug entrapment efficiency, showed decreased drug release rate and act as a controlled delivery system (Iliescu et al., 2014). ALGs form sol/gel transition in presence of multivalent cations (Ca^{2+})

independent of temperature which make it ideal immobilization matrix for living cells (Draget and Taylor, 2011). ALG forms stable irreversible gels (hydrogel) in presence of divalent cations which cross-links functional groups of ALG chains. ALGs form high viscosity acid gel at low pH compared to pKa value of uronic acid residues and pendent acid group's (COO⁻, COOH) ability to accept and release protons on change in pH makes ALG as pH sensitive (Yang et al., 2011). In some recent advancement, ALGs are used as metal sequestering agents in water treatment as gel casting and biocatalyst. ALG pellets which are fungus entrapped used in sewage for waste water treatment systems discriminative toward toxic metallic ions (Goh et al., 2012). ALG can be used for wound dressings as positive approach for the treatment of wounds as ALG has good water absorption capacity, optimal water transmission rate and mild antiseptic along with nontoxic and biodegradability. Kaltostat® Alginate dressings suggested as fast wound healing dressing by stimulating monocytes to produce wound healing cytokines; this is believed due to presence of endotoxin in ALGs (Sun and Tan, 2013).

10.2   CHEMICAL NATURE OF ALGINATES (ALGS)

Structurally, it is linear blocks of $(1 \rightarrow 4)$-linked β-D-mannuronic acid (M) and α-L-guluronic acid (G) monomers (Figure 10.1). These blocks consist three different forms of polymer segments; consecutive G residues, consecutive M residues, and alternative MG residues. The copolymer composition, molecular weight, and sequences depend on the source and species used for ALG extraction. In addition, the viscosity depends on molecular size and guluronic acid residue in block structure decides affinity for cations and gel-forming properties (Zia et al., 2015).

ALGs differ in M- and G-block content, length based on the source, G-blocks of ALG are responsible for cross-linking with divalent cations, that is, composition, sequence, and G-block length which affect physical properties of hydrogels formed (Tonnesen and Karlsen, 2002; George and Abraham, 2006). On fractionation of ALG shows soluble, insoluble fractions, whereas soluble portion constitutes of high MG block residues insoluble portion is either rich in M-block or G-block residues (Haug et al., 1966, 1967).

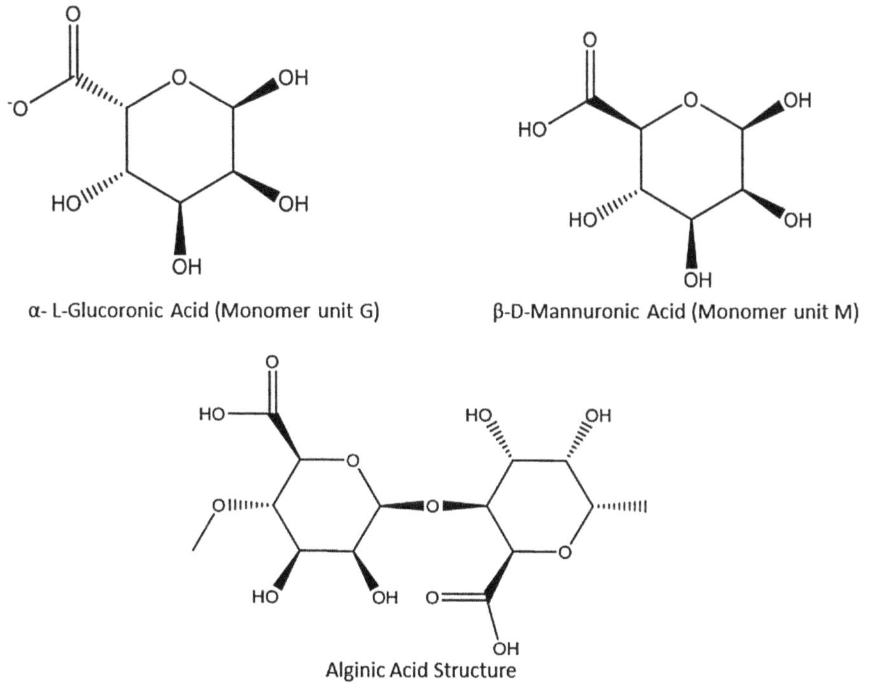

α- L-Glucoronic Acid (Monomer unit G)   β-D-Mannuronic Acid (Monomer unit M)

Alginic Acid Structure

FIGURE 10.1 Structure of alginic acid and its monomer units (α-L-Glucoronic acid, β-D-mannuronic acid).

10.3 ALG MODIFICATION

ALGs are chemically modified to alter solubility and other properties to increase its applications in biomedical, pharmaceutical, and tissue engineering. ALGs can be modified in its solubility by altering secondary –OH positions at C-2 and C-3 positions or- one –COOH at C-6 position through covalent attachment of long alkyl chains or aromatic groups to the polymer backbone. To decrease ALG dissolution and erosion, ALG hydrophobicity is increased by modifications in functional groups. ALGs are modified by grafting with different substances such as polyacrylamide, methacrylate, galactose, lectin, sulfate, cysteine, cyclodextrins, propylene glycol, and dodecylamine (Pawar and Edgar, 2012; Wong, 2011). Some examples for ALG-modified dosage forms and applications are mentioned in Table 10.1.

TABLE 10.1   Alginate (ALG) Modifications and its Applications.

Type of modification	Application	Dosage form
Oxidation	Improvement of corneal wound healing therapy, sustained oral delivery	Hydrogel, beads
Reductive-amination of oxidized ALG	Specific cell microencapsulation	Microspheres
Sulfation	Anticoagulant therapy, reduction of secretion inflammatory cytokines, improvement of the biocompatibility	Microspheres
Phosphorylation	Mineralization of hydroxyapatite and participation in the chelation process for tissue engineering	Gel
Esterification	Protein encapsulation with a sustained release	Microparticles
Na ALG-co-polyacrylamide	Sustained release gastroretentive carrier	Hydrogel
Starch-poly (acrylic acid)-NaALG	pH-sensitive matrices for the oral drug delivery	Hydrogel beads
ALG-glycidyl Methacrylate	Thermal polymerizable injectable hydrogel for tissue engineering, especially for myocardial repair	Hydrogel
Galactosylated ALG	Cell carrier with mechanical stability and selective permeability	Microcapsules
Cyclodextrin-ALG conjugate	Immobilization of bacteria	Beads
Cyclodextrin-ALG conjugate	Controlled drug delivery systems	Gel

Source: Adapted from Szekalska et al. (2016), Pawar and Edgar (2012), Wong (2011).

10.4   SOLUBILITY NATURE OF ALGS

ALGs are soluble when the carboxylic acid groups are deprotonated and pH of the medium is above certain critical value. Alginic acid is not soluble to the full extent when its carboxylic groups are protonated in water. Sodium ALG dissolved in water but not entirely soluble in the organic medium, whereas tetrabutylammonium salt forms of ALG (TBA-alginate) is completely soluble in water, ethylene glycol, and polar aprotic solvents. The solubility of ALGs depends on pH, the ionic strength of the medium, the presence of cations in the medium as divalent cations in medium leads to gelation of ALGs (Pawar and Edgar, 2011, 2012).

10.5   CROSS-LINKING OF ALGS: MECHANISM OF GEL FORMATION

Divalent cations induce cross-linking of sodium ALG in aqueous solution where sol-to-gel transformation occurs. Cross-linking mechanism of ALG for gel conversion includes gelation by external cations, gelation by internal cations, and gelation by cooling. External gelation mechanism involves the addition of ALG solution to the cationic solution by atomization. The external cationic solution is the ambiance where cross-linking of ALG leads to gel formation. Gelation by internal mechanism requires the addition of insoluble calcium salt (calcium carbonate) into ALG solution and pH is adjusted with glacial acetic acid for gelation. Acidic pH liberates calcium cations from insoluble salt which cross-link with ALG for gel formation. To reduce the further interaction of ALGs with free calcium ions trisodium citrate can be added as a sequestering agent, which competes with ALGs for free calcium. Concentration of calcium salt, particle size, and pH condition affect the release rate of cations and gel formation (Chan et al., 2006). In the cooling mechanism, ALG is dissolved in a hot medium of 90°C along with calcium salt and sequestering agent (preferably calcium) then this composition is allowed to cool which leads to gel formation. The intra-molecular bonding of ALGs are non-covalent with neighboring chains which are destabilized irreversibly due to high temperature, which also (high thermal energy) prevents polymeric alignment of ALG chains. Cooling promotes homogeneous gel formation, re-establishment of inter-molecular bonds in between polymeric chains forms ordered tertiary structure on cooling (Papageorgiou et al., 1994; Zheng, 1997).

Recent investigation also revealed that the ionic interaction plays important role in gel formation. Gaumann et al. reported ionic interaction of guluronic acid groups in ALGs is the result of G-residue chelation. The Van der Waals forces in the ALG segments induce three-dimensional (3D) gel structure in ALGs (Gaumann et al., 2000). It is also reported that based on the ion valence, radius, coordination number of the interacting ions, the binding affinity varies with ALGs. Divalent cations which include Ca^{2+}, Ba^{2+}, Sr^{2+}, and so forth, show more affinity toward GG segments, whereas trivalent ions which include La^{3+}, Pr^{3+}, Nd^{3+}, and so forth, show an affinity toward GG and MM segments. The water surrounding the trivalent ions affects the cross-linking of ALGs (Braccini et al., 1999; DeRamos et al., 1997).

Calcium is required for cross-linking of ALG solution, slow release of calcium ions assist homogeneous ALG matrix formation. Sequestering agents are added to chelate with free calcium cations and the complex formed by sequestering agent release free calcium ions in low concentration which assist in homogeneous matrix formation. Commonly used sequestering agent in cross-linking of ALG is trisodium citrate which chelates with the free calcium ions for adequate cross-linking (Papageorgiou et al., 1994). The cross-linking quality of ALGs depends on the guluronic segment composition which affects the quality of the matrices formed. ALG gelling is mainly depended on the proportions of M-blocks, G-block, and MG blocks. The increased amount of repeating G-block units result in the stiffer, brittle, and mechanically more stable form of ALG gels. The high amount of M-blocks forms soft and gradually elastic ALG gels, whereas MG blocks determine shrinkage and high flexible ALG gels. ALGs with the high amount of M-blocks results in high water uptake, ion exchange capacity compared to ALGs with G-blocks residues (Szekalska et al., 2016).

10.6   ALG APPLICATION IN TISSUE IMPLANTATION

ALGs have wide use in protein delivery, gene delivery, and other biomaterials. In combination with ALGs various body organs regeneration can be exploited in tissue engineering. ALGs have a high range of applications due to specific features such as gelling ability, bio adhesion, and biodegradation behavior. Various ALG based commercial products are reported in Table 10.2, which indicate the broad application and acceptability of ALGs.

TABLE 10.2   ALGs-Based Commercial Products.

Product	Indications
Oral administration	
Gastrotuss® baby syrup (Ummarino et al., 2015)	Used in children and infants
Algicid® suspension/tablets (Jakaria et al., 2015)	To treat acid reflux in adults
Gaviscon Double Action Liquid® (De Ruigh et al., 2014)	
Gaviscon Double Action Tablets® (Thomas et al., 2014)	
Dermal application	
Flaminal Forte® gel (Rashaan et al., 2016)	Burns, wounds, diabetic ulcers and pressure sores
Purilon Gel®, Saf-Gel® (Calo et al., 2015)	Abrasions, skin tear, dry necrotic wounds and venous ulcers
Hyalogran® dressing (Sussman et al., 2007)	Used in diabetic foot ulcers to absorb exudates

TABLE 10.2 *(Continued)*

Product	Indications
SeaSorb® dressing (Carella et al., 2013)	Cavity wounds and second-degree burns
Tromboguard® dressing (Ausili et al., 2013)	To control postoperative wounds and traumatic bleeding
Fibracol Plus® dressing (Bale et al., 2001)	Ulcers due to vascular etiologies, exuding wounds and diabetic ulcers
Algivon® dressing (Porter and Kelly, 2014)	Necrotic, malodorous wounds
Guardix-SG® (Sohn et al., 2013; Park et al., 2013)	Reduction of incidence in postoperative adhesions
Rectal administration	
Natalsid® Suppositories (Abramowitz et al., 2010)	Chronic hemorrhoids, anal fissures after surgical interventions in rectum
Periodontal application	
Progenix putty® injection, Progenix plus® injection (Gruskin et al., 2012)	Bony voids or gaps of the skeletal system
Emdogain® gel (Al Machot et al., 2014; Yan et al., 2014; Sculean et al., 2001)	Recession defects, minimal interproximal bone defects
Arthroscopic application	
ChondroArt 3D® injection (Barzegari and Saei, 2012)	Osteoarthrosis, osteochondrosis
Cell culture application	
AlgiMatrix® (Andersen et al., 2015)	Cell and tissue culture
NovaMatrix® (Andersen et al., 2015)	

Source: Adapted from Szekalska et al. (2016).

10.6.1 BLOOD VESSELS

Formation of the new blood vessel is crucial in wound healing and organ formation of the embryo. New blood vessel formation is decisive in case of tissue engineering as the formed new cells require enough nutrients and oxygen for their survival and replication which can be overcome by new blood vessel formation (Carmeliet et al., 2005). Patients suffering from coronary and peripheral arterial disease suffer from inadequate or occlude blood flow; alternative propitious approach to treat a patient is by new blood vessel formation (neovascularization). New blood vessel formation required recombinant proteins, genes alone or in combination, along with transplantation of various cell types into the body. Angiogenic molecules are delivered using ALG gel as a drug delivery vehicle; spatiotemporal control became a special attraction for therapeutic drug delivery of molecules related to neovascularization (Cao and Mooney, 2007). For delivery of heparin-binding blood vessel growth factors (VEGF) in a sustained and confine release for the formation of the new blood vessel was obtained using ALG gels (Gu et al., 2004; Jay and Saltzman, 2009). Delivery of VEGF into the ischemic muscle tissue relieves the tissue ischemia by the formation of new blood capillaries due to increased VEGF gradient in neighboring tissues. Injection of ALGs gels shows prolonged release of VEGF factor in ischemic muscle (Lee and Mooney, 2003). Delivery of VEGF followed by platelet-derived growth factor-BB (PGDF-BB) sequentially to enhance maturation of new blood vessel formation in ischemic hind limbs and myocardial infarc-tion site utilizing ALGs gel injection resulted in a proliferation of new blood vessel, maturation and function in ischemic cells (Lee and Mooney, 2003). Sun et al. developed injectable polymeric system in which PDGF encapsu-lated in poly (lactide-co-glycolide) microspheres. These microspheres along with free VEGF encapsulated in ALG gels. The combination collectively improves new blood vessel formation as VEGF exhibits its action by initiating angiogenesis to form new blood cells, whereas PDGF exhibits its action in the maturation of capillaries. Encapsulation of VEGF and PGDF in free form into ALG gel, comparative to VEGF release, PGDF release is decreased due to heparin binding (Sun et al., 2010). Increase in neovascular-ization and smooth muscle cell invested was reported in mice, when VEGF and monocyte chemotactic protein-1 delivered by ALG microparticles composite with endothelial cell transplantation. It is a progressive access to promote neovascularization by transplantation to make cells respond to growth factor (Jay et al., 2010).

10.6.2   BONE REGENERATION

Reconstructive surgery is the major challenge in the field of bone regenera-tion. An important strategy to repair bone tissue is to induce osteogenesis in situ. ALGs gels are used as potential delivery systems of factors which induce bone formation and bone-forming cells in bone regeneration. Mesenchymal stem cells (MSCs) and ALG-based injectable scaffold have been utilized for bone regeneration and adequate bone tissue formation was observed (Chen et al., 2012, Tang et al., 2012). Injectable scaffolds combining ALG-based hydrogels or microspheres which were mixed with undifferentiated MSCs or adipose-derived stem cells reported bone regeneration (Xia et al., 2012; Brun et al., 2011). A peptide-modified ALG hydrogel with a hybrid growth factor delivery system consists of electrospun nanofibre mesh tube is used for guiding bone regeneration by injecting inside the tube for sustained recombinant BMP2 (rhBMP-2) release. The sustained release of rhBMP-2 is required for substantial regeneration to occur (Kolambkar et al., 2011). In another study, osteosarcoma cells adhesion was enhanced by alginate/hydroxyapatite conglomerate. Hydroxyapatite is the inorganic material along with ALG a porous structure is formed by phase separation technique which promotes bone tissue formation (Lin and Yeh, 2004). β-tricalcium phosphate encapsulated in ALG gels also showed excellent potential to proliferate and differentiate in vitro conditions prior to implantation in presence and absence of collagen (Lawson et al., 2004).

10.6.3 CARTILAGE REPAIR

Tissue engineering became an important part heath improvement. There is a need for tissue-engineered cartilage which is having an immense and great clinical application. Degenerative and traumatic lesions of articular cartilage may be leading to cause of disability. Over 100 million Chinese it is estimated that currently suffer from osteoarthritis. ALG-associated advanced tissue engineering methods can improve cartilage repair and regeneration will therefore provide high clinical impact. The physicomechanical properties of the ALG hydrogel can be best utilized to design a scaffold with the native tissue to match the articular cartilage. The major advantage of injectable therapies for cartilage repair is that it allows immediate weight bearing due to its strength and stiffness that is achieved instantly and the implant is maintained within the defect (Sun and Tan, 2013). ALG-based injectable hydrogels, solid microspheres, and gel microspheres have been used in cartilage regeneration. The combination of the both ALG-based microspheres and hydrogels are used for controlled growth factor delivery in tissue engineering (Lubiatowski et al., 2006; Ghahramanpoor et al., 2011). ALG gel-encapsulated beads of human MSCs cultured in serum-free medium for more than 1 week with the addition of transforming growth factor (TGF-β1), dexamethasone and ascorbate 2-phosphate and determined to form cartilage in extensive osteochondral defects (Ma et al., 2003). Human adipose-derived stem cells are suggested as a possible cell source for cartilage regeneration, and chondrogenic differentiation. Human adipose-derived stem cells encapsulated in ALG gels immensely improved in the presence of TGF-β1 (Awad et al., 2004; Jin et al., 2007). Bian et al. (2011) investigated an implantable construct for cartilage repair; the report states that co-encapsulation of TGF-β-containing ALG microspheres with human MSCs in hyaluronic acid hydrogels. A composite carrier which helps to retain TGF-β bioactivity in the scaffold and promote chondrogenesis of MSCs when loaded to TGF-β with ALG microspheres combined with hydrogels. Literature also revealed the positive effect of immobilizing arginylglycylaspartic acid (RGD) to a macro-porous ALG scaffold in promoting TGF-β-induced human MSC differentiation (Ma et al., 2012; Re'em et al., 2010). The interactions in cell matrix which allow better cell accessibility to the chondrogenic inducing molecule by facilitating the immobilized RGD peptide which is an essential feature of the cell microenvironment (Re'em et al. 2010; Wang et al., 2012).

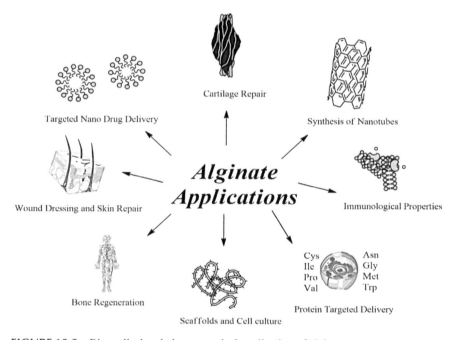

FIGURE 10.2   Biomedical and pharmaceutical application of alginates.

10.7   PHARMACEUTICAL APPLICATIONS

ALGs are having an extensive and important role in pharmaceutics in various applications such as a tablet-binding agent, alginic acid as disintegrant, stabilizer, gelling, thickening agents and can play a key role in controlled release drug formulations (Leonard et al., 2004). In the recent decades, the application knowledge of ALGs has been explored in the department of biomedical devices as well with the higher impact of chemical composition and its sequential arrangement of ALG on biological systems as well as pharmaceuticals (Figure 10.2) (Dornish et al., 2001).

10.7.1   DELIVERY OF SMALL CHEMICAL DRUGS

When drug and ALGs form a primary or secondary bond between them, it can be used to regulate the release of the drug thereby plays a key role in the kinetics of drug release. ALG gels have been explored for the controlled delivery of various low molecular weight drugs. These are typically nanoporous (with a pore size ~5 nm), promoting to faster diffusion of small molecules through gel formation. For example, the release of ionically cross-linked flurbiprofen, partially oxidized ALG gels are almost complete in 1.5 h. However, for maintaining prolonged release, increase in the number of cross-links, in the ALG incorporated beads by the combination of covalent and ionic cross-linking leads to sustained release due to the increased number of cross-links which resultants in reduced swelling. By using partially oxidized agents in the formulation of small chemical drugs, one can achieve the controlled and localized delivery. Simultaneous codelivery or multiple drug molecules can be encapsulated into ALG-based gels, as the chemical structure of the molecules and mode of encapsulation will dramatically alter the release of kinetics. Drugs with non-interactive loaded ALG will be released rapidly by diffusion process, whereas drugs covalently attached to the ALG will be released through chemical hydrolysis of the cross-linker and drugs with ionically complex to ALG will be released only after the dissociation of the ALG gel (Lee and Mooney, 2012).

10.7.2   ALG APPLICATION IN ORAL DRUG DELIVERY

10.7.2.1   HYDROPHILIC MATRIX SYSTEM

ALGs have a long and proven history of use in the hydrophilic matrix system. Sodium ALGs can be used alone or with other hydrophilic polymers to give sustained drug release with acidic, basic, and neutral drugs. Unlike other commonly used hydrophilic polymers, sodium ALG forms porous insoluble alginic acid covering in the gastric fluid that suppresses release in the stomach. Such systems protect acid-sensitive drugs or prevent a burst release of highly soluble drugs in the stomach. After passing into the higher pH of the intestinal fluid, sodium ALG erodes slowly to release the drug. When the sodium ALG is used with pH-sensitive hydrophilic polymers, such as xanthan gums or hydroxyl propyl methyl cellulose (HPMC), the release profile is further modified (Wang et al., 2009).

Sriamornsak et al. reported the effect of ALG grades on matrix system. In acidic pH, hydrated ALG layer is low viscous and less adhesive, the texture of matrix system found rubbery. This may be due to the conversion of sodium ALG into alginic acid. Compared to neutral medium ALG erosion is lesser in the acidic medium this is due to formation of tough and rubbery gel. The drug release from ALG matrix depends on the pH of the dissolution medium, in acidic medium ALG system fits into Korsmeyer-Peppas model which indicates drug release follows diffusion and erosion mechanism. The release in neutral medium follows zero-order release (Sriamornsak et al., 2007). The ALG grade used in the matrix formation has an important role in the drug release; it alters with the ALG composition. Drug physicochemical properties solely affect the drug release mechanism from the matrix. Hydrophilic drugs follow diffusion mechanism of drug release from ALG matrix, whereas hydrophobic drugs release depends on the erosion of ALG matrix. In addition, the porosity of ALG matrix also affects the drug release. The concentration of ALG is directly proportional to porosity which increases with increase in ALG concentration. This porosity of ALG matrix governs the drug release mechanism. Increased pore structure in the matrix leads to diffusion limited drug release and reduced pore size cause high degree of swelling and shrinkage of matrix.

10.7.2.2   ALG IN GASTRIC REFLUX: ANTACID FORMULATIONS

ALGs are one of the most important components in the antacid formulations; it is used as adjuvant or itself used as active agent is gastroesophageal reflex (Gaviscon®) in antacid formulations. ALGs exhibit unique mechanism as antacid it forms gel in presence of gastric acid. ALG is used in raft forming antacid formulations in combination with sodium bicarbonate or potassium bicarbonate. These formulations when come in contact with gastric fluid ALG form gel, whereas carbonate salts evolve carbon dioxide which gets entrapped in gel and the gel appears as foam and floats on gastric content similar to raft on water. The ALG raft reduces oesophageal acid reflux by acting as a physical barrier on the gastric content. ALGs are considered to be fast relief providing antacids as it form raft within the few seconds of dosing, the formed raft retains for longer duration time these are considered in long-lasting relief. The ALG raft strength depends on the carbon dioxide entrapped in it, properties of ALG that used in the formulation and presence of other antacid components like aluminium/calcium in the formulation. ALG-based antacid formulations are used in infants, during pregnancy in management of heartburn and reflux disorder (Chatfield et al., 1999; Mandel et al., 2000). In pregnancy, ALGs are prescribed against heartburn due to being reasonably safe with minor or no adverse effects, such as anti-reflux formulations such as Gaviscon (Lindow et al., 2003; Chatfield et al., 1999).

10.7.2.3   SPECIFIC GASTRO TARGETING DRUG DELIVERY SYSTEMS

ALG can be used for design of floating drug delivery systems of various drugs for prolong action at upper part of gastrointestinal tract (GIT). Shishu et al. reported 5-fluorouracil calcium ALG floating beads by ionotropic gelation method using sodium ALG and calcium carbonate. These floating beads were optimized with different ratios of ALG and calcium carbonate and beads were found with extended floating time upto 24 h. ALG is also used with vegetable oils and chitosan for sustain release of drugs and targeting the gastric mucosa (Iwamoto et al., 2005). Further, the buoyancy and gelling strength of ALGs beads can be increased with some gas generating agents such as $CaCO_3$ or $NaHCO_3$ (Choi et al., 2002).

ALG can be utilized for delayed release (enteric coated), sustained release and colonic drug delivery. Rastogi et al. reported isoniazid microsphere prepared with sodium ALG as a hydrophilic carrier which exhibited pH-mediated drug release. Prolog drug release in alkaline pH and γ-scintigraphy indicated the enteric protection of drug and delayed release of ALG microspheres (Rastogi et al., 2007). Encapsulation of mesoporous silica material with ALG with ionic interaction can be utilized for sustained release (Hu et al., 2014). Microsphere prepared with ALG is also reported for colon targeting to treat inflammatory bowel diseases by decreasing drug release in upper gastrointestinal tract (Samak et al., 2017). The specific particles size range of microsphere can be produced with different preparation methods such as aerosolization and homogenization for high drug loading, minimum drug release in upper GIT part, and maximum drug release at colonic site (Samak et al., 2017).

ALG is also used for buccal drug delivery with combination of hydrophilic polymers such as HPMC. A Choi et al. developed omeprazole buccal adhesive tablets, using sodium ALG, HPMC, magnesium oxide, and cros-carmellose sodium. Results indicated that the concentration ratios of ALG to HPMC is controlling factor for drug release. ALG form stronger interaction with drug which influence the overall drug release rate (Choi et al., 2000).

10.7.3   ALGS AS NANOPARTICLES

Recently, alginates have been investigated for nanoformulation for bioavail-ability enhancement, drug targeting to cancer cells, and multiple drug delivery. Antituberculosis drugs loaded ALG nanoparticles prepared by cation-induced gelification method exhibited enhanced oral bioavailability compared to oral administered free drug. In addition, these encapsulated nanoparticles caused complete clearance of bacteria from organs in 15 days, whereas oral adminis-tration of free drug had 45 conventional doses (Ahmad et al., 2006).

Zhang et al. reported developed nanoparticles of doxorubicin-loaded glycyrrhetinic acid (GA) modified with ALG to target liver in cancer therapy, exhibited enhanced liver targeting due to enhanced permeation rate, and it retention time was improved to larger extent due to targeting ability of GA. Free doxorubicin exhibit high cardiovascular effect. The report indi-cated that ALG-based nanoparticles have less or reduced cardiotoxic effect compared to free doxorubicin. There was induced cell death in majority of tumor cells, the normal cells which are found to be unaffected suggest that ALG nanoparticles are effective in liver targeting (Zhang et al., 2012).

ALG nanoparticles can be used for encapsulation of multidrugs such as hydrophilic and hydrophobic drugs. Wu et al. prepared ALG–calcium carbonate nanoparticles for combination therapy using co-precipitation method in aqueous solution. The dual drug-loaded nanoparticles were found with significant enhanced cell uptake and nuclear localization compared to single drug-loaded nanoparticles. In addition, cell inhibitory effect in tumor cells was significantly enhanced with dual drug-loaded nanoparticles (Wu et al., 2014). This indicated that ALG can be explored as multidrug delivery system against drug resistance diseases.

10.7.4   PROTEIN DELIVERY

Protein delivery of drugs has been rapidly growing with respect to its market also. ALG is a perfect candidate for the delivery of drugs along with proteins. ALG can encapsulate the proteins with maintaining their 3D structure and this can minimize their denaturation and protect from degradation in external biological environment. Various strategies such as delivery of DNA, enzymes, and hormones have been explored to control the rate of protein release from ALG gels (Gombotz and Wee, 2012).

10.7.5   OPHTHALMIC DRUG DELIVERY

The unique gelling property and fraction of G-residues of ALG can be used for modified ophthalmic drug delivery. Cohen et al. developed in situ gel-forming ALG ophthalmic drug delivery system of pilocarpine using different grade of ALG of FMC BioPolymer without addition of calcium ions/divalent ions in the formulation. The report concludes that Manugel DMB (ALGs with more than 65% of G-residues) form gel as it gets in contact with simulated lacrimal fluid, whereas Kelton LV formed weak gel as it consist less G-residues. In vitro studies of pilocarpine ALG gels revealed diffusion controlled drug release in 24-h release study. The extent of pilocarpine effect on intraocular pressure reduction was for high duration by ALG formulation (i.e., Manugel DMB) compared to pilocarpine nitrate solution in rabbits suggest as suitable biodegradable drug delivery vehicle for extended ophthalmic preparations. Report also concluded that Kelton LV ALG eye drop formulations has no difference in drug release compared to pilocarpine nitrate solution (Cohen et al., 1997).

10.7.6   WOUND DRESSINGS

Use of wound dressings are difficult in exuding wounds such as ulcers, pressure sores, and burns produce ample volumes of exudates, the sticky nature of exudates make critical use of the synthetic/semi synthetic wound dressings. ALG-based wound dressings have many advantageous and significant in the treatment of acute and chronic wounds in many facets of medical injuries. ALGs wound dressings which form soft gel when come in contact with exudates and can be easily removed by washing. The ALGs are proved better wound dressings in terms of wound healing and damaging friable tissue on removal (Lalau et al., 2002).

ALG dressings are mainly manufactured by ionic cross-linking of an ALG solution with calcium or sodium ions to form a gel, followed by performing to allow freeze-dried porous sheets and fibrous non-woven dressings as well. Another type of ALG dressings which are in dry form and absorb the wound fluid to re-gel and this gel can release the water to a dry wound for maintaining a physiologically moist environment so that bacterial infection can be minimized at the wound site. These advantageous can also promote to granulation tissue formation, rapid epithelialization, and healing. Different types of ALG dressings including Algicell, Comfeel Plus, Sorbsan, AlgiSite M, Kaltostat, Tegagen, and so forth are commercially available (Lee and Mooney, 2012).

Some other types of ALG dressing such as non-woven ALG fiber wound dressings, for example, Sorbsan, SeaSorb, and Kaltostat have been used in the treatment of epidermal and dermal wounds. In case of diabetic patients, wound healing is the major problem for healing, to overcome that calcium-ALG dressing appears to be a suitable topical treatment of foot lesions with respect to both tolerance and healing (Lalau et al., 2002). Lalau et al. (2002) have studied ALG fiber wound dressings such as non-woven, Sorbsan, SeaSorb, Kaltostat, and so forth. Since many years ALG fibers have been extensively used for the management of epidermal and dermal wounds. In case of diabetic foot lesions as well calcium ALGs can also be used for the topical treatment. Lansdown et al. (2002) studied ALG property with respect to dressing and wound healing. It was observed that ALG itself has a positive tendency for wound healing and demonstrate that ALG can be an effective delivery vehicle and scaffold for wound healing.

10.7.7   MODIFIED/CONJUGATE ALG IN DRUG DELIVERY

Recently, modified or conjugated ALGs are widely used in drug delivery. A pressure responsive nanogel prepared of cross-linking ALG with β-cyclodextrin was found to be effective for colon drug targeting. In vitro cell line evaluation on HT-29 cells of conjugated ALG nanoformulation indicated rapid uptake, high accumulation, and high cell death by apoptosis mechanism compared to free drug. Results conclude that ALG-cyclodextrin cross-linked nanoformulation can be employed in cancer treatment (Hosseinifar et al., 2018). Zidovudine-loaded nanoperticles prepared with Amide derivative of ALG also proved as efficient in antiviral drug delivery (Joshy et al., 2017). ALG conjugation with poly(N-isopropylacrylamide) (PNIPAAm) can be used to produce a thermoresposive hydrogel.

Liu et al. developed similar injectable thermoresposive drug delivery for anticancer drug doxorubicin. The developed ALG-conjugated formulations indicated sustained drug release, high cellular uptake and cancer cell death. Thermoresposive ALG-g-PNIPAAm can be considered as a better approach for drug resistance cancer therapy (Liu et al., 2017).

ALG covalently attached with propylene glycol backbone and modified with maleimide is also reported for enhancement for mucoadhesion compared to unmodified polymer. ALG-PEG-maleimide found to be non-toxic in human dermal fibroblast cells by viability studies (Shtenberg et al., 2017).

10.7.8   ALG IN CELL CULTURE STUDIES

In the biomedical field, as well ALG gels are being increasingly utilized for a model selection in mammalian cell culture studies. ALG gels can be readily used to study either 2D or more physiologically similar 3D culture systems. When these are combined with the low protein adsorption which allows these to serve in many ways as an ideal blank due to the lack of mammalian cell receptors for ALG and quantitative modes for cell adhesion can be incorporated (e.g., for specific cellular adhesion to receptors coupling of synthetic peptides may be used). Studies which have been performed in vitro studies can be readily translated to the in vivo, due to having their biocompatibility and simple to inject of ALG into the body (Ruvinov et al., 2016).

3D culture systems, macroporous structures prepared using natural, synthetic polymers, or their composites, with the ability to reflect the native extracellular matrix and natural physiological conditions have been regarded as advanced technology for complex cellular physiology investigations, drug evaluation, and tissue engineering. Among natural polymers, ALGs with regard to gel formation ability, mechanical strength, and interactions with cell through bioadhesive bonds are considered to be promising material for cell and tissue culture and have been employed as 3D systems. 3D material based on ionically gelled and dried ALG macroporous scaffolds creates favorable conditions for cellular attachment, proliferation, and differentiation (Astashkina et al., 2014). ALG scaffolds are able to turn into hydrogels upon rehydration following cell seeding. At present, two ALG-based 3D products for cell culture AlgiMatrix (Thermo Fisher Scientific/ Life Technologies, USA) and NovaMatrix 3-D (NovaMatrix, Norway) are commercially available in different formats of a standard cell culture well plates. AlgiMatrix is a lyophilized sponge prepared of pharmaceutical-grade ALG extracted from brown seaweed. After application of the cell suspension on the top surface of porous ALG platform, the lyophilizate becomes hydrated and entraps cells inside its porous structure. The unopened product is stable at room temperature up to 12 months. In contrary, NovaMatrix 3D comprises sterile ALG foam structure, a source of gel-forming ions to initiate polymer gelation, and a vial of lyophilized ALG to be dissolved in a culture medium. Once the pores are filled with the ALG solution, in situ hydrogels is formed which enables fast and gentle cell immobilization under physiological conditions (Sun and Tan, 2013).

10.8   ALG APPLICATIONS IN FOOD INDUSTRY

ALGs are used as a potential additive in a variety of food applications in the food industry. Specific properties of ALGs such as gelling at low temperature, thermostable nature make them ideal to use in food applications. ALGs are indigestible, as they are unchanged in the human stomach and small intestine, they fit as dietary fiber.

10.8.1   GELLING AGENTS

Restructured food is common in the food industry for increasing the aesthetic quality of products and offer unique products that meet consumer's requirements. Restructured foodstuffs are more uniform and its aesthetic nature can be produced in required shape or size and texture. Its structural properties can be controlled to produce desired products. The shelf life of fruits and products can be developed after postharvesting to desirable stability so that they can be sold throughout the year. ALGs are suitable to form gels at low temperature for foods which get damaged under low temperatures such as meat products, fruits, and vegetables. ALGs have been used for restructured application as a gelling agent in meat, fruit, vegetable, and some extruded food products such as pasta and noodles (Chen et al., 2006; Suklim et al., 2004; Grizotto et al., 2006; Grizotto et al., 2007).

10.8.2   THICKENING, STABILIZING, AND EMULSIFYING AGENTS

ALGs are used in conjunction with other thickening agents such as pectin, propylene glycol, to produce improved and acceptable low-fat processed food. ALG in combination with pectin produces a heat reversible and viscous system which can be used in jams, marmalades, and fruit sauces as a thickening agent. Propylene glycol ALG used in low concentrations, compared to regular salt and produce highly stable and relative low viscous products (Mancini et al., 2002; Brownlee et al., 2005). ALG is used as a hydrocolloid in food products as it improves organoleptic properties, aids moisture retention, and improves the texture of food. ALG used in bakery creams enriches the cream reducing separation of the solid and liquid as stability is induced due to freeze/thaw of creams. ALG is used in ice creams conjunction with other hydrocolloids to stabilize ice cream to maintain product viscosity, increase heat-shock resistance, reduces crystal formation and shrinkage. Propylene glycol ALG is one of the best emulsifiers for simple food emulsions and is also used as mayonnaise and other dressings (Kumar et al., 2007; Paraskevopoulou et al., 2005).

10.8.3 FOOD COATINGS

Food products are coated with edible thin films for the effective protective barrier to protect from moisture, temperature, and atmospheric gases apart from packaging material. ALGs and carrageenan are good barriers as a film coat for fats and oils mostly provide protection against oxygen, but a poor barrier against moisture as it is hydrophilic (Varela and Fiszman, 2011). ALGs and carrageenan film coating on fruits delay ripening of fruits and extend shelf life. Edible coatings on food minimally processed products such as fresh cut fruits prevent microbial proliferation and delay respiration to control microbial spoilage (Mastromatteo et al., 2012).

10.9 ALG APPLICATIONS IN AGRICULTURE

10.9.1 SLOW RELEASE FERTILIZERS

ALG in combination with acrylic acid, acrylamide, and clinoptilolite using N, N-methylene bisacrylamide, ammonium persulfate as an initiator hydrogel nanocomposite have been investigated for slow release of fertilizer. Hydrogels prepared with clinoptilolite showed pH-dependent swelling and in salt solutions (NaCl, KCl, $CaCl_2$, and $FeCl_3$) the swelling was lower compared to swelling in distilled water. Hydrogels with clinoptilolite zeolite had good water adsorption capacity, this formulation was found to be potential to use as nutrient carrier vehicle (Azam et al., 2014).

10.9.2 SOIL CONDITIONER

Sodium-ALG cross-linked with polyacrylamide can be used as soil conditioner. The addition of sodium-ALG/polyacrylamide copolymer in sandy soil increases the water retaining ability of the soil. The growth of the faba bean cultivated in sodium-ALG/polyacrylamide-treated soil was better compared to soil treated only with polyacrylamide. Increased faba bean plant performance in sodium-ALG/polyacrylamide compared to polyacrylamide is due to degradation of ALG into oligo-ALG growth factor. Sodium-ALG/polyacrylamide copolymer was suggested as soil conditioner and growth promoter in agriculture field (Abd El-Rehim et al., 2006).

10.10   ALG APPLICATIONS IN TEXTILE INDUSTRY

Environmental pollution due to extensive use of synthetic dyes in the textile industry is a serious problem as synthetic dyes are least biodegradable. Dalel et al. prepared immobilized partially purified acid fungal laccase extracted from *Coriolopsis gallica* by calcium ALG beads and applied for decolorization of synthetic dyes. Immobilization of *Coriolopsis gallica* laccase by 2% w/v of sodium ALG, 2% w/v $CaCl_2$, and 1:4 enzyme/ALG (v/v) was found to be optimal. Immobilized laccase was found stable with increased temperature and pH conditions, high efficiency to de-colorization toward anthraquinone dye and metal textile dye observed using both free and immobilized laccase. Immobilized laccase after four successive de-colorization cycles retained 70% of its activity except for Bismark Brown R which shows immobilized laccase potential application in dyestuff treatment (Dalel et al., 2014)

10.11   CONCLUSION

ALGs have been explored for many decades in various fields of pharmaceutical and biomedical devices. Recently, ALGs applications in the area of tissue engineering have been extensively increased in scaffolds preparations. The most important features of ALG for these applications include non-toxicity, biocompatibility, mild gelation, and easy modification technique. ALG has a brad acceptability and wider application in biomedical and pharmaceutical field. In addition, ALGs have been proved one of the most utilized items in food industry as well. There is extensive research have been carried out for ALG properties such as chemical modification, cross-linking strategy, establish the structure activity relationship, conjugation, cross-linking, and so forth for the improvement of physicochemical properties of

ALG for enlarging its application. In future, further new classes of ALGs with precisely designed physical and chemical properties can be designed for its extensive application to meet the human demand.

SUMMARY

Recently, the uses of natural and biodegradable ingredients are increasing in pharmaceutical formulations, biotechnology products, and cosmetics. Among various natural polymers, ALG, a naturally occurring anionic and unbranched polysaccharide processed from seaweeds (brown algae) and bacterial stains. ALG is most widely used in biomedical, pharmaceutical, food industries, tissue engineering, and cosmetic application due to its biocompatibility, low toxicity, and inexpensive in availability. The conventional use of ALG as an excipient in various drug delivery systems as thickening agent, gel-forming agent, stabilizer, and so forth have been reported since many decades. In the current advanced drug delivery scenario, there is always a need for prolonged and programmed controlled drug delivery systems using modified natural polymers. Compare to neutral macromolecules, ALG has unique ability to form pH dependent gel which makes it more versatile for various kinds of tailor-made drug delivery systems. As biodegradable hydrocolloids, ALG can be utilized for design and development of various modified drug release products with low cost. ALG has also been reported as excellent carriers for biomolecules such as DNA, proteins, and cells. ALG can entrap biomolecules and cells into its polymeric matrices with the retention of their biological activity. The current book chapter will introduce various aspects and applications of ALG in design of conventional drug delivery, nanocarriers' preparation, biomolecules delivery, and tailor-made for a number of applications.

KEYWORDS

- alginate
- drug delivery
- pharmaceutical applications
- tissue implantation

REFERENCES

Abd El-Rehim, H. A. Characterization and Possible Agricultural Application of Polyacrylamide/Sodium Alginate Crosslinked Hydrogels Prepared by Ionizing Radiation. *J. Appl. Polym. Sci.* **2006,** *101,* 3572–3580.

Abramowitz, L.; Weyandt, G. H.; Havlickova, B.; Matsuda, Y.; Didelot, J. M.; Rothhaar, A.; Sobrado, C.; Szabadi, A.; Vitalyos, T.; Wiesel, P. The Diagnosis and Management of Haemorrhoidal Disease from a Global Perspective. *Aliment. Pharmacol. Ther.* **2010,** *31,* 1–58.

Ahmad, Z.; Pandey, R.; Sharma, S.; Khuller, G. K. Alginate Nanoparticles as Antituberculosis Drug Carriers: Formulation Development, Pharmacokinetics and Therapeutic Potential. *Indian J. Chest Dis. Allied Sci.* **2006,** *48,* 171–176.

Al Machot, E.; Hoffmann, T.; Lorenz, K.; Khalili, I.; Noack, B. Clinical Outcomes After Treatment of Periodontal Intrabony Defects with Nanocrystalline Hydroxyapatite (Ostim) or Enamel Matrix Derivatives (Emdogain): A Randomized Controlled Clinical Trial. *BioMed. Res. Int.* **2014,** *2014,* 9, Article ID 786353.

Andersen, T.; Auk-Emblem, P.; Dornish, M. 3D Cell Culture in Alginate Hydrogels. *Microarrays* **2015,** *4,* 133–161.

Astashkina, A.; Grainger, D. W. Critical Analysis of 3-D Organoid in Vitro Cell Culture Models for High-Throughput Drug Candidate Toxicity Assessments. *Adv. Drug Delivery Rev.* **2014,** *69,* 1–18.

Ausili, E.; Paolucci, V.; Triarico, S.; Maestrini, C.; Murolo, D.; Focarelli, B.; Rendeli, C. Treatment of Pressure Sores in Spina Bifida Patients with Calcium Alginate and Foam Dressings. *Eur. Rev. Med. Pharmacol. Sci.* **2013,** *17,* 1642–1647.

Awad, H. A.; Wickham, M. Q.; Leddy, H. A.; Gimble, J. M.; Guilak, F. Chondrogenic Differentiation of Adipose-Derived Adult Stem Cells in Agarose, Alginate, and Gelatin Scaffolds. *Biomaterials* **2004,** *25,* 3211–3222.

Azam, R.; Ali, O.; Dariush, S.; Adel, R. On the Preparation and Swelling Properties of Hydrogel Nanocomposite Based on Sodium Alginate-g-Poly (Acrylic Acid-Co-Acrylamide)/Clinoptilolite and its Application as Slow Release Fertilizer. *J. Polym. Res.* **2014,** *21,* 1–15.

Bale, S.; Baker, N.; Crook, H.; Rayman, A.; Rayman, G.; Harding, K. G. Exploring the Use of an Alginate Dressing for Diabetic Foot Ulcers. *J. Wound Care* **2001,** *10,* 81–84.

Barzegari, A.; Saei, A. A. An Update to Space Biomedical Research: Tissue Engineering in Microgravity Bioreactors. *BioImpacts* **2012,** *2,* 23–32.

Bian, L.; Zhai, D. Y.; Tous, E.; Rai, R.; Mauck, R. L.; Burdick, J. A. Enhanced MSC Chondrogenesis Following Delivery of TGF-β3 from Alginate Microspheres within Hyaluronic Acid Hydrogels in Vitro and in Vivo. *Biomaterials* **2011,** *32*(27), 6425–6434.

Braccini, I.; Grasso, R. P.; Perez, S. Conformational and Configurational Features of Acidic Polysaccharides and Their Interactions with Calcium Ions: A Molecular Modeling Investigation. *Carbohydr. Res.* **1999,** *317*(1–4), 119–130.

Brownlee, I. A.; Allen, A.; Pearson, J. P.; Dettmar, P. W.; Havler, M. E.; Atherton, M. R.; Onsoyen, E. Alginate as a Source of Dietary Fiber. *Crit. Rev. Food Sci. Nutr.* **2005,** *45,* 497–510.

Brun, F.; Turco, G.; Accardo, A.; Paoletti, S. Automated Quantitative Characterization of Alginate/Hydroxyapatite Bone Tissue Engineering Scaffolds by Means of Micro-CT Image Analysis. *J. Mater. Sci. Mater. Med.* **2011,** *22,* 2617–2629.

Calo, E.; Khutoryanskiy, V. V. Biomedical Applications of Hydrogels: A Review of Patents and Commercial Products. *Eur. Polym. J.* **2015,** *65,* 252–267.

Cao, L.; Mooney, D. J. Spatiotemporal Control Over Growth Factor Signaling for Therapeutic Neovascularization. *Adv. Drug Delivery Rev.* **2007,** *59,* 40–50.

Carella, S.; Maruccia, M.; Fino, P.; Onesti, M. G. An Atypical Case of Henoch-Shonlein Purpura in a Young Patient: Treatment of the Skin Lesions with Hyaluronic Acid-Based Dressings. *In Vivo* **2013,** *27,* 147–151.

Carmeliet, P. Angiogenesis in Life, Disease and Medicine. *Nature* **2005,** *438,* 932–936.

Chan, L. W.; Lee, H. Y.; Heng, P. W. S. Mechanisms of External and Internal Gelation and Their Impact on the Functions of Alginate as a Coat and Delivery System. *Carbohydr. Polym.* **2006,** *63*(2), 176–187.

Chatfield, S. A Comparison of the Efficacy of the Alginate Preparation, Gaviscon Advance, with Placebo in the Treatment of Gastro-Oesophageal Reflux Disease. *Curr. Med. Res. Opin.* **1999,** *15*(3), 152–159.

Chen, C.-G.; Gerelt, B.; Jiang, S. T.; Nishiumi, T.; Suzuki, A. Effects of High Pressure on pH, Water-Binding Capacity and Textural Properties of Pork Muscle Gels Containing Various Levels of Sodium Alginate. *Asian-Australas. J. Anim. Sci.* **2006,** *19,* 1658–1664.

Chen, W.; Zhou, H.; Weir, M. D.; Bao, C.; Xu, H. Umbilical Cord Stem Cells Released from Alginate-Fibrin Microbeads Inside Macroporous and Biofunctionalized Calcium Phosphate Cement for Bone Regeneration. *Acta Biomater.* **2012,** *8,* 2297–2306.

Choi, H. G.; Jung, J. H.; Yong, C. S.; Rhee, C. D.; Lee, M. K.; Han, J. H.; Park, K. M.; Kim, C. K. Formulation and in Vivo Evaluation of Omeprazole Buccal Adhesive Tablet. *J. Controlled Release* **2000,** *68,* 405–412.

Choi, B. Y.; Park, H. J.; Hwang, S. J.; Park, J. B. Preparation of Alginate Beads for Floating Drug Delivery System: Effects of CO_2 Gas-Forming Agents. *Int. J. Pharma.* **2002,** *239,* 81–91.

Cohen, S.; Lobel, E.; Trevgoda, A.; Peled, Y. A Novel in Situ-Forming Ophthalmic Drug Delivery System from Alginates Undergoing Gelation in the Eye. *J. Controlled Release.* **1997,** *44,* 201–208.

Dalel, D.; Susana, R. C.; Moncef, N.; Tahar, M. Biodegradation of Textile Dyes by Immobilized Laccase from *Coriolopsis gallica* into Ca-Alginate Beads. *Int. Biodeterior. Biodegrad.* **2014,** *90,* 71–78.

De Ruigh, A.; Roman, S.; Chen, J.; Pandolfino, J. E.; Kahrilas, P. J. Gaviscon Double Action Liquid (Antacid & Alginate) is More Effective than Antacid in Controlling Post-Prandial Oesophageal Acid Exposure in GERD Patients: A Double-Blind Crossover Study. *Aliment. Pharmacol. Ther.* **2014,** *40,* 531–537.

DeRamos, C. M.; Irwin, A. E.; Nauss, J. L.; Stout, B. E. 13C NMR and Molecular Modeling Studies of Alginic Acid Binding with Alkaline Earth and Lanthanide Metal Ions. *Inorg. Chim. Acta* **1997,** *256*(1), 69–75.

Dornish, M.; Kaplan, D.; Skaugrud, Ø. Standards and Guidelines for Biopolymers in Tissue-Engineered Medical Products. *Ann. N. Y. Acad. Sci.* **2001,** *944*(1), 388–397.

Draget, K. I.; Taylor, C. Chemical, Physical and Biological Properties of Alginates and Their Biomedical Implications. *Food Hydrocolloids* **2011,** *25,* 251–256.

Gaumann, A.; Laudes, M.; Jacob, B.; Pommersheim, R.; Laue, C.; Vogt, W.; Schrezenmeir, J. Effect of Media Composition on Long-Term in Vitro Stability of Barium Alginate and Polyacrylic Acid Multilayer Microcapsules. *Biomaterials* **2000,** *21*(18), 1911–1917.

George, M.; Abraham, T. E. Polyionic Hydrocolloids for the Intestinal Delivery of Protein Drugs. *J. Controlled Release* **2006,** *114,* 1–14.

Ghahramanpoor, M. K.; Najafabadi, S. A.; Abdouss, M.; Bagheri, F.; Eslaminejad, B. M. A Hydrophobically-Modified Alginate Gel System: Utility in the Repair of Articular Cartilage Defects. *J. Mater. Sci. Mater. Med.* **2011,** *22,* 2365–2375.

Goh, C. H.; Heng, P. W. S.; Chan, L. W. Alginates as a Useful Natural Polymer for Microencapsulation and Therapeutic Applications. *Carbohydr. Polym.* **2012,** *88,* 1–12.

Gombotz, W. R.; Wee, S. F. Protein Release from Alginate Matrices. *Adv. Drug Delivery Rev.* **2012,** *64,* 194–205.

Grizotto, R. K.; Berbari, S. A. G.; DeMoura, S. C. S. R.; Claus, M. L. Estudo da vida-de-prateleira de fruta estruturada e desidratada obtida de polpa concentrada de mamao (Shelf life studies of restructured and dried fruit made from concentrated papaya pulp). *Cienc. Tecnol. Aliment.* **2006,** *26,* 709–714.

Grizotto, R. K.; Bruns, R. E.; De Aguirre, J. M.; De Menezes, H. C. Technological Aspects for Restructuring Concentrated Pineapple Pulp. *LWT Food Sci. Technol.* **2007,** *40,* 759–765.

Gruskin, E.; Doll, B. A.; Futrell, F. W.; Schmitz, J. P.; Hollinger, J. O. Demineralized Bone Matrix in Bone Repair: History and Use. *Adv. Drug Delivery Rev.* **2012,** *64,* 1063–1077.

Gu, F.; Amsden, B.; Neufeld, R. Sustained Delivery of Vascular Endothelial Growth Factor with Alginate Beads. *J. Controlled Release* **2004,** *96,* 463–472.

Haug, A.; Larsen, B.; Smidsrød, O. A Study of the Constitution of Alginic Acid by Partial Hydrolysis. *Acta Chem. Scand.* **1966,** *20,* 183–190.

Haug, A.; Larsen, B.; Smidsrød, O. Studies on the Sequence of Uronic Acid Residues in Alginic Acid. *Acta Chem. Scand.* **1967,** *21,* 691–704.

Haugstad, K. E.; Hati, A. G.; Nordgard, C. T.; Adl, P. S.; Maurstad, G.; Sletmoen, M.; Draget, K. I.; Dias, R. S.; Stokke, B. T. Direct Determination of Chitosan-Mucin Interactions Using a Single Molecule Strategy: Comparison to Alginate-Mucin Interactions. *Polymers* **2015,** *7,* 161–185.

Hosseinifar, T.; Sheybani, S.; Abdouss, M.; Hassani, N. S. A.; Shafie, A. M. Pressure Responsive Nanogel Base on Alginate- Cyclodextrin with Enhanced Apoptosis Mechanism for Colon Cancer Delivery. *J. Biomed. Mater. Res.* **2018,** *106*(2), 349–359.

Hu, L.; Sun, C.; Song, A.; Chang, D., Zheng, X.; Gao, Y.; Jiang, T.; Wang, S. Alginate Encapsulated Mesoporous Silica Nanospheres as a Sustained Drug Delivery System for the Poorly Water-Soluble Drug Indomethacin. *Asian J. Pharm. Sci.* **2014,** *9,* 183–190.

Iwamoto, M.; Kurachi, M.; Nakashima, T.; Kim, D.; Yamaguchi, K.; Oda, T.; et al. Structure-Activity Relationship of Alginate Oligosaccharides in the Induction of Cytokine Production from RAW264.7 Cells. *FEBS Lett.* **2005,** *579*(20), 4423–4429.

Jakaria, M.; Zaman, R.; Parvez, M.; Islam, M.; Haque, A. M.; Sayeed, M. A.; Ali. M. H. Comparative Study Among the Different Formulation of Antacid Tablets by Using Acid-Base Neutralization Reaction. *Global J. Pharmacol.* **2015,** *9,* 278–281.

Jay, S. M.; Saltzman, W. M. Controlled Delivery of VEGF via Modulation of Alginate Microparticle Ionic Cross-Linking. *J. Controlled Release* **2009,** *134,* 26–34.

Jay, S. M.; Shepherd, B. R.; Andrejecsk, J. W.; Kyriakides, T. R.; Pober, J. S.; Saltzman, W. M. Dual Delivery of VEGF and MCP-1 to Support Endothelial Cell Transplantation for Therapeutic Vascularization. *Biomaterials* **2010,** *31,* 3054–3062.

Jin, X. B.; Sun, Y. S.; Zhang, K.; Wang, J.; Shi, T. P.; Ju, X. D.; Lou, S. Q. Ectopic Neocartilage Formation from Predifferentiated Human Adipose Derived Stem Cells Induced by Adenoviral-Mediated Transfer of hTGF-Beta2. *Biomaterials* **2007,** *28,* 2994–3003.

Joshy, K. S.; Susan, M. A.; Snigdha, S.; Nandakumar, K.; Laly, A. P.; Sabu, T. Encapsulation of Zidovudine in PF-68 Coated Alginate Conjugate Nanoparticles for Anti-HIV Drug Delivery. *Int. J Biol. Macromol.* **2018,** *107,* 929–937.

Kolambkar, Y. M.; Dupont, K. M.; Boerckel, J. D.; Huebsch, N.; Mooney, D. J.; Hutmacher, D. W.; Guldberg, R. E. An Alginate-Based Hybrid System for Growth Factor Delivery in the Functional Repair of Large Bone Defects. *Biomaterials* **2011,** *32,* 65–74.

Kumar, M.; Sharma, B. D.; Kumar, R. R. Evaluation of Sodium Alignate as a Fat Replacer on Processing and Shelf-Life of Low-Fat Ground Pork Patties. *Asian-Australas. J. Anim. Sci.* **2007,** *20,* 588–597.

Lalau, J. D.; Bresson, R.; Charpentier, P.; Coliche, V.; Erlher, S.; Ha Van, G.; et al. Efficacy and Tolerance of Calcium Alginate Versus Vaseline Gauze Dressings in the Treatment of Diabetic Foot Lesions. *Diabetes Metab.* **2002,** *28,* 223–229.

Lansdown, A. B. Calcium: A Potential Central Regulator in Wound Healing in the Skin. *Wound Repair Regener.* **2002,** *10*(5), 271–285.

Lawson, M. A.; Barralet, J. E.; Wang, L.; Shelton, R. M.; Triffitt, J. T. Adhesion and Growth of Bone Marrow Stromal Cells on Modified Alginate Hydrogels. *Tissue Eng.* **2004,** *10,* 1480–1491.

Lee, K. Y.; Mooney, D. J. Alginate: Properties and Biomedical Applications. *Prog. Polym. Sci.* **2012,** *37,* 106–126.

Lee, K. Y.; Peters, M. C.; Mooney, D. J. Comparison of Vascular Endothelial Growth Factor and Basic Fibroblast Growth Factor on Angiogenesis in SCID Mice. *J. Controlled Release* **2003,** *87,* 49–56.

Leonard, M.; De Boisseson, M. R.; Hubert, P.; Dalencon, F.; Dellacherie, E. Hydrophobically Modified Alginate Hydrogels as Protein Carriers with Specific Controlled Release Properties. *J. Controlled Release* **2004,** *98*(3), 395–405.

Lin, H. R.; Yeh, Y. J. Porous Alginate/Hydroxyapatite Composite Scaffolds for Bone Tissue Engineering: Preparation, Characterization, and in Vitro Studies. *J. Biomed. Mater. Res. Part B* **2004,** *71,* 52–65.

Lindow, S. W.; Regnell, P.; Sykes, J.; Little, S. An Open-Label, Multicentre Study to Assess the Safety and Efficacy of a Novel Reflux Suppressant (Gaviscon Advance) in the Treatment of Heartburn During Pregnancy. *Int. J. Clin. Pract.* **2003,** *57*(3), 175–179.

Liu, M.; Song, X.; Wen, Y.; Zhu, J. L.; Li, J. Injectable Thermoresponsive Hydrogel Formed by Alginate-g-Poly(N-isopropylacrylamide) Releasing Doxorubicin-Encapsulated Micelles as Smart Drug Delivery System. *ACS Appl. Mater. Interfaces* **2017,** *9*(41), 35673–35682.

Lubiatowski, P.; Kruczynski, J.; Gradys, A.; Trzeciak, T.; Jaroszewski, J. Articular Cartilage Repair by Means of Biodegradable Scaffolds. *Transplant. Proc.* **2006,** *38,* 320–322.

Ma, H. L.; Hung, S. C.; Lin, S. Y.; Chen, Y. L.; Lo, W. H. Chondrogenesis of Human Mesenchymal Stem Cells Encapsulated in Alginate Beads. *J. Biomed. Mater. Res. Part A* **2003,** *64,* 273–281.

Ma, K.; Titan, A. L.; Stafford, M.; Zheng, C. H.; Levenston, M. E. Variations in Chondrogenesis of Human Bone Marrow-Derived Mesenchymal Stem Cells in Fibrin/Alginate Blended Hydrogels. *Acta Biomater.* **2012,** *8*(10), 3754–3764.

Mancini, F.; Montanari, L.; Peressini, D.; Fantozzi, P. Influence of Alginate Concentration and Molecular Weight on Functional Properties of Mayonnaise. *LWT Food Sci Technol.* **2002,** *35,* 517–525.

Mandel, K. G.; Daggy, B. P.; Brodie, D. A.; Jacoby, H. I. Review article: Alginate-Raft Formulations in the Treatment of Heartburn and Acid Reflux. *Aliment. Pharmacol. Ther.* **2000,** *14,* 669–690.

Mastromatteo, M.; Conte, A.; Del Nobile, M. A. Packaging Strategies to Prolong the Shelf Life of Fresh Carrots (*Daucus carota* L.). *Innovative Food Sci. Emerging Technol.* **2012,** *13,* 215–220.

Papageorgiou, M.; Kasapis, S.; Gothard, M. G. Structural and Textural Properties of Calcium-Induced, Hot-Made Alginate Gels. *Carbohydr. Polym.* **1994,** *24*(3), 199–207.

Paraskevopoulou, A.; Boskou, D.; Kiosseoglou, V. Stabilization of Olive Oil–Lemon Juice Emulsion with Polysaccharides. *Food Chem.* **2005,** *90,* 627–634.

Park, S. O.; Han, J.; Minn, K. W.; Jin, U. S. Prevention of Capsular Contracture with Guardix-SG® After Silicone Implant Insertion. *Aesthetic Plast. Surg.* **2013,** *37,* 543–548.

Pawar, S. N.; Edgar, K. J. Chemical Modification of Alginates in Organic Solvent Systems. *Biomacromolecules* **2011,** *12,* 4095-4103.

Pawar, S. N.; Edgar, K. J. Alginate Derivatization: A Review of Chemistry, Properties and Applications. *Biomaterials* **2012,** *33*(11), 3279–3305.

Porter, M.; Kelly, J. Pressure Ulcer Treatment in a Patient with Spina Bifida. *Nurs. Stand.* **2014,** *28,* 60–69.

Rashaan, Z. M.; Krijnen, P.; van den Akker-van Marle, M. E.; van Baar, M. E.; Vloemans, A. F. P.; Dokter, J.; Tempelman, F. R. H.; van der Vlies, C. H.; Breederveld, R. S. Clinical Effectiveness, Quality of Life and Cost-Effectiveness of Flaminal® Versus Flamazine® in the Treatment of Partial Thickness Burns: Study Protocol for a Randomized Controlled Trial. *Trials* **2016,** *17,* 1–9.

Rastogi, R.; Sultana, Y.; Aqil, M.; Ali, A.; Kumar, S.; Chuttani, K.; Mishra, A. K. Alginate Microspheres of Isoniazid for Oral Sustained Drug Delivery. *Int. J. Pharm.* **2007,** *334,* 71–77.

Re'em, T.; Tsur-Gang, O.; Cohen, S. The Effect of Immobilized RGD Peptide in Macroporous Alginate Scaffolds on TGFβ1-Induced Chondrogenesis of Human Mesenchymal Stem Cells. *Biomaterials.* **2010,** *31*(26), 6746–6755.

Ruvinov, E.; Cohen, S. Bioengineering Alginate for Regenerative Medicine Applications. In *Biomaterials from Nature for Advanced Devices and Therapies;* Neves, N. M., Reis, R. L., Eds.; John Wiley & Sons, Inc. 2016; 274–306. doi:10.1002/9781119126218.ch17.

Iliescu, R. I.; Andronescu, E.; Ghitulica, C. D.; Voicu, G.; Ficai, A.; Hoteteu, M. Montmorillonite–Alginate Nanocomposite as a Drug Delivery System – Incorporation and in Vitro Release of Irinotecan. *Int. J. Pharm.* **2014,** *463,* 184–192.

Samak, Y. O.; El Massik, M.; Coombes, A. G. A. A Comparison of Aerosolization and Homogenization Techniques for Production of Alginate Microparticles for Delivery of Corticosteroids to the Colon. *J. Pharm. Sci.* **2017,** *106,* 208–216.

Sculean, A.; Auschill, T. M.; Donos, N.; Brecx, M.; Arweiler, N. B. Effect of an Enamel Matrix Protein Derivative (Emdogain) on ex Vivo Dental Plaque Vitality. *J. Clin. Periodontol.* **2001,** *28,* 1074–1078.

Shtenberg, Y.; Goldfeder, M.; Schroeder, A.; Bianco-Peled, H. Alginate Modified with Maleimide-Terminated PEG as Drug Carriers with Enhanced Mucoadhesion. *Carbohydr. Polym.* **2017,** *175,* 337–346.

Sohn, E. J.; Ahn, H. B.; Roh, M. S.; Ryu, W. Y.; Kwon, Y. H. Efficacy of Temperature-Sensitive Guardix-SG for Adhesiolysis in Experimentally Induced Eyelid Adhesion in Rabbits. *Ophthalmic Plast. Reconstr. Surg.* **2013,** *29,* 458–463.

Sriamornsak, P.; Thirawong, N.; Korkerd, K.; Swelling, Erosion and Release Behavior of Alginate-Based Matrix Tablets. *Eur. J. Pharm. Biopharm.* **2007,** *66,* 435–450.

Suklim, K.; Flick, G. J., Jr.; Marcy, J. E.; Eigel, W. N.; Haugh, C. G.; Granata, L. A. Effect of Cold-Set Binders: Alginates and Microbial Transglutaminase on the Physical Properties of Restructured Scallops. *J. Texture Stud.* **2004,** *35,* 634–642.

Sun, J.; Tan, H. Alginate-Based Biomaterials for Regenerative Medicine Applications. *Materials* **2013,** *6,* 1285-1309.

Sun, Q. H.; Silva. E. A.; Wang, A. X.; Fritton, J. C.; Mooney, D. J.; Schaffler, M. B.; Grossman, P. M.; Rajagopalan, S. Sustained Release of Multiple Growth Factors from Injectable Polymeric System as a Novel Therapeutic Approach Towards Angiogenesis. *Pharm Res.* **2010,** *27,* 264–271.

Sussman, C.; Bates-Jensen, B. Management of the Wound Environment with Dressings and Topical Agents. In *Wound Care: A Collaborative Practice Manual for Health Professionals*, 3rd ed.; Lippincott Williams & Wilkins: Philadelphia, PA, 2007; p 254.

Szekalska, M.; Puciłowska, A.; Szymańska, E; Ciosek, P.; Winnicka, K. Alginate: Current Use and Future Perspectives in Pharmaceutical and Biomedical Applications. *Int. J. Polym. Sci.* **2016**, *2016*, 1–17.

Tang, M.; Chen, W.; Weir, M. D.; Thein-Han, W.; Xu, H. Human Embryonic Stem Cell Encapsulation in Alginate Microbeads in Macroporous Calcium Phosphate Cement for Bone Tissue Engineering. *Acta Biomater.* **2012**, *8*, 3436–3445.

Thomas, E.; Wade, A.; Crawford, G.; Jenner, B.; Levinson, N.; Wilkinson, J. Randomised Clinical Trial: Relief of Upper Gastrointestinal Symptoms by an Acid Pocket-Targeting Alginate – Antacid (Gaviscon Double Action) a Double-Blind, Placebocontrolled, Pilot Study in Gastro-Oesophageal Reflux Disease. *Aliment. Pharmacol. Ther.* **2014**, *39*, 595–602.

Tonnesen, H. H.; Karlsen, J. Alginate in Drug Delivery Systems. *Drug Dev. Ind. Pharm.* **2002**, *28*, 621–630.

Ummarino, D.; Miele, E.; Martinelli, M.; Scarpato, E.; Crocetto, F.; Sciorio, E.; Staiano, A. Effect of Magnesium Alginate Plus Simethicone on Gastroesophageal Reflux in Infants. *J. Pediatr. Gastroenterol. Nutr.* **2015**, *60*, 230–235.

Varela, P.; Fiszman, S. M. Hydrocolloids in Fried Foods. A Review. *Food Hydrocolloids* **2011**, *25*, 1801–1812.

Wang, Q.; Zhang, J.; Wang, A. Preparation and Characterization of a Novel pH-Sensitive Chitosan-g-Poly (Acrylic Acid)/Attapulgite/Sodium Alginate Composite Hydrogel Bead for Controlled Release of Diclofenac Sodium. *Carbohydr Polym.* **2009**, *78*(4), 731–737.

Wang, C. C.; Yang, K. C.; Lin, K. H.; Liu, Y. L.; Liu, H. C.; Lin, F. H. Cartilage Regeneration in SCID Mice Using a Highly Organized Three-Dimensional Alginate Scaffold. *Biomaterials* **2012**, *33*, 1, 120–127.

Wong, T. W. Alginate Graft Copolymers and Alginate-Coexcipient Physical Mixture in Oral Drug Delivery. *J. Pharm. Pharmacol.* **2011**, *63*, 1497–1512.

Wu, J. L.; Wang, C. Q.; Zhuo, R. X.; Cheng, S. X. Multi-Drug Delivery System Based on Alginate/Calcium Carbonatehybrid Nanoparticles for Combination Chemotherapy. *Colloids Surf. B* **2014**, *123*, 498–505.

Xia, Y.; Mei, F.; Duan, Y.; Gao, Y.; Xiong, Z.; Zhang, T.; Zhang, H. Bone Tissue Engineering Using Bone Marrow Stromal Cells and an Injectable Sodium Alginate/Gelatin Scaffold. *J. Biomed. Mater. Res. Part A* **2012**, *100*, 1044–1050.

Yan, X. Z.; Rathe, F.; Gilissen, C.; van der Zande, M.; Veltman, J.; Junker, R.; Yang, F.; Jansen, J. A.; Walboomers, X. F. The Effect of Enamelmatrix Derivative (Emdogain®) on Gene Expression Profiles of Human Primary Alveolar Bone Cells. *J. Tissue Eng. Regener. Med.* **2014**, *8*, 463–472.

Yang, J. S.; Xie, Y. J.; He, W. Research Progress on Chemical Modification of Alginate: A Review. *Carbohydr. Polym.* **2011**, *84*, 33–39.

Zhang, C.; Wang, W.; Liu, T.; Wu, Y.; Guo, H.; Wang, P.; Tian, Q.; Wang, Y.; Yuan, Z. Doxorubicin-Loaded Glycyrrhetinic Acid-Modified Alginate Nanoparticles for Liver Tumor Chemotherapy. *Biomaterials* **2012**, *33*, 2187–2196.

Zheng, H. Interaction Mechanism in Sol-Gel Transition of Alginate Solutions by Addition of Divalent Cations. *Carbohydr. Res.* **1997**, *302*(1–2), 97–101

Zia, K. M.; Zia, F.; Zuber, M.; Rehman, S.; Ahmad, M. N. Alginate Based Polyurethanes: A Review of Recent Advances and Perspective. *Int. J. Biol. Macromol.* **2015**, *79*, 377–387.

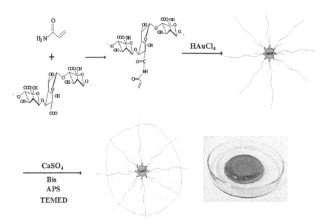

FIGURE 6.6   Schematic illustration of the preparation of the hydrogel/gold nanocomposites.

Source: Adapted from Zhang (2014).

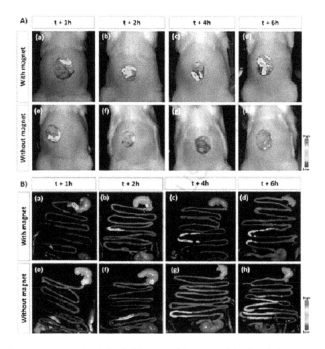

FIGURE 6.9   Fluorescence and bright-field merged images of the beads in the rats intestine (A) under the magnet position, after skin removal and (B) after unfolding the intestine from stomach to caecum at time (a) and (e) 1 h, (b) and (f) 2 h, (c) and (g) 4 h, (d) and (h) 6 h after administration of the beads in the stomach of the rats for animal (a) to (d) with magnet and (e) to (h) without magnet.

Source: Adapted from Seth (2017).

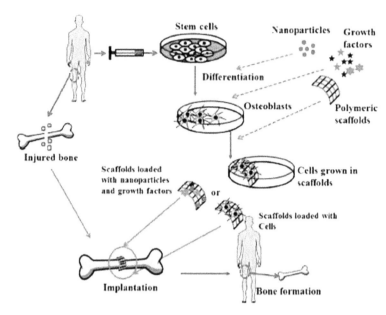

FIGURE 8.1 Bone tissue engineering involves the use of cells and biomaterials or a combination of cells loaded onto biodegradable scaffolds to treat critical-sized bone defects. Mesenchymal stem cells isolated from the patient donor are differentiated into osteoblasts in vitro prior to its loading into scaffolds. The cell-free construct is also used along with bioactive molecules and nanoparticles for enhancing bone formation.

Source: Reprinted with permission from Saravanan et al., 2016b. © 2016 Elsevier.

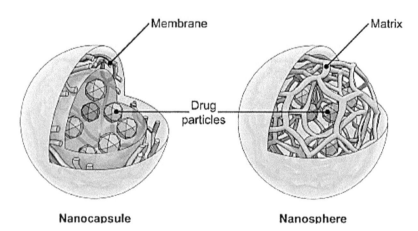

FIGURE 12.13 A schematic representation of the structure of a nanocapsule and a nanosphere.

Source: Suffredini et al. (2014).

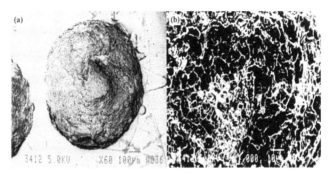

FIGURE 16.2 Scanning electron microscopy photographs of the calcium alginate–poly(vinyl pyrrolidone)/nano-HAp composite beads of diclofenac sodium at lower magnification (60x) and bead surface topography at higher magnification (1000x).

Source: Adapted from Hasnain et al. (2016) (Copyright © 2014 Elsevier B. V.).

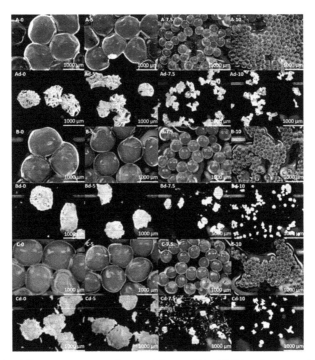

FIGURE 20.2 Microscope photos of wet and freeze-dries ALG beads prepared under various voltages. A-0, A-5, A-7.5, and A-10 are the blank wet ALG beads prepared with voltage of 0, 5, 7.5, and 10 kV, respectively, while Ad-0, Ad-5, Ad-7.5, and Ad-10 are the blank freeze dried ALG beads prepared with the same conditions, respectively; photos numbered with B stands for 50% ALG beads and C is 33% ALG beads loaded with of gallic acid (numbers are voltages applied and d means freeze-dried form, scale bar is 1000 μm).

Source: Adapted from Li et al. (2016).

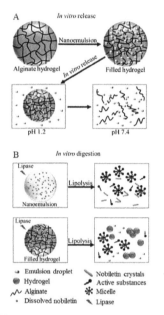

FIGURE 20.5 Schematic illustrations of (A) in vitro release behavior and (B) in vitro digestion behavior for nanoemulsions and filled ALG hydrogels.

Source: Reprinted with permission from Lei et al., 2017. © 2017 Elsevier.

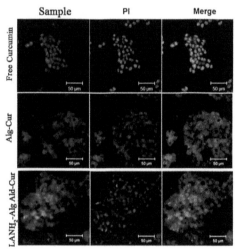

FIGURE 20.6 Cellular uptake of free curcumin (row 1) Alg-Cur (row 2) and LANH$_2$-Alg Ald-Cur (row 3) by HepG2 cells observe under CLSM signal from curcumin (column 1) and PI (column 2) was separately obtained and merged (column 3). LANH$_2$-Alg Ald-Curcumin shows higher intensity as a result of increased level of particle internalization compared to Alg-Curcumin and free curcumin.

Source: Adapted from Sarika et al. (2016a).

CHAPTER 11

CHEMICAL AND PHYSICAL MODIFICATIONS OF ALGINATES TO IMPROVE THEIR USE AS CARRIERS IN DELIVERY SYSTEMS

GABRIELA VALLADARES[1,2], KARINA BIERBRAUER[2,3], and MIRIAM STRUMIA[*,4,5]

[1]Departamento de Sanidad Vegetal, Universidad Nacional de Tucumán, Facultad de Agronomía y Zootecnia, Tucumán, Argentina

[2]CONICET, Consejo Nacional de Investigaciones Científicas y Técnicas, Buenos Aires, Argentina

[3]Centro de Excelencia en Productos y Procesos de Córdoba, Gobierno de la Provincia de Córdoba, Pabellón CEPROCOR, Santa María de Punilla, Córdoba, Argentina

[4]Departamento de Química Orgánica, Universidad Nacional de Córdoba, Facultad de Ciencias Químicas, Córdoba, Argentina

[5]Conicet-Instituto de Investigación en Ingeniería de Procesos y Química Aplicada (IPQA), Córdoba, Argentina

*Corresponding author. E-mail: mcs@fcq.unc.edu.ar

11.1 INTRODUCTION

The design of biomaterials is based mainly on the mimicking of specific functions pertaining to the extracellular matrices of body tissues. The resulting materials are able to regulate the responses to various stimuli in a controlled manner. Natural polymers are highly sought after for the preparation of biomaterials due to their inherent biocompatibility and high adaptability to different forms and uses (Ratner and Bryant, 2004; Williams, 2009).

Alginate is an anionic and linear polysaccharide of natural origin obtained from brown seaweeds such as *Laminaria hyperborea*, *Macrocystis pyrifera*, and *Ascophyllum nodosum*. This biopolymer is composed of alternating blocks of (1, 4)-linked-d-mannuronate (M) and l-guluronate (G) residues. The blocks consist of consecutive G residues (GGGGGG), consecutive M residues (MMMMMM) and alternating M and G residues (GMGMGM) (Lee and Mooney, 2012) (Figure 11.1). Alginates extracted from different sources differ in M and G content as well as in the length of each block. More than 200 different alginates are currently being manufactured (Rinaudo, 2008) and extensively studied for a wide range of potential biomedical and engineering applications, taking advantage of their favorable properties such as biocompatibility, low toxicity, relatively low cost, and easy gelation capacity to obtain hydrogels (Cardoso et al., 2016; Larsen et al., 2015; Caetano et al., 2016; Agüero et al., 2017).

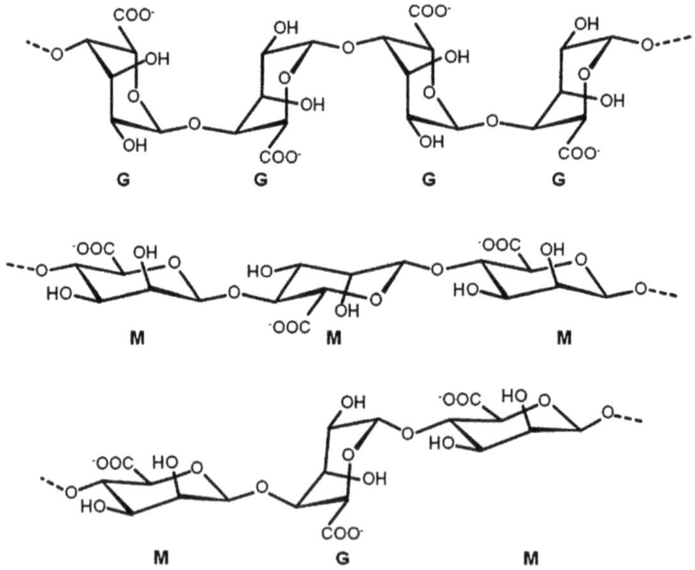

FIGURE 11.1 Chemical structures of G-block, M-block, and alternating block in alginate.

Source: Reprinted with permission from Lee and Mooney, 2012. © 2012 Elsevier.

Hydrogels are three-dimensional, hydrophilic, polymeric networks capable of retaining large amounts of water or biological fluids and characterized by a soft and rubbery consistency. Hydrogels are classified as chemical or physical, the former being synthesized by covalently cross-linked reactions to create stable networks with a permanent form (Dragan, 2014) and the latter being "reversible" gels obtained by molecular entanglements and/or secondary forces including ionic, H-bonding, or hydrophobic interactions (Hoffman, 2002; Peppas et al., 2000). "Ionotropic" hydrogels are formed by the interaction between a polyelectrolyte and an oppositely charged multivalent ion, and the polyelectrolyte complexes formed by the interaction between two oppositely charged polyelectrolytes (Bierbrauer et al., 2014). Physical or ionotropic gels can be disintegrated by changes in environmental conditions such as ionic strength, pH, and temperature. Both physical and chemical hydrogels have numerous biomedical applications in drug delivery; wound dressing, tissue engineering, and related fields.

Another type of hydrogel is the so-called "smart" hydrogels, which are able to significantly change their volume/shape in response to small alterations in certain environmental parameters (Figure 11.2). Responsive hydrogels have numerous applications, mostly related to biological, therapeutic (Agüero et al., 2017; Bajpai et al., 2008; Peak et al., 2013; Peng et al., 2008), and sensing applications (Richter et al., 2008).

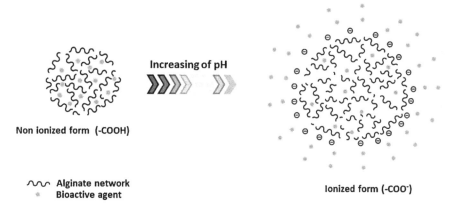

Increasing of pH

Non ionized form (-COOH)

Ionized form (-COO⁻)

∿∿ Alginate network
＊ Bioactive agent

FIGURE 11.2 Schematic illustration of pH stimuli-responsiveness of smart alginate microparticles.

Source: Reprinted with permission from Agüero et al., 2017. © 2017 Elsevier.

In addition to the advantages already mentioned, because of their chemical structure alginate biopolymers can be used to create all the hydrogel types described above: physical, chemical, ionotropic, and smart. However, only the G-blocks of alginate are believed to participate in intermolecular cross-linking with divalent cations (e.g., Ca^{2+}) to form hydrogels. Composition (i.e., M/G ratio), sequence, G-block length, and molecular weight are thus critical factors affecting the physical properties of alginate and its resultant hydrogels (George and Abraham, 2006).

The mechanical properties of alginate gels can typically be enhanced by increasing the length of the G-block and molecular weight. However, an alginate solution formed from high molecular weight polymer becomes greatly viscous, often an undesirable feature in processing (Lee and Mooney, 2012; LeRoux et al., 1999).

Alginate hydrogels have a particular appeal for drug delivery applications because they retain their structural stability and can be manipulated to perform a number of critical functions (Wu 2013). The porous structure of the alginate network allows drug molecules, from small chemical drugs to macromolecular proteins, to be incorporated and released in a controlled manner, depending on the cross-linker type and cross-linking method.

In order to understand how alginates can be optimized as useful delivery systems for therapeutic applications, this chapter focuses on the following factors impacting on drug release from alginate matrices: type or cross-linking reaction for networks formation, stability of alginate matrices, pH effect, alginate composition, chemical characteristics of encapsulated drugs, and modification of the functional groups in alginates.

11.2 DIFFERENT SYNTHETIC PATHWAYS TO OBTAIN ALGINATE NETWORKS

11.2.1 PHYSICAL NETWORKS

The formation of networks for alginate delivery systems through non-covalent bonds involves synthetic strategies including ionic interaction and interpenetrating polymer networks (IPNs). The advantage of using physical gels is their easy disintegration in response to changes in environmental conditions such as ionic strength, pH, and temperature, making them particularly suitable for biological, therapeutic (Peak et al., 2013) and sensing applications (Ritcher, 2008). However, single-network hydrogels have weak mechanical properties and slow response at swelling. One way to enhance their mechanical strength and swelling/deswelling response is the formation of multicomponent networks such as IPNs.

11.2.1.1   IONIC CROSS-LINKING

The most common method for preparing hydrogels from an aqueous algi-nate solution is to combine the solution with ionic cross-linking agents such as divalent cations such as Ca^{2+}, Cu^{2+}, Zn^{2+}, or Mn^{2+}. The affinity of alginates to polyvalent ions increases in the order of $Mg^{2+} \ll Mn^{2+} < Ca^{2+} < Sr^{2+} < Ba^{2+} < Cu^{2+} < Pb^{2+}$ ions (Grøndhal et al., 2010). Divalent cations preferentially bind to the G-block rather than the M-block (Goh et al., 2012). Alginates, which are rich in G-residues, generally form hard, brittle gels with high porosity, whereas M-rich samples form soft, elastic gels (Khotimchenko et al., 2001). The guluronate/mannuronate blocks of one polymer then form junctions with the guluronate/mannuronate blocks of adjacent polymer chains in what is termed the egg-box model of cross-linking (Gombotz and Wee, 1998), resulting in the gel structure shown in Figure 11.3.

Calcium chloride ($CaCl_2$) is one of the most frequently used agents to ionically cross-link alginate. However, it typically leads to rapid and poorly controlled gelation due to its high solubility in aqueous solutions. The gelation rate is a critical factor in controlling gel uniformity and strength when using divalent cations, and slower gelation produces more uniform structures and greater mechanical integrity (Kuo and Ma, 2001). The gelation temperature also influences the gelation rate and the resulting mechanical properties of the gels. At lower temperatures, the reactivity of ionic cross-linkers (e.g., Ca^{2+}) is reduced, and cross-linking becomes slower. The resulting cross-linked network structure is more ordered, leading to enhanced mechanical properties (Augst et al., 2006). In addi-tion, the mechanical properties of ionically cross-linked alginate gels can vary significantly depending on the chemical structure of the alginate. For example, gels prepared from alginate with a high content of G-residues exhibit higher stiffness than those with a low amount of G-residues (Drury et al., 2004). One critical drawback of ionically cross-linked alginate gels is their limited long-term stability under physiological conditions: the release of divalent ions into the surrounding media as a result of exchange reactions with monovalent cations can cause the gels to dissolve. The last-mentioned feature may be beneficial or detrimental, depending on the particular circumstances. In order to circumvent such biological reactions and more general limitations of ionically cross-linked gels, there is growing interest in covalently cross-linked alginate hydrogels.

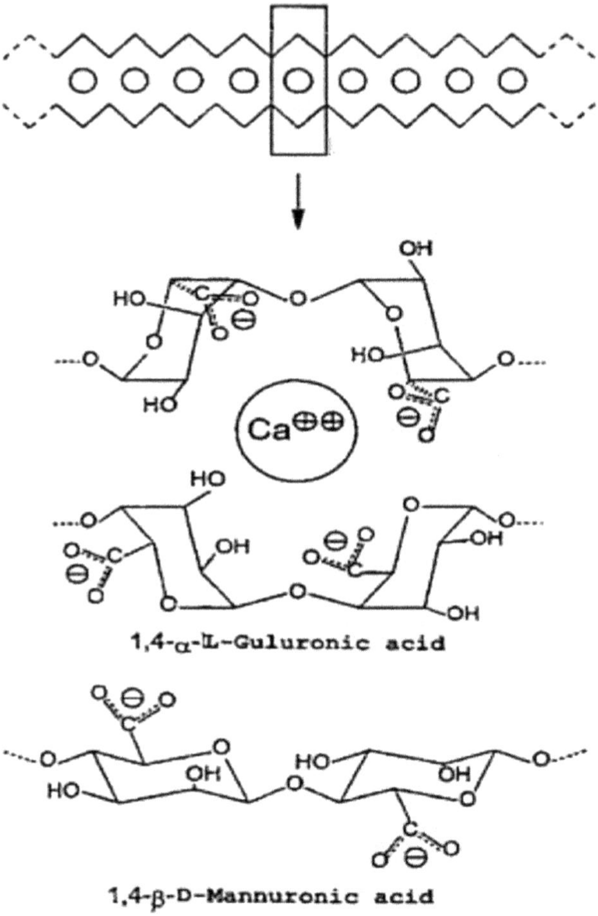

FIGURE 11.3 Schematic representation of an egg-box model showing the mechanism of the reaction between calcium ion and alginate that leads to gelation.

Source: Reprinted with permission from Gomes et al., 2014. © 2014 John Wiley.

In the case of beads prepared with alginate and cross-linked with Cu^{2+}, the ion is used both for gelation of the polymer and for its intrinsic antimicrobial activities against *Staphylococcus aureus, Escherichia coli, Pseudomonas aeruginosa, Enterococcus faecalis, Candida albicans*, and so forth. The spherical alginate beads prepared with this ion release sufficient Cu^{2+} for therapeutic purposes. After contact with an aqueous medium, the hydrophilic polymer starts to swell rapidly, adheres to the site of action (e.g., the vaginal mucosa) and Cu^{2+} ions are released from the polymer matrix through diffusion (Pavelková et al., 2016).

11.2.1.2 INTERPENETRATING POLYMER NETWORKS

Multicomponent networks known as IPNs have been designed to enhance the mechanical strength and swelling/deswelling response of single-network hydrogels that have weak mechanical properties and slow swelling response. IPNs are a combination of cross-linked polymers, at least one of them being synthesized and/or cross-linked within the immediate presence of the other, without any covalent bonds between them, and which cannot be separated unless the chemical bonds are broken (Myung et al., 2008). The combination of polymers must effectively produce an advanced multicomponent polymeric system, with a new profile of the desired activity (Lohani et al., 2014). Depending on the chemistry of preparation, IPN hydrogels can be classified as simultaneous or sequential. In the case of the former, the precursors of both networks are mixed and the two networks are synthesized at the same time by independent, noninterfering routes such as chain and stepwise polymerization (Kim et al., 2004a). In the latter case, the hydrogel is typically formed by the swelling of a single-network hydrogel in a solution containing a mixture of monomer, initiator, and activator, with or without a cross-linker. If a cross-linker is present, the outcome is a fully IPN hydrogel; in the absence of a cross-linker, a network having linear polymers embedded within the first network is formed (semi-IPN) (Chivukula et al., 2006; Hoare and Kohane, 2008) (Figure 11.4).

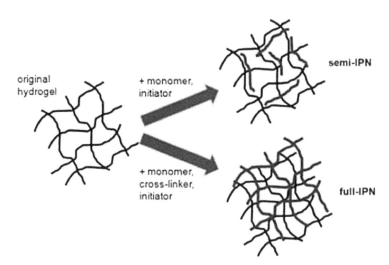

FIGURE 11.4 Formation and structure of semi- and fully interpenetrating polymer networks.

Source: Reprinted with permission from Hoare et al., 2008. © 2008 Elsevier.

The advantageous characteristics of sodium alginate (SA) have led to its wide use in the conditioning of fabrics, in foods and in various drug delivery systems. Several IPN composite hydrogels composed of SA and synthetic polymers containing carboxylic groups, with novel properties such as super porous (Yin et al., 2007), electrical sensitivity (Kim et al., 2004b), drug controlled release (Wang et al., 2009), and multi-responsive (Dumitriu et al., 2011), have been designed through physical interactions including solvent casting (Kulkarni et al., 2010a), freeze thawing (Martínez-Gómez et al., 2017), and chemical cross-linking methods such as free radical polymerization (Anwar et al., 2017). Super porous IPN composite hydrogels were prepared by Yin et al. through sequential cross-linking, by fast cross-linking polymerization of acrylamide and sodium acrylate in the presence of SA as entrapped polymer and sodium bicarbonate as blowing agent. $CaCl_2$ was applied to cross-link of the SA chains in semi-IPN gels. Owing to their high porosity, the IPN hydrogels thus prepared had fast swelling and a high swelling ratio, this being affected by the external pH and ionic strength. The IPN hydrogels had a high mechanical strength and a good biocompatibility.

Alginate-based IPNs have gained widespread appeal for industrial applications as actuators or muscle-like materials. In order to make such materials, polymer gels with fast electric response and a high mechanical strength were required. IPN composite hydrogels based on poly(methacrylic acid) and SA showed significant and rapid bending when subjected to an electric field in HCl solution (Kim et al., 2004b). Poly(N-isopropylacrylamide) (PNIPAAm) is one of the most widely studied thermoresponsive polymers and has a slow response rate to temperature changes. Synthesis of multi-responsive IPN composite hydrogels, based on SA and PNIPAAm, constitutes one of the strategies adopted by numerous research groups to increase the porosity of the gels and thus achieve gels with a faster response rate as required for drug release systems. The pH/temperature-sensitive release of indomethacin (IM) from semi-IPN hydrogel beads composed of Ca-alginate and previ-ously synthesized PNIPAAm has been reported by Shi et al. A drastic change in the drug release was achieved by alternating the pH of the buffer solution between 2 and 7. The drug release was higher at 37°C than at 25°C and showed that the Ca-alginate/PNIPAAm beads had potential as an effective pH/temperature responsive delivery system for bioactive agents. The pulsatile swelling/deswelling behavior of semi-IPN hydro-gels composed of cross-linked PNIPAAm and linear SA revealed that the process was repeatable by alternating both temperature and pH, their mechanical strength making them suitable for stimuli-responsive drug release systems (Zhang et al., 2005) (Figure 11.5).

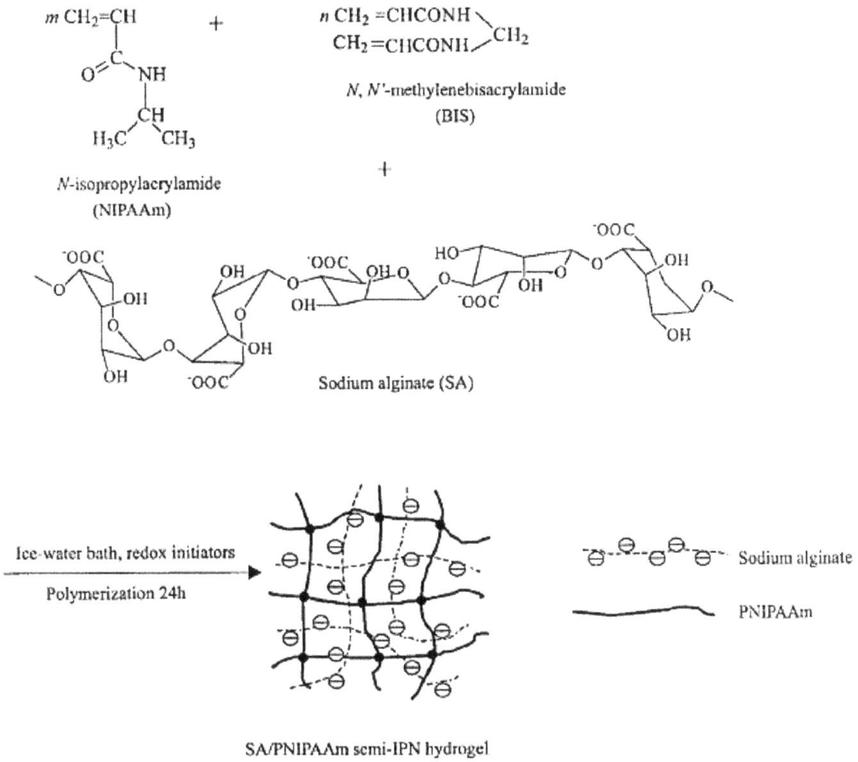

FIGURE 11.5   Synthesis scheme of SA/PNIPAAm semi-IPN hydrogel.

Source: Reprinted with permission from Zhang et al., 2005. © 2005 John Wiley.

11.2.2   CHEMICAL MODIFICATIONS

The chemical modification of alginate furnishes it with different functionalities, thus expanding the number of potential applications and improving its mechanical properties in delivery systems. Covalent modifications can be carried out mainly through cross-linking reactions or grafting reactions. This section details the main modification mechanisms as well as the most relevant applications of the materials obtained.

11.2.2.1 COVALENT CROSS-LINKING

The objective of alginate covalent cross-linking is an improvement in physical properties, making a material not easily influenced by environmental variables such as pH, ionic strength, temperature, and so forth (Lee and Mooney, 2012; Alvarez-Lorenzo et al., 2013).

In this context, one of the physical properties that are modified is the hydrogel's response to stress. The stress applied to an ionically cross-linked alginate gel relaxes as the cross-links dissociate and reform elsewhere, and water is lost from the gel, leading to plastic deformation. While water migration also occurs in covalently cross-linked gels, leading to stress relaxation, the inability to dissociate and reform bonds lead to significant elastic deformation (Isıklan and Kucukbalcı, 2012). Within the range of available cross-linking agents, glutaraldehyde (GA) is most commonly used to cross-link alginate. In this case, the reaction that occurs is between the hydroxyl groups of the polymer and aldehyde groups of GA (Figure 11.6) (Zhao et al., 2010). The advantage of using this cross-linker is that it leaves other functional polymer groups free to interact with other compounds or give rise to a certain physical response. Such is the case with alginate beads cross-linked with GA; they show a higher degree of swelling at pH 7.8 (Murat et al., 2008) than calcium cross-linked alginate, leaving the carboxylic acid moieties free for pH-responsiveness, whereas in the presence of calcium ions some carboxylic moieties cooperatively participate in the binding of the ions (Chan and Neufeld, 2010). In the first example, the formation of the SA beads is carried out by dropping aqueous sodium alginate into GA and HCl as a catalyst mixture solution. Beads prepared in this way were used to deliver a model nonsteroid, anti-inflammatory drug, indomethacin, IM. In this study, IM release from the beads was found to be much higher at high pH values than at low pH values and decreased with increasing exposure times to GA, the concentration of GA, drug/polymer ratio, and percentage of HCl.

Another example of GA utilization is in beads made with alginate mixed with other polymers (Sanlı et al., 2007). In this case, polymeric blend beads of polyvinyl alcohol (PVA)-g-PAAm and PVA with SA were prepared by cross-linking with GA and used to deliver a model anti-inflammatory drug, diclofenac sodium (DS). The advantage obtained from this combination is that blending of PVA with SA polymers leads to a decrease in the release rate of DS, whereas it increases the entrapment efficiency. It was also observed that release of DS is much higher at high pH values than at low pH values, suggesting that the release system is of interest as a controlled release system for colon-specific drug delivery. Further DS release from the beads increases with the increase in acrylamide grafting onto PVA, whereas it decreases with the increase in exposure time to GA, the concentration of GA, PVA/SA ratio, and drug/polymer ratio.

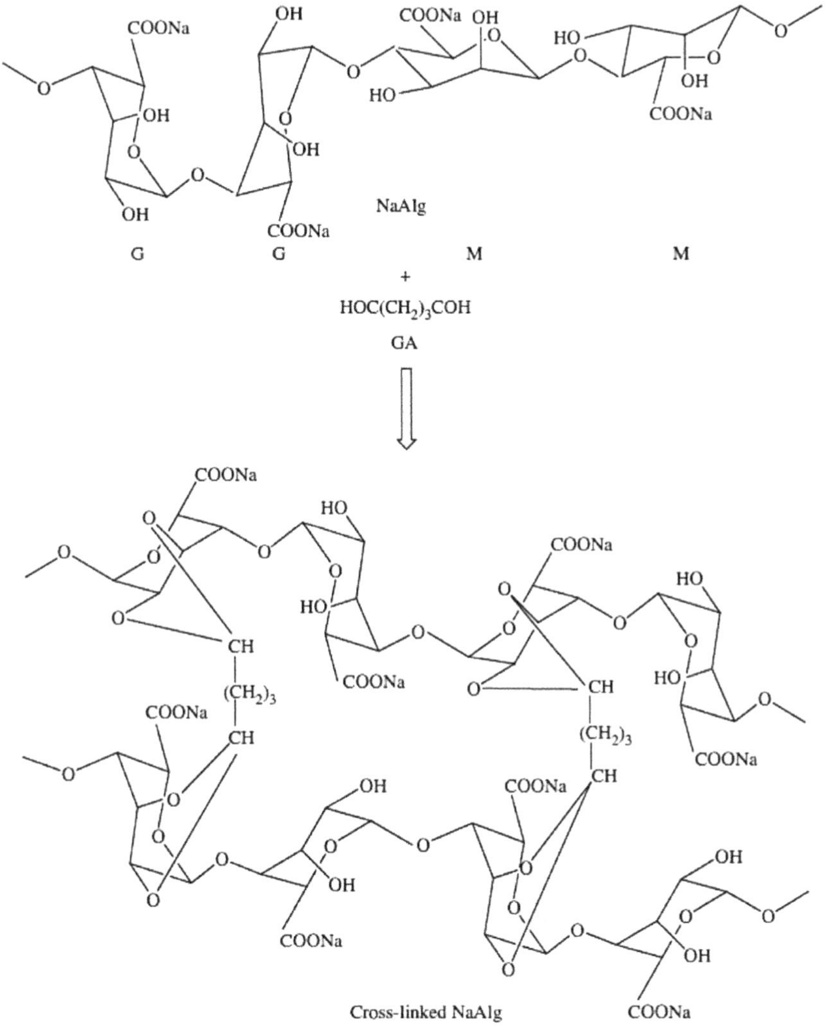

FIGURE 11.6   Postulated cross-linking reaction between sodium alginate (SA) and GA.

Source: Reprinted with permission from Işıklan and Küçükbalcı, 2012 © 2012 Elsevier.

The combination of ionic and chemical cross-linking through the prior formation of a hydrogel with alginate and calcium, forming a semisynthetic network alginate polymer has also been studied (Chan and Neufeld, 2010). This semisynthesis enables fine-tuned gel pore size through the use of kinetic and thermodynamic reaction control for tissue engineering application and a universal oral drug delivery vehicle for protein therapeutics such as insulin.

11.2.2.2   GRAFTING REACTIONS

Another type of alginate modification is through grafting reactions, which as mentioned earlier, provide alginate with improvements in its mechanical properties in drug delivery applications, adding different functionalities to produce materials with responses to changes in pH, luminous intensity, temperature, magnetically or electric fields.

A wide variety of methodologies are used, depending on the required response of the material to be obtained. Throughout the following paragraphs, we present the most commonly used reactions to produce the relevant modifications: reactions with carbodiimides, radical reactions, and oxidation reactions.

Reactions with carbodiimides are used to activate the alginate to then interact with another polymer which confers additional properties to those of alginate alone. For example, the addition of thiol groups to the alginate increases its interaction with the mucus layer through disulfide bridges improving its properties as a drug delivery carrier through this interaction (Davidovich-Pinhas et al., 2009). In this case, the alginate is conjugated with cysteine through 1-ethyl-3-(3-dimethylaminopropyl) carbodiimide hydrochloride, EDAC (Figure 11.7). In this scheme, it can be observed that alginate-thiol forms intermolecular disulfide interactions, as well as intramolecular interactions with mucin molecules.

Also of interest is the formation of amphiphilic derivatives of SA by covalent fixation of poly(ε-caprolactone) (PCL) pendant chains onto the polysaccharide backbone through ester links (Colinet et al., 2009a). These polymers exhibit viscometric properties markedly different from those of the parent polymer and resulting from intra and intermolecular hydrophobic associations. In this case, due to the differences in solubility between the two components, the reaction takes place in a heterogeneous medium (water/dichloromethane) between hydroxyl groups of PCL (dichloromethane soluble) and carboxylate groups of alginate (water soluble). Hydroxyl groups of PCL cannot easily react on carboxylate groups of alginate, which are, therefore "activated" by EDCI (Figure 11.8).

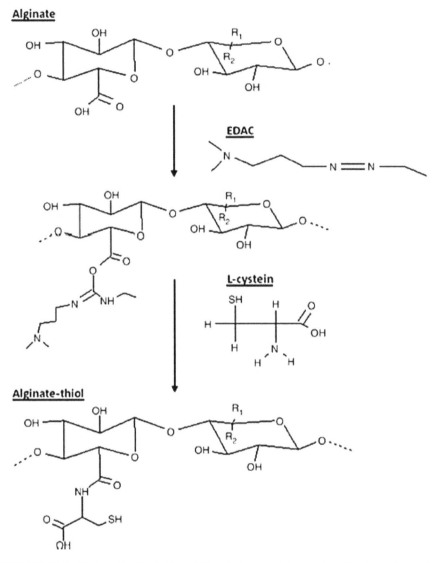

FIGURE 11.7 Schematic illustration of the alginate-cysteine conjugation through amide bond between the primary amino group of L-cysteine and carboxylic acid group of alginate mediated by EDAC.

Source: Reprinted with permission from Davidovich-Pinhas et al., 2009. © 2009 Elsevier.

This hydrogel, with characteristics such as pH-sensitivity, amphiphilicity, and biocompatibility based on alginate-g-PCL, was prepared for controlled delivery of poorly water-soluble drugs such as theophylline (TPH). This bioactive compound belongs to a class of medications called bronchodilators used in treating asthma and other airway diseases (Colinet et al., 2009b). Swelling profiles obtained indicate that these hydrogels swell slightly (10–14%) in a simulated gastric fluid (SGF) (pH 1.2) and strongly (700–1300% before disintegration) in a simulated intestinal fluid (SIF) (pH 6.8).

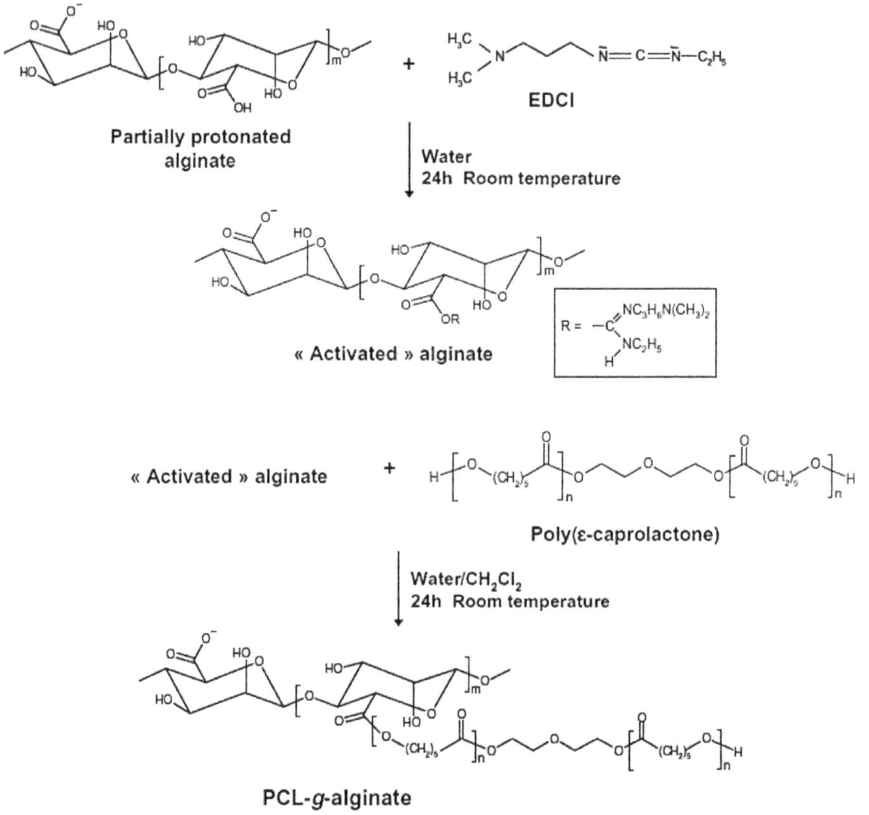

FIGURE 11.8   Synthesis of PCL-g-alginate.

Source: Reprinted with permission from Colinet et al., 2009a. © 2009 Elsevier.

With radical reactions, the first step of the reaction mechanism is the formation of a macroradical, as in the case of the reaction with ammonium peroxydisulfate (APS) (Abd El-Ghaffar et al., 2012). SA grafted with polyglycidyl methacrylate hydrogels (PGMA-g-SA) is prepared as a pH-sensitive drug delivery matrix for riboflavin (RF) delivery (Figure 11.9). It was observed that the in vitro release of RF from this formulation was superior to the others and the release was able to be maintained for ~3 and 4 days for SIF and SGF, respectively. In general, it has been shown that GMA grafted onto SA enhances drug entrapment efficiency and decreases the swelling and degradation behaviors of the carrier. It also slowed and controlled the release of RF from the PGMA-g-SA hydrogel compared with pure SA beads cross-linked with Ca^{2+} ions alone, thereby providing a simple and effective method of improving drug delivery systems.

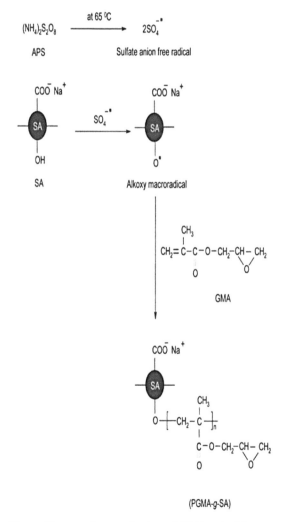

FIGURE 11.9   The grafting reaction mechanism of GMA onto SA.

Source: Reprinted with permission from El-Ghaffar et al., 2012. © 2012 Elsevier.

Another example of grafting mediated by APS is hydrolyzed polyacryl-amide-grafted SA (H-PAAm-g-SA) copolymer for pH-sensitive oral drug delivery application (Kulkarni et al., 2010b). This graft copolymer has the additional characteristic of an electrically responsive transdermal system: it possesses large numbers of ionizable-COO⁻ groups responsible for electrical sensitivity and large polymeric side chains that can entrap higher drug load-ings, both of importance in transdermal systems and implants. In this case, ketoprofen is used as a model nonsteroidal anti-inflammatory drug which acts in musculoskeletal and joint disorders such as ankylosing spondylitis, osteoarthritis, and rheumatoid arthritis.

A further type of radical initiator commonly used is azobisisobutyroni-trile (AIBN). An example of this is grafting SA with N-vinyl-2-pyrrolidone (Figure 11.10). The graft copolymers (SA-g-PVP) are prepared by the cross-linking method using GA as a cross-linker in the hydrochloric acid catalyst

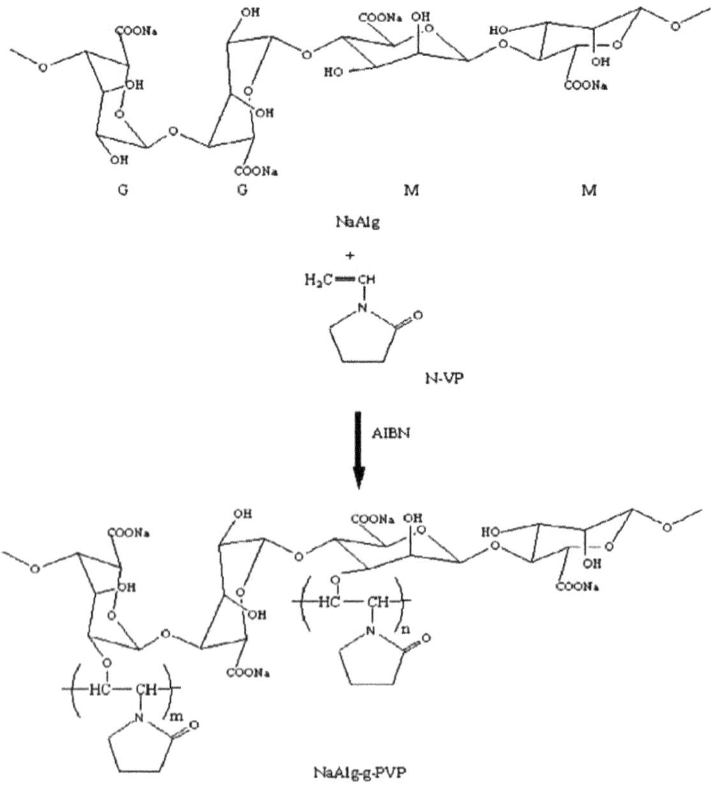

FIGURE 11.10   Postulated grafting reaction mechanism of SA with N-VP.

Source: Reprinted with permission from Isıklan et al., 2008. © 2008 John Wiley.

(HCl) and these beads are used to deliver the anti-inflammatory drug, IM. It is observed that release of IM is much higher at high pH values compared to low pH values, showing that the release system is of interest as a controlled release system for colon-specific drug delivery. Furthermore, IM release from the beads decreases with the increase in exposure time to GA, the concentration of GA, drug/polymer ratio and concentration of HCl.

IM has been also been entrapped in another structure built by graft copolymerization of SA with NIPAAm by microwave irradiation using CAN, CAN/TEMED or AIBN as radical initiators (Isıklan and Kucukbalcı, 2012). This graft copolymer has been used for the development of dual-stimuli responsive hydrogels especially for delivery vehicles that respond to localized conditions of pH and temperature in the human body. In this composition, PNIPAM is the thermal-responsive polymer because of its unique phase transition at a lower critical solution temperature in the water at around 32°C, which is close to the human body temperature.

In the oxidation reactions, the first step is the formation of oxidized SA (OSA). As an example of this type of reaction, we can mention oxidation with periodate to form OSA (Gao et al., 2009). In this case, graft copolymerization of amino group-terminated poly(2-dimethylamino) ethyl methacrylate (PDMAEMA-NH$_2$) onto OSA was reacted without using a catalyst through Schiff's base formation between aldehyde group in OSA and amino group in PDMAEMA-NH$_2$ (Figure 11.11).

The results showed that the oral delivery of proteins (Bovine serum albumin) can be controlled by adjusting the graft percentage (G, %), pH, and ionic strength.

11.3 NANOPARTICLES

A vast amount of literature is available today on the development and application of alginate macro and microparticles (Thakur and Singha, 2015; Valladares et al., 2016). As mentioned in numerous of these publications, interest in these biopolymers is due to their innumerable advantages for a variety of applications, largely in the pharmaceutical industry as carriers of controlled release. In parallel with these developments, there is also growing interest in learning more about the advantages that nanoscience offers in different areas of application, more specifically in nanomedicine (Martinelli and Strumia, 2017; Rimondino et al., 2017), opening up a new challenge little explored to date: obtaining nanoparticles of alginate. Achieving this goal would further enhance the already known advantages of this biopolymer for its use as a nanocarrier in specific therapies, such as cancer, arthritis, and so forth. It is therefore of great interest to optimize preparation methodologies to obtain nanoscale alginate particles much smaller than 200 nm.

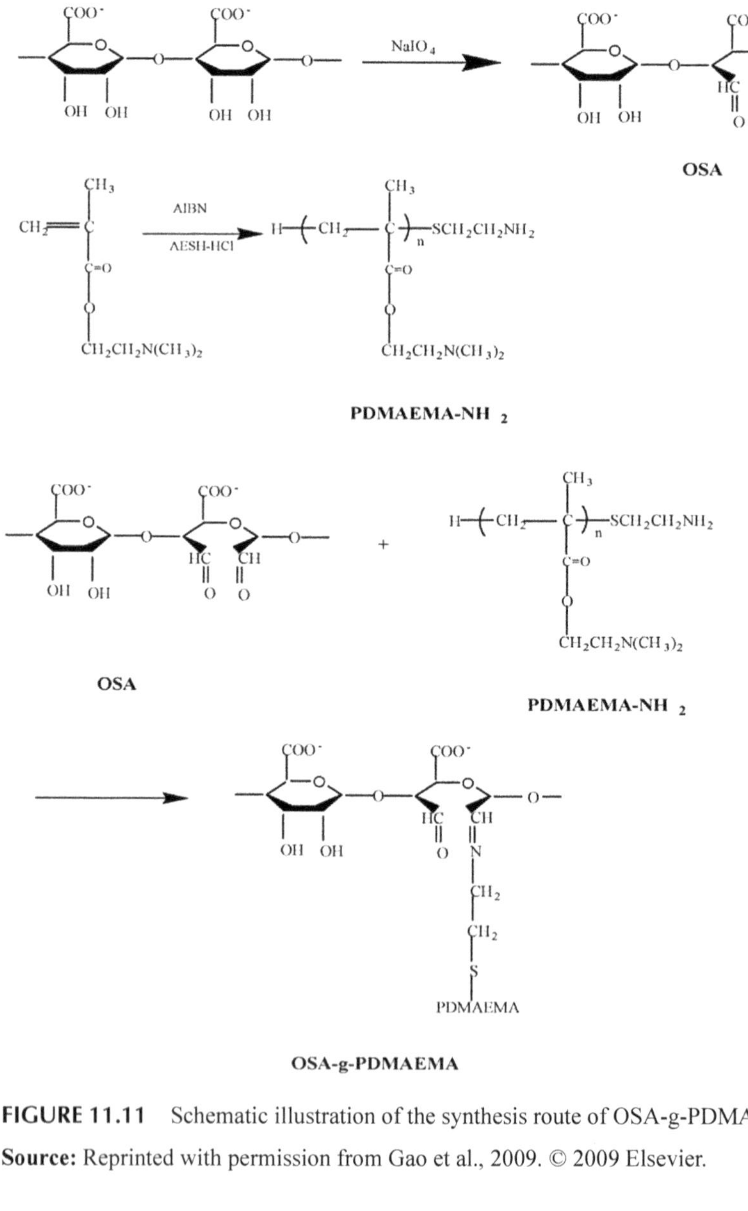

FIGURE 11.11 Schematic illustration of the synthesis route of OSA-g-PDMAEMA.

Source: Reprinted with permission from Gao et al., 2009. © 2009 Elsevier.

The uniquely advantageous properties of nanoscale size particles are obviously of fundamental importance to their enhanced application in medicine (Ficai and Grumezescu, 2017). The following are some of the already known advantages of nano with respect to macrosizes:

- Long-circulating characteristics with low immunogenicity
- Good biocompatibility and bioavailability, averting efflux transport
- Protection of the therapeutic cargo from enzymatic degradation
- Higher mechanical strength and larger specific surface area
- Easy flow through narrow nozzles and channels which would be blocked by larger particles
- Furthermore, the choice of polymer that forms part of the nanoparticle is decisive in achieving additional properties for enhanced application as nanocarriers such as:
- Ease of preparation and handling (for example,self-assembly)
- Easy incorporation of hydrophobic drugs
- High encapsulation efficiency (%) of hydrophobic drugs
- Easily sterilized
- Presence of a hydrophilic shell for preventing non-specific interactions with plasma proteins or uptake by reticuloendothelial system (inherited stealth property)
- Possibility of surface modification by determined ligands for specific and efficient targeting

It is therefore important to know which synthetic methodologies permit the formation of nanoparticles with good yields. The ease with which alginate forms gels indicates that the methodologies can be optimized to achieve nanosize gel particles. On the whole, such methodologies ensure that the formation of the gel particle occurs under strict control of the progress of the cross-linking conditions. In general, the most widely used methods for controlling size involve working with a low concentration of physical or covalent cross-linking agent and high shearing conditions (Paques et al., 2014).

Chemical cross-linked nanogels are usually obtained by inverse emulsion polymerization (Landfester, 2006; Moya-Ortega et al., 2012), precipitation polymerization (Cuggino et al., 2016) or inverse mini-emulsion (Oh et al., 2006), using some cross-linked reactions (covalent or physical) (Biglione et al., 2015) and also by liposomal template (Hong et al., 2008). Specifically, alginate nanogels are prepared in an aqueous solution by cross-linking alginate chains and contraions or other polymeric chains such

as chitosan (Yang et al., 2014) or polylysine, with oppositely charged polyelectrolyte, giving rise to nanoaggregates. Grafting reactions or chemical
modifications of the functional groups of alginate permit the introduction
of vinyl or methacrylic groups, enabling radical cross-linking as applied for
the production of nanogels.

It is possible to obtain different forms of nanoparticles (Mora-Huertas
et al., 2010) and the method of preparation determines whether nanoaggregates, nanocapsules, nanospheres, or nanocapsules with a structured interior
are obtained (Figure 11.12).

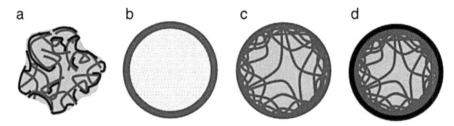

FIGURE 11.12   Schematic representation of a nanoaggregate (a), nanocapsule (b),
nanosphere with the structured interior (c) and nanocapsule with the structured interior (d).
The nanocapsule has an oily or aqueous liquid core surrounded by a shell and nanospheres
are spherical matrix systems. The nanocapsule with the structured interior is a combination of
a nanosphere and a nanocapsule.

Source: Reprinted with permission from Paques et al. 2014. © 2014 Elsevier.

Some authors have used their ingenuity to adapt classical methodologies
for obtaining macrogels to render nanoparticles. There are several examples
of obtaining nanoaggregates merely by combining chitosan or calcium
ions with a sodium alginate solution. The alginate and cationic polymer
concentration, their molecular weight, the calcium chloride concentration,
and the order of addition of calcium chloride and cationic polymer to the
sodium alginate solution were found to have a great impact on the size and
properties of the obtained nanoparticles. Some were studied in vitro for their
application as nanocarriers of different drug types and have shown promising
results (Amiri et al., 2017; Anirudhan et al., 2017).

Several examples of ingeniously adapted methodologies for obtaining
nanogels are given below. For example, Chang et al. (2012) developed
the synthesis of alginate nanoaggregates through self-assembly. These
authors did not require calcium-induced aggregation of alginate or cationic
polymers to form a polyelectrolyte complex with alginate; instead, they

synthesized amphiphilic thiolated SA and the oxidation reaction of the thiol groups facilitated by sonication-induced self-assembly of the alginate into nanoaggregates.

A different strategy to produce a controlled delivery device is layer-by-layer (LbL) microcapsule formation by a combination of alginate and chitosan. In this case, the chitosan/alginate multilayer microcapsules are fabricated by a template-assisted assembly in an LbL manner, followed by core removal (Zhao et al., 2006). The $CaCO_3$ (CMC) colloidal particles are incubated in chitosan/NaCl solution (pH 5.0–5.5) and the excess polysaccharides removed by washings with NaCl (pH 5.0–5.5) solution. The microparticles are then incubated in SA/NaCl solution (pH 5.0–5.5), followed by new washings. This deposition cycle is repeated for the desired number of layers to yield chitosan/alginate multilayers on the $CaCO_3$ (CMC) microparticles. The core–shell particles are subsequently cross-linked by 2% GA at room temperature for 12 h and the $CaCO_3$ particles finally dissolved in 0.2M disodium ethylenediamine tetraacetic acid solution. These capsules show a strong ability to spontaneously load the positively charged daunorubicin (DNR), as proved by quantitative analysis with Ultra–visible spectroscopy and qualitative analyses with confocal laser scanning microscopy and transmission electron microscopy. The accumulation of DNR from its solution can be hundreds of times higher than the feeding concentration. The encapsulated DNR can be released again, following a diffusion-controlled procedure at the initial stage. In vitro BEL-7402, culture confirms the efficacy of the encapsulated DNR on induction of cell apoptosis, as evidenced by phase contrast microscopy. Finally, the encapsulated DNR has been applied to treat tumors in BALB/c/nu mice, revealing greater efficacy at tumor inhibition than the same dosage of free DNR. Thermoresponsive polymer complex micelles were prepared by Yu et al. (2016) by electrostatic interaction between divalent cationic metal ions (Ba^{2+}, Zn^{2+}, Co^{2+}) and anionic SA previously grafted with NIPAM (SA-g-PNIPAM) in aqueous medium. The products showed regular nanosized spheres and morphology of the complex micelles with good polydispersity and with a cloud point temperature of M2+/SA-g-PNIPAM of 32.5°C. The drug-loading experiment using 5-fluorouracil indicated excellent drug entrapment and release ability based on the core-corona structure. The release rate of 5-FU was controlled by changing external conditions. These metal ion-induced micelles demonstrated promising properties for use as carriers of controlled drug release (Figure 11.13).

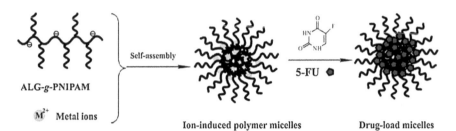

FIGURE 11.13 Schematic illustrations of metal ion-induced complex micelles for drug encapsulation.

Source: Reprinted with permission from Yu et al., 2016. © 2016 Elsevier.

Another important aim in nanomedicine is the synthesis of theranostic nanoparticles. These new nanosystems combine therapeutic and diagnostic capabilities in one platform and are considered a step forward in personalized medicine. They can be used for tracing the delivery of a drug to the targeted organ. Podgórna et al. (2017) have successfully synthesized 110-nm gadolinium alginate nanogels which show great potential for use in theranostic applications. They prepared gadolinium alginate gel nanoparticles (gadolinumnanogels–GdNG) by the reverse microemulsion and physical cross-linking method. The surface of the nanogel particles was modified by the LbL technique using bio-polyelectrolytes such as chitosan as the polycation and alginate as the polyanion. The cytotoxicity and encapsulation model developed by these authors involving a fluorescent dye shows promising theranostic properties for application in nanomedicine.

SUMMARY

Alginate is a biopolymer of anionic nature with numerous applications as a biomaterial and in biomedical science owing to its advantageous properties, the main ones being biocompatibility, biodegradability, low toxicity, and ease of gelation. To date, alginate polymers and derivatives have had particular attraction in wound healing, drug delivery, and tissue engineering applications. It is known that drug molecules, from small chemical drugs to macromolecular proteins, can be released from alginate gels in a controlled manner, depending on the specific characteristics of the network. In order to understand how alginates can be optimized as a useful delivery system for therapeutic applications, however, it is necessary to know more about the various factors affecting drug release from alginate matrices, such as network porosity, pH effect, composition, and modification of the functional groups in alginates; these can then be controlled through their structure/ property relationships, which closely dependent on the type of cross-linker and cross-linking methods. Several synthetic strategies have been employed to improve the behavior of alginates, including covalent and non-covalent bonds. In this chapter, we present the different methodologies for the forma- tion of networks: ionic interaction, covalent cross-linking, grafting reac- tions, interpenetrating and semi-IPNs and amphiphilic structures formed by association or conjugation. In each case, we show their advantages and main applications deriving from the synthetic pathway employed. In summary, this chapter provides a comprehensive overview of synthetic ways to improve the physical-chemical properties of alginate hydrogels in relation to their biomedical applications as alginate carriers in delivery systems. Lastly, we present the advantages and preparation of alginate nanogels and their potential application in nanomedicine.

KEYWORDS

- alginate
- physical networks
- ionic crosslinkig
- chemical modifications
- nanoparticles

REFERENCES

Abd El-Ghaffar, M. A.; Hashem, M. S.; El-Awady, M. K.; Rabie, A. M. pH-Sensitive Sodium Alginate Hydrogels for Riboflavin Controlled Release. *Carbohydr. Polym.* **2012,** *89,* 667–675.

Agüero, L.; Zaldivar-Silva, D.; Peña, L.; Dias, M. L. Alginate Microparticles as Oral Colon Drug Delivery Device: A Review. *Carbohydr. Polym.* **2017,** *168,* 32–43.

Alvarez-Lorenzo, C.; Blanco-Fernandez, B.; Puga, A. M.; Concheiro, A. Crosslinked Ionic Polysaccharides for Stimuli-Sensitive Drug Delivery. *Adv. Drug. Delivery Rev.* **2013,** *65,* 1148–1171.

Amiri, M.; Salavati-Niasari, M.; Pardakhty, A.; Ahmadi, M.; Akbari, A. Caffeine: A Novel Green Precursor for Synthesis of Magnetic $CoFe_2O_4$ Nanoparticles and pH-Sensitive Magnetic Alginate Beads for Drug Delivery. *Mater. Sci. Eng. C* **2017,** *76,* 1085–1093.

Anirudhan, T. S.; Anila, M. M.; Franklin, S. Synthesis Characterization and Biological Evaluation of Alginate Nanoparticle for the Targeted Delivery of Curcumin. *Mater. Sci. Eng. C* **2017**, *78*, 1125–1134.

Anwar, H.; Ahmad, M.; Minhas, U. M.; Rehmani, S. Alginate-Polyvinyl Alcohol Based Interpenetrating Polymer Network for Prolonged Drug Therapy, Optimization and in-Vitro Characterization. *Carbohydr. Polym.* **2017**, *166*, 183–194.

Augst, A. D.; Kong, H. J.; Mooney, D. J. Alginate Hydrogels as Biomaterials. *Macromol. Biosci.* **2006**, *6*, 623–633.

Bajpai, A. K.; Shukla, S. K.; Bhanu, S.; Kankane, S. Responsive Polymers in Controlled Drug Delivery. *Prog. Polym. Sci.* **2008**, *33*, 1088–1118.

Bierbrauer, K. L.; Alasino, R. V.; Strumia, M. C.; Beltramo, D. M. Cationic Cellulose and its Interaction with Chondroitin Sulfate. Rheological Properties of the Polyelectrolyte Complex. *Eur. Polym. J.* **2014**, *50*, 142–149.

Biglione, C.; Sousa-Herves, A.; Menger, M.; Wedepohl, S.; Calderon, M.; Strumia M. C. Facile Ultrasonication Approach for the Efficient Synthesis of Ethylene Glycol-Based Thermos Responsive Nanogels. *RSC Adv.* **2015**, *5*, 15407.

Caetano, L. A.; Almeida, A. J.; Gonçalves, L. M. D. Effect of Experimental Parameters on Alginate/Chitosan Microparticles for BCG Encapsulation *Mar. Drugs.* **2016**, *14*(5), 90.

Cardoso, M. J.; Costa, R. R.; Mano, J. F. Marine Origin Polysaccharides in Drug Delivery Systems. *Mar. Drugs* **2016**, *14*, 34.

Chan, A. W.; Neufeld, R. J. Tuneable Semi-Synthetic Network Alginate for Absorptive Encapsulation and Controlled Release of Protein Therapeutics. *Biomaterials* **2010**, *31*, 9040–9047.

Chang, D.; Lei, J.; Cui, H.; Lu, N.; Sun, Y.; Zhang, X. Disulfide Cross-Linked Nanospheres from Sodium Alginate Derivative for Inflammatory Bowel Disease: Preparation, Characterization, and in Vitro Drug Release Behavior. *Carbohydr. Polym.* **2012**, *88*, 663–669.

Chivukula, P.; Dusek, K.; Wang, D.; Duskova-Smrckova, M.; Kopeckova P.; Kopecek J. *Biomaterials* **2006**, *27*, 1140.

Colinet, I.; Dulong, V.; Hamaide, T.; Le Cerf, D.; Picton, L. New Amphiphilic Modified Polysaccharides with Original Solution Behavior in Salt Media. *Carbohydr. Polym.* **2009a**, *75*, 454–462.

Colinet, V.; Dulong, G.; Mocanu, L.; Picton, D.; Le Cerf, D. New Amphiphilic and pH-Sensitive Hydrogel for Controlled Release of a Model Poorly Water-Soluble Drug. *Eur. J. Pharm. Biopharm.* **2009b**, *73*, 345–350.

Cuggino, J. C.; Molina, M.; Wedepohl, S.; Alvarez Igarzabal, C. I.; Calderón M.; Gugliotta, L. M. Responsive Nanogels for Application as Smart Carriers in Endocytic pH-Triggered Drug Delivery Systems. *Eur. Polym. J.* **2016**, *78*, 14–24.

Davidovich-Pinhas, M.; Harari, O.; Bianco-Peled, H. Evaluating the Mucoadhesive Properties of Drug Delivery Systems Based on Hydrated Thiolated Alginate. *J. Controlled Release* **2009**, *136*, 38–44.

Dragan, E. S. Design and Applications of Interpenetrating Polymer Network Hydrogels. A Review. *Chem. Eng. J.* **2014**, *243*, 572–590.

Drury, J. L.; Dennis, R. G.; Mooney, D. J. The Tensile Properties of Alginate Hydrogels. *Biomaterials* **2004**, *25*, 3187–3199.

Dumitriu, R. P.; Mitchell, G. R.; Vasile, C. Multi-Responsive Hydrogels Based on Nisopropylacrylamide and Sodium Alginate. *Polym. Int.* **2011**, *60*, 222–233.

Ficai, D.; Grumezescu A. M. *Nanostructures for Novel Therapy: Synthesis, Characterization and Applications,* 1st ed.; Elsevier: Amsterdam, 2017.

Gao, C.; Liu, M.; Chen, S.; Jin, S.; Chen, J. Preparation of Oxidized Sodium Alginate-Graft-Poly((2-Dimethylamino) Ethyl Methacrylate) Gel Beads and in Vitro Controlled Release Behavior of BSA. *Int. J. Pharm.* **2009,** *371,* 16–24.

George, M.; Abraham, T. E. Polyionic Hydrocolloids for the Intestinal Delivery of Protein Drugs. *J. Controlled Release.* **2006,** *114,* 1–14.

Goh, C. H.; Heng, P. W. S.; Chan, L. W. Alginates as a Useful Natural Polymer for Microencapsulation and Therapeutic Applications. *Carbohydr. Polym.* **2012,** *88*(1), 1–12.

Gombotz, W. R.; Wee, S. F. Protein Release from Alginate Matrices. *Adv. Drug. Delivery Rev.* **1998,** *31*(3), 267–285.

Gomes, A. P.; Mano, J. F.; Queiroz, J. A.; Gouveia, I. C. New Biomaterial Based on Cotton with Incorporated Biomolecules. *J. Appl. Polym. Sci.* **2014,** *131,* 40519.

Grøndhal, L.; Lawrie, G.; Jejurikar, A. Alginate-Based Drug Delivery Devices. In *Biointegration of Medical Implant Materials: Science and Design;* Sharma, C. P., Ed.; Woodhead Publishing Limited: Cambridge, 2010; Vol. 1, p 239.

Hoare, T. R.; Kohane, D. S. Hydrogels in Drug Delivery: Progress and Challenges. *Polymer* **2008,** *49*(8), 1993–2007.

Hoffman, A. S. Hydrogels for Biomedical Applications. *Adv. Drug Delivery Rev.* **2002,** *54,* 3–12.

Hong, J. S.; Vreeland, W. N.; DePaoli Lacerda, S. H.; Locascio, L. E.; Gaitan, M.; Raghavan, S. R. Liposome-Templated Supramolecular Assembly of Responsive Alginate Nanogels. *Langmuir* **2008,** *24,* 4092–4096.

Işıklan, N.; Kucukbalcı, G. Microwave-Induced Synthesis of Alginate–Graft-Poly(*N*-Isopropylacrylamide) and Drug Release Properties of Dual pH- and Temperature-Responsive Beads. *Eur. J. Pharm. Biopharm.* **2012,** *82,* 316–331.

Işıklan, N.; Inal, M.; Yiğitoğlu, M. Synthesis and Characterization of Poly (*N*-Vinyl-2-Pyrrolidone) Grafted Sodium Alginate Hydrogel Beads for the Controlled Release of Indomethacin. *J. App. Polym. Sci.* **2008,** *110,* 481–493.

Khotimchenko, Y. S.; Kovalev, V. V.; Savchenko, O. V.; Ziganshina, O. A. Physical-Chemical Properties, Physiological Activity, and Usage of Alginates, the Polysaccharides of Brown Algae. *Russ. J. Mar. Biol.* **2001,** *27*(1), 853–864.

Kim, S. J.; Yoon, S. G.; Lee, Y. H.; Kim, S. I. Bending Behavior of Hydrogels Composed of Poly(Methacrylic Acid) and Alginate by Electrical Stimulus. *Polym. Int.* **2004a,** *53,* 1456–1460.

Kim, S. J.; Yoon, S. G.; Lee, S. M.; Kim S. I. Electrical Sensitivity Behavior of a Hydrogel Composed of Polymethacrylic Acid/Poly(Vinyl Alcohol). *J. App. Polym. Sci.* **2004b,** *91*(6), 3613–3617.

Kulkarni, R. V.; Sreedhar, V.; Mutalik, S.; Setty, C. M.; Sa, B. Interpenetrating Network Hydrogel Membranes of Sodium Alginate and Poly (Vinyl Alcohol) for Controlled Release of Prazosin Hydrochloride Through Skin. *Int. J. Biol. Macromol.* **2010a,** *47,* 520–527.

Kulkarni, R. V.; Setty, C. M.; Sa, B. Polyacrylamide-g-Alginate Based Electrically Responsive Hydrogel for Drug Delivery Application: Synthesis, Characterization, and Formulation Development. *J. App. Polym. Sci.* **2010b,** *115,* 1180–1188.

Kuo, C. K., Ma, P. X. Ionically Crosslinked Alginate Hydrogels as Scaffolds for Tissue Engineering. Biomaterials **2001,** *22,* 511–521.

Landfester, K. Synthesis of Colloidal Particles in Miniemulsions. *Annu. Rev. Mater. Res.* **2006,** *36*(1), 231–279.

Larsen, B. E.; Bjørnstad, J.; Pettersen, E. O.; Tønnesen, H. H.; Melvik, J. E. Rheological Characterization of an Injectable Alginate Gel System. *BMC Biotechnol.* **2015,** *15,* 29.

Lee, K. Y.; Mooney, D. J. Alginate: Properties and Biomedical Applications. *Prog. Polym. Sci.* **2012,** *37,* 106–126.

LeRoux, M. A.; Guilak, F.; Setton, L. A. Compressive and Shear Properties of Alginate Gel: Effects of Sodium Ions and Alginate Concentration. *J. Biomed. Mater. Res.* **1999,** *47,* 46–53.

Lohani, A.; Singh, G.; Bhattacharya, S. S.; Verma, A. Interpenetrating Polymer Networks as Innovative Drug Delivery Systems. *J. Drug Delivery* **2014,** *2014,* e583612.

Martinelli, M.; Strumia, M. C. Multifunctional Nanomaterials: Design, Synthesis and Application Properties. *Molecules* **2017,** *22,* 243.

Martínez-Gómez, F.; Guerrero, J.; Matsuhiro, B.; Pavez, J. In Vitro Release of Metformin Hydrochloride from Sodium Alginate/Polyvinyl Alcohol Hydrogels. *Carbohydr. Polym.* **2017,** *155,* 182–191.

Mora-Huertas, C. E.; Fessi, H.; Elaissari, A. Polymer-Based Nanocapsules for Drug Delivery. *Int. J. Pharm.* **2010,** *385*(1), 13–42.

Moya-Ortega, M. D; Alvarez-Lorenzo, C.; Concheiro, A.; Loftsson, T. Cyclodextrin-Based Nanogels for Pharmaceutical and Biomedical Applications. *Int. J. Pharm.* **2012,** *428*(1–2), 152–163.

Murat, I.; Yiğitoğlu, M.; Işiklan, N. Controlled Release of Indomethacin from Crosslinked Alginate Beads. *E-Polymers* **2008,** *8,* 17.

Myung, D.; Waters, D.; Wiseman, M. Progress in the Development of Interpenetrating Polymer Network Hydrogels. *Polym. Adv. Technol.* **2008,** *19,* 647–657.

Oh, J. K.; Drumright, R.; Siegwart, D. J.; Matyjaszewski, K. The Development of Microgels/Nanogels for Drug Delivery Applications. *Prog. Polym. Sci.* **2006,** *33*(4), 448–477.

Paques, J. P.; van der Linden, E.; van Rijn, C. J. M.; Sagis, L. M. C. Preparation Methods of Alginate Nanoparticles. *Adv. Colloid Interface Sci.* **2014,** *209,* 163–171.

Pavelková, M.; Kubová, K.; Vysloužil, J.; Kejdušová, M.; Vetchý, D.; Celer, V.; Molinková, D.; Lobová, D.; Pechová, A.; Vysloužil, J.; Kulich P. Biological Effects of Drug-Free Alginate Beads Cross-Linked by Copper Ions Prepared Using External Ionotropic Gelation. *AAPS PharmSciTech.* **2016,** *18*(4), 1343–1354.

Peak, C. W.; Wilker, J. J.; Schmidt, G. A Review on Tough and Sticky Hydrogels. *Colloid Polym. Sci.* **2013,** *291,* 2031–2047.

Peng, H. T.; Martineau, L.; Shek, L. P. N. Hydrogel–Elastomer Composite Biomaterials: 3. Effects of Gelatin Molecular Weight and Type on the Preparation and Physical Properties of Interpenetrating Polymer Networks. *J. Mater. Sci. Mater. Med.* **2008,** *19,* 997–1007.

Peppas, N. A.; Bures, P.; Leobandung, W.; Ichikawa, H. Hydrogels in Pharmaceutical Formulations. *Eur. J. Pharm. Biopharm.* **2000,** *50,* 27–46.

Podgórna, K.; Szczepanowicz, K.; Piotrowski, M.; Gajdošová, M.; Štěpánek, F.; Warszyński, P. Gadolinium Alginate Nanogels for Theranostic Applications. *Colloids Surf. B* **2017,***153,* 183–189.

Ratner, B. D.; Bryant S. J. Biomaterials: Where We have been and Where We are Going? *Ann. Rev. Biomed. Eng.* **2004,** *6,* 41–75.

Richter, A.; Paschew, G.; Klatt, S.; Lienig, J.; Arndt, K. F.; Adler, H. J. P. Review on Hydrogel-Based pH Sensors and Microsensors. *Sensors* **2008,** *8,* 561–581.

Rimondino, G. N.; Oksdath, G.; Brunetti, V.; Strumia, M. C. More than Just Size: Challenges and Opportunities of Hybrid Dendritic Nanocarriers. *Curr. Pharm. Des.* **2017,** *23*(21), 3142–3153.

Rinaudo, M. Main Properties and Current Applications of some Polysaccharides as Biomaterials. *Polym. Int.* **2008,** *57,* 397–430.

Sanlı, O.; Ay, N.; Isıklan, N. Release Characteristics of Diclofenac Sodium from Poly(Vinyl Alcohol)/Sodium Alginate and Poly(Vinyl Alcohol)-Grafted-Poly(Acrylamide)/Sodium Alginate Blend Beads. *Eur. J. Pharm. Biopharm.* **2007,** *65,* 204–214.

Thakur, V. K.; Singha, A. S. *Surface Modification of Biopolymers;* Wiley: New York, 2015.

Wu, J., Kong, T., Yeung, K. W., Shum, H. C., Cheung, K. M., Wang, L., To, M. K. *Acta Biomate.* **2013,** *9,* 7410–7419.

Valladares, G. A.; Gonzalez Audino P.; Strumia M. C. Preparation and Evaluation of Alginate/ Chitosan Microspheres Containing Pheromones for Pest Control of *Megaplatypus mutatus* (Platypodinae: Platypodidae). *Polym. Int.* **2016,** *65*(2), 216–223.

Wang, Q.; Li, S.; Wang, Z.; Li, C. Preparation and Characterization of a Positive Thermoresponsive Hydrogel for Drug Loading and Release. *J. Appl. Polym. Sci.* **2009,** *111*(3), 1417–1425.

Williams, D. F. On the Nature of Biomaterials. *Biomaterials* **2009,** *30,* 5897–5909.

Yang, X.; Sun, Y.; Kootala, S.; Hilborn, J.; Heerschap, A.; Ossipov, D. Injectable Hyaluronic Acid Hydrogel for 19F Magnetic Resonance Imaging. *Carbohydr. Polym.* **2014,** *101,* 95–99.

Yin, L.; Fei, L.; Cui, F.; Tang, C.; Yin, C. Synthesis, Characterization, Mechanical Properties and Biocompatibility of Interpenetrating Polymer Network Superporous Hydrogel Containing Sodium Alginate. *Polym. Int.* **2007,** *56,* 1563–1571.

Yu, N.; Li, G.; Gao, Y.; Jiang, H.; Tao, Q. Thermo-Sensitive Complex Micelles from Sodium Alginate-Graft-Poly(N-Isopropylacrylamide) for Drug Release. *Int. J. Biol. Macrom.* **2016,** *86,* 296–301.

Zhang, G. Q.; Zha, L. S.; Zhou, M. H.; Ma, J. H.; Liang, B. R. Preparation and Characterization of pH- and Temperature Responsive Semi-Interpenetrating Polymer Network Hydrogels Based on Linear Sodium Alginate and Crosslinked Poly(N-Isopropylacrylamide). *J. Appl. Polym. Sci.* **2005,** *97,* 1931–1940.

Zhao, Q.; Mao, Z.; Gao C.; Shen, J. Assembly of Multilayer Microcapsules on $CaCO_3$ Particles from Biocompatible Polysaccharides. *J. Biomater. Sci. Polym.* **2006,** *17*(9), 997–1014.

Zhao, X.; Huebsch, N.; Mooney, D. J.; Suo, Z. Stress-Relaxation Behavior in Gels with Ionic and Covalent Crosslinks. *J. Appl. Phys.* **2010,** *107,* 063509, 1–5.

CHAPTER 12

UPDATES ON ALGINATE-BASED INTERPENETRATING POLYMER NETWORKS FOR SUSTAINED DRUG RELEASE

IBRAHIM M. EL-SHERBINY[1,*] and KHOLOUD ARAFA[2]

Center for Materials Science, University of Science and Technology (UST), Zewail City of Science and Technology, 6th of October City, Giza, Egypt

Center for Aging and Associated Disease (CAAD), Zewail City of Science and Technology, 6th of October, Giza, Egypt

Corresponding author. E-mail: ielsherbiny@zewailcity.edu.eg

12.1 INTRODUCTION

Controlled drug release technology emerged during the 1980s as a commercial approach to expand the available possibilities of administering pharmaceutical therapies. Considerable attention in drug delivery field has been paid to adding novel dimensions to the development and application of the controlled release drug delivery systems (CDDSs). CDDSs have proved to be superior at different aspects over conventional immediate release dosage forms including lower risk of dose dumping and side effects, decreased dosing frequency, improved bioavailability, and better patient compliance (du Toit et al., 2016; Liu et al., 2007). Various approaches have been attempted to monitor and sustain the release of drugs through the utilization of suitable biocompatible carriers, where drugs are either dispersed or incorporated into inert matrices. Various natural, semi-synthetic, and synthetic biocompatible biopolymers have been extensively employed in the designing of polymer-based carriers for the prolonged release of different drugs. Among innumerable biopolymers available, natural polymers, including the widely used sodium alginate polymer, are being preferred in designing of CDDS because they are nontoxic, biodegradable, freely available, eco-friendly, and inexpensive (Lohani et al., 2014). However, natural polymers still exhibit some processing limitations that need to be addressed. Overcoming these limitations can be achieved through various chemical modifications like cross-linking, polymer grafting, carboxymethylation, cyanomethylation, thiolation, esterification, polyelectrolyte complexation, or incorporation into interpenetrating polymer networks (IPNs) (Nayak and Pal, 2015). IPNs are formed by two different polymer networks that are cross-linked conferring versatility in terms of properties and performances. In lights of the above discussion, the present chapter deals with a comprehensive description and discussion of various IPNs made of alginate, a nontoxic natural polysaccharide, and its derivatives for use in sustained drug release applications.

12.2   INTERPENETRATING POLYMER NETWORKS (IPNS)

The concept of IPN dates back as far as 1914 and the first IPN was invented by Aylsworth, and the term IPN was firstly coined by Miller in 1960s in a scientific study about polystyrene network. An IPN may be defined as any material which contains two or more polymers concatenated in the network form. The IUPAC definition of IPN is: "A polymer comprising two or more networks, which are at least partially interlocked on a molecular scale, but not covalently bonded to each other and cannot be separated unless chemical bonds are broken. A mixture of two or more preformed polymer networks is not an IPN" (Work et al., 2004). If only one component of the assembly is cross-linked leaving the other in a linear form, the system is referred to as a semi-IPN. The following conditions should be existing during the fabrication of IPNs for a successful process (Margaret et al., 2013; Somya et al., 2015):

- At least two polymers must be synthesized and cross-linked in the immediate presence of each other.
- Both polymers need to have similar kinetics.
- Phase separation between polymers should not be drastic.
- An IPN is distinctive from other polymer blends in a couple of ways (Kudela, 1987; Lohani et al., 2014):
- IPNs swell without dissolution in the solvent.
- They prevent the action of creep and flow.

IPNs can be distinguished from other multiple polymeric systems through their bicontinuous structure ideally formed by cross-linking of two polymers that are in intimate contact but without any chemical contact and yield a material with improved properties depending on their composition and degree of cross-linking. Adopting this perspective specifically, IPNs can be generally named as "polymer alloys" (Work et al., 2004).

As previously mentioned, IPNs are not prepared by merely mixing the two or more polymers and are also not produced from copolymers. IPNs-based drug delivery system (DDS) may follow zero-order pattern with lesser degree of fluctuation (Jain et al., 2011). IPNs are regarded as novel biomaterials. A combination of polymers, that is, synthetic and natural polymers, is useful in developing sustained release DDSs of short half-lived drug under physiological condition. As IPNs possess more complicated network structures and improved mechanical properties, the extent of cross-linking can be manipulated for preparing microsphere for controlled drug delivery. The chemical and physical combination methods as well as properties of multi-polymers are the key determinants controlling the release rate of the drug that can be monitored by tailoring the final IPNs properties to meet specific needs. Among these methods, IPNs-based DDSs are one of the newly developed methods for designing novel CDDS.

12.3 POLYMERS USED IN PREPARATION OF IPNS

A diverse arsenal of polymers or their precursors has been deployed to synthesize IPNs as apparent in Figure 12.1. A plausible categorization relays on the source to which polymers belong. Thus, IPNs constituting polymers can be classified into either natural polymers and their derivatives (particularly, polysaccharides and proteins) or synthetic polymers.

Natural polymers are considered favorable model for scientists to work with due to their innate biocompatibility. In addition, the versatility of chemical structures allows the development of advanced functionalized materials for biomedical applications including drug delivery. In the biomedical field, the degradation of natural polymers into physiological metabolites makes them potential biomaterials. The most commonly used natural polymers in the application of pharmaceutical DDS include chitosan and alginate among others in combination with either natural origin or synthetic polymers (Karan et al., 2016).

Second are the synthetic polymers where the edge of which is the spontaneous ability to devise the polymers' properties according to the desired specifications with high degree of reproducibility. In the following sections, we aim at shedding the light on the alginate-based IPNs that are fabricated to ensure the controlled release of the pharmacological moieties.

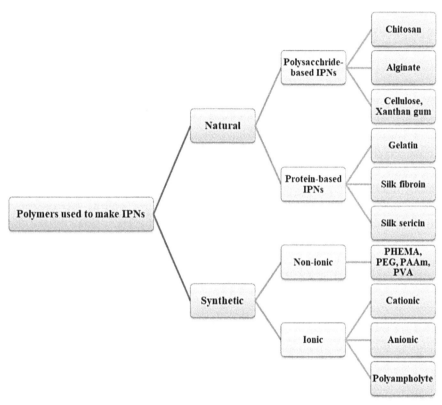

FIGURE 12.1   A schematic illustration of polymers used to synthesize interpenetrating polymer networks (IPNs).

12.4   USE OF ALGINATE-BASED IPNS IN CONTROLLED RELEASE DRUG DELIVERY SYSTEMS

Given the unique traits IPNs inherent to its composition, a duel control over its physicochemical properties can be practiced, an advantage nominating IPNs to be employed for diverse purposes. The pertinent role of polymers in progressing drug delivery technologies to great heights is evident due to their potential to provide controlled bioactive release, either as sustained levels over prolonged periods, pulsatile or cyclic dosage, or tunable release, of both hydrophilic and hydrophobic drugs. Innovative DDS design now focuses on tailor-made polymer networks for explicit drug loads, with stimulus-responsive mechanisms for more patient-specific care. The design of a truly intelligent polymeric network for controlled drug delivery should ultimately achieve definitive targeting, intracellular transport, and biocompatibility, with integration of responsive components and feedback control recognition.

The aim of the increasingly intricate design of controlled release polymeric systems is the enhancement of drug therapy. The rationale for developing controlled release systems is manifold, dependent partly on the incorporated drug, and includes (du Toit et al., 2016):

- Controlling temporal drug exposure
- Enhancing drug permeability through various physiological barriers
- Hindering premature drug elimination
- Targeting drug specifically to the desired site of action
- Boosting patient compliance through reduction in administration frequency
- Reducing drug release inconsistency and dose dumping

Recently, biodegradable polymers deemed attractive as biomaterials particularly, for tissue engineering, gene therapy, wound healing, and controlled DDSs. The most important advantage of biodegradable polymers is the disappearance of xeno-materials from the body as a result of their biodegradation, lowering the probability of toxicity as a side effect.

Conventionally, alginate-based DDSs belong to the biodegradable class of polymeric networks (Figure 12.2). Another property accounting for the favorability of alginates is the relative ease with which they can undergo gelation via forming a reticulate structure with divalent cations under the very mild conditions suitable for biomacromolecules and living cells (Dragan, 2014). However, alginate-based DDS possess a limited mechanical stability under physiological conditions, which is a crucial attribute of successful biomedical systems aimed at in vivo studies. Moreover, compromised chemical stability, uncontrolled rate of hydration, and reduction in viscosity on storage shall be counted as well. Hence, IPNs offer a novel platform that added a dimension of versatility to the chemical and mechanical properties indigenous to alginates. This is chiefly achieved by the incorporation of other polymers in the IPN system, thus endowing the entire system with the privileges of both polymers.

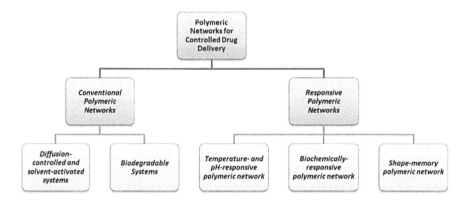

FIGURE 12.2   A schematic illustration of polymeric networks for controlled release drug delivery system.

Source: du Toit et al. (2016).

Various IPN composites composed of alginate and synthetic polymers containing carboxylic groups, with novel properties like super-porous, electrical sensitivity, drug-controlled release, and multi-responsive nature, have been designed. Their physical and biological characteristics such as enhanced solubility of hydrophobic drugs, excellent swelling capacity, and imparting drug stability during formulation step, in addition to their biodegradability, biocompatibility, weak antigenicity, and targeting of drug in a specific tissue, make hydrogels of IPNs suitable for the controlled release of drugs. In the following subsections, the use of alginate-based IPNs as DDS will be discussed with the focus on recent researches developing various formulations.

12.5   OVERVIEW OF IPNS CHARACTERISTICS WITH HIGHLIGHTS ON ALGINATE-BASED IPNS

12.5.1   CLASSIFICATION OF IPNS

Multicomponent polymer materials are the result of mixing two or more polymers. The end result varies according to the structural and chemical composition of the final product (Figure 12.3).

IPNs can be classified according to various facets relevant to network structure, method of synthesis, and network type (Figure 12.4).

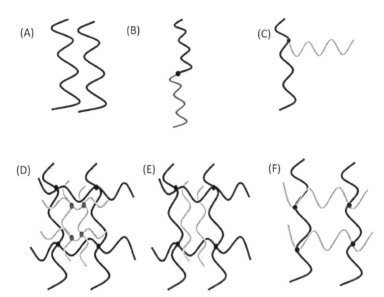

FIGURE 12.3 A schematic illustration of diverse combinations of two polymers: (A) polymer blend, where no bonding between chains; (B) block copolymers; (C) graft copolymers; (D) full-IPN; (E) semi-IPN; (F) AB-graft copolymers. Structures A–C are thermoplastic; structures D–F are thermosets.

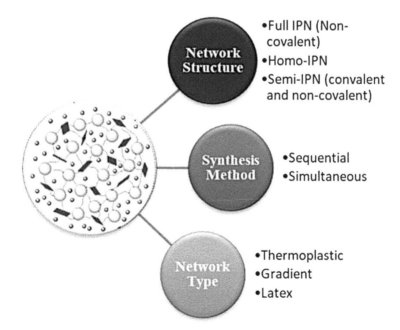

FIGURE 12.4 A schematic illustration of classifications of IPN.

12.5.1.1   BASED ON CHEMICAL BONDING

12.5.1.1.1   Non-covalent full-IPN

A non-covalent full-IPN is formed when two independently cross-linked polymers are juxtaposed, leading to the occurrence of various entanglements and interactions between the networks (Figure 12.3D). Homo-IPNs are a special class of full-IPNs, where both polymers used in the networks are the same. They are usually sequential IPNs. They were one of the earliest types of IPNs to be commercialized and they are used as model materials for theoretical work (Yin et al., 2007).

12.5.1.1.2   Non-covalent semi-IPN

In non-covalent semi-IPN, only one of the polymer systems is cross-linked, while the other remains linear (Figure 12.3E). It shall be taken into consideration that the linear component of the IPN can be removed from the network if the material is swollen in the appropriate solvent. These types of IPNs can be formed by either a sequential or simultaneous process. To further complicate the issue, IPNs of this type that are made by a sequential process are called semi-IPN and the ones made by a simultaneous process are pseudo-IPNs.

12.5.1.1.3   Covalent semi-IPN

When two distinct polymer systems that are cross-linked form a single polymer network, it is called covalent semi-IPN. Irreversible covalent cross-linking leads to formation of permanent network-structured hydrogels. This type of linkage allows absorption of water and/or bioactive compounds without dissolution and permits drug release by diffusion.

12.5.1.2   BASED ON METHOD OF SYNTHESIS

IPNs can be fabricated by innumerable techniques (Sperling et al., 1996; Sperling et al., 1981). The in situ synthesis of IPNs and semi-IPNs involves the mixing of reactants prior to triggering polymerization reaction or cross-linking.

12.5.1.2.1 Sequential IPNs

In sequential IPNs, the first cross-linked polymer network is swollen by all the precursors of the second polymer that is polymerized and/or cross-linked afterward. In this class, an IPN is formed by allowing the first mixture of monomer (I), cross-linker, and initiator to polymerize forming a network. Afterward, in situ polymerization is deployed to polymerize the second polymer network within the first polymer network, forming an IPN. Sequential IPNs are easy to synthesize. The key step is that monomer (II) and co-reactants swell properly into polymer network I. Usually, network I is made of elastomers because they swell easily compared to glassy network (Figure 12.5).

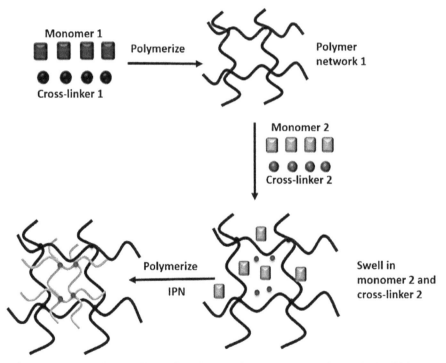

FIGURE 12.5 A schematic illustration of sequential polymerization for synthesis of full-IPN.

Double-network (DN) gels also obtained from IPNs, and they are characterized by a special network structure consisting of two types of polymer components with opposite physical natures: the first rigid brittle network (minor component), densely cross-linked strong polyelectrolyte gels are

always used. Due to their large osmotic pressure derived from dense counterions, the gels swell so much, and their polymer chains are in stretched
state. As a result, the gels show brittle nature. In contrast, the second ductile
network (major component), sparsely cross-linked neutral polymer gels are
mainly used due to their high stretchability. DNs are generally synthesized
through a two-step procedure: the first step involves the formation of a covalently cross-linked first network (Figure 12.6). Then, the first polyelectrolyte
gel is immersed and swelled in a precursor solution containing second
network monomers, initiators, and cross-linkers (Haque et al., 2012).

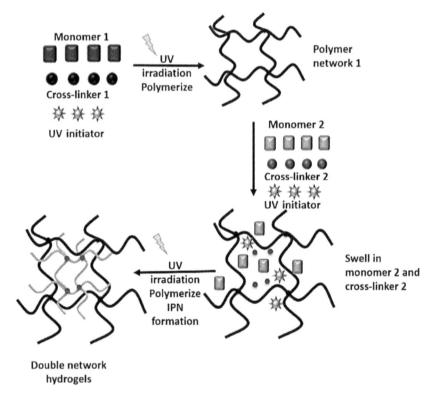

FIGURE 12.6 A schematic illustration of the synthesis of double gel network.

12.5.1.2.2 Simultaneous IPN

The monomers along with the cross-linkers and activators of both networks
are mixed. This process necessitates that the two components polymerize
simultaneously by noninterfering routes (Figure 12.7).

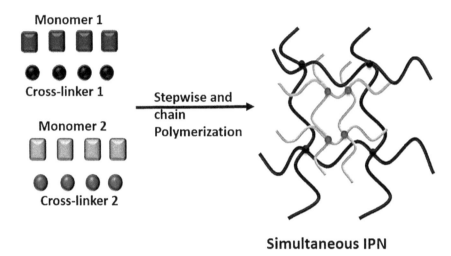

FIGURE 12.7 A schematic illustration of simultaneous polymerization process.

A study was implemented to prepare alginate-/acrylamide-based IPN using both simultaneous and sequential polymerization procedures. Upon comparison, it was concluded that the two-step sequential procedure of IPN formation improved the homogeneous combination of the two highly cross-linked networks, yielding a more uniform product (Demianenko et al., 2016).

12.5.1.3 BASED ON FINAL NETWORK TYPE

12.5.1.3.1 Latex IPNs

Most IPNs are considered as thermosets meaning having the difficulty in molding once formed. One way to overcome this problem is to use latex IPNs. They are also called interpenetrating elastomeric networks, especially when both polymers are above the glass transition temperature (Tg). In latex type IPN, both networks are encompassed in a single latex particle, usually by polymerization of the second monomer together with the cross-linking agent and activator in the initial seed latex of the first cross-linked monomer. The final IPN morphology relies on how was the polymerization process. If the second monomer diffuses swiftly into the first polymer latex, a homogeneous morphology is produced. In contrast, if the second diffuses slowly, it reacts mostly near the surface of the first polymer latex consequently; core–shell morphology is achieved. Cytocompatible alginate-/gelatin-based

IPN-structured elastomeric hybrid hydrogels have been developed recently. Unlike, pristine, the highly elastic tough IPN-structured alginate hydrogels possessed full shape recovery post large strains and long-term cyclic strain loading (Jeon et al., 2017).

12.5.1.3.2 Thermoplastic IPNs

Unlike the abovementioned IPNs, physical cross-linking is used in this subtype, thermoplastic elastomers. The thermoplastic IPNs are hybrids between polymer blends that are physically cross-linked (Jaisankar et al., 2013). Thus, these materials flow at elevated temperatures similar to the thermoplastic elastomers, while acting like conventional thermoset IPNs at their application temperature. Usually, at least one component is a block copolymer and the other one is a semicrystalline or glassy polymer. Depending on the continuity and proportion of phases, this kind of IPNs can exhibit a wide range of properties, from reinforced rubber to high impact plastics.

12.5.1.3.3 Gradient IPNs

IPNs have compositions which vary as a function of spatial orientation in the sample. They are formed as a result of the swelling of the first monomer network in the network of the second monomer. Before equilibrium is established, swelling is terminated, and polymerization subsequently takes place to produce the IPN. In this system, the concentration of second monomer network has a gradient over the first monomer network. IPN is one of the other forms, which is formed when the film made with a network of one polymer on the one surface and the network of another polymer on the other surface, there is a gradient inside the film.

12.5.2 PREPARATION OF IPNS

12.5.2.1 CASTING EVAPORATION

This method has been used extensively to form cross-linked polymer networks. In this method, each polymer constituent is heated until it is dissolved and then in turn added to a cross-linker solution. This can be done either by sequential or simultaneous procedure, and in either case, the solution is heated and mixed, and then casted and dried. IPN gels can be prepared by this technique (Lohani et al., 2014). Among numerous studies, the successful development of sodium alginate/polyethylene oxide-based membranes for the controlled release of valganciclovir employing this method of preparation was recently reported (Mallikarjuna et al., 2013).

12.5.2.2 EMULSIFICATION CROSS-LINKING

This method is based on phase separation. Usually, single-emulsion cross-linking technique is based on water-in-oil (w/o) emulsion. First, the water-soluble materials are dissolved in aqueous phase at specific temperature. Continuous stirring is applied to assure the formation of homogenous solution. This aqueous phase is in turn added to oil phase to prepare w/o emulsion. This method is mainly employed to prepare microsphere IPNs. For instance, this approach was adopted for the synthesis of sodium alginate/polyvinyl alcohol (PVA)-based IPN microspheres for controlled delivery of naproxen (Solak, 2011).

Recently, water-in-water (w/w) emulsion method has also been developed to form IPNs. The main privilege of w/w emulsion method is that organic solvents are omitted, thus evading any probable biological incompatibility. In w/w emulsion technique, an aqueous solution of water-soluble polymers is emulsified as a dispersed phase in an aqueous solution of another polymer that acts as continuous phase. Then, the dispersed polymer phase is cross-linked to form IPN network (Lohani et al., 2014).

12.5.2.3 MINIEMULSION/INVERSE MINIEMULSION TECHNIQUE

This technique utilizes high shear stress to create small stable droplets in a continuous phase (Landfester, 2006). Miniemulsion polymerization relies on the initiation of polymer formation in each of the small stabilized droplets. In order to hinder miniemulsion coalescence, a surfactant and a costabilizer that are soluble in dispersed phase but insoluble in continuous phase are employed. This process of IPNs formation can be divided into three steps. In the first step, constituent polymers are obtained by sonication using specific initiator. In the second step, one of the constituent polymers is polymerized and cross-linked using a cross-linking agent. As a result, a semi-IPN is formed until the second stage. In the third step, a full-IPN is formed, polymerizing and cross-linking the second constituent polymer by the addition of a second cross-linker. Figure 12.8 represents the formation of IPN particles by the process of direct (oil-in-water) miniemulsion polymerization.

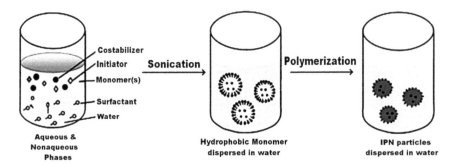

FIGURE 12.8   A schematic illustration of the miniemulsion polymerization process to synthesize IPNs.

Source: Reprinted from Lohani et al, 2014. https://creativecommons.org/licenses/by/3.0/

In the case of inverse miniemulsion (w/o), hydrophilic monomers can be easily polymerized. In this IPN class, the monomer solution is miniemulsified in a continuous hydrophobic phase. The polymerization process can be initiated either from the continuous phase or from the droplet (Koul et al., 2011).

12.5.3   ADVANTAGES AND DISADVANTAGES OF IPNS

IPNs possess some features that impart their superior performance and stability (Bhardwaj et al. 2012; Hou and Siow, 2001; Qadri et al. 2015) as follows:

- The effect of IPN formation on tensile strength is nonlinear, as the maximum strength is many times higher than that of a copolymer. The elastic moduli and tensile strength can be modified by varying the molecular weight of constituent polymers. Nagarjuna et al reported that sodium alginate/karaya gum blend membranes exhibited a higher degree of stiffness compared to pure alginate membrane (Nagarjuna et al., 2016), therefore allowing for the provisional use of alginate-based structures in tissue engineering applications. The developed formulation was effective in controlling release of flutamide, an antiandrogenic drug.
- Superior oxygen permeability.

- Shape memory: Materials that possess shape memory effect can be deformed and fixed into a temporary shape and recover to their original permanent shape only on the exposure of external stimuli such as heat, light, etc. Porous alginate scaffold with shape memory properties was employed for tissue repair and it attained the capacity to spontaneously revert back to its original geometry upon hydration (Guillaume et al., 2014). Figure 12.9 depicts the phenomenon of shape memory.

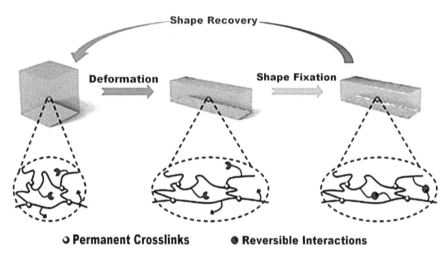

FIGURE 12.9   A schematic illustration depicting shape memory concept.

Source: del Valle et al., 2017. https://creativecommons.org/licenses/by/4.0/

- Equilibrium water content, where IPNs can swell in solvent without dissolving. Mainly, swelling characteristics depend upon the amount and the nature of polymer as well as the degree of cross-linking. Sodium alginate-/acrylamide-grafted hydroxyethyl cellulose-based IPN was investigated. The equilibrium swelling (%) of the developed microspheres decreased with increasing the amount of cross-linker in the IPN matrix. Moreover, the hydrophilic nature of both the graft copolymer and sodium alginate increased the degree of IPN swelling due to their higher water uptake (AL-Kahtani and Sherigara, 2014).
- IPN systems are known to increase the phase stability of the final product. IPN hydrogels developed from two polymers at a given temperature show negligible risk of physical phase separation between the component polymers due to the infinite zero viscosity of the produced gel.

- When the blends are subjected to stress, they can keep the separate phases together.
- Thermodynamic incompatibility can be overcome due to the permanent interlocking of the network segments.
- High thermal stability.

On the other hand, the main disadvantage associated with the use of the IPN is that sometimes the polymers are highly interpenetrated, thus hampering the release of active moieties from the polymer matrix. Moreover, the quality of the final product is extremely sensitive to various in-process parameters like the reaction mechanism, reactor type, and reactor operating conditions (Somya et al., 2015). Furthermore, the lack of effective interface is observed which stems mainly from the absence of molecular interaction between phases (Qadri et al., 2015).

12.6 INSIGHTS INTO THE USE OF ALGINATE-BASED IPNS DRUG DELIVERY SYSTEMS

Development of suitable carrier systems for delivery of active pharmaceuticals always remains a major challenge. New technological advances have put forward many innovative DDSs. A variety of approaches have been investigated for the controlled release of drugs and their targeting to selective sites, including the use of hydrogels, IPNs, microspheres, nanoparticles, tablets, beads, capsules, and films (Hou and Siow, 2001). Some widely studied IPNs-based DDSs are discussed here.

12.6.1 BEADS

A recent study involved preparation of dual-responsive IPN hydrogel microbeads from sodium alginate and functionally modified guar gum (GG) (Eswaramma and Rao, 2017). GG was modified via graft copolymerization using N-vinylcaprolactam (NVCL). The GG-g-PNVCL graft copolymer was blended with sodium alginate to form hydrogel microbeads via emulsion cross-linking method using glutaraldehyde (GA) as a crosslinker. Then, zidovudine, an anti-HIV drug, was encapsulated with 68% encapsulation efficiency (EE%). FTIR, ^{1}H NMR spectroscopy, SEM, DSC, and XRD studies justified the grafting reaction, structure, morphology, and polymer–drug interactions, respectively. Swelling studies ascertained that microbeads were potentially sensitive to both pH and temperature. The in vitro release studies were performed at both pH 1.2 and 7.4 at 25 and 37°C, which confirmed that the maximum% of drug release was achieved for 34 h through diffusion controlled non-Fickian transport.

Optimum drug–resin complexes of ofloxacin, which were prepared for taste masking, got entrapped with different biopolymers (Rajesh and Popat, 2017). Sodium alginate and sodium carboxymethyl cellulose were utilized in the presence of ferric chloride ($FeCl_3$) and GA as cross-linkers to form IPN beads. FTIR studies proved that IPNs beads were cross-linked with Fe^{3+} and GA. The study also revealed that the release of drug was prolonged at gastric pH to reach only $65.86 \pm 1.29\%$ over duration of 10 h. The kinetics of release study showed Fickian diffusion for ionically cross-linked beads and zero-order release for GA cross-linked beads.

Controlled release of chlorpheniramine maleate drug through sodium alginate-g-methylmethacrylate (NaALG-g-MMA) IPN beads has been reported (Reddy et al., 2010). Beads were prepared by precipitating the viscous solution of NaALG-g-MMA in acetone with subsequent cross-linking with GA. DSC studies confirmed the molecular-level distribution of drug in the polymer matrix. Furthermore, FTIR of beads confirmed the successful grafting and cross-linking. Moreover, SEM of the beads suggested that they attained a spherical shape. The drug was released in a controlled manner up to 12 h (Figure 12.10).

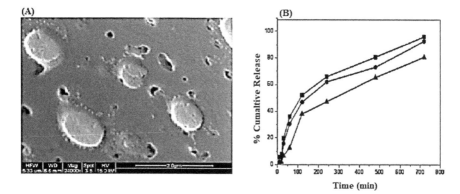

FIGURE 12.10   (A) SEM images of the developed sodium alginate-g-methylmethacrylate beads, (B) percent cumulative release of CPM at different amounts of cross-linker, GA.

Source: Reprinted with permission from Reddy et al., 2010. © 2010 John Wiley.

12.6.2 HYDROGELS

In recent decades, hydrogels have been extensively used as a smart bioma-terial in many biomedical applications such as drug delivery and tissue engineering because of their excellent physicochemical properties. IPNs hydrogels deemed outstanding in the field of drug delivery due to their use in the development of smart (stimuli-sensitive) drug delivery systems (SDDS). The concept of SDDS is based on tunability of physicochemical properties of polymer systems according to a certain environmental stimulus (Figure 12.11). The spectrum of such stimuli encompasses physical (temper-ature, electricity, light, and mechanical stress), chemical (pH, ionic strength), or biological (enzymes) signals. Such stimuli can be either internal signals (as a result of changes in the physiological conditions of a living subject) or external signals (artificially induced). This sensitive behavior of hydrogels has sparked particular interest in their use as drug delivery vehicles that are capable of controlling drug release and drug targeting (Bajpai et al., 2008).

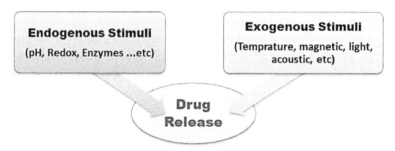

FIGURE 12.11 A schematic illustration of different stimuli affecting drug delivery from SDDS.

Novel grafted pH-sensitive IPNs composites composed of sodium algi-nate/acrylic acid (AA) for colonic controlled delivery of analgesic, diclofenac potassium, were recently developed (Jalil et al., 2017). The highly porous polymeric composites were synthesized by free-radical polymerization using ethylene glycol dimethacrylate as cross-linking agent. Selected samples were loaded with diclofenac potassium. It was concluded that the sodium alginate/ AA IPNs hydrogels are pH-sensitive and modulate their swelling and drug release behavior according to the surrounding medium. Drug release from all the formulations follows non-Fickian pattern. Structural, morphological, and thermal properties of the developed IPNs hydrogels were studied by FTIR, XRD, DSC, and SEM. Therefore, these polymeric formulations were found to be promising for CDDS applications.

Extended-release delivery IPN system for tramadol HCl was prepared, utilizing sodium alginate and PVA (Anwar et al., 2017). Free-radical polymerization through grafting of 2-acrylamido-2-methylpropane sulfonic acid onto the polymeric backbone was the selected method of preparation. Results showed that drug release was pH-independent at both pH 1.2 and 7.4. Moreover, pH-independent swelling occurred with diffusion being the major mechanism of drug release. However, varying polymer ratio and concentration of monomer to higher level resulted in prolonged drug delivery. Concluding that, such polymeric blend might serve as a promising system for the prolonged drug delivery. In another study, multifunctional injectable thermo-/pH-responsive IPN hydrogels as release systems for the oral delivery of small molecule drugs and the local delivery of protein were recently presented (Zhao et al., 2014). The injectable IPN hydrogels are based on poly(ethylene glycol) methacrylate, N-isopropylacrylamide (NIPAAm), and methacrylated alginate polymers. Ammonium persulfate and N,N,N′,N′-tetramethylethylenediamine were used as a redox initiator system at physiological temperature. The rheometric analysis of hydrogels showed good mechanical strength. Moreover, swelling test results affirmed that the developed IPN exhibited temperature and pH sensitivity. Diclofenac sodium (DCS) and bovine serum albumin (BSA) were used as model molecules that were encapsulated in situ in the hydrogel. DCS release from hydrogel at pH 2.1 was low which increased radically at pH 7.4. The aforementioned results highlighted the potential application of the prepared IPNs for the oral delivery of molecules. BSA release from the hydrogel at pH 7.4 took place for 13 days, signifying that the matrix is a promising system for sustained protein release. Finally, cell viability and proliferation studies proved that the developed IPNs are noncytotoxic.

Zhang et al. developed highly porous IPN hydrogel (Figure 12.12), comprising interwoven sericin (natural protein and a major component of silkworm silk) and alginate DNs (Zhang et al., 2015). IPNs' mechanical strength was inversely proportional to alginate ratio, thus tunable to various sericin-to-alginate ratios, to reach the desired stiffness properties. Moreover, high sericin content IPNs showed higher stability relative to pristine alginate hydrogels. Regardless of pH and composition, tested IPNs showed a high swelling ratio which is advantageous in many biomedical applications. Conceptually, employing horseradish peroxidase as a model compound, results showed that the developed IPNs sustained a 24 h controlled release with the adjustable rates which was positively correlated to the fractions of sericin within the IPNs. Furthermore, these IPNs are adhesive to cells, supporting cell proliferation, long-term survival, and migration. Notably, the IPNs inherit sericin's photoluminescent property, enabling bioimaging in vivo. Conclusively, the study indicated that the sericin–alginate IPN hydrogels may have a great utility in the field of tissue engineering and drug delivery.

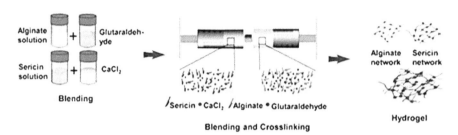

FIGURE 12.12 Synthesis scheme of sericin–alginate porous IPN hydrogels and an SEM image illustrating its surface morphology.

Source: Zhang et al. (2015).

12.6.3 MICROSPHERES

IPN microspheres are considered a multipurpose carrier for controlled release and drug targeting applications due to their capability to encapsulate a wide variety of drugs and confer sustained release characteristics amongst other favorable attributes.

Blend microspheres of sodium alginate/PVA were prepared by w/o emulsion method using GA as a cross-linker (Swamy et al., 2012). Metformin hydrochloride (MHC) was employed as the model drug. In vitro characterization experiments including FTIR, DSC, and XRD analysis were carried out for the drug-loaded microspheres. Furthermore, SEM analysis showed the formation of spherical microspheres with rough surfaces. Drug EE% and release pattern were dependent on the microspheres' composition, drug loading, and degree of cross-linking. The EE% as well as the drug release rate were negatively correlated to the GA concentration used. On the other hand, the EE% was directly proportional to PVA concentration; however, increasing the PVA concentration from 20 to 60% hindered the drug release. Taken together, results indicated that the blend microspheres controlled the release of the loaded drug, MHC and extended its release up to 10 h.

Reddy et al. (2008) prepared semi-IPN microspheres constituted from sodium alginate and NIPAAm. The synthesis was performed via w/o emulsification method with 5-fluorouracil (5-FU) being the model drug. The release of 5-FU lasted for 12 h in a controlled manner which was caused by the presence of the NIPAAm component in the matrix. The swelling behavior was dependent on buffer media pH as well as temperature variation at 25 and 37°C. Delayed drug release from the semi-IPN microspheres at 37°C confirmed the thermosensitive nature by in vitro dissolution. Noteworthy that the synthesis of multi-responsive IPN composite hydrogels, composed of alginate and NIPAAm, has been approached repeatedly to increase the porosity of the gels and thus hasten their respective response rate in order to modulate drug release profiles. NIPAAm is one of the most intensively investigated thermoresponsive polymers which exhibit a slow response rate with temperature changes.

12.6.4 NANOPARTICLES

Recently, there has been increased interest in IPNs nanoparticles for utilization as the smart DDS in the field of controlled drug release, to meet the demand for better control of drug administration. The idea of IPNs nanoparticles as drug carriers may be employed to modify or to control the drug distribution at the tissue, cellular, or subcellular levels. IPNs nanoparticles can be either nanospheres or nanocapsules, depending on the method of preparation (Figure 12.13). Nanospheres are polymeric matrix systems in which the drug is dispersed within the polymer throughout the particle. On the other hand, nanocapsules are vesicular systems, which are made of a drug-containing liquid inner core (aqueous or lipophilic) surrounded by an outer polymeric membrane; hence, nanocapsules can be considered a reservoir system.

The development of multifunctional intelligent hydrogels has been achieved via the development of sodium alginate and poly(acrylamide-co-N-vinylcaprolactam-co-acrylamidoglycolic acid) (NaALG/PAVA)-based dual-responsive semi-IPN hydrogels (Rao et al., 2014). The preparation method was based on free-radical redox polymerization, where N, N'-methylene-bis-acrylamide was used as a cross-linker and 5-FU drug was loaded onto these semi-IPN hydrogels via equilibrium swelling method. The hydrogels were also used as model systems for the entrapment of silver nanoparticles (AgNPs) by the in situ reduction of Ag^+ ions using $NaBH_4$ as a reducing agent. The study confirmed that NaALG/PAVA IPN hydrogel network possessed controlled release pattern of drug over 25 h, which was dependent on solution pH, temperature, and degree of cross-linking (Figure 12.14). Hence, it was concluded that the synthesized hydrogels and hydrogel/AgNPs are potential candidates for drug delivery and antimicrobial applications, respectively.

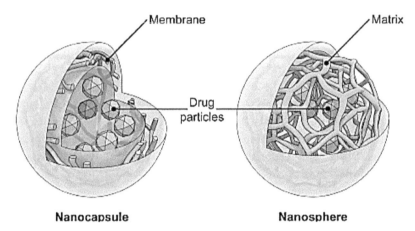

FIGURE 12.13 (See color insert.) A schematic representation of the structure of a nanocapsule and a nanosphere.

Source: Suffredini et al. (2014).

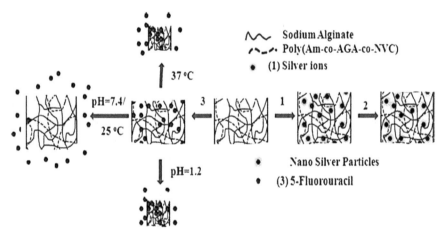

FIGURE 12.14 A schematic representation of the development of sodium alginate and poly(acrylamide-co-N-vinylcaprolactam-co-acrylamidoglycolic acid) semi-IPN hydrogels.

Source: Reddy et al. (2014).

12.7 CONCLUSION

In this chapter, the properties and applications of alginate-based IPNs were reviewed. First, the classification and fabrication of diverse types of IPNs were discussed. Afterward, the advantages of CDDS were mentioned.

Special focus on the superiority of IPN systems utilization in the arena of controlled drug release was highlighted. Finally, recent studies that extensively employed alginate-based IPNs biomaterials in controlled drug delivery at different scales were summarized.

SUMMARY

Alginate, a naturally occurring biocompatible polymer, has offered an interesting model in various biomedical applications such as wound healing, drug delivery, and tissue engineering. Structurally, alginate-based hydrogels serve as mimetics to the extracellular matrices in tissues, thus malleable to manipulations to serve in diverse biomedical application. Recently, alginate has been heavily deployed as a backbone component of vast IPN hydrogel systems. IPN systems are synthesized via the interweaving of two independent polymers in a cross-linked form. In general, the IPNs, prepared utilizing a natural polymer along with a synthetic one, are imparted the synergistic advantageous properties of both polymers, and hence evading their drawbacks. Subsequently, incorporation of alginate into IPN hydrogel system endues it with the superior robustness and mechanical stability which deemed attractive approach recently. In this chapter, particular attention is devoted to tackling all aspects, highlighting the advantages of alginate-based IPNs. Comprehensively, this chapter will also touch upon the facets of alginate-based IPNs properties, stimuli-sensitive swelling, and cytocompatibility. Moreover, the fabrication techniques used to develop different alginate-based IPNs will be discussed. The second part of this contribution is focused on the biomedical utilization of alginate IPN hydrogels as a versatile platform for delivering various drugs.

KEYWORDS

- alginate
- IPN
- drug delivery
- hydrogel
- biomedical

REFERENCES

AL-Kahtani, A. A.; Sherigara, B. Controlled Release of Diclofenac Sodium through Acrylamide Grafted Hydroxyethyl Cellulose and Sodium Alginate. *Carbohydr. Polym.* **2014,***104,* 151–157.

Anwar, H.; Ahmad, M.; Minhas, M. U.; Rehmani, S. Alginate-Polyvinyl Alcohol Based Interpenetrating Polymer Network for Prolonged Drug Therapy, Optimization and in-Vitro Characterization. *Carbohydr. Polym.* **2017,** *166,* 183–194.

Bajpai, A.; Shukla, S. K.; Bhanu, S.; Kankane, S. Responsive Polymers in Controlled Drug Delivery. *Prog. Polym. Sci. 33*(11), **2008,** 1088–1118.

Bhardwaj, V.; Harit, G.; Kumar, S. Interpenetrating Polymer Network (IPN): Novel Approach in Drug Delivery. *Int. J. Drug Dev. Res.* **2012,** *4*(3), 41–54.

del Valle, L. J.; Díaz, A.; Puiggalí, J. Hydrogels for Biomedical Applications: Cellulose, Chitosan, and Protein/Peptide Derivatives. *Gels* **2017,** *3*(3), 27.

Demianenko, P.; Minisini, B.; Lamrani, M.; Poncin-Epaillard, F. Stiff IPN Hydrogels of Poly (Acrylamide) and Alginate: Influence of the Crosslinking Ion's Valence on Hydrogel's Final Properties. *J. Chem. Eng. Process Technol.* **2016,** *7,* 304.

Dragan, E. S. Design and Applications of Interpenetrating Polymer Network Hydrogels. A Review. *Chem. Eng. J.* **2014,** *243,* 572–590.

du Toit, L. C.; Choonara, Y. E.; Kumar, P.; Pillay, V. Polymeric Networks for Controlled Release of Drugs: A Patent Review. *Expert Opin. Ther. Pat.* **2016,** *26*(6), 703–717.

Eswaramma, S.; Rao, K. S. Synthesis of Dual Responsive Carbohydrate Polymer Based IPN Microbeads for Controlled Release of Anti-HIV Drug. *Carbohydr. Polym.* **2017,** *156,* 125–134.

Guillaume, O.; Daly, A.; Lennon, K.; Gansau, J.; Buckley, S. F.; Buckley, C. T. Shape-Memory Porous Alginate Scaffolds for Regeneration of the Annulus Fibrosus: Effect of TGF-β3 Supplementation and Oxygen Culture Conditions. *Acta Biomater.* **2014,** *10*(5), 1985–1995.

Haque, M. A.; Kurokawa, T.; Gong, J. P. Super Tough Double Network Hydrogels and their Application as Biomaterials. *Polymer* **2012,** *53*(9), 1805–1822.

Hou, X.; Siow, K. S. Novel Interpenetrating Polymer Network Electrolytes. *Polymer* **2001,** *42*(9), 4181–4188.

Jain, N.; Sharma, P. K.; Banik, A.; Gupta, A.; Bhardwaj, V. Pharmaceutical and Biomedical Applications of Interpenetrating Polymer Network. *Curr. Drug Ther.* **2011,** *6*(4), 263–270.

Jaisankar, S. N.; Sankar, R. M.; Meera, K. S.; Mandal, A. B. Thermoplastic Interpenetrating Polymer Networks Based on Polyvinyl Chloride and Polyurethane Ionomers for Damping Application. *Soft Mater.* **2013,***11*(1), 55–60.

Jalil, A.; Khan, S.; Naeem, F.; Haider, M. S.; Sarwar, S.; Riaz, A.; Ranjha, N. M. The Structural, Morphological and Thermal Properties of Grafted pH-Sensitive Interpenetrating Highly Porous Polymeric Composites of Sodium Alginate/Acrylic Acid Copolymers for Controlled Delivery of Diclofenac Potassium. *Des. Monomers Polym.* **2017,** *20*(1), 308–324. DOI:10.1080/15685551.2016.1259834.

Jeon, O.; Shin, J.-Y.; Marks, R.; Hopkins, M.; Kim, T.-H.; Park, H.-H.; Alsberg, E. Highly Elastic and tough IPN-Structured Hybrid Hydrogels for Cyclic Mechanical Loading-Enhanced Tissue Engineering. *Chem. Mater.* **2017,** *29*(19), 8425–8432.

Karan, S.; Pal, R.; Ruhidas, B.; Banerjee, S.; Chatterjee, T. K. Comparative Pharmacokinetic Study and Quantification of Ibuprofen Released from Interpenetrating Polymer Network Beads of Sodium Carboxymethyl Xanthan and Sodium Alginate. *Indian J. Pharm. Educ.* **2016,** *50*(3), 442–450.

Koul, V.; Mohamed, R.; Kuckling, D.; Adler, H.-J. P.; Choudhary, V. Interpenetrating Polymer Network (IPN) Nanogels Based on Gelatin and Poly (acrylic acid) by Inverse Miniemulsion Technique: Synthesis and Characterization. *Colloids Surf. B* **2011**, *83*(2), 204–213.

Kudela, V. Hydrogels. In *Encyclopedia of Polymer Science and Engineering;* Kroschwitz, J. I., Ed., John Wiley & Sons: New York and Chichester 1987; Vol 7, pp 703–807.

Reddy, C. L. N.; Swamy, B. Y.; Prasad, C. V.; Subha, M.; Rao, K. C. Controlled Release of Chlorpheniramine Maleate through IPN Beads of Sodium Alginate-g-Methylmethacrylate. *J. Appl. Polym. Sci.* **2010,***118*(4), 2342–2349.

Landfester, K. Synthesis of Colloidal Particles in Miniemulsions. *Annu. Rev. Mater. Res.* **2006,** *36,* 231–279.

Liu, Y.-F.; Huang, K.-L.; Peng, D.-M.; Ding, P.; Li, G.-Y. Preparation and Characterization of Glutaraldehyde Cross-Linked O-Carboxymethylchitosan Microspheres for Controlled Delivery of Pazufloxacin Mesilate. *Int. J. Biol. Macromol.* **2007,** *41*(1), 87–93.

Lohani, A.; Singh, G.; Bhattacharya, S. S.; Verma, A. Interpenetrating Polymer Networks as Innovative Drug Delivery Systems. *J. Drug Delivery* **2014a,** *2014,* 102–112.

Rao, K. M.; Rao, K. S.; Ramanjaneyulu, G.; Rao, K. C.; Subha, M. C.; Ha, C. S. Biodegradable Sodium Alginate-Based Semi-Interpenetrating Polymer Network Hydrogels for Antibacterial Application. *J. Biomed. Mater. Res. A* **2014,***102*(9), 3196–3206.

Mallikarjuna, B.; Madhusudana Rao, K.; Siraj, S.; Chandra Babu, A.; Chowdoji Rao, K.; Subha, M. Sodium Alginate/Poly(ethylene Oxide) Blend Hydrogel Membranes for Controlled Release of Valganciclovir Hydrochloride. *Des. Monomers Polym.* **2013,** *16*(2), 151–159.

Reddy, K. M.; Ramesh Babu, V.; Krishna Rao, K.; Subha, M.; Chowdoji Rao, K.; Sairam, M.; Aminabhavi, T. Temperature Sensitive Semi-IPN Microspheres from Sodium Alginate and N-Isopropylacrylamide for Controlled Release of 5-Fluorouracil. *J. Appl. Polym. Sci.* **2008,***107*(5), 2820–2829.

Margaret, T.; Brahmaiah, B.; Krishna, V.; Revathi, B.; Nama, S. Interpenetrating Polymer Network (IPN) Microparticles an Advancement in Novel Drug Delivery System: A Review. *Int. J. Pharm. Res. Bio-Sci.* **2013,** *2*(3), 215–224.

Nagarjuna, G.; Babu, P. K.; Maruthi, Y.; Parandhama, A.; Madhavi, C.; Subha, M.; Chowdojirao, K. Interpenetrating Polymer Network Hydrogel Membranes of Karayagum and Sodium Alginate for Control Release of Flutamide Drug. *J. App. Pharm. Sci.* **2016,** *6*(12), 11–19.

Nayak, A. K.; Pal, D. Chitosan-Based Interpenetrating Polymeric Network Systems for Sustained Drug Release. In *Advanced Theranostic Materials;* Patra, H. K., Tiwari, A., Choi, J.-W., Eds.; John Wiley & Sons, Inc.: Hoboken, NJ, USA, 2015; pp 183–208.

Qadri, M. F.; Malviya, R.; Sharma, P. K. Biomedical Applications of Interpenetrating Polymer Network System. *Open Pharm. Sci. J.* **2015,** *2*(1), 21–30.

Rajesh, A. M.; Popat, K. M. In Vivo and in Vitro Taste Masking of Ofloxacin and Sustained Release by Forming Interpenetrating Polymer Network Beads. *Pharm. Dev. Technol.* **2017,** *22*(1), 26–34.

Reddy, P. R. S.; Rao, K. M.; Rao, K. K.; Shchipunov, Y.; Ha, C.-S.; Synthesis of Alginate Based Silver Nanocomposite Hydrogels for Biomedical Applications. *Macromol. Res.* **2014,** *22*(8), 832–842.

Solak, E. K. Preparation and Characterization of IPN Microspheres for Controlled Delivery of Naproxen. *J. Biomater. Nanobiotechnol.* **2011,** *2*(04), 445.

Somya, G.; Nayyar, P.; Akanksha, B.; Kumar, S. P. Interpenetrating Polymer Network-Based Drug Delivery Systems: Emerging Applications and Recent Patents. *Egypt. Pharm. J.* **2015,** *14*(2), 75.

Sperling, L. H.; Mishra, V. The Current Status of Interpenetrating Polymer Networks. *Polym. Adv. Technol.* **1996,** *7*(4), 197–208.

Sperling, L. H. (1981). Synthesis of IPNs and Related Materials. In *Interpenetrating Polymer Networks and Related Materials;* Plenum Press: New York,, pp 65–103.

Suffredini, G.; East, J. E.; Levy, L. M. New Applications of Nanotechnology for Neuroimaging. *Am. J. Neuroradio* **2014,** *35*(7), 1246–1253.

Swamy, B. Y.; Prasad, C. V.; Reddy, C. L. N.; Sudhakara, P.; Chung, I.; Subha, M. S. C.; Chowdoji Rao, K. Preparation of Sodium Alginate/Poly(vinyl Alcohol) Blend Microspheres for Controlled Release Applications. *J. Appl. Polym. Sci.* **2012,** *125*(1), 555–561.

Work, W. J.; Horie, K.; Hess, M.; Stepto, R. F. T. Definition of Terms Related to Polymer Blends, Composites, and Multiphase Polymeric Materials (IUPAC Recommendations 2004). *Pure Appl. Chem.* **2004,** *76*(11), 1985–2007.

Yin, L.; Fei, L.; Tang, C.; Yin, C. Synthesis, Characterization, Mechanical Properties and Biocompatibility of Interpenetrating Polymer Network–Super-Porous Hydrogel Containing Sodium Alginate. *Polym. Int.* **2007,** *56*(12), 1563–1571.

Zhang, Y.; Liu, J.; Huang, L.; Wang, Z.; Wang, L. Design and Performance of a Sericin-Alginate Interpenetrating Network Hydrogel for Cell and Drug Delivery. *Sci. Rep.* **2015,** *5,* 12374.

Zhao, J.; Zhao, X.; Guo, B.; Ma, P. X. Multifunctional Interpenetrating Polymer Network Hydrogels Based on Methacrylated Alginate for the Delivery of Small Molecule Drugs and Sustained Release of Protein. *Biomacromolecules* **2014,** *15*(9), 3246–3252.

CHAPTER 13

ALGINATE NANOPARTICLES

ISRA DMOUR[1] and MUTASEM TAHA[2,*]

[1]Facuty of Pharmacy, Al-Ahliyya Amman University, Amman, Jordan

[2]Department of Pharmaceutical Sciences, Faculty of Pharmacy, University of Jordan, Amman 11942, Jordan

*Corresponding author. E-mail: mutasem@ju.edu.jo

13.1 INTRODUCTION

One of the most innovative approaches in human medicine in the last decades is the development of nanoparticles (NPs) to deliver drugs to cells. The concept of nanotechnology has a wide range of applications in human health including tissue engineering, gene delivery, and imaging studies. The principal goals of nanotechnology research in drug delivery includes enhanced drug targeting and delivery, reduction in toxicity while maintaining therapeutic effects, greater safety and biocompatibility, and accelerated development of new safe medicines (Chan et al., 2010; De Jong and Borm, 2008). NPs are colloidal particles consisting of macromolecular substances that vary in size from 10 to 1000 nm (Singh and Lillard, 2009.). Depending on the method of preparation, NPs can be constructed to possess different properties and release characteristics for the best delivery or encapsulation of the therapeutic agent. NPs can be used to deliver enzymes, drugs, and other compounds by dissolving or entrapping them in, or attaching them to the particle's matrix (Masood, 2016; Paques et al., 2014).

Polysaccharides such as chitosan, alginate, dextran, and so forth, have been extensively investigated for the production of natural polymer-based NP carriers. They offer great potential in nanoscale science and technology, including drug delivery systems and medical devices. Polysaccharides offer several advantages such as biocompatibility, biodegradablity, and the facile control of NP size and surface properties through chemical modification (Hamidi et al., 2008; Wilczewsk et al., 2012). Polysaccharide NPs proved to be effective in stabilizing and protecting biologically active components including proteins, vaccines, DNA, and so forth from various environmental hazards and degradation (Elzoghby et al., 2016; Jahangirian et al., 2017). Moreover, polysaccharide NPs tend to adhere to target tissues due to the presence of reactive functional groups at their surfaces, leading to enhanced residence time and consequently improved drug uptake (Anwunobi and Emeje, 2011; Nait Mohamed and Laraba-Djebari, 2016).

Alginate (ALG) is a polysaccharide that is obtained from algae and has been extensively used as a food additive and thickener in salad dressings. In the pharmaceutical industry, ALG has been widely used due to its abundance, low price, nontoxicity, mucoadhesivity, and biocompatibility. These properties together with its high functionality made ALG promising biopolymer material for use in biomedical applications, such as tissue engineering, immobilization of cells, and controlled drug release devices (Masood, 2016; Shaikh et al., 2011). ALG is easily chemically modifiable polymer due to the presence of several reactive groups within its structure. Moreover, ALG hydrophilic groups, such as hydroxyl and carboxyl groups, enhance bioadhesion to biological tissues, like mucous membranes, forming noncovalent bonds that improve the bioavailability of drugs incorporated in ALG drug delivery systems. ALG can be gelled with cations such as calcium and magnesium under mild conditions, enabling the entrapment of various drugs (Paques et al., 2014; Sosnik, 2014).

This chapter reviews the physicochemical properties of alginic acid and its derivatives investigated so far for nanodrug delivery and a brief discussion will be included to cover their application as nanocarriers, their limitations, and future standpoint on how to enhance their utilization in pharmaceutical nanotechnology.

13.2 PHYSICOCHEMICAL PROPERTIES OF ALGINATE (ALG)

Alginic acid/ALG is a naturally occurring polysaccharide and it is the most abundant marine biopolymer and the second most abundant biopolymer (next to cellulose) in the world. ALG is extracted from brown seaweed (Phaeophyceae), including *Laminaria hyperborea*, *Laminaria digitata*, *Laminaria japonica*, *Ascophyllum nodosum*, and *Macrocystis pyrifera*. The extract is treated with aqueous alkali (typically NaOH) and it can be transformed back into alginic acid using dilute mineral acids. ALG and its calcium and sodium salts are available in over than 200 different grades depending on the percentage of its monomers (Ahmad and Khuller, 2008;

Mushollaeni, 2011). ALG can be obtained commercially in an ultrapure form and may be prepared in neutral/charged forms which make it compatible with broad range of substances (Hecht and Srebnik, 2016; Tønnesen and Karlsen, 2002).

ALG is a linear unbranched anionic copolymer of homopolymeric blocks of (1–4)-linked β-D-mannuronate (M) and α-L-guluronate (G) residues (Figure 13.1). The monomers can appear in homopolymeric blocks of consecutive G residues (GGGGGG), consecutive M residues (MMMMMM), and alternating M and G residues (GMGMGM), or randomly organized blocks.

ALG monomer composition greatly affects drug release properties. High "M"-content ALG are suitable for thickening applications, whereas those with high "G" content are best for gelation. In addition, composition (i.e., M/G ratio), sequence, G-block length, and molecular weight are critical factors affecting the physical properties of ALG and its resultant hydrogels. Bacterial epimerases are currently used to develop designer ALG involving the 5-epimerization of β-(1→4)-linked "M" residues to α-(1→4)-linked "G" residues in algal ALG (Guarino et al., 2015; Lee and Mooney, 2012).

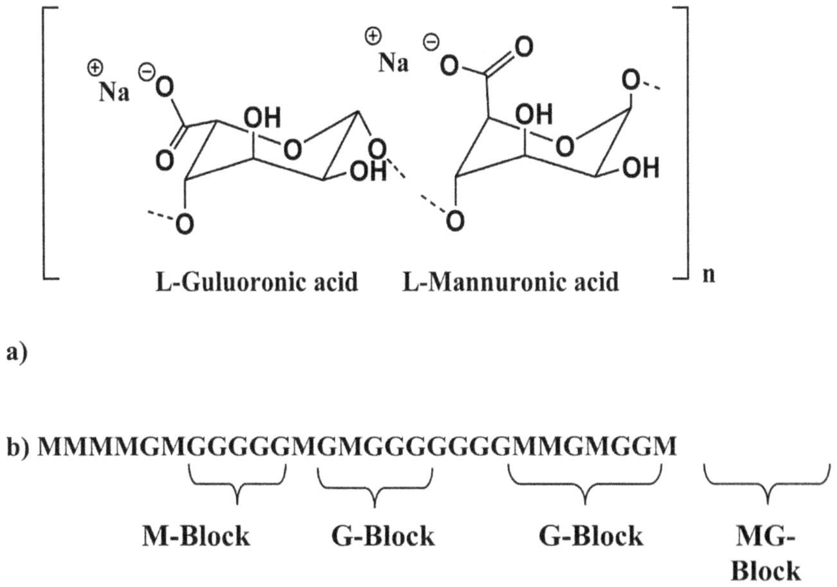

a)

b) **MMMMGMGGGGGMGMGGGGGGGGMMGMGGM**

| M-Block | G-Block | G-Block | MG-Block |

FIGURE 13.1   (a) Representative alginate (ALG) structure and (b) block distribution.

The molecular weight of commercially available ALG range between 32,000 and 400,000 g/mol. Increasing ALG molecular weight can physically improve its gelling properties. However, solutions of high-molecular-weight ALG are greatly viscous, which is often undesirable for pharmaceutical processing. Manipulation of the molecular weight and its distribution can independently control the pre-gel solution viscosity and post-gelling stiffness (Lee and Mooney, 2012).

ALG aqueous solutions have pH-dependent viscosities: viscosity increases at low pH value and vice versa. It reaches a maximum around pH = 3–3.5 as carboxylate groups in the ALG backbone become protonated and form hydrogen bonds (Lee and Mooney, 2012).

Monovalent metal ions form soluble salts with ALG, whereas divalent and multivalent cations (except Mg^{2+}) form gels or precipitates. Only the G-blocks of ALG are believed to participate in intermolecular cross-linking with divalent cations (e.g., Ca^{2+}) to form hydrogels. The high affinity of ALG for alkaline multivalent cations is in order $Mg^{2+} \ll Ca^{2+} < Sr^{2+} < Ba^{2+}$, with the selectivity increases with increasing content of α-L-guluronate residues, and independent from poly-mannuronate blocks (Jain and Bar-Shalom, 2014; Smidsørdh and Haug, 1968). The ionotropic gelation process is usually described by the "egg-box" model (Figure 13.2) (Braccini and Pérez, 2001).

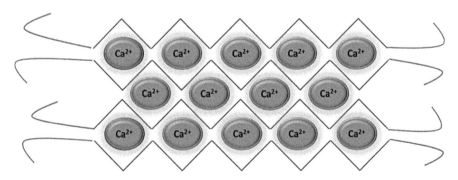

FIGURE 13.2   Egg-box model of calcium ALG.

ALG solubility is influenced by solution pH and ionic strength, and the presence of gelling ions in the solvent. Every ALG has its own pKa value depending on its chemical composition, concentration, and ionic strength of the gelling solvent. Alginic acid is not completely soluble in any solvent including water, while Na-ALG is soluble in water (Guarino et al., 2015; Kakita and Kamishima, 2008).

13.3 BIODEGRADABILITY AND SAFETY OF ALG

ALG lyases are present in marine algae, marine animals, Gram-negative and Gram-positive soil bacteria, marine fungi, and viruses, while they are absent in humans. In marine organisms, ALG lyases cleave the polymeric chains via β-elimination mechanism. Most lyases have a preference for poly(M) substrates, although few G-specific lyases have been identified. ALG is degraded and metabolized by brown algae cell wall as carbon source and for energy (Szekalska et al., 2016; Zhu and Yin, 2015). Accordingly, ALG is inherently nondegradable in mammals; however, ionically cross-linked ALG gels can dissolve under physiological conditions by exchanging the cross-linking divalent ions with monovalent cations such as sodium ions (Forster et al., 2010).

The average molecular weights of many commercially available ALG are higher than renal clearance threshold of the kidneys, and likely will not be completely removed from the body. Nevertheless, ALG biodegradability under physiological conditions can be enhanced by partial oxidation of ALG chains through partial oxidation by sodium periodate. The periodate oxidation cleaves the carbon–carbon bond of the cis-diol group in the uronate residue and alters the chair conformation to an open-chain adduct, which enables degradation of the ALG backbone. However, partial oxidation of ALG does not significantly interfere with its gel-forming capability in the presence of divalent cations. The resulting degradation rate of the gels is strongly dependent on the degree of oxidation, as well as on the pH and temperature of the media (Balakrishnan et al., 2005; Kristiansen et al., 2010).

The safety of ALG as dietary supplement was studied in healthy volunteers following ingestion of ALG at a high level for 23 days. There were no adverse physiological effects as evident by the unchanged enzymatic and other parameters that serve as sensitive indicators of adverse toxicological effects. No allergenic or other untoward subjective manifestations were reported by, nor observed in, any of the volunteers during the period (Anderson et al., 1991).

13.4 PHARMACEUTICAL APPLICATIONS OF ALG

ALG forms high-viscosity aqueous solutions of mucoadhesive properties. These properties made ALG widely used in food, cosmetics, and pharmaceutical industries (Abulateefeh and Taha, 2015; Ching et al., 2015). Alginic acid, sodium and potassium ALG have been extensively used as mucoadhesive biomaterials owing to their very good biocompatibility, biodegradation, solgel transition properties, and chemical versatility that make possible further modifications to tailor its properties (Sosnik, 2014). ALG have been used as a binding and disintegrating agent in tablets, suspending and release-modifying agent, taste-masking agent, thickener, viscosity-increasing agent, and stabilizer (Mandal et al., 2010; Szekalska et al., 2016; Taha et al., 2008).

As a drug delivery vehicle, ALG was formulated in several forms including hydrogels, beads, and microsphere (Figure 13.3). It has been investigated to deliver low-molecular-weight drugs such as methotrexate and mitoxantrone, through a primary or secondary bond between the drug and the ALG to regulate the kinetics of drug release (Santhi et al., 2005). ALG has also been widely exploited in many drug delivery applications in combination with chitosan, as the combination forms ionic complexes. These complexes have been used to deliver triamcinolone, metronidazole, and other drugs. Amphiphilic ALG gel beads have also been prepared to modulate the release of poorly water-soluble drugs like theophylline. Magnetic ALG–chitosan beads loaded with albendazole were also prepared for passive targeting to the gastrointestinal tract using physical capture mechanisms (e.g., magnetic field, pH). The beads showed unique pH-dependent swelling behaviors and a continuous release of albendazole (Wang et al., 2010; 2011).

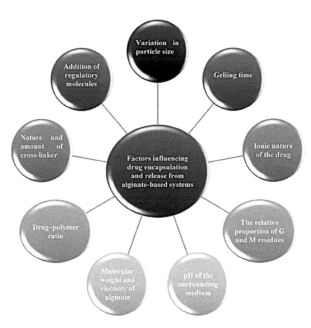

FIGURE 13.3   Factors influencing drug encapsulation and release from ALG-based systems.

In addition, ALG has been investigated extensively for delivery of protein drugs such as lysozyme and chymotrypsin as the fabrication conditions are relatively mild to affect protein denaturation, while the resulting gels can protect proteins from degradation until their release. In general, the release rate of proteins from ALG gels is rapid due to the inherent porosity and hydrophilic nature of the gels. For example, heparin-binding growth factors such as vascular endothelial growth factor or basic fibroblast growth factor exhibit reversible binding to ALG hydrogels, enabling their sustained and localized release (Gu et al., 2004). Insulin-loaded ALG-microspheres have also shown enhanced release following coating with chitosan in order to protect insulin at gastric pH and obtain its sustained release at intestinal pH. The gels protected acid-labile proteins such as insulin from denaturation in the gastric environment (pH 1.2), while releasing the loaded protein at near zero-order kinetics in neutral pH (Lee and Mooney, 2012; Silva et al., 2006; Tønnesen and Karlsen, 2002).

13.5   CHEMICAL MODIFICATIONS OF ALG AS A NANOCARRIER

Different chemical modifications have been performed on ALG including acetylation, thiolation, phosphorylation, covalent cross-linking, and graft copolymerization (Guarino et al., 2015; Pawar and Edgar, 2012). Some of the modified ALG polymers were investigated for the delivery of proteins, antitumors, and genes as described below.

The hydroxyls of ALG can undergo acetylation, phosphorylation, and thiolation reactions. It was observed that a higher degree of acetylation generates more flexible polymers of better swellabilities, while phosphorylated ALG hydrogels have enhanced resistance to degradation (Pawar and Edgar, 2012). The carboxylic group of ALG is another site for ALG chemical modifications, for example, by esterification, thiolation, and amidation. Grafting ALG with fatty alcohols (e.g., octanol, dodecanol, or hexadecanol) generates amphiphilic ALG esters that were reported as carriers for protein and hydrophobic drugs. Amidation of carboxylic groups with amine-containing molecules have been alternatively proposed to form more hydrophilic derivatives of ALG (Leone et al., 2008; Yang et al., 2011).

ALG hydrophilicity has been a drawback for its use in NP formulation. Attachment of the hydrophobic segments on the ALG backbone is one way to enhance drug loading and controlled release. The hydrophobic substitution was reported to form multimolecular cluster by undergoing intermolecular association. For example, alkyl-chain-grafted sodium ALG showed controlled released properties and high encapsulation yields as in the case of curcumin-loaded ALG–oleate NPs (Raja et al., 2015). Oleoyl ALG ester was also used to fabricate NP by self-assembly as nanocarrier for liposoluble nutraceuticals such as vitamin D3 with the controlled release in gastrointestinal fluid (Li et al., 2011; Sun et al., 2012). In a similar manner, phenylalanine–ALG conjugates were used to fabricate vitamin B2-loaded ALG NPs. It was observed that the drug loading increased with increasing degree of phenylalanine ester substitution. Phenylalanine–ALG conjugates NPs released their contents through biphasic release profile over 50 h (Zhang et al., 2016). The conjugation of glycyrrhetinic acid (a liver-targeting molecule) to ALG was successfully used to fabricate doxorubicin-loaded NPs. The drug release was shown to last 20 days with a distinct killing effect on hepatocellular carcinoma cells (Zhang et al., 2009).

The preparation of amphiphilic self-assembled NPs through conjugation of a variety of alkyl chains to ALG with hydrophobic character resulted in enhanced stability in the presence of various concentrations of sodium chloride (Chen et al., 2017). Cholersteryl–ALG conjugates were reported to enhance the photodynamic therapy of photofrin-loaded NPs against human pancreatic cancer (Panc-1) cells. These NPs have the advantage of increased tumor selectivity by the enhanced permeability and retention effect as well as avoiding rapid renal clearance and unwanted uptake by the reticuloendothelial system (Yu et al., 2014). Amphiphilic self-assembled NPs of ALG were also fabricated by coupling phytosterols to ALG through esterification reaction. These NPs were successfully used for targeting folate-receptor-overexpressing cancer cells (Wang et al., 2015).

Thiolated ALG-based NPs were prepared by ALG–cysteine conjugation through covalent cross-linking using carbodiimide-mediated coupling. Varying reaction conditions, thiol content, amount and proportion of reactants enabled the manipulation of NP characteristic. The resulting NPs were used to deliver tamoxifen with sustained release up to 75 h (Martínez et al., 2011; Martínez et al., 2012). The attachment of folate moiety to cysteine-conjugated ALG NPs allowed enhanced tamoxifen targeting and cellular uptake using different cancer cell lines (Martínez et al., 2014). Hauptstein et al. (2015) reported the conjugation of cysteine to ALG by carbodiimides to obtain thiolated residues with more efficient controlled drug release, mucoadhesiveness, swelling behavior, and cohesive properties.

The use of covalent cross-linking of ALG is another method to chemically modify the mechanical and chemical properties of ALG. The reactions involve polymeric hydroxyl or carboxylic acid functionalities. Different cross-linking agents may be used including epichlorohydrin, glutaraldehyde, hexamethylene diisocyanate, adipic acid hydrazide, and carbodiimide. For example, glutar-aldehyde was used to covalently cross-link ALG and gelatin NPs to deliver doxorubicin (Lee et al., 2014). It was also used to cross-link ALG–chitosan NPs to deliver paclitaxel and folate to cancer cells (Wang et al., 2016). In addition, controlled exposure of ALG to ultraviolet light was reported to be less invasive and more rapid cross-linking and can be performed under physiological conditions in situ (Jeon and Alsberg, 2013; Jeon et al., 2012).

13.6 METHODS OF FABRICATIONS OF ALG NANOPARTICLES (NPS)

ALG-based NPs are fabricated by two main methods, either the ionic gelation or by oil-in-water emulsification (Paques et al., 2014):

13.6.1 IONIC GELATION USING A CROSS-LINKER OR BY POLYELECTROLYTE COMPLEXATION

Divalent cations like calcium (calcium chloride) or cationic polyelectrolytes such as polylysine or chitosan can be used as complexing agents to prepare ALG NPs. Rajaonarivony et al. (1993) were the first to describe the formation of ALG nano-aggregates as drug carrier first by adding calcium chloride solution followed by poly-L-lysine. The concentrations of ALG and calcium chloride were lower than those required for typical ALG gel formation. Hence, by mixing low concentrations of ALG and calcium chloride, a pre-gel state was formed consisting of nanosized aggregates dispersed in a water continuous phase. Polylysine is toxic and immunogenic when injected into the human body and was later substituted by chitosan owing to its nontoxicity, bioadhesiveness, and lower cost. It is believed that ionotropic gelation occurs through coordination between calcium ions and guluronic acid blocks of ALG polymers, leading to the characteristic egg-box model (Figure 13.4) (Ching et al., 2015; Hassan et al., 2013).

ALG NP size range depends on ALG and calcium chloride concentrations, the molecular weight of chitosan, and the order of addition of calcium chloride and cationic polymer to the sodium ALG solution. The use of high-energy stirring conditions like ultrasonication during nano-aggregate formation was also reported to achieve tunable NP size (Abulateefeh and Taha, 2015; Lopes et al., 2017). Examples of ALG-based NPs prepared by ionic gelation are listed in Table 13.1.

TABLE 13.1   List of Alginate (ALG)-Based Nanoparticles (NPs) Applications in Drug, Gene, and Vaccine Delivery.

Disease	Polymer	Drug	Studies	NP fabrication method	Reference
Diabetes	ALG–chitosan	Insulin	In vivo oral	Ionic gelation	Mukhopadhyay et al. (2015)
	Alginic acid	Insulin	In vivo sublingual	Ionic gelation	Patil and Devarajan (2016)
	ALG–chitosan	Insulin	*	Ionic gelation	Sarmento et al. (2006)
	ALG–chitosan	Insulin	In vivo oral	Emulsion–cross-linking	Goswami et al. (2014)
	Sodium ALG	Metformin	In vivo parenteral	Emulsion–cross-linking	Kumar et al. (2017)
	Sodium ALG	Insulin	In vivo oral	Emulsification and spraying	Rovshandeh et al. (2016)
	ALG and dextran sulfate/ chitosan	Insulin	Cell lines	Ionotropic gelation	Woitiski et al. (2011)
Cancer therapy	Alginic Acid	Doxorubicin	In vivo parenteral	Counterion complexation	Cheng et al. (2012)
	Oleate ALG ester	Curcumin	Cell lines	Ionic gelation	Raja et al. (2015)
	Calcium ALG	Curcumin and resveratrol	Cell lines	Emulsification and cross-linking process	Saralkar and Dash (2017)
	ALG	BSA—model drug	Cell lines	Emulsion/reticulation technique	Ciofani et al. (2008)
	ALG–chitosan	Curcumin	Cell lines	Ionic gelation	Das et al. (2010)
	Chitosan–ALG	Paclitaxel	Cell lines	Double emulsion cross-linking electrostatic attraction method	Wang et al. (2016)
	Phytosterols–ALG	Doxorubicin	Cell lines	Self-assembly	Wang et al. (2015)
	Sodium ALG	BSA—model drug	*	Microemulsion	Nesamony et al. (2012)
	ALG–chitosan	Doxorubicin	Cell lines	Ionic gelation	Katuwavila et al. (2016)
	Sodium ALG	Doxorubicin	In vivo parenteral	Stirring method	Zhang et al. (2017)

TABLE 13.1 (Continued)

Disease	Polymer	Drug	Studies	NP fabrication method	Reference
	ALG-gelatin	Doxorubicin	Cell lines	Emulsion–cross-linking	Lee et al. (2014)
	ALG-chitosan	Legumain DNA vaccine	In vivo oral	Stirring method	Liu et al. (2013)
	ALG	Exemestane	Cell lines	Ionic gelation	Jayapal and Dhanaraj (2017)
	Sodium ALG	Venom-derived peptides	Cell lines	Ionic gelation	Moradhaseli et al. (2013)
	Glycyrrhetinic acid modified ALG	Doxorubicin	Cell lines	Microemulsion	Zhang et al. (2009)
	ALG-chitosan	Cisplatin	*	Ionic gelation	Maan et al. (2016)
	Sodium ALG	Doxorubicin	Cell lines/zebrafish	Ionic gelation	Gao et al. (2017a)
	ALG-cysteine conjugate	Tamoxifen	*	Coacervation	Martínez et al. (2011)
	ALG-cysteine conjugate	Tamoxifen	Cell lines	Coacervation	Martínez et al. (2014)
	ALG-cysteine conjugate	Tamoxifen	Cell lines	Coacervation	Martínez et al. (2012)
	Sodium ALG	Methotrexate	Cell lines	Ionic gelation	Santhi et al. (2005)
	Chitosan-sodium ALG	Curcumin	*	Ionic gelation	Putra et al. (2016)
	Sodium ALG	Curcumin	Cell lines	Ionic gelation	Anirudhan et al. (2017)
Gene delivery	Sodium ALG	GFP-encoding plasmids	Cell lines	Water-in-oil microemulsion	You and Peng (2005)
	Alginate-chitosan	DNA	Cell lines	Water-in-oil microemulsion	You et al. (2006)
	Sodium ALG	Plasmid DNA	Cell lines	Ionic gelation	Jain and Amiji (2012)
	ALG	siRNA	*	Ionic gelation	Wang et al. (2017)
	Polyethyleneimine (PEI)–ALG	siRNA and DNA	Cell lines	Ionic gelation	Wang et al. (2017)

TABLE 13.1 *(Continued)*

Disease	Polymer	Drug	Studies	NP fabrication method	Reference
Vascular diseases	ALG-chitosan	Nefidipine	*	Ionic gelation	Li et al. (2008)
	Calcium ALG	Diltiazem HCl	*	Ionic gelation	Abulateefeh and Taha (2014)
	ALG-chitosan	Enoxaparin	In vivo oral	Ionic gelation with tripolyphosphate	Bagre et al. (2013)
Antioxidant	ALG-chitosan	Trans-cinnamaldehyde	*	Ionic gelation	Loquercio et al. (2015)
Dietary supplement	phenylalanine ethyl ester–ALG	Vitamin B$_2$	Cell lines	Self-assembly	Zhang et al. (2016)
Anti-oxidant	Chitosan-ALG	Quercetin	In vivo oral	Ionic gelation	Aluani et al. (2017)
Parasite infection	Sodium ALG	Quinapyramine sulfate	In vivo parenteral	Emulsion–cross-linking	Manuja et al. (2014)
	Sodium alginate	Isometamidium-ALG	Cell lines	Covalent cross-linking	Singh et al. (2016)
Tuberculosis	Sodium ALG	Isoniazid (INH), rifampicin (RIF) and pyrazinamide (PZA)	In vivo Inhalation	Ionotropic gelation	Ahmad et al. (2005)
	Sodium alginate	RIF, INH, PZA and ethambutol	In vivo oral	Ionic gelation	Ahmad et al. (2006)
	Sodium ALG	Econazole, INH, RIF, ethambutol, and PZA	In vivo oral	Ionic gelation	Ahmad et al. (2007)

TABLE 13.1 (Continued)

Disease	Polymer	Drug	Studies	NP fabrication method	Reference
Infections	ALG-chitosan	Levofloxacin	*	Ionic gelation	Balaji et al. (2015)
	ALG-chitosan	Gatifloxacin	*	Ionic gelation	Motwani et al. (2008)
	Alginic acid	Tetracycline	Cell lines	Ionic gelation	Ghosh et al. (2011)
Rheumatic diseases	Chitosan-sodium ALG	Aceclofenac	In vivo topical	Ionic gelation	Katakam and Chary (2016)
Analgesia	Sodium ALG	Ibuprofen	*	Desolvation technique covalent cross-linking	Sailaja and Swathi (2015)
Hyperthermia	ALG/Fe$_3$O$_4$	Iron oxide	Cell lines	Ionic gelation and coprecipitation method	Liao et al. (2015)
Vaccine	Sodium ALG	Chicken immunoglobulin (IgY)	Cell lines	Ionic gelation	Bakhshi et al. (2017)
	Calcium ALG	Androctonus australis hector (Aah) venom	In vivo parenteral	Ionic gelation	Nait Mohamed and Laraba-Djebari (2016)
	Sodium alginate	Diphtheria toxoid	In vivo parenteral	Ionic gelation	Sarei et al. (2013)
Osteoporosis	Amphiphilic ALG	Vitamin D$_3$	*	Self-assembly	Li et al. (2011)
	Oleoyl ALG ester	Vitamin D$_3$	In vivo oral	Self-assembly	Sun et al. (2012)
Photodynamic therapy	Chitosan-ALG	Temoporfin	*	Ionic gelation	Brezaniova et al. (2017)
	Sodium ALG derivative	Photosan	Cell lines	Self-assembly	Yu et al. (2014)

*In vitro release study only

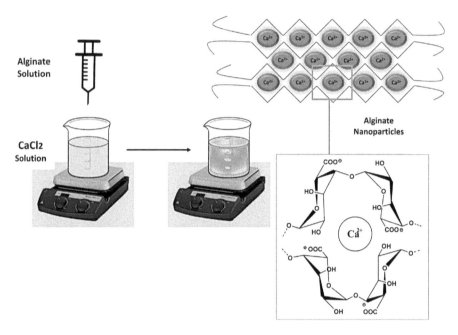

FIGURE 13.4 Formation of ALG nanoparticles (NPs) by calcium cations, resulting in "egg-box" calcium-linked junctions.

13.6.2 ALG NP FABRICATION USING EMULSIFICATION METHODS

This method involves the deposition of ALG on the interface of a template droplet, stabilization by physical or covalent intermolecular cross-linking followed by solvent removal. The interior oil phase will consist of an organic solvent containing the drug or components that are to be encapsulated (Daemi and Barikani, 2012; Paques et al., 2014). The mixture is slowly added to an aqueous solution of ALG, containing a surfactant, such as Tween 80 with sonication to enhance the formation of an oil-in-water (o/w) emulsion. The formed NPs are stabilized by the gradual addition of calcium chloride (with or without chitosan) solution to the emulsion. Finally, the NPs aqueous suspension is allowed to equilibrate for a certain time prior to solvent removal. It was found that the combined addition of chitosan and calcium chloride results in significantly larger NPs compared to NPs prepared without chitosan (Lopes et al., 2017; Natrajan et al., 2015).

Factors that influence the size and drug-loading capacities of these NPs include type of oil phase, order of addition of chitosan and calcium chloride solutions, addition of surfactant, and the use of high mixing energy during fabrication, that is, sonication and ultrasonication (Lopes et al., 2015; Masalova et al., 2013).

A modification of this method involves dispersing calcium carbonate in ALG aqueous phase as internal calcium source (instead of external calcium chloride) (Shilpa et al., 2003). The ALG solution is then emulsified in an oil phase and an oil-soluble acid or glacial acetic acid is then added to the oil phase where it solubilizes the calcium carbonate, allowing the formation of gelled spheres. The ALG NPs are gelled before they are transferred into the aqueous phase, which makes them more robust compared to external gelation using calcium chloride.

Other coatings such as silica have been used on ALG particles (Lopes et al., 2017). Alternating the deposition of cationic polymers with anionic polymers allows the stacking of multiple shell layers on top of each other, a so-called layer-by-layer assembly. Using multiple shell layers can significantly reduce the permeability of the entire shell and can also give additional mechanical strength to the NP (Paques et al., 2014).

ALG NPs can also be functionalized by adding shell layers, either by adsorbing functional compounds in the shell (folate), or by modifying shell polymers by chemically attaching specific functional groups (glycyrrhizic acid). Particle charge can also be modified, hence influencing the interaction with its environment (Martínez et al., 2014; Zhang et al., 2013). Examples of ALG-based NPs produced by water-in-oil emulsification are listed in Table 13.1.

Other methods have been used to prepare ALG-based NPs; these include microfluidic emulsification (through nozzle). In this method, microfluidic "chip" reactors offer the advantage of NP uniformity, high reproducibility, sterility, and good manufacturing practice compliance. However, emulsion-based methods for NP formation are relatively easy and can be scaled up to industrial sizes better than nozzle-based methods (Lopes et al., 2017; Tapia-Hernández et al., 2015).

Advanced methods for fabricating ALG NPs, for example, high-energy stirring (ultrasonication) and spray-drying, offer considerable advantages over conventional methods with respect to size control and polydispersity of the final sample (Daemi and Barikani, 2012; Liu et al., 2013; Paques et al., 2014).

Finally, ALG NPs fabrication can be induced simply through self-assembly, without calcium or polyelectrolyte sonication-induced aggregation using amphiphilic ALG (conjugated to cysteine, phytosterols, etc.) (Paques et al., 2014; Wang et al., 2015).

13.7   DRUG RELEASE CHARACTERISTICS OF ALG NPS

In general, drug encapsulation and release from ALG-based systems are affected by polymer properties, encapsulated drug, fabrication conditions, release medium, extent of cross-linking, polymer morphology, size and density of the particulate system, as well as the presence of adjuvants. In addition, in vitro release also depends on the pH, polarity, and presence of enzymes in the dissolution media (Ahmad and Khuller, 2008). Drug release from ALG NPs is described by several mechanisms including erosion, diffusion, and swelling-diffusion of the NPs matrices (Jayapal and Dhanaraj, 2017). In general, drug release from ALG NPs exhibit biphasic release profile: an initial rapid release of drug over a short period, followed by a stable "plateau." The initial burst release effect is due to the rapid release of surface-bound drug molecules to the large surface of the ALG NPs, while the second phase (steady controlled release) is related to drug diffusion across the hydrophilic matrix of ALG (Kamaly et al., 2016; Santhi et al., 2005).

The burst effect has been minimized by decreasing the hydrophilicity of the polymeric matrix to reduce water entry into the system, thus minimizing the rate of outward mobility of the drug load. Covalent cross-linking or addition of bridging agents (tannic acid) has also been attempted to minimize initial burst effect from ALG NPs (Abulateefeh and Taha, 2015, Katuwavila et al., 2016; Lee and Mooney, 2012).

The steady controlled release phase seems to be triggered by the conversion of calcium ALG into soluble form in the presence of aqueous sodium ions, allowing water to penetrate ALG NPs matrices. Subsequent drug release from ALG NPs involves the absorption of water into the NP matrix and dissolution of drug into the imbibed water with simultaneous release of drug via diffusion, as governed by Fick's law (Kumar et al., 2017; Maan et al., 2016). In this model, drug release is basically determined by the process of relaxation of macromolecular chains and the diffusion of the entrapped drug molecules into the exterior medium. In other words, a swollen NP may be imagined as strands of three-dimensional polymer network structures intervened by permeation channels filled with water. While the polymeric chains relax, the loaded dissolved drug passes into the external-receiving medium, crossing the swollen polymeric layer formed around the matrix. The rate of swelling process decides the Fickian or non-Fickian nature of the released drug (Emami et al., 2014; Maan et al., 2016).

Additionally, drug release from ALG NPs could also be affected by disintegration/erosion mechanism of ALG matrices coupled with diffusion (Abulateefeh and Taha, 2015; Motwani et al., 2008). The efficiency of drug encapsulation/loading depends on the type of drug, the resultant drug–polymer interactions and solvent–drug interaction. Higher drug loading observed in ALG NPs can be attributed to their inherent ability to withstand higher drug-to-polymer ratio (Cheng et al., 2012). It should be noted that the use of ALG–chitosan NPs has the advantage of sustained release enhancement of the encapsulated drugs due to the bioadhesive characteristics of these two polymers which prolong adhesion of the formulation to the intestinal mucosa, thereby increasing the time period available for its absorption. Besides, chitosan itself is known to modulate the intestinal tight junctions, thereby extending the paracellular transport process (Ahmad and Khuller, 2008; Kamaly et al., 2016).

13.8   APPLICATIONS OF ALG IN PHARMACEUTICAL NANOTECHNOLOGY

Recently, ALG-based nanosystems have received great interest because of their mucoadhesivity, biocompatibility, and biodegradability. The ability to tailor their physicochemical properties and their mild fabrication conditions allowed application of ALG NPs in nonconventional drug delivery settings, for example, ocular, transdermal, parenteral, and sublingual routes (Ching et al., 2015; Jahangirian et al, 2017).

Abundance of carboxyl groups at the surface of the alginic acid NPs ensures that they have negatively charged surface in blood circulation, and therefore can escape adsorption to negatively charged proteins in physiological media (Cheng et al., 2012; Tønnesen and Karlsen, 2002). The prolonged systemic circulation of ALG NPs, their targeted drug delivery, and enhanced cellular uptake prompted extensive studies to explore their use to control the release rate of delivered drugs, proteins, DNA, and antigens to targeted specific sites (Sarei et al., 2013; Sosnik, et al., 2014).

ALG NPs received particular interest as candidate for protein and gene delivery because of their mild fabrication conditions that reduce possibility of protein or gene denaturation during fabrication, as well as their excellent abilities to protect their load from degradation until release (Ghosh et al., 2011; Patil and Devarajan, 2016; Sarei et al., 2013). For example, ALG NPs were successfully used to deliver insulin and venom peptides (Moradhaseli et al., 2013; Patil and Devarajan, 2016), transfection by DNA and siRNA (Jain and Amiji, 2012; Wang et al., 2017), deliver vaccines including Androctonus australis hector (Aah) venom and diphtheria toxoid (Nait Mohamed and Laraba-Djebari, 2016).

Moreover, ALG NPs have been investigated as carriers for low-molecular-weight drugs, for example, doxorubicin, paclitaxel, tamoxifen, cisplatin (Cheng et al., 2012; Maan et al., 2016; Wang et al., 2016), for the delivery of phytomaterials, for example, curcumin and resveratrol (Raja et al., 2015, Saralkar and Dash, 2017) as well as diverse antibacterial and anti-tubercular agents (Ahmad et al., 2006; Balaji et al., 2015).

A detailed list of published work on drug, vaccine, and gene delivery using ALG NPs is presented in Table 13.1.

13.9   MODERN ADVANCES IN USING ALG AS POLYMERIC NANOCARRIER IN DRUG TARGETING

On-demand controlled drug delivery and targeted drug nanocarriers are becoming feasible with the design of systems that recognize their microenvironment and deliver their drug load in response to certain stimuli (Crucho, 2015). Stimuli-responsive design is capable of conformational and chemical changes in response to environmental stimuli, and these changes are subsequently accompanied by variations in their physical properties including drug release (Lu et al., 2014).

Magnetic-responsive ALG NPs been fabricated as safe and effective means of delivering drugs to specific organs, tissues, or cellular targets. These NPs are composed of magnetic core material (usually iron or iron oxide) treated to retain drugs on its surface or internally. Ciofani et al. (2008) reported the use of ALG NPs that are suitable for sustained release (of about 5–6 days, after the initial burst). In vitro assays using NIH/3T3 cells performed under dynamic conditions demonstrated that these NPs can effectively drive the drug delivery toward an external magnetic field source. In addition, core–shell NPs consisting of inorganic iron oxide (Fe_3O_4) as core and ALG as shell with cell-targeting ligands (i.e., D-galactosamine) were prepared by combining pre-gel method and coprecipitation in aqueous solution. These NPs showed significant potential as an effective and visually observable transmembrane heat nanogenerators (Liao et al., 2015).

ALG has been also used to fabricate nanogels (NGs) which are cross-linked NPs that can swell by absorption (uptake) of large amounts of solvent, but are not dissolved due to the constituent structure of the polymeric network. NGs can undergo change from a polymeric solution (swell form) to a hard particle (collapsed form) in response to (i) physical stimuli such as temperature, ionic strength, magnetic or electric fields; (ii) chemical stimuli such as pH, ions, and specific molecules; or (iii) biochemical stimuli such as enzymatic substrates or affinity ligands (Vicario-de-la-Torre and Forcada, 2017). Pan et al. (2012) reported the preparation of ALG-based NG that was functionalized with methacrylic acid using a cystamine derivative as cross-linker to provide a pH/redox dual responsiveness. This system was successfully used to release doxorubicin dependent on both pH and the presence of reducing conditions. The resulting NG yielded good cytotoxic effects against HT-29 cells.

Redox-sensitive drug release was also implemented using a novel disulfide cross-linked ALG NPs triggered by the presence of glutathione in tumor cells. The resulting doxorubicin-loaded cross-linked ALG NPs illustrated selective intracellular drug release and cellular uptake in the presence of glutathione. They exhibited selective and remarkable cytotoxic effects against Hep-G2 and HeLa cells, while leaving healthy human liver cells unharmed. The in vivo test of these NPs showed them to be totally devoid of cardiotoxicity commonly observed in doxorubicin NPs (Gao et al., 2017a).

In the same manner, conjugation of a peptide sequence containing tuftsin to ALG NPs enabled enhanced gene transfection by efficient delivery of plasmid DNA and sustained in vitro gene expression in macrophages (Jain and Amiji, 2012).

On the other hand, a simple and efficient platform selective to tumor cells was investigated using pH-sensitive ALG-based NPs for co-delivery of doxorubicin and curcumin into tumor cells. Doxorubicin was covalently conjugated to oxidized ALG through Schiff base reaction to produce amphiphilic macromolecular prodrug responsive to the acidic environment within tumor cells. Curcumin was also encapsulated in the core of these NPs through hydrophobic effects. These NPs exhibited efficient release of doxorubicin and curcumin in acidic media. Further studies of their intracellular uptake and drug release confirmed their enhanced uptake by cells and selective drug release in human breast cancer cell line MCF-7. The in vivo studies of these NPs confirmed their improved cardiotoxicity profile in comparison with free doxorubicin (Gao et al., 2017b).

The potential of ALG NPs in brain drug delivery was demonstrated using venlafaxine-loaded NPs for the treatment of depression through the intranasal route. Behavioral studies on albino Wistar rats showed improved behavioral parameters, that is, swimming, climbing, and immobility in the group treated with intranasal ALG NPs in comparison to venlafaxine tablets given orally. Additionally, intranasal ALG NPs improved locomotor activity when compared with intramuscular or oral venlafaxine dosage forms. Confocal laser scanning fluorescence microscopy studies performed on isolated rat organs after treatment indicated the superiority of ALG NPs for direct intranasal delivery to the brain (Elzoghby et al., 2016; Haque et al., 2014).

13.10   LIMITATIONS FOR USE OF ALG IN PHARMACEUTICAL NANOTECHNOLOGY

Although ALG has been widely investigated as a nanocarrier, its use is limited by its batch-to-batch variability and broad molecular weight distributions, making it less attractive than synthetic polymers that are more reproducible and versatile (Ige et al., 2012). In addition, the hydrophilicity of ALG resulted in NPs instability at biological pH and low drug encapsulation due to drug leakage (Boontheekul et al., 2005; Lee and Mooney, 2012). In many instances, the hydrophilicity of ALG leads to swelling and more rapid release (burst effect) when compared with synthetic polymers (especially for water-soluble drugs) due to extensive leaching of drug molecules from ALG NPs to the surrounding media during preparation (Kamaly et al., 2016). Some NP fabrication conditions like the use of organic solvents, high processing temperatures, long fabrication time, decreased yield, and complex purification conditions have also limited the use of ALG as nanocarrier (Lopes et al., 2017).

To overcome these limitations, several approaches have been implemented. The most successful approach used was to enhance the hydrophobic character of ALG through chemical modifications, resulting in enhanced encapsulation efficiency of these NPs as the described in Section 13.5. The use of chemical cross-linking can enhance the mechanical strength of ALG NPs despite the safety concern in this regard (Hennink and Van Nostrum, 2002; Nitta and Numata, 2013). Covalent cross-linking approach involves chemical conjugation of ALG polymers (within Ca–ALG matrices) to cross-linking reagents such as aldehydes (Chan et al., 2002; Kulkarni et al., 2000). Apparently, this approach requires complicated synthetic steps as compared with the ionic cross-linking method beside the use of toxic chemical reagents that necessitates extensive cleaning procedures before any medical use (Lee and Mooney, 2012). In addition, covalent cross-linking reactions may require anhydrous conditions (organic solvents) which would adversely affect labile active drugs such as proteins or genes (Kulkarni et al., 2000).

The use of bridging cross-linking aid agent such as tannic acid enhanced the encapsulation and release of ALG-based NPs. The method is based on strengthening the coordinate bonds in calcium–ALG by tannic acid within the NP, leading to more stable particles with more resistance to attack by surrounding water molecules and reduced burst effect. Consequently, calcium–ALG–tannic acid NPs showed lower drug leakage upon preparation, leading to higher drug encapsulation (Abulateefeh and Taha, 2015). It should be noted that NPs can accumulate inside cells and lead to intracellular changes, such as disruption of organelle integrity or gene alterations, which cause severe toxicity. This factor combined with the unexpected release behavior of ALG (and other natural polymers) and their high fabrication costs contributed to the vague clinical future of ALG NPs vis-à-vis achieving regulatory approvals (Zhang et al., 2013).

13.11 FUTURE PERCEPTIVE IN USING ALG AS A NANOCARRIER

Nanocarriers based on natural polymers will continue to attract researchers working in drug delivery. These NPs can be engineered to meet specific requirements such as decreasing immune system recognition. ALG as natural polymer offers great opportunity as nanocarrier due to its ability to be chemically modified, its intrinsic properties of being safe, biocompatible, and biodegradable. ALG has been evaluated for several types of drugs including antibiotics, anticancers, vaccines, and genes albeit none was evaluated in clinical trials.

Research efforts should progress toward understanding more about ALG NP cellular uptake mechanisms. It should be pointed out that most of the targeted delivery systems mechanisms do well in vitro studies but fails in in vivo testing. Hence, more extensive in vivo evaluation is warranted to understand this apparent discrepancy.

Targeted delivery has been achieved successfully by stimuli-triggered release of ALG-based NPs as in the case of cancer, but more effort is needed on other pathologies including immune and genetic diseases. From the chemical point of view, ALG modification will continue to enrich the field of NP fabrication by generating new derivatives with optimal physicochemical properties. In addition, the fields of stimuli-triggered release NPs can have a very good impact on achieving targeted delivery of many drugs. This can also enhance the localized effect of many drugs (Muhamad et al. 2014).

Among all future advancements in polymeric nanocarriers, the use of ALG NP as nonviral gene delivery systems seems to be a critical area in future research. Finally, designing a nanoparticulate delivery system at an industrial production scale with effective control on particle size, surface character, and release of therapeutically active agents is still challenging and not comprehensively investigated. More effort is needed to be taken to improve the fabrication costs of NPs in order to reach population scale. Thus, it may be concluded that despite the great advancement demonstrated by persistent efforts of researchers, there exist numerous challenges that have to be addressed.

13.12   CONCLUSION

From the foregoing, it is obvious that natural polymers such as ALG are no longer used only as binders, disintegrant, or diluents but are now being used as nanocarriers for drugs and genes. The efficiency of delivery and release of bioactive molecules from ALG-based NPs is influenced by factors such as ALG chemical modifications, cross-linking agent, drug loading, particle size, interactions between the drug and polymer, and several other technological and pharmacotechnical factors. Natural polymers like ALG may not enjoy the same robustness and easy amenability to formulation of synthetic polymers. Nevertheless, the low cost, excellent biocompatibility and safety profiles of ALG render its corresponding NPs of prominent potential as drug delivery system. The physicochemical properties of ALG depend largely on their botanical or biological sources; therefore, there is a greater need for scientists to search for more homogeneous pharmaceutical ALG. Finally, the challenge for regulatory approval of NP-based drug delivery systems is a significant hurdle that needs to be dealt with in the near future.

SUMMARY

Nanoparticulate systems based on biopolymers have promising properties as carriers and adjuvants for drug delivery. ALG is one of the most widely investigated biomaterials in the field of nano-drug delivery due to its biodegradability, biocompatibility, low toxicity, and adhesivity. ALG NPs are fabricated by two main methods: ionotropic gelation and microemulsion. This nanoparticulate system offered a valuable tool to controlled drug delivery using various routes of administration, such as oral, nasal, ocular, parenteral, and mucosal drug delivery. These systems have been reported to deliver wide range of drugs, enzymes, vaccines, and genes. The present chapter describes the physicochemical properties of ALG which enabled its use as a pharmaceutical excipient and its applications as a nanocarrier. The various chemical modifications and the fabrication methods of ALG-based NPs are also discussed. A special insight is given to the modern advances in drug targeting to certain biological function. In addition, limitations of ALG as nanosystems are reviewed.

KEYWORDS

- **alginate/alginic acid**
- **nanocarrier**
- **nanoparticle**
- **natural polymer**

REFERENCES

Abulateefeh, S. R.; Taha, M. O. Enhanced Drug Encapsulation and Extended Release Profiles of Calcium-Alginate Nanoparticles by Using Tannic Acid as a Bridging Cross-Linking Agent. *J. Microencapsulation* **2015,** *32*(1), 96–105.

Ahmad, Z.; Khuller, G. K. Alginate-Based Sustained Release Drug Delivery Systems for Tuberculosis. *Expert Opin. Drug Delivery* **2008,** *5*(12), 1323–1334.

Ahmad, Z.; Sharma, S.; Khuller, G. K. Inhalable Alginate Nanoparticles as Antitubercular Drug Carriers Against Experimental Tuberculosis. *Int. J. Antimicrob. Agents* **2005,** *26*(4), 298–303.

Ahmad, Z.; Pandey, R.; Sharma, S., Khuller, G. K. Alginate Nanoparticles as Antituberculosis Drug Carriers: Formulation Development, Pharmacokinetics and Therapeutic Potential. *Indian J. Chest Dis. Allied Sci.* **2006,** *48*(3), 171–176.

Ahmad, Z.; Sharma, S.; Khuller, G. K. Chemotherapeutic Evaluation of Alginate Nanoparticle-Encapsulated Azole Antifungal and Antitubercular Drugs Against Murine Tuberculosis. *Nanomedicine* **2007,** *3*(3), 239–243.

Aluani, D.; Tzankova., V.; Kondeva-Burdina, M.; Yordanov, Y.; Nikolova, E.; Odzhakov, F.; Apostolov, A.; Markova, T.; Yoncheva, K. Evaluation of Biocompatibility and Antioxidant Efficiency of Chitosan-Alginate Nanoparticles Loaded with Quercetin. *Int. J. Biol. Macromol.* **2017,** *103,* 771–782.

Anderson, D. M.; Brydon, W. G.; Eastwood, M. A.; Sedgwick, D. M. Dietary Effects of Sodium Alginate in Humans. *Food Addit. Contam.* **1991,** *8*(3), 237–248.

Anirudhan, T. S.; Anila, M. M.; Franklin, S. Synthesis Characterization and Biological Evaluation of Alginate Nanoparticle for the Targeted Delivery of Curcumin. *Mater. Sci. Eng. C Mater. Biol. Appl.* **2017,** *78,* 1125–1134.

Anwunobi, A. P.; Emeje, M. O. Recent Applications of Natural Polymers in Nanodrug Delivery. *J. Nanomed. Nanotechnol* **2011,** S4:002. DOI: 10.4172/2157-7439.S4-002.

Bagre, A. P.; Jain, K.; Jain, N. K. Alginate Coated Chitosan Core Shell Nanoparticles for Oral Delivery of Enoxaparin: in Vitro and in Vivo Assessment. *Int. J. Pharm.* **2013,** *456*(1), 31–40.

Bakhshi, M.; Ebrahimi, F.; Nazarian, S.; Zargan, J.; Behzadi, F.; Gariz, D. S. Nano-Encapsulation of Chicken Immunoglobulin (IgY) in Sodium Alginate Nanoparticles: In Vitro Characterization. *Biologicals* **2017,** *49,* 69–75.

Balaji, R.; Raghunathan, S.; Revathy R. Levofloxacin: Formulation and in-Vitro Evaluation of Alginate and Chitosan Nanospheres. *Egypt. Pharm. J.* **2015,** *14*(1), 30–35.

Balakrishnan, B.; Lesieur, S.; Labarre, D.; Jayakrishnan, A. Periodate Oxidation of Sodium Alginate in Water and in Ethanol–Water Mixture: A Comparative Study. *Carbohydr. Res.* **2005,** *340*(7), 1425–1429.

Boontheekul, T.; Kong, H.; Mooney, D. Controlling Alginate Gels Degradation Utilizing Partial Oxidation and Bimodal Molecular Weight Distribution. *Biomaterials* **2005,** *26,* 2455–2465.

Braccini, I.; Pérez S. Molecular Basis of Ca²⁺-Induced Gelation in Alginates and Pectins: The Egg-Box Model Revisited. *Biomacromolecules* **2001,** *2,* 1089–1096.

Brezaniova, I.; Trousil, J.; Cernochova, Z.; Kral V.; Hruby, M.; Stepanek, P.; Slouf M. Self-Assembled Chitosan-Alginate Polyplex Nanoparticles Containing Temoporfin. *Colloid Polym. Sci.* **2017,** *295,* 1259.

Chan, L; Jin, Y; Heng, P. Cross-Linking Mechanisms of Calcium and Zinc in Production of Alginate Microspheres. *Int. J. Pharm.* **2002,** *242*(1–2), 255–258.

Chan, J. M.; Valencia, P. M.; Zhang, L.; Langer, R.; Farokhzad, O. C. Polymeric Nanoparticles for Drug Delivery. *Methods Mol. Biol.* **2010,** *624,* 163–175.

Chen, K.; Li, J.; Feng, Y.; He, F.; Zhou, Q.; Xiao, D.; Tang, Y. Structural and Rheological Characterizations of Nanoparticles of Environment-Sensitive Hydrophobic Alginate in Aqueous Solution. *Mater. Sci. Eng. C* **2017,** *70*(Pt. 1), 617–627.

Cheng, Y.; Yu, S.; Zhen, X; Wang, X.; Wu, W.; Jiang, X. Alginic Acid Nanoparticles Prepared Through Counterion Complexation Method as a Drug Delivery System. *ACS Appl. Mater. Interfaces* **2012,** *4*(10), 5325–5332

Ching, S. H.; Bansal. N.; Bhandari, B. Alginate Gel Particles-A Review of Production Techniques and Physical Properties. *Crit. Rev. Food Sci. Nutr.*. **2015,** *57*(6), 1133–1152.

Ciofani, G.; Raffa, V.; Obata, Y.; Menciassi; A., Dario, P.; Takeoka, S. Magnetic Driven Alginate Nanoparticles for Targeted Drug Delivery. *Curr. Nanosci.* **2008,** *4,* 212–218.

Crucho, C. I. Stimuli-Responsive Polymeric Nanoparticles for Nanomedicine. *ChemMedChem* **2015,** *10,* 24–38.

Daemi, H.; Barikani, M. Synthesis and Characterization of Calcium Alginate Nanoparticles, Sodium Homopolymannuronate Salt and its Calcium Nanoparticles. *Sci. Iran.* **2012,** *19*(6), 2023–2028.

Das, R. K.; Kasoju, N.; Bora, U. Encapsulation of Curcumin in Alginate-Chitosan-Pluronic Composite Nanoparticles for Delivery to Cancer Cells. *Nanomedicine* **2010,** *6*(1), 153–160.

De Jong, W. H.; Borm, P. J. Drug Delivery and Nanoparticles: Applications and Hazards. *Int. J. Nanomed.* **2008,** *3*(2), 133–149.

Elzoghby, A. O.; Abd-Elwakil, M. M.; Abd-Elsalam, K.; Elsayed, M. T.; Hashem, Y.; Mohamed, O. Natural Polymeric Nanoparticles for Brain-Targeting: Implications on Drug and Gene Delivery. *Curr. Pharm. Des.* **2016,** *22*(22), 3305–3323.

Emami, J.; Boushehri, M. S. S.; Varshosaz, J. Preparation, Characterization and Optimization of Glipizide Controlled Release Nanoparticles. *Res. Pharm. Sci.* **2014,** *9*(5), 301–314.

Forster, R. E. J.; Thürmer, F.; Wallrapp, C.; Lloyd, A. W.; Macfarlane, W.; Phillips, G. J.; Boutrand, J. P.; Lewis, A. L. Characterisation of Physico-Mechanical Properties and Degradation Potential of Calcium Alginate Beads for Use in Embolization. *J. Mater. Sci. Mater. Med.* **2010,** *21*(7), 2243–2251.

Gao, C.; Tang, F.; Zhang, J.; Lee S. M. Y.; Wang, R. Glutathione-Responsive Nanoparticles from a Sodium Alginate Derivative for Selective Release of Doxorubicin in Tumor Cells. *J. Mater. Chem. B* **2017a,** *5,* 2337–2346.

Gao, C.; Tang, F.; Gong, G.; Zhang, J.; Hoi, M.; Lee, S.; Wang, R. pH-Responsive Prodrug Nanoparticles Based on a Sodium Alginate Derivative for Selective Co-Release of Doxorubicin and Curcumin in Tumor Cells. *Nanoscale* **2017b,** *9,* 12533–12542.

Ghosh, D.; Pramanik, A.; Sikdar, N.; Pramani P. Synthesis of Low Molecular Weight Alginic Acid Nanoparticles Through Persulfate Treatment as Effective Drug Delivery System to Manage Drug Resistant Bacteria. *Biotechnol. Bioprocess Eng.* **2011,** *16,* 383.

Goswami, S.; Bajpai, J.; Bajpai, A. K. Calcium Alginate Nanocarriers as Possible Vehicles for Oral Delivery of Insulin. *J. Exp. Nanosci.* **2014,** *9*(4), 337–356.

Gu, F.; Amsden, B.; Neufeld, R. Sustained Delivery of Vascular Endothelial Growth Factor with Alginate Beads. *J. Controlled Release* **2004,** *96*(3), 463–472.

Guarino, V.; Caputo, T.; Altobelli, R.; Ambrosio, L. Degradation Properties and Metabolic Activity of Alginate and Chitosan Polyelectrolytes for Drug Delivery and Tissue Engineering Applications. *AIMS Mater. Sci.* **2015,** *2*(4), 497–450.

Hamidi, M.; Azadi, A.; Rafiei, P. Hydrogel Nanoparticles in Drug Delivery. *Adv. Drug Delivery Rev.* **2008,** *60*(15), 1638–1649.

Haque, S.; Md, S.; Sahni, J. K.; Ali, J.; Baboota, S. Development and Evaluation of Brain Targeted Intranasal Alginate Nanoparticles for Treatment of Depression. *J. Psychiatr. Res.* **2014,** *48*(1), 1–12.

Hassan, R.; Gobourib, A.; Zaafarany I. Kinetics and Mechanism of Sol-Gel Transformation Between Sodium Alginate Anionic Polyelectrolyte and Some Alkaline Earth Metal Ions with Formation of Coordination Biopolymer Ionotropic Polymembrane Hydrogels of Capillary Structures. *Adv. Biosens. Bioelectron.* **2013,** *2*(3), 47–56.

Hauptstein, S.; Dezorzi, S.; Prufert, F.; Matuszczak, B.; Bernkop-Schnurch, A. Synthesis and in Vitro Characterization of a Novel S-Protected Thiolated Alginate. *Carbohydr. Polym.* **2015,** *124,* 1–7.

Hecht, H.; Srebnik, S. Structural Characterization of Sodium Alginate and Calcium Alginate. *Biomacromolecules* **2016,** *17*(6), 2160–2167.

Hennink, W. E.; van Nostrum, C. F. Novel Crosslinking Methods to Design Hydrogels. *Adv. Drug Delivery Rev.* **2002,** *54*(1), 13–36.

Ige, O.; Umoru, L. E.; Aribo, S. Review Article Natural Products: A Minefield of Biomaterials. *ISRN Mater. Sci.* **2012,** *2012,* 20, Article ID 983062.

Jahangirian, H.; Lemraski, E. G.; Webster, T. J.; Rafiee-Moghaddam, R.; Abdollahi, Y. A Review of Drug Delivery Systems Based on Nanotechnology and Green Chemistry: Green Nanomedicine. *Int. J. Nanomed.* **2017,** *12,* 2957–2978.

Jain, S.; Amiji, M. Tuftsin-Modified Alginate Nanoparticles as a Noncondensing Macrophage-Targeted DNA Delivery System. *Biomacromolecules* **2012,** *13*(4), 1074–1085.

Jain, D.; Bar-Shalom, D. Alginate Drug Delivery Systems: Application in Context of Pharmaceutical and Biomedical Research. *Drug Dev. Ind. Pharm.* **2014,** *40*(12), 1576–1584.

Jayapal, J. J.; Dhanaraj, S. Exemestane Loaded Alginate Nanoparticles for Cancer Treatment: Formulation and in Vitro Evaluation. *Int. J. Biol. Macromol.* **2017,** *105,* 416–421.

Jeon, O.; Alsberg, E. Photofunctionalization of Alginate Hydrogels to Promote Adhesion and Proliferation of Human Mesenchymal Stem Cells. *Tissue Eng. Part A* **2013,** *19*(11–12), 1424–1432.

Jeon, O.; Alt, D. S.; Ahmed, S. M.; Alsberg; E. The Effect of Oxidation on the Degradation of Photocrosslinkable Alginate Hydrogels. *Biomaterials* **2012,** *33*(13), 3503–3514.

Kakita, H.; Kamishima, H. Some Properties of Alginate Gels Derived from Algal Sodium Alginate. In *Nineteenth International Seaweed Symposium. Developments in Applied*

Phycology; Borowitzka, M. A., Critchley, A. T., Kraan, S., Peters, A., Sjøtun, K., Notoya, M., Eds.; Springer: Dordrecht, 2008; Vol. 2, pp 93–99.

Kamaly, N.; Yameen, B.; Wu, J.; Farokhzad, O. C. Degradable Controlled-Release Polymers and Polymeric Nanoparticles: Mechanisms of Controlling Drug Release. *Chem. Rev.* **2016,** *116*(4), 2602–2663.

Katakam, P.; Chary, T. N. Development of Nano Particle Encapsulated Pemulen Gel for Aceclofenac Topical Delivery. *Afr. J. Pharm. Pharmacol.* **2016,** *10*(40), 854–864.

Katuwavila, N. P.; Perera, A. D. L. C.; Samarakoon, S. R.; Soysa, P.; Karunaratne, V.; Amaratunga, G. A.; Karunaratne, D. N. Chitosan-Alginate Nanoparticle System Efficiently Delivers Doxorubicin to MCF-7 Cells. *J. Nanomater.* **2016,** *2016,* 15.

Kristiansen, K. A.; Potthast A.; Christensen, B. E. Periodate Oxidation of Polysaccharides for Modification of Chemical and Physical Properties. *Carbohydr. Res.* **2010,** *345*(10), 1264–1271.

Kulkarni, A. R.; Soppimath, K. S.; Aralaguppi, M. I.; Aminabhavi, T. M.; Rudzinski, W. E. Preparation of Cross-Linked Sodium Alginate Microparticles Using Glutaraldehyde in Methanol. *Drug Dev. Ind. Pharm.* **2000,** *26*(10), 1121–1124.

Kumar, S.; Bhanjana, G.; Verma, R. K.; Dhingra, D.; Dilbaghi, N.; Kim, K. H. Metformin-Loaded Alginate Nanoparticles as an Effective Antidiabetic Agent for Controlled Drug Release. *J. Pharm. Pharmacol.* **2017,** *69*(2), 143–150.

Lee, K. Y.; Mooney, D. J. Alginate: Properties and Biomedical Applications. *Prog. Polym. Sci.* **2012,** *37*(1), 106–126.

Lee, E. M.; Singh, D.; Singh, D.; Choi, S. M.; Zo, S. M.; Park, S. J.; Han, S. S. Novel Alginate Gelatin Hybrid Nanoparticle for Drug Delivery and Tissue Engineering Applications. *J. Nanomater.* **2014,** *2014,* 147. DOI: 10.1155/2014/124236.

Leone, G.; Torricelli, P.; Chiumiento, A.; Facchini, A.; Barbucci, R. Amedic Alginate Hydrogel for Nucleus Pulposus Replacement. *J. Biomed. Mater. Res. A* **2008,** *84,* 391–401.

Li, P.; Dai, Y. N.; Zhang, J. P.; Wang, A. Q.; Wei, Q. Chitosan-Alginate Nanoparticles as a Novel Drug Delivery System for Nifedipine. *Int. J. Biomed. Sci.* **2008,** *4*(3), 221–228.

Li, Q.; Liu, C. G.; Huang, Z. H.; Xue, F. F. Preparation and Characterization of Nanoparticles Based on Hydrophobic Alginate Derivative as Carriers for Sustained Release of Vitamin D3. *J. Agric. Food Chem.* **2011,** *59*(5), 1962–1967.

Liao, S. H.; Liu, C. H.; Bastakoti, B. P.; Suzuki, N.; Chang, Y.; Yamauchi, Y.; Wu, K. C. W. Functionalized Magnetic Iron Oxide/Alginate Core-Shell Nanoparticles for Targeting Hyperthermia. *Int. J. Nanomed.* **2015,** *10,* 3315–3328.

Liu, Z; Lv, D.; Liu, S.; Gong, J.; Wang, D.; Xiong, M.; Chen, X.; Xiang, R.; Tan, X. Alginic Acid-Coated Chitosan Nanoparticles Loaded with Legumain DNA Vaccine: Effect Against Breast Cancer in Mice. *PLoS One* **2013,** *8*(4), e60190.

Lopes, M. A.; Abrahim-Vieira, B.; Oliveira, C.; Fonte, P.; Souza, A. M.; Lira, T.; Sequeira, J. A.; Rodrigues, C. R.; Cabral, L. M.; Sarmento, B.; Seiça, R.; Veiga, F.; Ribeiro, A. J. Probing Insulin Bioactivity in Oral Nanoparticles Produced by Ultrasonication-Assisted Emulsification/Internal Gelation. *Int. J. Nanomed.* **2015,** *10,* 5865–5880.

Lopes, M.; Abrahim, B.; Veiga, F.; Seiça; R.; Cabral, L. M.; Arnaud, P.; Andrade, J. C.; Ribeiro, A. J. Preparation Methods and Applications Behind Alginate-Based Particles. *Expert Opin. Drug Delivery* **2017,** *14*(6), 769–782.

Loquercio, A.; Castell-Perez, E.; Gomes, C.; Moreira, R. G. Preparation of Chitosan-Alginate Nanoparticles for Trans-Cinnamaldehyde Entrapment. *J. Food Sci.* **2015,** *80*(10), N2305–2315.

Lu, Y.; Sun, W.; Gu, Z. Stimuli-Responsive Nanomaterials for Therapeutic Protein Delivery. *J. Controlled Release* **2014**, *194*, 1–19.

Maan, G. K.; Bajpai, J.; Bajpai, A. K. Investigation of In Vitro Release of Cisplatin from Electrostatically Crosslinked Chitosan-Alginate Nanoparticles. *Synth. React. Inorg. Met.-Org. Nano-Met. Chem.* **2016**, *46*(10), 1532–1540.

Mandal, S.; Kumar, S. S.; Krishnamoorthy, B.; Basu, S. K. Development and Evaluation of Calcium Alginate Beads Prepared by Sequential and Simultaneous Methods. *Braz. J. Pharm. Sci.* **2010**, *46*, 785–793.

Manuja, A.; Kumar, S.; Dilbaghi, N.; Bhanjana, G.; Chopra, M.; Kaur, H.; Kumar, R.; Manuja, B. K.; Singh, S. K.; Yadav, S. C. Quinapyramine Sulfate-Loaded Sodium Alginate Nanoparticles show Enhanced Trypanocidal Activity. *Nanomedicine* **2014**, *9*(11), 1625–1634.

Martínez, A.; Iglesias, I.; Lozano, R.; Teijón, J. M.; Blanco, M. D. Synthesis and Characterization of Thiolated Alginate-Albumin Nanoparticles Stabilized by Disulfide Bonds. Evaluation as Drug Delivery Systems. *Carbohydr. Polym.* **2011**, *83*, 1311–1321.

Martínez, A.; Benito-Miguel, M.; Iglesias, I.; Teijón, J. M.; Blanco, M. D. Tamoxifen-Loaded Thiolated Alginate-Albumin Nanoparticles as Antitumoral Drug Delivery Systems. *J. Biomed. Mater. Res. Part A* **2012**, *100*, 1467–1476.

Martínez, A.; Olmo, R.; Iglesias, I.; Teijón J.; M. Blanco, M. D. Folate-Targeted Nanoparticles Based on Albumin and Albumin/Alginate Mixtures as Controlled Release Systems of Tamoxifen: Synthesis and in Vitro Characterization. *Pharm. Res.* **2014**, *31*, 182–193.

Masalova, O.; Kulikouskaya, V.; Shutava, T.; Agabekov, V. Alginate and Chitosan Gel Nanoparticles for Efficient Protein Entrapment. *Phys. Procedia* **2013**, *40*, 69–75.

Masood, F. Polymeric Nanoparticles for Targeted Drug Delivery System for Cancer Therapy. *Mater. Sci. Eng. C* **2016**, *60*, 569–578.

Moradhaseli, S.; Mirakabadi, A. Z.; Sarzaeem, A.; Dounighi, N. M.; Soheily, S.; Borumand M. R. Preparation and Characterization of Sodium Alginate Nanoparticles Containing ICD-85 (Venom Derived Peptides). *Int. J. Innovation Appl. Stud.* **2013**, *4*(3), 534–542.

Motwani, S. K.; Chopra, S.; Talegaonkar, S.; Kohli, K.; Ahmad, F. J.; Khar, R. K. Chitosan-Sodium Alginate Nanoparticles as Submicroscopic Reservoirs for Ocular Delivery: Formulation, Optimisation and in Vitro Characterisation. *Eur. J. Pharm. Biopharm.* **2008**, *68*(3), 513–525.

Muhamad, I. I.; Selvakumaran, S.; Md Lazim, N. A. Designing Polymeric Nanoparticles for Targeted Drug Delivery System. In *Nanomedicine;* Seifalian, A., de Mel, A., Kalaskar, D. M., Eds., One Central Press (OCP): Manchester, UK, 2014; pp 287–313.

Mukhopadhyay, P.; Chakraborty, S.; Bhattacharya S.; Mishra. R.; Kundu, P. P. pH-Sensitive Chitosan/Alginate Core-Shell Nanoparticles for Efficient and Safe Oral Insulin Delivery. *Int. J. Biol. Macromol.* **2015**, *72*, 640–648.

Mushollaeni, W. The Physicochemical Characteristics of Sodium Alginate from Indonesian Brown Seaweeds. *Afr. J. Food Sci.* **2011**, *5*, 349–352.

Nait Mohamed, F. A.; Laraba-Djebari, F. Development and Characterization of a New Carrier for Vaccine Delivery Based on Calcium-Alginate Nanoparticles: Safe Immunoprotective Approach Against Scorpion Envenoming. *Vaccine* **2016**, *34*(24), 2692–2699.

Natrajan, D.; Srinivasan, S.; Sundar, K.; Ravindran, A. Formulation of Essential Oil-Loaded Chitosan–Alginate Nanocapsules. *J. Food Drug Anal.* **2015**, *23*(3), 560–568.

Nesamony, J.; Singh, P. R.; Nada, S. E.; Shah, Z. A.; Kolling, W. M. Calcium Alginate Nanoparticles Synthesized Through a Novel Interfacial Cross-Linking Method as a Potential Protein Drug Delivery System. *J. Pharm. Sci.* **2012**, *101*(6), 2177–2184.

Nitta, S. K.; Numata, K. Biopolymer-Based Nanoparticles for Drug/Gene Delivery and Tissue Engineering. *Int. J. Mol. Sci.* **2013,** *14*(1), 1629–1654.

Pan, Y.; Chen, Y.; Wang, D.; Wei, C.; Guo, J.; Lu, D.; Chu, C.; Wang, C. Redox/pH Dual Stimuli-Responsive Biodegradable Nanohydrogels with Varying Responses to Dithiothreitol and Glutathione for Controlled Drug Release. *Biomaterials* **2012,** *33,* 6570–6579.

Paques, J. P.; van der Linden, E.; van Rijn, C. J.; Sagis., L. M. Preparation Methods of Alginate Nanoparticles. *Adv. Colloid Interface Sci.* **2014,** *209,* 163–171.

Patil, N.; Devarajan, P. Insulin-Loaded Alginic Acid Nanoparticles for Sublingual Delivery. *Drug Delivery* **2016,** *23*(2), 429–436.

Pawar, S. N.; Edgar, K. J. Alginate Derivatization: A Review of Chemistry, Properties and Applications. *Biomaterials* **2012,** *33*(11), 3279–3305.

Putra, P.; Siswanta, D; Suratman, A. Improving the Slow Release System Using Chitosan-Alginate Nanoparticles with Various Methods for Curcumin. *Am. Chem. Sci. J.* **2016,** *14*(4), 1–10, Article No. ACSJ.25989.

Raja, M. A.; Liu, C.; Huang, Z. Nanoparticles Based on Oleate Alginate Ester as Curcumin Delivery System. *Curr. Drug Delivery.* **2015,** *12*(5), 613–627.

Rajaonarivony, M.; Vauthier, C.; Couarraze, G.; Puisieux, F.; Couvreur, P. Development of a New Drug Carrier Made from Alginate. *J. Pharm. Sci.* **1993,** *82,* 912–917.

Rovshandeh, M. J.; Aghajamali, M.; Haghbin Nazarpak, M.; Toliyat, T. Evaluation of Insulin Release from Alginate Nanoparticles by Two Different Methods. *J. Pharm. Drug Delivery Res.* **2016,** *5*(3).

Sailaja, K.; Swathi, P. Preparation of Sodium Alginate Nanoparticles by Desolvation Technique Using Iso Propyl Alcohol as Desolvating Agent. *Int. J. Adv. Pharm.* **2015,** *4*(5), 60–71.

Saralkar, P. L.; Dash, A. K., Alginate Nanoparticles Containing Curcumin and Resveratrol: Preparation, Characterization, and in Vitro Evaluation Against Du145 Prostate Cancer Cell. *AAPS PharmSciTech* **2017,** *18,* 2814.

Sarei, F.; Dounighi, N. M.; Zolfagharian, H.; Khaki, P.; Bidhendi, S. M. Alginate Nanoparticles as a Promising Adjuvant and Vaccine Delivery System. *Indian J. Pharm. Sci.* **2013,** *75*(4), 442–449.

Sarmento, B.; Ferreira, D.; Veiga, F.; Ribeiro A. Characterization of Insulin-Loaded Alginate Nanoparticles Produced by Ionotropic Pre-Gelation Through DSC and FTIR Studies. *Carbohydr. Polym.* **2006,** *66,* 1–7.

Santhi, K.; Dhanraj, S. A.; Nagasamyvenkatesh, D.; Sangeetha, S.; Suresh, B. Preparation and Optimization of Sodium Alginate Nanospheres of Methotrexate. *Indian J. Pharm. Sci.* **2005,** *67,* 691–696.

Shaikh, R.; Raj Singh, T. R.; Garland, M. J.; Woolfson, A. D.; Donnelly, R. F. Mucoadhesive Drug Delivery Systems. *J. Pharm. Bioallied Sci.* **2011,** *3*(1), 89–100.

Shilpa, S. S.; Agrawal, A. R. R. Controlled Delivery of Drugs from Alginate Matrix. *J. Macromol. Sci. Polym. Rev C* **2003,** *43,* 187–221.

Silva, C. M.; Ribeiro, A. J.; Ferreira, D.; Veiga, F. Insulin Encapsulation in Reinforced Alginate Microspheres Prepared by Internal Gelation. *Eur. J. Pharm. Sci.* **2006,** *29*(2), 148–159.

Singh, R.; Lillard J. W. Nanoparticle-Based Targeted Drug Delivery. *Exp. Mol. Pathol.* **2009,** *86*(3), 215–223.

Singh, S.; Chopra, M.; Dilbaghi, N.; Manuja, B. K.; Kumar, S.; Kumar, R.; Rathore, N. S.; Yadav, S. C.; Manuja, A. Synthesis and Evaluation of Isometamidium-Alginate Nanoparticles on Equine Mononuclear and Red Blood Cells. *Int. J. Biol. Macromol.* **2016,** *92,* 788–794.

Smidsrød, O.; Haug, A. Dependence Upon Uronic Acid Composition of Some Ion-Exchange Properties of Alginates. *Acta Chem. Scand.* **1968**, *22,* 1989–1997.

Sosnik, A. Alginate Particles as Platform for Drug Delivery by the Oral Route: State-of-the-Art. *ISRN Pharma.* **2014**, *2014,* 17, Article ID 926157.

Sun, F.; Ju, C.; Chen, J.; Liu, S.; Liu, N.; Wang, K.; Liu, C. Nanoparticles Based on Hydrophobic Alginate Derivative as Nutraceutical Delivery Vehicle: Vitamin D3 Loading. *Artif. Cells Blood Substitutes Immobilization Biotechnol.* **2012**, *40*(1–2), 113–119.

Szekalska, M.; Puciłowska, A.; Szymańska, E.; Ciosek, P.; Katarzyna, W. Alginate: Current Use and Future Perspectives in Pharmaceutical and Biomedical Applications. *Int. J. Polym. Sci.* **2016**, *2016,* 1–17.

Taha, M. O.; Nasser, W.; Ardakani, A.; Alkhatib, H. S. Sodium Lauryl Sulfate Impedes Drug Release from Zinc-Crosslinked Alginate Beads: Switching from Enteric Coating Release into Biphasic Profile. *Int. J. Pharm.* **2008**, *350,* 291.

Tapia-Hernández, J. A., Torres-Chávez, P. I.; Ramírez-Wong, B.; Rascón-Chu, A.; Plascencia-Jatomea, M.; Barreras-Urbina, C. G.; Rangel-Vázquez, N. A.; Rodríguez-Félix, F. Micro- and Nanoparticles by Electrospray: Advances and Applications in Foods. *J. Agric. Food Chem.* **2015**, *63*(19), 4699–4707.

Tønnesen, H. H.; Karlsen, J. Alginate in Drug Delivery Systems. *Drug Dev. Ind. Pharm.* **2002**, *28*(6), 621–630.

Vicario-de-la-Torre, M.; Forcada, J. The Potential of Stimuli-Responsive Nanogels in Drug and Active Molecule Delivery for Targeted Therapy. *Gels* **2017**, *3,* 16.

Wang, F. Q.; Li, P.; Zhang, J. P.; Wang, A. Q.; Wei, Q. A Novel pH-Sensitive Magnetic Alginate-Chitosan Beads for Albendazole Delivery. *Drug Dev. Ind. Pharm.* **2010**, *36*(7), 867–877.

Wang, F. Q.; Li, P.; Zhang, J. P.; Wang, A. Q.; Wei, Q. pH-Sensitive Magnetic Alginate-Chitosan Beads for Albendazole Delivery. *Pharm. Dev. Technol.* **2011**, *16*(3), 228–236.

Wang, J.; Wang, M.; Zheng, M.; Guo, Q.; Wang, Y.; Wang, H.; Xie, X.; Huang, F.; Gong, R. Folate Mediated Self-Assembled Phytosterol-Alginate Nanoparticles for Targeted Intracellular Anticancer Drug Delivery. *Colloids Surf. B* **2015**, *129,* 63–70.

Wang, F.; Yang, S.; Yuan, J.; Gao, Q.; Huang, C. Effective Method of Chitosan-Coated Alginate Nanoparticles for Target Drug Delivery Applications. *J. Biomater. Appl.* **2016**, *31*(1), 3–12.

Wang, G. D.; Tan, Y. Z.; Wang, H. J.; Zhou, P. Autophagy Promotes Degradation of Polyethyleneimine-Alginate Nanoparticles in Endothelial Progenitor Cells. *Int. J. Nanomed.* **2017**, *12,* 6661–6675.

Wilczewska, A. Z.; Niemirowicz, K.; Markiewicz, K. H.; Car, H. Nanoparticles as Drug Delivery Systems. *Pharmacol. Rep.* **2012**, *64*(5), 1020–1037.

Woitiski, C. B.; Sarmento, B.; Carvalho, R. A.; Neufeld, R. J.; Veiga, F. Facilitated Nanoscale Delivery of Insulin Across Intestinal Membrane Models. *Int. J. Pharm.* **2011**, *412,* 123–131.

Yang, J. S.; Ren, H. B.; Xie, Y. J. Synthesis of Amidic Alginate Derivatives and Their Application in Microencapsulation of λ-Cyhalothrin. *Biomacromolecules* **2011**, *12*(8), 2982–2987.

You, J. O.; Peng, C. A. Calcium-Alginate Nanoparticles Formed by Reverse Microemulsion as Gene Carriers. *Macromol. Symp.* **2005**, *219,* 147–153.

You, J. O.; Liu, Y. C.; Peng, C. A. Efficient Gene Transfection Using Chitosan–Alginate Core-Shell Nanoparticles. *Int. J. Nanomed.* **2006**, *1*(2), 173–180.

Yu, Z.; Li, H.; Zhang, L. M.; Zhu, Z.; Yang, L. Enhancement of Phototoxicity Against Human Pancreatic Cancer Cells with Photosensitizer-Encapsulated Amphiphilic Sodium Alginate Derivative Nanoparticles. *Int. J. Pharm.* **2014**, *473*(1–2), 501–509.

Zhang, C.; Wang, W.; Wang, C.; Tian, Q.; Huang, W.; Yuan, Z.; Chen, X. Cytotoxicity of Liver Targeted Drug-Loaded Alginate Nanoparticles. *Sci. China Chem.* **2009**, *9*, 1382–1387.

Zhang, Y.; Chan, H.F.; Leong, K.W. Advanced materials and processing for drug delivery: the past and the future. *Adv. Drug Deliv. Rev.* **2013**, *65*(1), 104–120.

Zhang, P.; Zhao, S. R.; Li, J. X.; Hong, L.; Raja, M. A.; Yu, L. J.; Liu, C. G. Nanoparticles Based on Phenylalanine Ethyl Ester–Alginate Conjugate as Vitamin B2 Delivery System. *J. Biomater. Appl.* **2016**, *31*(1), 13–22.

Zhang, C.; Shi, G.; Zhang, J.; Niu, J.; Huang, P.; Wang, Z.; Wang, Y.; Wang, W.; Li C.; Kong, D. Redox- and Light-Responsive Alginate Nanoparticles as Effective Drug Carrier for Combinational Anticancer Therapy. *Nanoscale* **2017**, *9*(9), 3304–3314.

Zhu, B.; Yin, H. Alginate Lyase: Review of Major Sources and Classification, Properties, Structure-Function Analysis and Applications. *Bioengineered* **2015**, *6*(3), 125–131.

CHAPTER 14

ALGINATE-BASED NANOCARRIERS IN MODERN THERAPEUTICS

VANDANA SINGH* and ANGELA SINGH

Department of Chemistry, University of Allahabad, Allahabad, Uttar Pradesh 211002, India

Corresponding author. E-mail: vschemau@ gmail.com

14.1 INTRODUCTION

14.1.1 NANOSCIENCE AND NANOTECHNOLOGY

Advances in the field of nanoscience and nanotechnology have triggered several important breakthroughs in different therapeutic areas. Using this technology, drug delivery can be realized at the nanoscale level for meeting the therapeutic need of the patient while eliciting less adverse effect. This technology has the potential for reaching the outstanding therapeutic efficiency of drugs (Sahoo and Labhasetwar, 2003; Suri et al., 2007). From a biomedical perspective, nanotechnology has opened new vistas to control and manipulate the matter and enabled capitalization on novel properties of biomaterials. This has enhanced the prevention, diagnosis, and treatment of disease and emergence of new fields in the modern therapeutics (Couvreur et al., 2006; Sahoo et al., 2007; Forrest and Kwon, 2008).

The safety efficacy of drugs can be improved by addressing several factors, such as (Bhavsar and Amiji, 2008):

- Aggregation due to their low aqueous solubility
- Unequal absorption along the gastrointestinal (GI) tract
- Risk of degradation in the acidic media of the stomach
- Low permeation of the drugs in the upper GI tract
- Systematic side effects
- Systemic toxicity of cytotoxic drugs

- Short half-lives in blood circulation
- Undesirable pharmacokinetic behavior.

In simple terms, drug delivery can be defined as the procedure of releasing an active agent at a specific site without affecting the healthy organs or tissues. This can be achieved either through passive targeting of drugs to the site of action or by active targeting of the drug but in the current scenario, targeted drug delivery is a bottleneck that must be crossed to exploit the thousands of new therapeutics for a safe and effective administration. Therefore, one of the most desired areas of drug research is the development of techniques such that the drugs can be delivered at the specific site of disease.

The emergence of nanotechnology is expected to have a significant role in the field of nanomedicine as it focuses on the formulation of therapeutic agents using biocompatible nanocarriers. This ensures the carriage of drug to their action sites, which maximizes its desired pharmacological influence. This can overcome the usual limitations and drawbacks which normally hinder the required effectiveness of drugs (Juliano, 1978).

14.1.2 NANOCARRIERS

The prefix nano is derived from Greek word "nanos" which means "dwarf." These days, nano-size carriers have become the most promising vehicles for controlled drug delivery (Peer et al., 2007; Moghimi et al., 2005). Nano-carriers (Nicolas et al., 2013) can be defined as the systems which contain encapsulated, dispersed, adsorbed, or conjugated drugs with carriers having controlled size (preferably 1–1000 nm) and various morphologies such as nanoparticles (NPs), micelles, nanospheres, capsules, polymersomes, nanoliposomes, solid lipid NPs, nanotubes, nanowires, nanocages and dendrimers, and so forth (Figure 14.1) (Tang et al., 2016; Parveen et al., 2012).

14.1.2.1 REQUIRED PARAMETERS FOR IDEAL DRUG CARRIERS

The size of a nanocarrier is one of the most crucial factors to determine the effectiveness of drug delivery with fewer side effects. They should have the following properties for the effective biomedical application (Díaz and Vivas-Mejia, 2013):

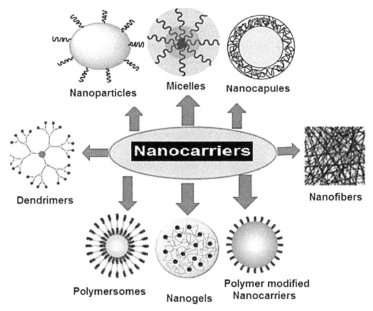

FIGURE 14.1 Polymeric nanocarriers for biomedical applications.

- Significant water solubility or dispersibility, well-controlled nano-size dimension to avoid fast clearance (10–200 nm), and preferred biodistribution
- Biodegradability to minimize side effects, nontoxic, nonimmunogenic, and fully biocompatible nature
- The ability to link with prodrug, targeting component, imaging element, and deliver the therapeutic molecules in a sustained fashion for the period of time that is required to cure the patient
- Steer therapeutic cargos to target tissues or specific cells, thus achieving maximum therapeutic efficiency with minimal toxic side effects under triggered conditions
- Cross the blood–brain barrier by incorporation of moieties which interact with endothelial/astrocytic cell receptors
- The ability to disintegrate in vivo such that its each component is flushed out through the body's clearance mechanism or it identifies the target, that is, the diseased tissue
- The ability to release the drug locally at the disease affected site at the same time releasing a disease-specific signal molecule that is detectable through microanalytical devices

- The ability to carry multiple drugs in a single formulation while maintaining the adequate drug concentration, and/or targeting a drug to a specific site while lowering its systemic levels
- The ability to overcome biological barriers with or without disturbing the immune system.

14.1.3 NANOPARTICLES (NPS) AS DRUG DELIVERY SYSTEMS

In conventional drug delivery, the drug concentration in blood first rises quickly and then declines. This limitation and drawback can be handled by controlling the drug delivery so that its concentration can be sustained for a longer time span (Pridgen et al., 2015; Hunter et al., 2012).

Drug delivery systems (DDSs) are based on interdisciplinary approaches that club polymer science with bioconjugate chemistry, pharmaceutics, and molecular biology. The controlled DDSs transport drug to the place of action where they influence only the diseased tissues, while the healthy tissues remain unaffected; so, there are minimal side effects. In addition, DDS protects the drug from rapid degradation or clearance and enhances the drug concentration in target tissues; therefore, lower doses of drug are now adequate. Nanomaterials-based targeted delivery systems (Salata, 2004) have emerged as area of current research.

At present, NP-based DDSs are considered as one of the largest groups of nanocarriers. Their size ranges from 1 to 1000 nm in diameter (Couvreur et al., 1995; Petros et al., 2010; Brigger et al., 2012; Salatin et al., 2015) and they possess high surface area. Many new therapeutic opportunities have emerged due to the development of new-age nanomaterials as these materials behave as efficient DDSs. The nanomaterials can influence both, the drug loading and the drug release. A number of procedures have been adopted for loading drugs onto the nanomaterials, such as encapsulation, surface attachment, or entrapment (Bertrand et al., 2014; Shi et al., 2009).

The main difficulties and limitations in drug delivery are the early drug release, delivery of relatively copious quantities of drug, release of drug over extended periods, and the rejection of nanocarrier from circulation by self-defense mechanisms of the body.

Biopolymers have diverse architecture, natural abundance, and nontoxicity (Nitta and Numata, 2013). They have been used to design NPs of unique shape and morphology and NP-based drug vehicles have shown an edge over traditional DDSs due to their unique properties (Sharma et al., 2015).

14.1.3.1 DEFINITION OF NPS

"Nanoparticles for pharmaceutical purposes can be defined as the solid colloidal particles consisting of macromolecular materials whose size range from1 to 1000 nm (1 μm) and which can dissolve, encapsulate, or entrap or adsorb or attach the active principle, the drug or the biologically active material."

14.1.3.2 ADVANTAGES OF NPS

NPs, due to their unique properties (Figure 14.2), have gained much attention in the last few decades particularly in the field of drug delivery. The advantages of NP-based DDSs include (Jung et al., 2000; Vauthier and Couvreur, 2000; Reis et al., 2006):

- NPs are capable of passing through the smallest capillary vessels due to their small size. Their rapid clearance by phagocytes is denied because of their ultratiny volume and this prolongs their duration in the bloodstream.
- The NPs easily penetrate cells and tissues for reaching the target organs as they possess subcellular and submicron size.
- They can show controlled release properties due to their biodegradability, pH and/or ion stability, and temperature sensibility.
- Their use has expanded the utility of drugs in terms of minimizing the drug toxicity, enhancing the solubility of hydrophobic drugs, and in providing sustained and controlled release systems for drugs.
- They act as a suitable vehicle to deliver therapeutic concentrations of drugs at the diseased sites of the living system, allowing, therefore, a sustained delivery of drug.
- They help to prevent the "burst release" of the encapsulated drug before reaching the target site in vivo conditions. This has significantly lowered the side effects of many drugs. The encapsulation of drugs in such systems can prevent the possible premature degradation/metabolization of the drug.

The characteristics of a carrier material can be modulated to control the release of a therapeutic agent so that the desired in vivo therapeutic activity of the drug can be sustained for the required duration of time.

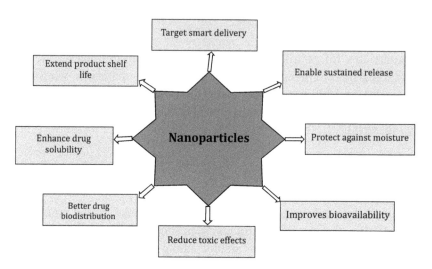

FIGURE 14.2   Advantages of nanoparticles (NPs)-based delivery systems.

14.1.4   POLYMERIC NPS

Polymeric NPs (El-Say and El-Sawy, 2017; Hans and Lowman, 2002) offer significant advantage over other nanocarrier platforms due to the following reasons:

- They can protect the encapsulated drugs from GI enzymes and pH gradients (Uzgiris, 2010) and therefore they can better survive the GI environment as compared to the other colloidal carriers.
- The particle surface of functional polymers can be easily modified through chemical modification (Kamaly et al., 2012). There is tremendous opportunity to ensure better biological interaction with the target organs and cells, and to design size, shape, hydrophobicity, degradation rate, and stimuli-responsiveness.
- The use of polymers allows the modulation of physicochemical characteristics (e.g., hydrophobicity, zeta potential), drug release properties (e.g., delayed, prolonged, triggered), and biological behavior (e.g., targeting, bioadhesion, improved cellular uptake) of the NPs (Lemarchand et al., 2004).

The polymeric NPs have been administered through every possible route: orally, parenterally, nasally, intravaginally, rectally, inhalationally, on the oral mucosa, topically, and in ophthalmic preparations. A drug can be physically entrapped during the formation of polymeric NPs, covalently attached to the precursor materials, or absorbed or adsorbed to the NPs post preparation. As synthetic polymers are toxic to the environment and living beings, only a handful of readily synthesizable polymers have gained regulatory approval for biomedical applications. Natural polysaccharides, because of their outstanding merits, have emerged as the good substitute for synthetic polymers in designing the nanometric drug carriers (Panyam and Labhasetwar, 2003; Herrero-Vanrell et al., 2005).

14.2 ALGINATE: AN OVERVIEW

14.2.1 STRUCTURE AND COMPOSITION

Alginate is a linear anionic polysaccharide sourced from brown algae such as *Laminaria hyperborea, Ascophyllum nodosum, and Macrocystis pyrifera* (Smidsrod and Skjak-Bræk, 1990; Draget et al., 2005). This polysaccharide contains linear blocks of $(1\rightarrow4)$-linked-β-D-mannuronic acid (M) and its C-5 epimer α-L-guluronic acid monomers. These units are linearly linked by 1,4-glycosidic linkages (Figure 14.3) (Caetano et al., 2016; Lee and Mooney, 2012).

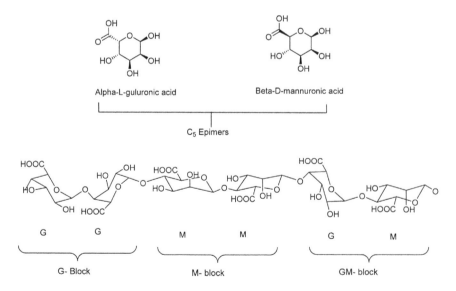

FIGURE 14.3 Chemical structures of alginate.

14.2.2   CHEMICAL AND PHYSICAL PROPERTIES

Alginate comprises different proportion and sequence of consecutive galactose (G) and mannose (M) residues which are arranged in an irregular block-wise pattern, consisting of one type of monomer (M-blocks or G-blocks) or an alternating sequence of M and G residues (MG-blocks) that determines the molecular weight (MW) and physical properties of the alginate and their derived structures (LeRoux and Setton, 1999; Kong et al., 2003). Commercially available alginates have MW ranging from 32,000 to 400,000 g/mol depending on from which source they are extracted. The distribution of alginate MW can control the pregel solution viscosity and gel rigidity which affect the choice of the adequate alginate for a specific use. The mechanical and physical stability of alginate gels depends on G content. Alginate with a high content of G-blocks gives gels of considerably higher strength than the alginates rich in M-blocks. This is due to G residues it exhibits a stronger affinity for divalent ions (Bajpai and Sharma, 2004; Sikorski et al., 2007). Hence, the arrangement of monosaccharide repeats and M/G ratio mainly alters the physicochemical properties of alginate (Lee and Mooney, 2012; Draget, 2005).

14.2.3   IMPORTANT CHARACTERISTICS OF ALGINATE POLYSACCHARIDES

Figure 14.4 summarizes some of the important characteristics of Alginates (Goh et al., 2012; Bidarra et al., 2014; Agüeroa and Zaldivar-Silva, 2017; Shilpa et al., 2003; Zimmermann et al., 2007). Though alginates possess many characteristics which suit a good drug carrier, it also has some inherent drawbacks such as poor mechanical strength, tendency for biodegradation, and extensive water-swelling properties.

14.2.4   AMPHIPHILIC ALGINATE

The multifunctional nature of alginate allows its easy modification through different chemical or physical techniques and therefore alginate-based NPs with diverse properties and miscellaneous structures have been designed. Amphiphilic alginate derivatives can be easily crafted as the NPs and have been extensively utilized for carrying the hydrophobic drugs (Tønnesen and Karlsen, 2002; Murtaza et al., 2011). It can be designed by introducing the hydrophobic groups within the hydrophilic alginate polysaccharide.

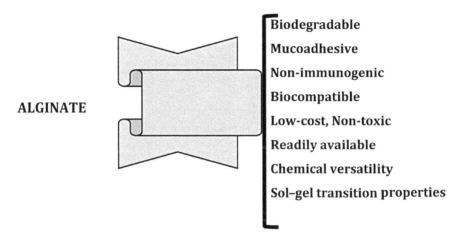

ALGINATE

- Biodegradable
- Mucoadhesive
- Non-immunogenic
- Biocompatible
- Low-cost, Non-toxic
- Readily available
- Chemical versatility
- Sol–gel transition properties

FIGURE 14.4   Important characteristics of alginate.

This has attracted the attention of researchers to use amphiphilic derivates of alginate as the drug carriers in different pharmaceutical and biomedical applications (Paques et al., 2014; Stevens et al., 2004). Alginate has four reactive sites: carboxylic acid and hydroxyl functional groups, and two relatively not sustainable bonds, that is, 1→4 glycosidic and internal glycolic bonds. These sites can be easily manipulated to introduce new functional groups for better performance in different applicability areas (Pawar and Edgar, 2012; Oliveira and Reis, 2011; Kuo and Ma, 2001; Ionita et al., 2013).

The existing properties of alginates such as ionic gel strength, hydrophilicity, and shelf life can be altered through chemical modification and completely new properties can be induced through such alterations. Carboxyl groups and hydroxyl groups on the alginate backbone have been diversely modified to tailor many properties of alginate such as physicochemical, biological, and mechanical (Figure 14.5) (Hua et al., 2010). In short, derivatization is the most convenient route for enhancing the inherent properties of alginate and also for the induction of new properties (Yang et al., 2011).

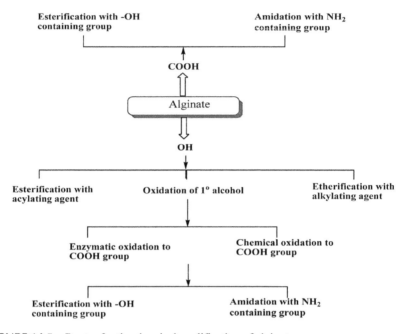

FIGURE 14.5   Routes for the chemical modification of alginates.

14.3   CRAFTING OF ALGINATE NPS

Polymeric NPs can be crafted through several techniques (Lopes et al., 2016) (Figure 14.6). Table 14.1 presents the techniques which have been adopted for the preparation of alginate NPs, specifically for drug delivery application (Ahmed et al., 2013; Chuah et al., 2009; Agüero et al., 2017).

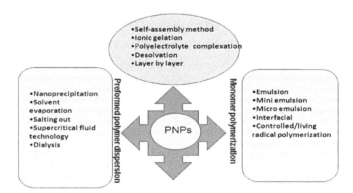

FIGURE 14.6   Summary of various techniques used in the preparation of polymer NPs.

TABLE 14.1 Methods used for the Preparation of Alginate-Based Nanoparticles (NPs).

Methods	Characteristics
Self-assembly method	Spontaneous formation of NPs by polymeric amphiphiles involving intra- and/or intermolecular association between the hydrophobic moieties
Polyelectrolyte (PE) complexation	Polysaccharides with opposite charge surface can form polysaccharides NPs by electrostatic attraction
Layer-by-layer self-assembly	Repeated deposition of oppositely charged polymers (e.g., negative-charged alginate and positive-charged chitosan in acid conditions) on material surfaces as PE multilayers
Covalent cross-linking	Chemical interaction
Ionic cross-linking	Polyanions/polycations with low molecular weight can act as ionic cross-linkers for charged polysaccharides
Emulsification method	Two immiscible phases are combined

14.3.1 SELF-ASSEMBLED NPS

Self-assembly is a ubiquitous process of NPs formation. It utilizes amphiphilic polymers which can be readily designed by covalently attaching the hydrophobic molecules onto the hydrophilic backbone (Figure 14.7) (Agüero et al., 2017; Hassani et al., 2012; Branco and Schneider, 2009). The introduction of hydrophobic segments in hydrophilic macromolecular backbone forms amphiphilic polymers which can form self-assembled nanostructures with unique rheological characteristics such as micelles, particles, and hydrogels (Alexis et al., 2010; Mei et al., 2013).

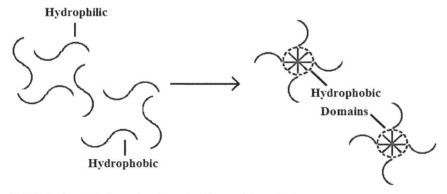

Hydrophilic

Hydrophobic

Hydrophobic Domains

FIGURE 14.7 NP formation through self-assembly method.

The self-assembly of amphiphilic molecules is an aqueous procedure and does not require any harsh reaction condition or solvents. The amphiphilic macromolecules spontaneously form self-aggregates by undergoing intra- and/or intermolecular hydrophobic association between hydrophobic moieties in an aqueous environment and form NPs to minimize the interfacial free energy (Kabanov et al., 1992; Hassani et al., 2012). The main driving forces in the self-assembly process are usually hydrophobic interactions, which originate from the rearrangement of water molecules as two nonpolar molecules come close to each other to avoid aqueous surroundings and electrostatic forces of interactions (Dalhaimer et al., 2004; Mortensen, 2001) that can be either repulsive or attractive depending on the surface charge of the interacting components. The self-assembly of alginate usually involves more than one driving forces. Hydrogen bonds are formed either intramolecularly or intermolecularly through specific binding sites on the backbone. In fact, the electrostatic interactions, hydrophobic interactions; hydrogen bonds, and van der Waals forces take their own roles simultaneously. The mechanism of self-assembly is a combined effect of these noncovalent forces and determined by the major driving force (Rotureau et al., 2005; Whitesides et al., 1991). The concentration at which the polymer aggregation starts is usually called the critical aggregation concentration (Ren et al., 2006). There are various hydrophobic molecules that can be attached to alginate in order to obtain these kind of systems, such as poly(ethylene glycol) derivatives, long-chain fatty acids, poly(ε-caprolactone), aliphatic alcohols (octanol or hexadecanol), pluronic copolymers, cholesterol, and poly(isobutyl cyanoacrylate) (Pelletier et al., 2001; Vallee et al., 2009).

Amphiphilic cholesteryl-grafted sodium alginate has been prepared in aqueous NaCl solution at room temperature using N,N-dicyclohexyl carbodiimide as a coupling agent and 4-dimethylaminopyridine as the catalyst (Yang et al., 2007). Sodium alginate with cholesteryl grafts (as the hydrophobic segments) possesses better biocompatibility as it can better interact with the cholesteryl receptors on the cell surface and also it has a stronger ability to form self-assembly. The major driving forces for self-assembly were intra- and intermolecular interactions which controlled the self-aggregation in aqueous NaCl solution. This included the hydrogen bonding among hydrophilic sodium alginate backbones and water molecules. As such the electrostatic repulsive interaction between anionic $-COO^-$ keeps the alginate main chains separated and inhibits the self-assembly of the macromolecules (Liu et al., 2004). Cholesteryl-grafted sodium alginate has been used in the controlled release of drugs and growth factors in pharmacology and tissue engineering applications (Yusa et al., 1998).

Zhang et al. (2012) studied doxorubicin-loaded glycyrrhetinic-acid-modified alginate NPs for liver tumor chemotherapy. The NPs showed strong liver-targeting efficiency owing to passive targeting through the enhanced permeability, retention effects, and the active targeting efficiency of glycyrrhetinic acid. Cardiac toxicity was reduced after the administration of the NPs (Guo et al., 2013).

Anirudhan et al. (2017) grafted polyethylene glycol (PEG) to polyethyleneimine (PEI) to form PEG-g-PEI (mPPS), which was then coupled with folic acid (FA) to form FA-PEG-g-PEI (PPF). PPF was then finally assembled with curcumin (CUR)-loaded alginate NP. These NPs were used in the targeted oral delivery of CUR. The FA acted as a targeting ligand, which selectively targeted the cancer cell lines with overexpressed folate receptors. The coupling of PEG and FA increased the cytocompatibility of PEI and the incorporation of PPF increased the stability of alginate NPs. The functionalization with FA also increased the targeting effect of the carrier. The cell viability of CUR-loaded carrier was less than 40%.

The biomedical application of NPs-based DDSs offers a new perspective for the treatment of tuberculosis. Zahoor et al. (2005) studied the pharmacokinetics and tissue distribution of free and alginate-encapsulated antitubercular drugs. Drugs such as isoniazid, rifampicin, pyrazinamide, and ethambutol were encapsulated in alginate NPs and were orally administered to mice. The average size of particles was found to be 235.5 ± 0.0 nm, with drug encapsulation abilities of 70–90, 80–90, and 88–95% for isoniazid, rifampicin, and ethambutol, respectively.

Amphiphilic conjugate nanostructures consisting of alginate and α-tocopherol were synthesized through esterification reaction. α-Tocopherol was entrapped in the hydrophobic microdomains of the nanostructures (Fayin et al., 2017). The aim of the study was to evaluate the ability of entrapped α-tocopherol in inhibiting lipid oxidation in an oil-in-water (o/w) emulsion. The percent entrapment and loading efficiency of α-tocopherol in the self-assembled nanostructures of the conjugate were 4.92–16.82 and 78.83–92.32%, respectively. The alginate–α-tocopherol conjugate nanostructures greatly increased the water dispersibility as well as antioxidant activity of α-tocopherol.

Amphiphilic alginate esters with a different degree of substitution have been synthesized by Yang et al. (2013). Hydrophobic alkyl length was introduced through the reaction between partially protonated sodium alginate and aliphatic alcohols (octanol, dodecanol, or hexadecanol). These amphiphilic alginate esters could easily self-aggregate into NPs in aqueous solution at room temperature. The morphology of the self-assembled particles of alginate esters was regular (spherical with the size about 100–200 nm).

Chang et al. (2012) developed amphiphilic thiolated sodium alginate. Its sonication facilitated the oxidation reaction of thiol groups, which induced the self-assembly of the alginate molecules into nano-aggregates. These alginate nano-aggregates were loaded with insulin (Sarmento et al., 2006) antisense oligonucleotide (Aynié et al., 1999), and anticancer drugs, such as methotrexate (Santhi et al., 2005) and 5-fluorouracil (Yu et al., 2008).

14.3.2   POLYELECTROLYTE (PE) COMPLEXATION METHOD

Polyelectrolytes (PEs) are macromolecules materials, which have multitudinous ionizable functional groups of different MWs and chemical compositions. They undergo partial or complete dissociation in aqueous solutions to create a charge on the macromolecules (Lankalapalli and Kolapalli, 2009; Liu, 1998). Polyelectrolyte complexes (PECs) are formed by simultaneous mixing of oppositely charged PEs in solution. Owing to intra- and/or intermolecular hydrophobic interactions, the amphiphilic polysaccharides can self-associate in aqueous solution to form NPs (Figure 14.8) (Deeksha, 2014). If any PE solution contains a positively charged electrolyte, it can be accompanied by small negatively charged ions, that is, charge on the repeating units of the PE is neutralized by oppositely charged smaller counterions that tend to preserve the electroneutrality (Dakhara and Anajwala, 2010).

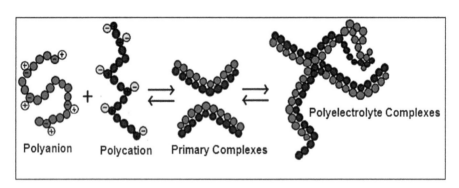

FIGURE 14.8   Schematic diagram for polyelectrolyte (PE) complexation.

In contrast to chemically cross-linked complexes, PEC is generally nontoxic, well-tolerated, and biocompatible as their formation does not involve the use of chemical cross-linkers. Such complexes present clear advantages as pharmaceutical excipients in controlling drug release.

The mechanism for particle formation involves noncovalent, cooperative electrostatic interactions, which are predominate, between polycations and polyanions. When the aqueous solutions of oppositely charged PEs are mixed, formation of a dense phase separates from the solvent when ionic strength, pH of the reaction medium, concentration of PEs, distribution of ionic groups, MW of the polymer, and the mixing ratio are controlled. The order of reacting PEs also influences the degree of ionization which in turn results in the NPs formation (Kuroiwa et al., 2015; Dakhara and Anajwala, 2010). PE complexation occurs mainly between the oppositely charged species, that is, PE–PE complexes, PE–drug complexes, PE–nucleic acid complexes, and PE–surfactant complexes (De Robertis, 2015).

14.3.2.1   PE–PE–PE COMPLEXES

14.3.2.1.1   Alginate–Chitosan PEC

PECs of chitosan and sodium alginate have been prepared by using various methods. A one-step process involves the gradual addition of alginate solution to a chitosan solution (with or without calcium ions) to induce the electrostatic interactions between the two polysaccharides to form the NPs (Daly and Knorr, 1988).

In an alternative method, alginate–calcium pre-gel is prepared before the addition of chitosan to ensure the strong polymeric network (Hackel et al., 1975; Skjåk-Br and Martinsen, 1991). The alginate–chitosan pluronic tripolymeric NPs have received much attention as these are usually prepared in low concentration (<0.1%) with a relatively small mass ratio (Das et al., 2010). The particles have been used as the carrier for CUR, which is a small molecule with poor water solubility. Pluronic was included in order to handle the solubility problem of CUR. Meanwhile, the drug release from the NPs was much faster than that of microparticles and beads. This better performance was assigned to the smaller particle size of the NPs, which have a large surface-area-to-mass ratio. The encapsulation efficiency of CUR in chitosan–alginate-pluronic tripolymeric NPs was 5–10 times greater than chitosan–alginate NPs (without pluronic) because, in the presence of pluronic, CUR had better solubility in aqueous calcium chloride. This novel tripolymeric delivery system is unique as it encapsulated hydrophobic drugs.

The alginate/chitosan NPs have been used as the platform for delivery of quercetin, which is a natural antioxidant that has anti-inflammatory, antiana-phylaxis, antiaging, and antiproliferative effects (Aluani et al., 2017). The NP formulations of different sizes and charges were prepared by varying the two polysaccharides. The antioxidant effects of quercetin-loaded NPs with higher chitosan content were superior to quercetin-encapsulated NPs which had higher sodium alginate content.

Alginate–chitosan NPs have been also used as the vehicle for oral delivery of crocin (Rahaiee et al., 2017). The NPs loaded with crocin behaved as the prospective candidates for the future anticancer therapeutics. The drug release was pH dependent. The swelling of these NPs was minimal at the acidic pH of the stomach; however, as they pass down the intestinal tract, the extent of swelling increased due to an increase in the pH. There was negligible release at pH 1.2, while it was maximum at pH 7.4.

The hybrid NPs of chitosan and alginate were shown to have muco-adhesive properties and they have been used as the drug carriers for the prolonged topical ophthalmic delivery of gatifloxacin. It has been found that the incorporation of alginate is an effective strategy for increasing the transfection efficiency of chitosan NPs as it modulates and improves the delivery of the associated plasmid (Motwani et al., 2008).

The alginate–chitosan hybrid NPs have also been used for encapsulating vitamin B_2 and the encapsulation efficiency and loading capacity of the material were investigated. Alginate and chitosan NPs, prepared by iono-tropic PE pre-gelation showed encapsulation efficiency and loading capacity values of 55.9 ± 5.6 and $2.2 \pm 0.6\%$, respectively (Maria et al., 2014). Fathi and Varshosaz (2013) carried out preservation and release study of hesper-etin flavonoid using chitosan–alginate nanocarriers. The results showed that above-mentioned two polymers well protected "hesperetin" against acidic conditions which resulted in about 11% release after 2 h of incubation. Also, the alginate–chitosan NPs were prepared by ionotropic pre-gelation for encapsulation of drug nifedipine. The encapsulation had not only protected "nifedipine" loss in acid environment but also controlled the drug release in the intestinal tract. The drug release was slow and this gastric protection against nifedipine release can be related to the more effective retention by a firm alginate matrix that was formed at low pH (Li et al., 2008).

Venlafaxine-loaded alginate NPs have been prepared in two-step proce-dures based on the ionotropic pre-gelation of alginate with calcium chloride followed by cross-linking by polycationic chitosan (Haque et al., 2014). Venlafaxine inhibited dual-action serotonin and norepinephrine reuptake inhibitor and increased their diminished levels in the synaptic cleft between neurons in the brain (Wilson et al., 2007). Brain uptake and pharmacokinetic studies were carried out by determining the venlafaxine concentration in blood and brain, respectively, using venlafaxine-loaded alginate NPs. The greater brain/blood ratios for the NPs in comparison to venlafaxine solution indicated the superiority of alginate NPs for the direct nose to brain transport of the drug. Sarmento et al. (2007a) designed insulin-loaded NPs using alginate ionotropic pre-gelation followed by chitosan PE complexations. The NPs could preserve the secondary structure of insulin which is needed for its bioactivity (Sarmento et al., 2007b; Sarmento et al., 2007c). The optimized NPs had high (92%) association efficiency and 14.3% loading degree. Moreover, the NPs could retain about 50% insulin for 24 h at gastric pH conditions, while 75% release was witnessed at the intestinal pH environment (Sarmento et al., 2007d).

14.3.2.1.2 Alginate-Poly-l-Lysine PEC

Alginate NPs were synthesized through a microfluidic mixing device by PE complexation between aqueous Ca–alginate pre-gels and cationic poly-l-lysine (PLL) solutions under mild aqueous environment. The NPs exhibited enhanced aggregation stability. Their size ranged from 380 to 520 nm depending on the flow rates of the Ca–alginate pre-gel and PLL solutions (Kim et al., 2015). The NPs were capable of encapsulating several types of drugs, such as antitumor agents and oligonucleotides (Rajaonarivony et al., 1993; Aynie et al., 1999).

Rajaonarivony et al. (1993) synthesized alginate poly-l-lysine NPs (250–850 nm) for doxorubicin delivery by adding calcium chloride in a sodium alginate solution that pre-contained doxorubicin. Finally, polylysine was added to obtain the NPs.

14.3.2.1.3 Alginate-Gelatin PEC

Oxidized alginate and gelatin complex was produced using periodate-oxidized sodium alginate of appropriate MW and degree of oxidation. It rapidly cross-linked with gelatin in the presence of small concentration of sodium tetraborate (borax) to give injectable NPs for tissue engineering, drug delivery, and other medical applications (Balakrishnan et al., 2005). CUR-loaded cationized gelatin/alginate hybrid PE (CG/Alg) complex NPs have been prepared from cationically modified gelatin and sodium alginate. Ethylenediamine was used to derive cationized gelatin from gelatin CG–alginate complex NPs that showed anticancer activity in MCF-7 cells and thus the NPs can find use in promising therapy (Sarika and James, 2016).

14.3.2.1.4   Alginate–Albumin PEC

Bovine serum albumin (BSA) and thiolated alginate (alginate–cysteine conjugate) NPs have been prepared by coacervation method. These were loaded with tamoxifen (TMX) drug. The administration of 10 μm TMX by TMX-NPs was effective in both MCF-7 and HeLa cell and the effect of the drug-loaded systems on MCF-7 cell cycle showed the efficacy of the TMX-loaded NPs (Martinez et al., 2011).

14.3.2.2   PE–DRUG BASED PECS

14.3.2.2.1   Alginate–Exemestane PEC

Exemestane (EXE) is an oral chemotherapeutic drug that is used for the treatment of breast cancer. The drug's side effects were significantly reduced by using it in the form of alginate–EXE PEC and the release of the drug took place in a controlled manner. The drug was loaded by simple gelation method and was evaluated in vitro to study the performance of alginate–EXE in delivering the drug EXE. The in vitro evaluations of the EXE-loaded alginate NPs proved the successful loading and sustained release profile of alginate NPs (Jayapal and Dhanaraj, 2017).

14.3.2.3   PE–SURFACTANT PEC

14.3.2.3.1   Alginate–Aerosol OT PEC

Alginate Aerosol OT™ NPs (Chavanpatil et al., 2007) of 40–70 nm size were prepared for the sustained release of water-soluble drugs. In vitro release studies with basic drug molecules such as methylene blue, doxorubicin, rhodamine, verapamil, and clonidine indicated that the NPs were able to release 60–70% of the encapsulated drug over the duration of 4 weeks. The release was near-zero order during first 15 days. The NPs had poorer drug encapsulation efficiency for anionic drug molecules, while it was rapid for the basic drugs.

14.3.3   COVALENTLY CROSS-LINKED NPS

NP preparation by covalent cross-linking method involves the introduction of covalent bonds between the PEs polysaccharides chains such as polyanions or polycations, which are present in ionic form in aqueous media at mild alkaline and at low pH (Figure 14.9) (Nesamony et al., 2012). However, this method is often avoided due to possible undesired side reactions with the active ingredient and the toxicity of the cross-linking agents (Goh et al., 2012).

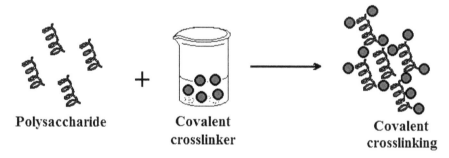

Polysaccharide   **Covalent crosslinker**   **Covalent crosslinking**

FIGURE 14.9   Covalent cross-linking method.

The carboxylic acid groups at alginate can ionize to make the polysaccharide surface negative. This anionic PE aggregates with cationic PE such as chitosan and after subsequent cross-linking with micromolecular substances of opposite charge, NPs are obtained through electrostatic interaction, for example, alginate gelation can be induced by cross-linking of the guluronic acid units with di- or polyvalent cations.

Thiolated alginate and modified albumin have been cross-linked through a disulfide bond to form NPs. To obtain the sulfhydryl group at albumin, it was reduced and was subsequently cross-linked with the polysaccharide using carbodiimide reaction. The size of the NPs varied from 42 to 388 nm depending on the pH (Martínez et al., 2012).

A nanoformulation based on sodium alginate/gum acacia and isometamidium hydrochloride (ISMM) was synthesized. ISMM is an effective drug for the treatment of trypanosomiasis. The formulation had better efficacy than the neat drug and it released the drug in a sustained way with minimum side effects (Chopra et al., 2012).

14.3.4 IONIC CROSS-LINKED NPS

Physical cross-linking of polysaccharides is based on ionic interactions between charged polysaccharides and oppositely charged cross-linkers (Figure 14.10). This can be done at room temperature under mild conditions without using any organic solvents (Patil et al., 2010; Kuo and Ma, 2001).

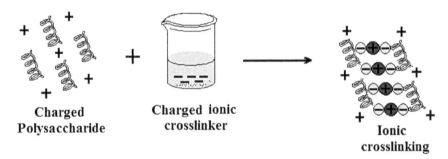

Charged Polysaccharide   Charged ionic crosslinker   Ionic crosslinking

FIGURE 14.10   Ionic cross-linking method.

Ionically cross-linked NPs are generally pH sensitive, and therefore they are very useful in designing stimuli-sensitive controlled release systems. They are promising agents for the encapsulation of fragile drugs (e.g., peptides and proteins) as they preserve their therapeutic function. The low-MW cations and anions can be used as the cross-linkers for charged polysaccharides.

The carboxylic acid groups at alginate can be cross-linked through bivalent calcium ions (Aslani and Kennedy, 1996; Bystricky et al., 1990). The clusters formed in the pre-gel phase can be subsequently stabilized with polycations such as polylysine and chitosan (Lertsutthiwong et al., 2009). Alginate has been cross-linked with polylysine through the formation of PEC with or without the previous formation of the pre-gel phase with calcium. The concentration and MW of alginate showed significant impact on the size of the NPs. NPs with an average size ranging from 194 nm to 1.6 μm were obtained and have been utilized as drug carriers. In general, the carboxylic acid group containing polysaccharides can be easily cross-linked by bivalent calcium ion to form the NPs (Fundueanu, 1999).

Zahoor et al. (2005) prepared Ca–alginate NPs (235.5±0 nm in size) through ion-induced gelification method. The NPs encapsulated isoniazid, pyrazinamide with 70–90% efficiency, while rifampicin was encapsulated with 80–90% efficiency. The relative bioavailabilities of all the encapsulated drugs were significantly higher than the oral free drugs. These inhalable NPs could serve as an ideal carrier for the controlled release of antitubercular drugs.

Chen et al. (2012) blended alginate with N,O-carboxymethyl chitosan cross-linked with genipin. The material showed pH-dependent release of Bovine Serum Albumin (BSA). Only 20% of the drug was released at pH 1.2, while rest of the 80% drug was released at pH 7.4. Rajaonarivony et al. (1993) added calcium chloride and polylysine in a sodium alginate solution that pre-contained doxorubicin for obtaining alginate NPs (250–850 nm) for drug delivery. The synthesis of nanocarrier having high drug encapsulation efficiency ranging from 70% to 90% was achieved by alginate-based NPs, which were prepared by the controlled cation-induced gelification method and administered orally.

In a similar study, alginate NPs have been used for the encapsulation of the antifungal drugs clotrimazole and econazole and the antituberculosis drugs (rifampicin, ethambutol, isoniazid, and pyrazinamide) using a modified cation-induced controlled gelification. The average size of particles was found to be 235.5±0.0 nm, with drug encapsulation abilities of 70–90%, 80–90%, and 88–95% for isoniazid, rifampicin, and ethambutol, respectively.

Alginate/chitosan NPs have been evaluated for mucopenetration during the release of amoxicillin, a drug used for treating infection caused by *Helicobacter pylori*, a pathogen that colonizes the deep gastric mucosa lining. Lower mucoadhesiveness was witnessed for the combination though it had greater mucopenetration than pure chitosan (Arora et al., 2011).

Goycoolea et al. (2009) developed the NPs by ionic gelation of chitosan hydrochloride with pentasodium tripolyphosphate (TPP) and complexing with sodium alginate. The material was used for the transmucosal delivery of macromolecules. The nanoparticles have shown enhanced systemic absorption of insulin after nasal administration to conscious rabbits.

14.3.5   EMULSIFICATION METHOD

Emulsification is a regular method which is often used for the preparation of polymer NPs. In this process, two immiscible phases are combined where the dispersed phase is spread as small droplets within the continuous phase. This method involves two steps: (i) preparation of an emulsified system (Vauthier and Bouchemal, 2009) using high-energy emulsification techniques such as ultrasonication, high-speed homogenization, and mechanical shearing. The narrowly dispersed emulsion can be formulated by using the techniques such as capillary, microchannel emulsification, straight-through microchannel emulsification and microfluidic approach; (ii) the formation of NPs (Desgouilles et al., 2003) and preformed polymer dispersion (Quintanar-Guerrero et al.,1999) which is executed by solvent evaporation, salting-out, supercritical fluid technology, and dialysis techniques (Figure 14.11) or by monomer polymerization (Kulkarni et al., 1971) using different mechanisms of polymerization such as controlled radical polymerization, emulsion, surfactant-free emulsion, mini-emulsion, microemulsion, and interfacial polymerization. In addition, NPs can be fabricated through an inter/intramolecular cross-linking processes. These systems can be classified as single (one interface) emulsion, for example, o/w, (Wu et al., 2015) water-in-oil (w/o), (Quintanar-Guerrero et al., 1998) liquid-in-liquid or solid-in-liquid emulsions (Jeong et al., 2008; Han et al., 2009). Apart from the simple o/w emulsion systems, double/multiple (more than one interface) emulsions having multiple components such as water-in oil-in water, water-in-oil-in-oil, and solid-in-oil-in-oil may be used. Furthermore, mini-emulsions, nano-emulsions, and microemulsions are also used in place of classical emulsions (Anton et al., 2008; Bouchemal et al., 2004).

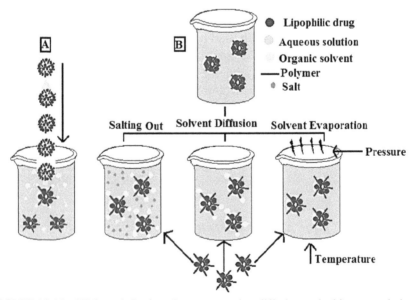

FIGURE 14.11   NP formulation by solvent evaporation, diffusion, and salting-out techniques.

Alginate NPs have been successfully prepared using the emulsification/internal gelation method by creating ideal conditions for the formulation and have recently been extended to the field of nanotechnology (Khdair et al., 2010; Akbari et al., 2014).

Entrapment of silk sericin into alginate NPs (Khampieng et al., 2015) provided several advantages which have been exploited for a wide range of applications such as antioxidant, anticoagulant, and anti-wrinkle. The NPs were prepared by using an emulsification method which was followed by internal cross-linking. When sericin loading was increased from 20 to 80%, the thermal stability of the material increased above 240°C.

Calcium alginate NPs of approximately 200 nm were synthesized by w/o emulsion using tetraethylene glycol monododecyl ether as a nonionic surfactant (Machado et al., 2012). Alginate NPs developed through a w/o emulsion method and physical cross-linking with calcium ions showed more than 71% encapsulation efficiency for insulin. It was demonstrated that at high calcium ion concentrations, more calcium ions are free to react with the M and G of alginate monomers and more rigid alginate polymer chains resulted which allowed sustainable insulin release from the alginate NPs (Reis et al., 2006).

Chitosan–alginate NPs of size 200 nm was developed by an emulsion method to incorporate 5-Fluorouracil (5-FU) drug for cancer. In vitro release of 50% drug was observed in 12 h (Xing et al., 2010).

Alginate–chitosan NPs have been used for the effective delivery of BSA. Low-MW alginate and chito-oligosaccharide NPs were developed using a microemulsion method. The average size of the NPs was ~136 nm and the encapsulation efficiency reached approximately 88.4% (Wang and He, 2010).

Using the same microemulsion method, alginate NPs were developed using aqueous $CaCl_2$, dioctyl sodium sulfosuccinate, and isopropyl myristate for sustained release of BSA. The loading efficiency of BSA was approximately 40% (Nesamony et al., 2012).

14.3.6 LAYER BY SELF-ASSEMBLY METHOD

The layer-by-layer technique, also referred to as electrostatic self-assembly, is a commonly employed method that produces NPs made of PE multilayers at solid substrates, where cationic and anionic PEs are alternately deposited onto a charged solid substrate (e.g., particles) such as alginate and chitosan or polylysine (Figure 14.12). The charge–charge interaction between the substrate and the monolayers of PEs creates multiple-layered NPs which are held together by electrostatic force (Zhou et al., 2010).

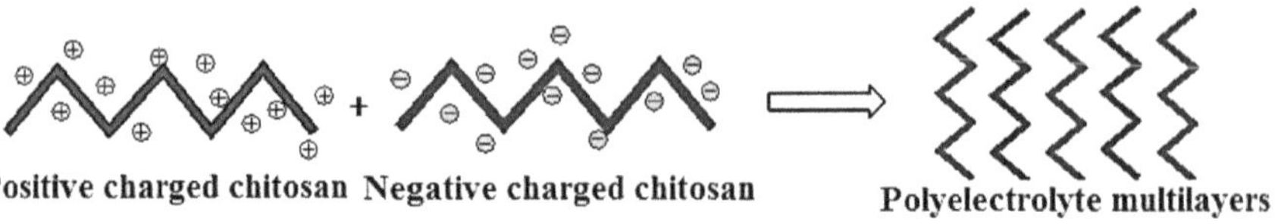

Positive charged chitosan Negative charged chitosan   **Polyelectrolyte multilayers**

FIGURE 14.12   Layer-by-layer self-assembly method.

Core–shell hybrid NPs have been designed by Haidar et al. (2008) by layer-by-layer assembly of alginate and chitosan on liposomes and have been used for the delivery of BSA. The delivery system had a spherical, monodisperse shape, and was sufficiently stable. It had a cumulative size of 383 ± 11.5 nm and zeta potential surface charge of 44.61 ± 3.31 mV for five bilayered liposomes. The system offered numerous compartments for encapsulation and showed good entrapment and sustained linear release of a model protein, BSA, in vitro. This delivery system exhibited an extended shelf life and could be loaded just before the administration and therefore no protein was lost.

Hong et al. (2008) utilized the core of liposomes with a high bilayer melting temperature as the reaction vessels to template the assembly of alginate. In this procedure, alginate was encapsulated in the liposomal core and exposed to a calcium chloride solution at a temperature above the melting point of the bilayer. This enabled the passage of calcium ions into the core followed by the gradual gelation of alginate. Finally, the liposome was removed with surfactants to form 120–200-nm-sized NPs of alginate.

14.3.7   SPRAY-DRYING METHOD

Spray-drying is a well-known process, which has been used to convert the NP suspensions in dry powder. Erdinc and Neufeld (2011) prepared alginate-based NPs with spherical shapes and high encapsulation efficiency by this technique. Alginate NPs associated with silica were prepared with the incorporation of magnetic iron oxide colloids for the development of multifunctional biocapsules (Boissière et al., 2007).

Ghaffari et al. (2012) developed ciprofloxacin-alginate–chitosan NPs. The loading efficiency of ciprofloxacin was 88%. A sustained release of ciprofloxacin was observed over 45 h. Chitosan–alginate NPs for strep-tomycin delivery are reported. Their drug encapsulation efficiency was 93.32% and the average size of the NPs was 328 nm (Chopra et al., 2012). Several other alginate–chitosan NPs encapsulating antimicrobial drugs have also been reported (Balaure et al., 2013; Zohri et al., 2010). Thus, the available literature revealed that alginate is a quite versatile natural polymer which has been used to design the NPs of various shapes, properties, and performances. Their tremendous use as DDS is based upon the favorable properties of alginate which include biocompatibility and ease of gelation. Alginate-based gels possess structural similarity to the extracellular matrices in tissues and thus has can be easily manipulated to entrap bioactive agents such as small chemical drugs and proteins to design nanomaterials for drug release. The NPs derived from alginate have played several critical roles in modern therapeutics. Drug molecules ranging from small chemical drugs to macromolecular proteins have been released from alginate-derived NPs in a controlled manner, depending on the nature of the method adopted for the NP preparation (Table 14.2).

The present understating of fundamental properties of alginate and developing new types of cell and tissue-interactive alginate NPs with improved properties may enable many future advances in modern therapeutics.

SUMMARY

The recent advances in nanotechnology have led to the development of many powerful drug delivery tools. Such drug carriers offer a suitable means of site-specific and/or time-controlled delivery of small- or large-molecular-weight drugs and other bioactive agents. Natural excipients seem to be the most promising materials for the preparation of micro- and nanometric carriers as they have several advantages over their synthetic counterparts, generally because they are safe, nontoxic, biocompatible, and biodegradable. Nevertheless, they are low cost, eco-friendly, and abundant materials. In general, the use of micro/nanoparticles (NPs) offers wide biomedical applications over other drug delivery systems (DDSs). They are used to enhance the solubility of highly hydrophobic drugs, sustained and controlled release of encapsulated drugs over prolonged periods, protection against premature drug degradation and reduction in drug toxicity and drug–drug interactions, increase in the stability of therapeutic agents by chemical or physical means, and delivery of drug in higher concentrations to target areas. Alginate, a promising natural polymer, has gained considerable attention as drug delivery vehicle owing to its ease of availability, compatibility with hydrophobic as well as hydrophilic molecules, high binding capacity, good absorption efficiency, controlled release as well as bioadhesive properties. It has an abundance of free hydroxyl and carboxyl groups along its

TABLE 14.2 Drug Delivery Applications of Alginate-Based NPs.

Materials	Methods	Drugs	Purpose	References
Alginate–glycyrrhetinic acid	Self-assembly method	Doxorubicin	Liver tumor chemotherapy	Zhang et al. (2012), Guo et al. (2013)
Alginate–polyethylene glycol and polyethylene amine	Self-assembly method	Curcumin (CUR)	Cancer therapy	Anirudhan et al. (2017)
Alginate–chitosan–pluronic	Polyelectrolyte complex (PEC)	CUR	Cancer therapy	Aluani et al. (2017)
Alginate–chitosan	PEC	Quercetin	Antioxidant	Rahaiee et al. (2017)
Alginate–chitosan	PEC	Crocin	Anticancer therapeutics	Motwani et al. (2008)
Sodium alginate–chitosan	Ionic gelation, PE	Gatifloxacin	Extraocular disease treatment	Azevedo et al. (2014)
Alginate–chitosan	Ionotropic pre-gelation and PE	Riboflavin	Essential for growth and development	Fathi and Varshosaz (2013)
Alginate–chitosan	PEC	Hesperetin flavonoid		Li et al. (2008)
Alginate–chitosan	PEC	Nifedipine	Delivery of hydrophobic drugs	Haque et al. (2014)
Alginate–chitosan	Ionic gelation, PE	Venlafaxine	Treatment of depression	Wilson et al. (2007), Sarmento et al. (2007a)
Alginate–chitosan	Ionotropic and PEC	Insulin	Antidiabetic oral formulation	Sarmento et al. (2007b), Sarmento et al. (2007c), Sarmento et al. (2007d), Kim et al. (2015)
Alginate–chitosan	PEC	Ciprofloxacin	Antimicrobial drugs	Ghaffari et al. (2012)
Alginate–chitosan	Ionotropic pre-gelation and PE	Streptomycin	Antimicrobial drugs	Chopra et al., 2012

TABLE 14.2 (*Continued*)

Materials	Methods	Drugs	Purpose	References
Alginate–chitosan	Gelification	Nisin	Antibiotic drug delivery	Balaure et al. (2013), Zohri et al. (2010)
Alginate–poly-l-lysine	Gelification with CaCl$_2$ and poly-l-lysine	Doxorubicin	Chemotherapy and photodynamic therapy	Sarika and James (2016)
Alginate–gelatin	PEC	CUR	Cancer therapy	Jayapal and Dhanaraj (2017)
Alginate–albumin	Coacervation method	Tamoxifen	Cancer therapy	Chavanpatil et al. (2007)
Alginate–exemestane (EXE)	Gelation method	EXE	Breast cancer	Nesamony et al. (2012)
Aerosol OT-alginate NPs	PEC	Methylene blue, doxorubicin, rhodamine, verapamil, and clonidine	Delivery of basic drugs	Martínez et al. (2012)
Sodium alginate/gum acacia	Covalent cross-linking	Isometamidium hydrochloride	Treatment of trypanosomiasis	Aslani and Kennedy (1996)
Alginate NPs	Ion-induced gelification method	Isoniazid, pyrazinamide, rifampicin	Antibiotic drug delivery	Vauthier and Bouchemal (2009)
Alginate–chitosan	Ion-induced gelification method	BSA	Protein drug delivery	Desgouilles et al. (2003)
Alginate–chitosan	Ion-induced gelification method	Amphiphloxin	Antibiotic drug delivery	Quintanar-Guerrero et al. (1999)
Alginate–chitosan	Gelification	Insulin	Antidiabetic oral formulation	Kulkarni et al. 1971
Alginate NPs	Emulsion method	Silk sericin	Antioxidant, anticoagulant, and anti-wrinkle	Nesamony et al. (2012)

TABLE 14.2 *(Continued)*

Materials	Methods	Drugs	Purpose	References
Alginate NPs	Water-in-oil emulsion method	Insulin	Antidiabetic oral formulation	Haidar et al. (2008)
Alginate–chitosan	Emulsion method	5-Fluorouracil	Cancer therapy	Hong et al. (2008)
Alginate–oligochitosan	Water-in-oil microemulsion method	BSA	Protein drug delivery	Erdinc and Neufeld (2011)
Alginate NPs	Microemulsion method	BSA	Protein drug delivery	Boissière et al. (2007)

backbone which can be easily modified to obtain tailor-made products for DDSs. Alginate-based nanocarriers have been used for various therapeutic purposes. These carriers with sizes ranging from 20 to 800 nm have been designed using ionic cross-linking, covalent cross-linking, precipitation, polymerization, self-assembly methods, and PE complexation. This chapter focuses on a comprehensive overview of the recent advances in the development of new alginate-based nanoparticles as DDSs through the manipulation of its chemical and structural properties.

KEYWORDS

- **alginate**
- **nanocarriers**
- **nanoparticles**
- **drug delivery**
- **therapeutics**

REFERENCES

Agüero, L.; Zaldivar-Silva, D. et al. Alginate Microparticles as Oral Colon Drug Delivery Device: A Review. *Carbohydr. Polym.* **2017,** *168,* 32–43.

Ahmed, M. M.; El-Rasoul, S. A.; Auda, S. H.; Ibrahim, M. A. Emulsification/Internal Gelation as a Method for Preparation of Diclofenac Sodium–Sodium Alginate Microparticles. *Saudi Pharm. J.* **2013,** *21,* 61–69.

Akbari, S.; Pirbodaghi, T. Microfluidic Encapsulation of Cells in Alginate Particles via an Improved Internal Gelation Approach. *Micro. Nano.* **2014,** *14,* 773–777.

Alexis, F.; Pridgen, E. M.; Langer, R.; Farokhzad, O. C. Nanoparticle Technologies for Cancer Therapy. In *Drug delivery;* Schafer-Korting M, Ed.; Springer: Heidelberg, Berlin, 2010; pp 55–86.

Aluani, D.; Tzankova, V.; Kondeva-Burdina, M.; Yordanov, Y.; Nikolova, E.; Odzhakov, F.; Apostolov, A.; et al. Evaluation of Biocompatibility and Antioxidant Efficiency of Chitosan-Alginate Nanoparticles Loaded with Quercetin. *Int. J. Biol. Macromol.* **2017,** *103,* 771–782.

Anirudhan, T. S.; Anila, M. M.; Franklin, S. Synthesis Characterization and Biological Evaluation of Alginate Nanoparticle for the Targeted Delivery of Curcumin. *Mat. Sci. Eng. C* **2017,** *78,* 1125–1134.

Anton, N.; Benoit, J. P.; Saulnier, P. Design and Production of Nanoparticles Formulated from Nano-Emulsion Templates – A Review. *J. Control. Release* **2008,** *128,* 185–199.

Arora, S.; Gupta, S.; Narang, R. K.; Budhiraja, R. D. Amoxicillin Loaded Chitosan–Alginate Polyelectrolyte Complex Nanoparticles as Mucopenetrating Delivery System for *H. Pylori. Sci. Pharm.* **2011,** *79,* 673–694.

Aslani, P.; Kennedy, R. A. Studies on Diffusion in Alginate Gels. I. Effect of Cross-Linking with Calcium or Zinc Ions on Diffusion of Acetaminophen. *J. Controlled. Release* **1996,** *42,* 75–82.

Aynié, I.; Vauthier, C.; Chacun, H.; Fattal, E.; Couvreur, P. Spongelike Alginate Nanoparticles as a New Potential System for the Delivery of Antisense Oligonucleotides. *Antisense Nucleic Acid Drug Delivery* **1999,** *9,* 301–312.

Bajpai, S. K.; Sharma, S. Investigation of Swelling/Degradation Behaviour of Alginate Beads Crosslinked with Ca^{2+} and Ba^{2+} ions. *React. Funct. Polym.* **2004,** *59,* 129–140.

Balakrishnan, B.; Mohanty, M.; Umashankar, P. R.; Jayakrishnan, A. Evaluation of an in Situ Forming Hydrogel Wound Dressing Based on Oxidized Alginate and Gelatin. *Biomaterials* **2005,** *26,* 6335–6342.

Balaure, P.C.; Andronescu, E.; Grumezescu, A. M.; Ficai, A.; Huang, K. S.; Yang, C. H.; Chifiriuc, C. M.; Lin, Y. S. Fabrication, Characterization and in Vitro Profile Based Interaction with Eukaryotic and Prokaryotic Cells of Alginate–Chitosan-Silica Biocomposite. *Int. J. Pharm.* **2013,** *441,* 555–561.

Bertrand, N.; Wu, J.; Xu, X.; Kamaly, N.; Farokhzad, O. C. Cancer Nanotechnology: the Impact of Passive and Active Targeting in the Era of Modern Cancer Biology. *Adv. Drug Delivery Rev.* **2014,** *66,* 2–25.

Bhavsar, M. D.; Amiji, M. M. Development of Novel Biodegradable Polymeric Nanoparticles-In-Microsphere Formulation for Local Plasmid DNA Delivery in the Gastrointestinal Tract. *AAPS PharmSciTech.* **2008a,** *9,* 288–294.

Bidarra, S. J.; Barrias, C. C.; Granja, P. L. Injectable Alginate Hydrogels for Cell Delivery in Tissue Engineering. *Acta Biomater.* **2014,** *10,* 1646–1662.

Boissière, M.; Allouche, J.; Chanéac, C. Potentialities of Silica/Alginate Nanoparticles as Hybrid Magnetic Carriers. *Int. J. Pharm.* **2007,** *344,* 128–134.

Bouchemal, K.; Briançon, S.; Perrier, E.; Fessi, H. Nano-Emulsion Formulation using Spontaneous Emulsification: Solvent, Oil and Surfactant Optimization. *Int. J. Pharm.* **2004,** *280,* 241–251.

Branco, M. C.; Schneider, J. P. Self-Assembling Materials for Therapeutic Delivery. *Acta Biomater.* **2009,** *5,* 817–831.

Brigger, I.; Dubernet, C.; Couvreur, P. Nanoparticles in Cancer Therapy and Diagnosis. *Adv. Drug Delivery Rev.* **2012,** *64,* 24–36.

Bystricky, S.; Malovíková, A.; Sticzay, T. Interaction of Alginates and Pectins with Cationic Polypeptides. *Carbohydr. Polym.* **1990,** *13,* 283–294.

Caetano, L. A.; Almeida, A. J.; Gonçalves, L. M. D. Effect of Experimental Parameters on Alginate/Chitosan Microparticle for BCG Encapsulation. *Mar. Drugs* **2016,** *14,* 90.

Chang, D.; Lei, J.; Cui, H.; Lu, N.; Sun, Y.; Zhang, X.; et al. Disulfide Cross-Linked Nanospheres from Sodium Alginate Derivative for Inflammatory Bowel Disease: Preparation, Characterization, and in Vitro Drug Release Behaviour. *Carbohydr. Polym.* **2012,** *88,* 663–669.

Chen, S.-C.; Wu, Y.-C.; Mi, F.-L.; Lin, Y.-H.; Yu, L.-C.; Sung, H.-W. A Novel pH-Sensitive Hydrogel Composed of N,O-Carboxymethyl Chitosan and Alginate Cross-Linked by Genipin for Protein Drug Delivery. *J. Controlled Release* **2004,** *96,* 285–300.

Chopra, M.; Kaur, P.; Bernela, M.; Thakur, R. Synthesis and Optimization of Streptomycin Loaded Chitosan-Alginate Nanoparticles. *Int. J. Sci. Technol. Res.* **2012,** *1,* 31–34.

Chuah, A. M.; Kuroiwa, T.; Kobayashi, I.; Zhang, X.; Nakajima, M. Preparation of Uniformly Sized Alginate Microspheres Using the Novel Combined Methods of Microchannel Emulsification and External Gelation. *Colloids. Surf. A* **2009,** *351,* 9–17.

Couvreur, P.; Dubernet, C.; Puisieux, F. Controlled Drug Delivery with Nanoparticles: Current Possibilities and Future Trends. *Eur. J. Pharm. Biopharm.* **1995,** *41,* 2–13.

Couvreur, P.; Gref, R.; Andrieux, K.; Malvy, C. Nanotechnologies for Drug Delivery: Application to Cancer and Autoimmune Diseases. *Prog. Solid State Chem.* **2006,** *34,* 231–235.

Dakhara, S. L.; Anajwala, C. C. Polyelectrolyte Complex: A Pharmaceutical Review. *Syst. Rev. Pharm.* **2010,** *1,* 121–127.

Dalhaimer, P.; Bermudez, H.; Discher, D. E. Biopolymer Mimicry with Polymeric Wormlike Micelles: Molecular Weight Scaled Xexibility, Locked-In Curvature, and Coexisting Microphases. *J. Polym. Sci. Part B Polym. Phys.* **2004,** *42,* 168–176.

Daly, M. M.; Knorr, D. Chitosan–Alginate Complex Coacervate Capsules – Effects of Calcium-Chloride, Plasticizers, and Poly-Electrolytes on Mechanical Stability. *Biotechnol. Prog.* **1988,** 4, 76–81.

Das, R. K.; Kasoju, N.; Bora, U. Encapsulation of Curcumin in Alginate-Chitosan-Pluronic Composite Nanoparticles for Delivery to Cancer Cells. *Nanomed. Nanotechnol. Biol. Med.* **2010,** *6,* 153–160.

De Robertis, S. Advances in Oral Controlled Drug Delivery: The Role of Drug-Polymer and Interpolymer Non-Covalent Interactions. *Expert Opin. Drug Delivery* **2015,** *12,* 441–453.

Deeksha; Malviya, R.; Sharma, P. K. Poly-Electrolyte Complex: A Novel System for Biomedical Applications and Recent Patents. *Recent Pat. Nanotechnol.* **2014,** *8,* 129–141.

Desgouilles, S.; Vauthier, C.; Bazile, D.; Vacus, J.; Grossiord, J. L.; Veillard, M.; Couvreur, P. The Design of Nanoparticles Obtained by Solvent Evaporation: a Comprehensive Study. *Langmuir* **2003,** *19,* 9504–9510.

Díaz, M. R.; Vivas-Mejia, P. E. Nanoparticles as Drug Delivery Systems in Cancer Medicine: Emphasis on RNAi-Containing Nanoliposomes. *Pharmaceuticals* **2013,** *6,* 1361–1380.

Draget, K. I.; Smidsrød, O.; Skjåk-Braek, G. Alginates from Algae. In *Polysaccharides and Polyamides in the Food Industry: Properties, Production and Patents;* Steinbüchel, E. A., Rhee, S. K., Eds.; Wiley-VCH Verlach GmbH, Weinheim, Germany, 2005; pp 1–30.

El-Say, K. M.; El-Sawy, H. S. Polymeric Nanoparticles: Promising Platform for Drug Delivery. *Int. J. Pharm.* **2017,** *528,* 675–691.

Erdinc, B.; Neufeld, R. J. Protein Micro and Nanoencapsulation within Glycol-Chitosan/ Ca^{2+}/Alginate Matrix by Spray Drying. *Drug Dev. Ind. Pharm.* **2011,** *37,* 619–627.

Fathi, M.; Varshosaz, J. Novel Hesperetin Loaded Nanocarriers for Food Fortification: Production and Characterization. *J. Funct. Foods* **2013,** *5,* 1382–1391.

Fayin, Y.; Carlos, E. A.; Sabliov, C. M. Entrapment and Delivery of α-Tocopherol by a Self-Assembled, Alginate-Conjugated Prodrug Nanostructure. *Food Hydrocolloids* **2017,** *72,* 62–72.

Forrest, M. L.; Kwon, G. S. Clinical Developments in Drug Delivery Nanotechnology. *Adv. Drug Delivery Rev.* **2008,** *60,* 861–862.

Fundueanu, G.; Nastruzz, C.; Carpov, A.; Desbrieres, J.; Rinaudo, M. Physico-chemical Characterization of Ca-Alginate Microparticles Produced with Different Methods. *Biomaterials* **1999,** *20,* 1427–1435.

Ghaffari, S.; Varshosaz, J.; Haririan, I.; Khoshayand, M. R.; Azarmi, S.; Gazori, T. Ciprofloxacin Loaded Alginate/Chitosan and Solid Lipid Nanoparticles, Preparation, and Characterization. *J. Dispersion Sci. Technol.* **2012**, *33*, 685–689.

Goh, C. H.; Heng, P. W. S.; Chan, L. W. Alginates as a Useful Natural Polymer for Microencapsulation and Therapeutic Applications. *Carbohydr. Polym.* **2012**, *88*, 1–12.

Goycoolea, F. M.; Lollo, G.; Remunán-López, C.; Quaglia, F.; Alonso, M. J. Chitosan-Alginate Blended Nanoparticles as Carriers for the TransMucosal Delivery of Macromolecules. *Biomacromolecules* **2009**, *10*, 1736–1743.

Guo, H.; Lai, Q.; Wang, W.; Wu, Y.; Zhang, C.; Liu, Y.; Yuan, Z. Functional Alginate Nanoparticles for Efficient Intracellular Release of Doxorubicin and Hepatoma Carcinoma Cell Targeting Therapy. *Int. J. Pharm.* **2013**, *451*, 1–11.

Hackel, U.; Klein, J.; Megnet, R.; Wagner, F. Immobilization of Microbial Cells in Polymeric Matrices. *Eur. J. Appl. Microbiol. Biotechnol.* **1975**, *1*, 291–293.

Haidar, Z. S.; Hamdy, R. C.; Tabrizian, M. Protein Release Kinetics for Core-Shell Hybrid Nanoparticles Based on the Layer-By-Layer Assembly of Alginate and Chitosan on Liposomes. *Biomaterials* **2008**, *29*, 1207–1215.

Han, Y.; Tian, H.; He, P.; Chen, X.; Jing, X. Insulin Nanoparticle Preparation and Encapsulation into Poly(lactic-co-glycolic acid) Microspheres by using an Anhydrous System. *Int. J. Pharm.* **2009**, *378*, 159–166.

Hans, M. L.; Lowman, A. M. Biodegradable Nanoparticles for Drug Delivery and Targeting. *Curr. Opin. Solid State Mater. Sci.* **2002**, *6*, 319–327.

Haque, S.; Md, S.; Sahni, J. K.; Ali, J.; Baboota, S. Development and Evaluation of Brain Targeted Intranasal Alginate Nanoparticles for Treatment of Depression. *J. Psychiatr. Res.* **2014**, *48*, 1–12.

Hassani, L. N.; Hendra, F.; Bouchemal, K. Auto-Associative Amphiphilic Polysaccharides as Drug Delivery Systems. *Drug Discovery Today* **2012**, *17*, 608–614.

Herrero-Vanrell, R.; Rincón, A. C.; Alonso, M.; Reboto, V.; Molina-Martinez, I. T.; Rodríguez-Cabello, J. C. Self-Assembled Particles of an Elastin-Like Polymer as Vehicles for Controlled Drug Release. *J. Control Release* **2005**, *102*, 113–122.

Hong, J. S.; Vreeland, W. N.; Lacerda, S. H.; Locascio, L. E.; Gaitan, M.; Raghavan, S. R. Liposome-Templated Supramolecular Assembly of Responsive Alginate Nanogels. *Langmuir* **2008**, *24*, 4092–4096.

Hua, S.; Ma, H.; Li, X.; Yang, H.; Wang, A. pH-Sensitive Sodium Alginate/Poly(vinyl alcohol) Hydrogel Beads Prepared by Combined Ca²⁺ Crosslinking and Freeze-Thawing Cycles for Controlled Release of Diclofenac Sodium. *Int. J. Biol. Macromol.* **2010**, *46*, 517–523.

Hunter, A. C.; Elsom, J.; Wibroe, P. P.; Moghimi, S. M. Polymeric Particulate Technologies for Oral Drug Delivery and Targeting: A Pathophysiological Perspective. *Nanomedicine* **2012**, *8*, 5–20.

Ionita, M.; Pandele, M. A.; Iovu, H. Sodium Alginate/Graphene Oxide Composite Films With Enhanced Thermal and Mechanical Properties. *Carbohydr. Polym.* **2013**, *94*, 339–344.

Jayapal, J. J.; Dhanaraj, S. Exemestane Loaded Alginate Nanoparticles for Cancer Treatment: Formulation and in Vitro Evaluation. *Int. J. Biol. Macromol.* **2017**, *105*, 416–421.

Jeong, Y. I.; Na, H. S.; Seo, D. H.; Kim, D. G.; et al. Ciprofloxacin-Encapsulated Poly(dl-lactide-co-glycolide) Nanoparticles and its Antibacterial Activity. *Int. J. Pharm.* **2008**, *352*, 317–323.

Juliano, R. L. Drug Delivery Systems: A Brief Review. *Can. J. Phys. Pharm.* **1978**, *56*, 683–690.

Jung, T.; Kamm, W.; Breitenbach, A.; Kaiserling, E.; Xiao, J. X.; Kissel, T. Biodegradable Nanoparticles for Oral Delivery of Peptides: Is there a Role for Polymers to Affect Mucosal Uptake? *Eur. J. Pharm. Biopharm.* **2000,** *50,* 147–160.

Kabanov, A.; Batrakova, E.; Melik-Nubarov, N.; Fedoseev, N.; Dorodnich, T.; Alakhov, V.; Chekhonin, V.; Nazarova, I.; Kabanov, V. J. *Controlled Release* **1992,** *22,* 141.

Kamaly, N.; Xiao, Z. Y.; Valencia, P. M.; Radovic-Moreno, A. F.; Farokhzad, O. C. Targeted Polymeric Therapeutic Nanoparticles: Design, Development and Clinical Translation. *Chem. Soc. Rev.* **2012,** *41,* 2971–3010.

Khampieng, T.; Aramwit, P.; Supaphol, P. Silk sericin Loaded Alginate Nanoparticles: Preparation and Anti-Inflammatory Efficacy. *Int. J. Biol. Macromol.* **2015,** *80,* 636–643.

Khdair, A.; Chen, D.; Patil, Y. Nanoparticle-Mediated Combination Chemotherapy and Photodynamic Therapy Overcomes Tumour Drug Resistance. *J. Control. Release* **2010,** *141,* 137–144.

Kim, K.; Kang, D.-H.; Kim, M.-S.; Kim, K.-S.; Park, K.-M.; Hong, S.-C.; Chang, P.-S.; Jung, H.-S. Generation of Alginate Nanoparticles through Microfluidics-Aided Polyelectrolyte Complexation. *Colloids. Surf. A* **2015,** *471,* 86–92.

Kong, H. J.; Smith, M. K.; Mooney, D. J. Designing Alginate Hydrogels to Maintain Viability of Immobilized Cells. *Biomaterials* **2003,** *24,* 4023–4029.

Kulkarni, R. K.; Bartak, D. E.; Leonard, F. Initiation of Polymerization of Alkyl 2-Cyanoacrylates in Aqueous Solutions of Glycine and Its Derivatives. *J. Polym. Sci. Polym. Chem.* **1971,** *9,* 2977–2981.

Kuo, C. K.; Ma, P. X. Ionically Crosslinked Alginate Hydrogels as Scaffolds for Tissue Engineering: Part 1. Structure, Gelation Rate and Mechanical Properties. *Biomaterials* **2001,** *22,* 511–521.

Kuroiwa, T.; Kobayashi, I.; Chuah, A. M.; Nakajima, M.; Ichikawa, S. Formulation and Stabilization of Nano-/Microdispersion Systems Using Naturally Occurring Edible Polyelectrolytes by Electrostatic Deposition and Complexation. *Adv. Colloid Interface Sci.* **2015,** *226,* 86–100.

Lankalapalli, S.; Kolapalli, V.R.M. Polyelectrolyte Complex: A Review of their Applicability in Drug Delivery Technology. *Indian J. Pharm. Sci.* **2009,** *71,* 481–487.

Lee, K. Y.; Mooney, D. J. Alginate: Properties and Biomedical Applications. *Prog. Polym. Sci.* **2012,** *37,* 106–126.

Lemarchand, C.; Gref, R.; Couvreur, P. Polysaccharide-Decorated Nanoparticles. *Eur. J. Pharm. Biopharm.* **2004,** *58,* 327–341.

LeRoux, M. A.; Guilak, F.; Setton, L. A. Compressive and Shear Properties of Alginate Gel: Effects of Sodium Ions and Alginate Concentration. *J. Biomed. Mater. Res.* **1999,** *47,* 46–53.

Lertsutthiwong, P.; Rojsitthisak, P.; Nimmannit, U. Preparation of Turmeric Oil-Loaded Chitosan-Alginate Biopolymeric Nanocapsules. *Mater. Sci. Eng. C* **2009,** *29,* 856–860.

Li, P.; Dai, Y.-N.; Zhang, J.-P.; et al. Chitosan-Alginate Nanoparticles as a Novel Drug Delivery System for Nifedipine. *Int. J. Biomed. Sci.* **2008,** *4,* 221–228.

Liu, H. Effect of Electrostatic Interactions on the Structure and Dynamics of a Model Polyelectrolyte, I. Diffusion. *J. Chem. Phys.* **1998,** *109,* 7556–7566.

Liu, X. M.; Pramoda, K. P.; Yang, Y. Y.; Chow, S. Y.; He, C. Cholesteryl-grafted Functional Amphiphilic Poly (N-isopropylacrylamide-co-N-hydroxylacrylamide): Synthesis, Temperature-Sensitivity, Self-Assembly and Encapsulation of a Hydrophobic Agent. *Biomaterials* **2004,** *25,* 2619–2628.

Lopes, M.; Abrahim, B.; Veiga, F.; Seiça, R.; Cabral, L. M.; Arnaud, P. Preparation Methods and Applications Behind Alginate-Based Particles. *Expert Opin. Drug Delivery* **2016**, *14,* 1–14.

Machado, A. H. E.; Lundberg, D.; Ribeiro, A. J.; Veiga, F. J.; Lindman, B.; Miguel, M. G.; Olsson, U. Preparation of Calcium Alginate Nanoparticles using Water-in-Oil (W/O) Nanoemulsions. *Langmuir* **2012**, *28,* 4131–4141.

Chavanpatil, M. D.; Khdair, A.; Patil, Y.; Handa, H.; Mao, G.; Panyam, J. Polymer-Surfactant Nanoparticles for Sustained Release of Water-Soluble Drugs. *J. Pharm. Sci.* **2007**, *96,* 3379–3389.

Maria, A.; Azevedo, M. A.; Bourbon, A. I.; Vicente, A. A.; Cerqueira, M. A. Alginate/Chitosan Nanoparticles for Encapsulation and Controlled Release of Vitamin B_2. *Int. J. Biol. Macromol.* **2014**, *71,* 141–146.

Martinez, A.; Iglesias, I.; Lozano, R.; Teijon, J. M.; Blanco, M. D. Synthesis and Characterization of Thiolated Alginate-Albumin Nanoparticles Stabilized by Disulfide Bonds. Evaluation as Drug Delivery Systems. *Carbohydr. Polym.* **2011**, *83,* 1311–1321.

Martínez, A.; Benito-Miguel, M.; Iglesias, I.; Teijón, J. M.; Blanco, M. D. Tamoxifen-Loaded Thiolated Alginate-Albumin Nanoparticles as Antitumoral Drug Delivery Systems. *J. Biomed. Mater. Res. A* **2012**, *6,* 1467–1476.

Mei, L.; Zhang, Z.; Zhao, L.; Huang, L.; Yang, X. L.; Tang, J.; Feng, S. S. Pharmaceutical Nanotechnology for Oral Delivery of Anticancer Drugs. *Adv. Drug Delivery Rev.* **2013**, *65,* 880–890.

Moghimi, S. M.; Hunter, A. C.; Murray, J. C. Nanomedicine: Current Status and Future Prospects. *FASEB J.* **2005**, *19,* 311–330.

Mortensen, K. Structural Properties of Self-Assembled Polymeric Aggregates in Aqueous Solutions. *Polym. Adv. Technol.* **2001**, *12,* 2–22.

Motwani, S. K.; Chopra, S.; Talegaonkar, S.; et al. Chitosan-Sodium Alginate Nanoparticles as Sub Microscopic Reservoirs for Ocular Delivery: Formulation, Optimisation and in Vitro Characterisation. *Eur. J. Pharm. Biopharm.* **2008**, *68,* 513–525.

Murtaza, G.; Waseem, A.; Nisarur, R.; Hussain, I. Alginate Microparticles for Biodelivery: A Review. *Afr. J. Pharm. Pharmacol.* **2011**, *5,* 2726–2737.

Nesamony, J.; Singh, P. R.; Nada, S. E.; Shah, Z. A.; Kolling, W. M. Calcium Alginate Nanoparticles Synthesized through a Novel Interfacial Cross-Linking Method as a Potential Protein Drug Delivery System. *J. Pharm. Sci.* **2012**, *101,* 2177–2184.

Nicolas, J.; Mura, S.; Brambilla, D.; Mackiewicz, N.; Couvreur, P. Design, Functionalization Strategies and Biomedical Applications of Targeted Biodegradable/Biocompatible Polymer-Based Nanocarriers for Drug Delivery. *Chem. Soc. Rev.* **2013**, *42,* 1147–1235.

Nitta, S. K.; Numata, K. Biopolymer-Based Nanoparticles for Drug/Gene Delivery and Tissue Engineering. *Int. J. Mol. Sci.* **2013**, *14,* 1629–1654.

Oliveira, J. T.; Reis, R. L. Polysaccharide-Based Materials for Cartilage Tissue Engineering Applications. *J. Tissue. Eng. Regener. Med.* **2011**, *5,* 421–436.

Panyam, J.; Labhasetwar, V. Biodegradable Nanoparticles for Drug and Gene Delivery to Cells and Tissue. *Adv. Drug Delivery Rev.* **2003**, *55,* 329–347.

Paques, J. P.; van der Linden, E.; van Rijn, C. J.; Sagis L. M. Preparation Methods of Alginate Nanoparticles. *Adv. Colloid. Interface Sci.* **2014**, *209,* 163–171.

Parveen, S.; Mishra, R.; Sahoo, S. K. Nanoparticles: A Boon to Drug Delivery, Therapeutics, Diagnostics and Imaging. *Nanomed. Nanotechnol. Biol. Med.* **2012**, *8,* 147–166.

Patil, J. S.; Kamalapur, M. V.; Marapur, S. C.; Kadam, D. V. Ionotropic Gelation and Polyelectrolyte Complexation: The Novel Techniques to Design Hydrogel Particulate

Sustained, Modulated Drug Delivery System: A Review. *Dig. J. Nanomater. Biostructures* *2010*, 5, 241–248.

Pawar, S. N.; Edgar, K. J. Alginate Derivatization: A Review of Chemistry, Properties and Applications. *Biomaterials* **2012**, *33*, 3279–3305.

Peer, D.; Karp, J. M.; Hong, S.; Farokhzad, O. C.; Margalit, R.; Langer, R. Nanocarriers as an Emerging Platform for Cancer Therapy. *Nat. Nanotechnol.* **2007**, *2*, 751–760.

Pelletier, S.; Hubert, P.; Payan, E.; Marchal, P.; Choplin, L.; Dellacherie, E. Amphiphilic Derivatives of Sodium Alginate and Hyaluronate for Cartilage Repair: Rheological Properties. *J. Biomed. Mat. Res.* **2001**, *54*, 102–108.

Petros, R. A.; DeSimone, J. M. Strategies in the Design of Nanoparticles for Therapeutic Applications. *Nat. Rev. Drug Discovery* **2010**, *9*, 615–627.

Pridgen, E. M.; Alexis, F.; Farokhzad, O. C. Polymeric Nanoparticle Drug Delivery Technologies for Oral Delivery Applications. *Expert Opin. Drug Deliv.* **2015**, *121*, 1459–1473.

Quintanar-Guerrero, D.; Allémann, E.; Fessi, H.; Doelker, E. Pseudo Latex Preparation Using a Novel Emulsion-Diffusion Process Involving Direct Displacement of Partially Water-Miscible Solvents By Distillation. *Int. J. Pharm.* **1999**, *188*, 155–164.

Quintanar-Guerrero, D.; Allemann, E.; Fessi, H.; Doelker, E. Preparation Techniques and Mechanisms of Formation of Biodegradable Nanoparticles from Preformed Polymers. *Drug Dev. Ind. Pharm.* **1998**, *24*, 1113–1128.

Rahaiee, S.; Hashemi, M.; Shojaosadat, S. A.; Moini, S.; Razavi, S. H. Nanoparticles Based on Crocin Loaded Chitosan-Alginate Biopolymers: Antioxidant Activities, Bioavailability and Anticancer Properties. *Int. J. Biol. Macromol.* **2017**, *99*, 401–408.

Rajaonarivony, M.; Vauthier, C.; Couarraze, G.; Puisieux, F.; Couvreur, P. Development of a New Drug Carrier Made from Alginate. *J. Pharm. Sci.* **1993**, *82*, 912–917.

Reis, C. P.; Neufeld, R. J.; Ribeiro, A. J.; Veiga, F. Nanoencapsulation I. Methods for Preparation of Drug-Loaded Polymeric Nanoparticles. *Nanomedicine* **2006**, *2*, 8–21.

Reis, C. P.; Neufeld, R.; Ribeiro, A. J.; Veiga, F. Design of Insulin-Loaded Alginate Nanoparticles: Influence of the Calcium Ion on Polymer Gel Matrix Properties. *Chem. Ind. Chem. Eng. Q.* **2006**, *12*, 47–52.

Ren, B.; Gao, Y. M.; Lu, L.; Liu, X. X.; Tong, Z. Aggregates of Alginates Binding with Surfactants of Single and Twin Alkyl Chains in Aqueous Solutions: Fluorescence and Dynamic Light Scattering Studies. *Carbohydr. Polym.* **2006**, *66*, 266–273.

Rotureau, E.; Chassenieux, C.; Dellacherie, E.; Durand, A. Neutral Polymeric Surfactants Derived from Dextran: A Study of their Aqueous Solution Behaviour. *Macromol. Chem. Phys.* **2005**, *206*, 2038–2046.

Sahoo, S. K.; Labhasetwar, V. Nanotech Approaches to Drug Delivery and Imaging. *Drug Discovery. Today* **2003**, *8*, 1112–1120.

Sahoo, S. K.; Parveen, S.; Panda, J. J. The Present and Future of Nanotechnology in Human Health Care. *Nanomedicine* **2007**, *3*, 20–31.

Salata, O. V. Applications of Nanoparticles in Biology and Medicine. *J. Nanobiotechnol.* **2004**, *2*, 1–6.

Salatin, S.; Maleki-dizaj, S.; Yari-khosroushahi, A. Effect of the Surface Modification, Size, and Shape on Cellular Uptake of Nanoparticles. *Cell Biol. Int.* **2015**, *39*, 881–890.

Santhi, K.; Dhanraj, S. A.; Venkatesh, D. N.; Sangeetha, S.; Suresh, B. Preparation and Optimization of Sodium Alginate Nanospheres of Methotrexate. *Indian J. Pharm. Sci.* **2005**, *67*, 691–696.

Sarika, P. R.; James, N. R. Polyelectrolyte Complex Nanoparticles from Cationised Gelatin and Sodium Alginate for Curcumin Delivery. *Carbohydr.Polym.* **2016**, *148*, 354–361.

Sarmento, B.; Ferreira, D.; Veiga, F.; Ribeiro, A. Characterization of Insulin-Loaded Alginate Nanoparticles Produced by Ionotropic Pre-Gelation through DSC and FTIR Studies. *Carbohyd. Polym.* **2006,** *66,* 1–7.

Sarmento, B.; Ferreira, D. C.; Jorgensen, L.; van de Weert, M. Probing Insulin's Secondary Structure after Entrapment into Alginate/Chitosan Nanoparticles. *Eur. J. Pharm. Biopharm.* **2007a,** *65,* 10–17.

Sarmento, B.; Martins, S.; Ferreira, D.; Souto, E. B. Oral Insulin Delivery by Means of Solid Lipid Nanoparticles. *Int. J. Nanomed.* **2007b,** *2,* 743–749.

Sarmento, B.; Ribeiro, A.; Veiga, F.; Ferreira, D.; Neufeld, R. Oral Bioavailability of Insulin Contained in Polysaccharide Nanoparticle. *Biomacromolecules* **2007c,** *8,* 3054–3060.

Sarmento, B.; Ribeiro, A.; Veiga, F.; Sampaio, P., Neufeld, R., Ferreira, D. Alginate/Chitosan Nanoparticles are Effective for Oral Insulin Delivery. *Pharm. Res.* **2007d,** *24,* 2198–2206.

Sharma, R.; Agrawal, U.; Mody, N.; Vyas, S. P. Polymer Nanotechnology Based Approaches in Mucosal Vaccine Delivery: Challenges and Opportunities. *Biotechnol. Adv.* **2015,** *33,* 64–79.

Shi, M.; Lu, J.; Shoichet, M. S. Organic Nanoscale Drug Carriers Coupled with Ligands for Targeted Drug Delivery in Cancer. *J. Mater. Chem.* **2009,** *19,* 5485.

Shilpa, A.; Agrawal, S. S.; Ray, A. R. Controlled Delivery of Drugs from Alginate Matrix. *J. Macromol. Sci. Polym. Rev. Part C* **2003,** *43,* 187–221.

Sikorski, P.; Mo, F.; Skjåk-Bræk, G.; Stokke, B. T. Evidence for Egg-Box-Compatible Interactions in Calcium−Alginate Gels from Fiber X-ray Diffraction. *Biomacromolecules* **2007,** *8,* 2098–2103.

Skjåk-Br, K.; Martinsen, A. Applications of Some Algal Polysaccharides in Biotechnology. In *Seaweed Resources in Europe: uses and Potential;* Guiry, M. D., Blunden, G., Eds.; John Wiley & Sons: Chichester, 1991; 219–257.

Smidsrød, O.; Skjåk-Braek, G. Alginate as Immobilization Matrix for Cells. *Trends Biotechnol.* **1990,** *8,* 71–78.

Stevens, M. M.; Qanadilo, H. F.; Langer, R.; Shastri, P. V. A Rapid-Curing Alginate Gel System: Utility in Periosteum-Derived Cartilage Tissue Engineering. *Biomaterials* **2004,** *25,* 887–894.

Suri, S. S.; Fenniri, H.; Singh, B. Nanotechnology-Based Drug Delivery Systems. *J. Occup. Med. Toxicol.* **2007,** *2,* 1–6.

Tang, Z.; He, C.; Tian, H.; Ding, J.; Hsiao, B. S.; Chu, B.; Chen, X. Polymeric Nanostructured Materials for Biomedical Applications. *Prog. Polym. Sci.* **2016,** *60,* 86–128.

Tønnesen, H. H.; Karlsen, J. Alginate in Drug Delivery Systems. *Drug Dev. Ind. Pharm.* **2002,** *28,* 621–630.

Uzgiris, E. E. Polymeric Nanoparticles for Medical Imaging. In *Polymer-Based Nanostructures: Medical Applications;* 1st ed.; Broz, P., Ed.; The Royal Society of Chemistry: Cambridge, United Kingdom, 2010; pp 173–236.

Vallée, F.; Muller, C.; Durand, A.; Schimchowitsch, S.; Dellacherie, E.; Kelche, C.; Cassel, J. C.; Leonard, M. Synthesis and Rheological Properties of Hydrogels Based on Amphiphilic Alginate-Amide Derivatives. *Carbohydr. Res.* **2009,** *344,* 223–228.

Vauthier, C.; Bouchemal, K. Methods for the Preparation and Manufacture of Polymeric Nanoparticles. *Pharm. Res.* **2009,** *26,* 1025–1058.

Vauthier, C.; Couvreur, P. Development of Nanoparticles Made of Polysaccharides as Novel Drug Carrier Systems. In *Handbook of Pharmaceutical Controlled Release Technology;* Wise D. L., Eds.; Marcel Dekker: New York, 2000; pp 413–429.

Wang, T.; He, N. Preparation, Characterization and Applications of Low-Molecular-Weight Alginate–Oligochitosan Nano Capsules. *Nanoscale* **2010,** *2,* 230–239.

Whitesides, G. M.; Mathias, J. P.; Seto, C. T. Molecular Self-Assembly and Nano Chemistry: a Chemical Strategy for the Synthesis of Nanostructures. *Science* **1991**, *254*, 1312–1319.

Wilson, A. D.; Howell, C.; Waring, W. S. Venlafaxine Ingestion is Associated with Rhabdomyolysis in Adults: A Case Series. *J. Toxicol. Sci.* **2007**, *32*, 97–101.

Wu, J.; Fan, Q. Z.; Xia, Y. F.; Ma, G. H. Uniform-Sized Particles in Biomedical Field Prepared by Membrane Emulsification Technique. *Chem. Eng. Sci.* **2015**, *125*, 85–97.

Xing, J.; Deng, L.; Dong, A. Chitosan/alginate nanoparticles stabilized by poloxamer for the controlled release of 5-fluorouracil. *J. Appl. Polym. Sci.* **2010**, *117*, 2354–2359.

Yang, L.; Zhang, B.; Wen, L.; Liang, Q.; Zhang, L.-M. Amphiphilic Cholesteryl Grafted Sodium Alginate Derivative: Synthesis and Self-Assembly in Aqueous Solution. *Carbohydr. Polym.* **2007**, *68*, 218–225.

Yang, J. S.; Xie, Y.-J.; He, W. Research Progress on Chemical Modification of Alginate: A Review. *Carbohydr. Polym.* **2011**, *84*, 33–39.

Yang, J. S.; Zhou, Q. Q.; He, W. Amphipathicity and Self-Assembly Behaviour of Amphiphilic Alginate Esters. *Carbohydr. Polym.* **2013**, *92*, 223–227.

Yu, C.-Y.; Jia, L.-H.; Yin, B.-C.; Zhang, X.-Z.; Cheng, S.-X.; Zhuo, R.-X. Fabrication of Nanospheres and Vesicles as Drug Carriers by Self-Assembly of Alginate. *J. Phys. Chem. C* **2008**, *112*, 16774–16778.

Yusa, S.; Kamachi, M.; Morishima, Y. Hydrophobic Self-Association of Cholesteryl Moieties Covalently Linked to Polyelectrolytes: Effect of Spacer Bond, *Langmuir* **1998**, *14*, 6059–6067.

Zahoor, A.; Sharma, S.; Khuller, G. K. Inhalable Alginate Nanoparticles as Antitubercular Drug Carriers Against Experimental Tuberculosis. *Int. J. Ant. Agents* **2005**, *26*, 298–303.

Zhang, C.; Wang, W.; Liu, T.; Wu, Y.; Guo, H.; Wang, P.; Tian, Q.; Wang, Y.; Yuan,Z. Doxorubicin-Loaded Glycyrrhetinic Acid-Modified Alginate Nanoparticles for Liver Tumor Chemotherapy. *Biomaterials* **2012**, *33*, 2187–2196.

Zhou, J.; Romero, G.; Rojas, E.; et al. Layer by Layer Chitosan/Alginate Coatings on Poly(Lactide-Co-Glycoside) Nanoparticles for Anti-Fouling Protection and Folic Acid Binding to Achieve Selective Cell Targeting. *J. Colloid Interface Sci.* **2010**, *345*, 241–247.

Zimmermann, H.; Shirley, S. G.; Zimmermann, U. Alginate-Based Encapsulation of Cells: Past, Present, and Future. *Curr. Diabetes Rep.* **2007**, *7*, 314–320.

Zohri, M.; Alavidjeh, M. S.; Haririan, I.; Ardestani, M. S.; Ebrahimi, S. E. S.; Sani, H. T.; Sadjadi, S. K. A Comparative Study between the Antibacterial Effect of Nisin and Nisin-Loaded Chitosan/Alginate Nanoparticles on the Growth of *Staphylococcus aureus* in Raw and Pasteurized Milk Samples. *Probiotics Antimicrob. Proteins* **2010**, *2*, 258–266.

CHAPTER 15

ALGINATE-BASED COMPOSITES IN DRUG DELIVERY APPLICATIONS

ANKITA TIWARI[1], ANKIT JAIN[2], AMIT VERMA[1],
PRITISH KUMAR PANDA[1], and SANJAY K. JAIN[1*]

[1]*Pharmaceutics Research Projects Laboratory, Department of
Pharmaceutical Sciences, Dr. Hari Singh Gour Vishwavidyalaya,
Sagar, Madhya Pradesh 470003, India*

[2]*Institute of Pharmaceutical Research, GLA University, NH-2,
Mathura-Delhi Road, Mathura, Uttar Pradesh 281406, India*

*Corresponding author. E-mail: drskjainin@yahoo.com;
drskjainin@gmail.com*

15.1 INTRODUCTION

Alginates (ALGs) are natural polysaccharides found in brown algae Phaeo-phyceae and having linear unbranched polymers consisting of β-(1,4)-linked D-mannuronic acid and α-(1,4)-linked L-guluronic acid residues which are ordered in the polymer chain in the form of blocks. The characteristics of ALG are determined by the cross-linking. Heat-stable gels are produced at room temperature. During gelling, the concentration of divalent cations massively influences the gel network and uniformity of the gel. The process of gelation and cross-linking of polymers are commonly consummated by the replacement of monovalent sodium ions with the divalent cations, from the guluronic acids and the assembling of these guluronic groups constitute to form the microspheres. ALGs have numerous properties such as low toxicity, less immunogenicity, hydrophilicity, porosity, adequate adsorption capability, stability, biodegradability, ease of accessibility, economic price and simple method of preparation due to which Food and Drug Administration has approved it for utilization in drug delivery. They possess mucoadhesive properties within the gastrointestinal track (GIT) epithelium. The controlled release attribute of dried ALG beads is imparted owing to their re-swelling property. pH susceptibility of re-swelling property prevents the loss of potency of the acid-sensitive drug in gastric juice. The biological activity can be restored by the mild gelation process which has alleviated proteins, cells and DNA to be consolidated into ALG matrices. Besides, the kinetics of drug release can be changed by considering the different varieties of ALG along with their coating agents, the pore size, and the decay rate (Domb and Kumar, 2011; Lee and Mooney, 2012). ALG is a natural biopolymer possessing numerous unique properties which make it a discrete polymer for fabrication with various composites of polymers which form different complexes for a diverse utility in drug delivery on account of their inbuilt characteristics such as excellent biocompatibility and biodegradability, economic accessibility, ease and natural availability, and sol-gel transition characteristics. Various technologies are employed for the formulation of microparticles, nanoparticles (NPs) and other composite systems which manifests a vast utility in the arena of drug delivery (Lopes et al., 2017). Figure 15.1 illustrates the various types of composite ALG systems for the delivery of drugs/active ingredients/biomolecules.

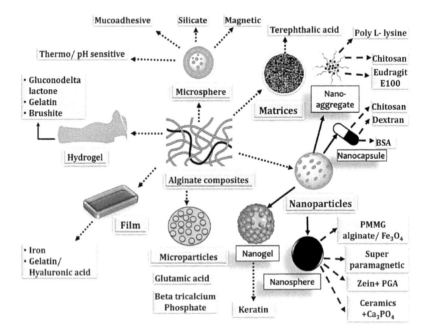

FIGURE 15.1   An illustration of several types of composite alginate (ALG) systems for the delivery of drugs/active ingredients/biomolecules: bovine serum albumin (BSA), poly(methyl methacrylate)-grafted, and β-tricalcium phosphate.

15.2 ALGINATE (ALG)-BASED COMPOSITE SYSTEMS EXPLOITED FOR DRUG DELIVERY

Numerous ALG-based composite carrier systems have been extensively studied for application in drug delivery. They are discussed under separate subheadings below.

15.2.1 ALG MICROSPHERES COMPOSITE SYSTEM

ALG microspheres are multipurpose systems for delivering a broad range of drugs and biomolecules. This biopolymer with a natural origin has numerous distinctive assets making it an ultimate applicant for adapting with diverse combinations of polymers heading to the construction of strong complexes for extensive uses. ALG-based composite microsphere systems show controlled drug delivery owing to their capability to entrap many drugs, enzymes, DNA, vaccines, proteins, growth factors, and so forth. Furthermore, this system will bestow more advantages in the domain of tissue engineering, stem cell researches and the evolution of different kinds of cancer-targeting approaches (Poojari and Srivastava, 2013).

15.2.2 ALG HYDROGELS COMPOSITE SYSTEM

ALG hydrogels are broadly acceptable biomaterials which have been applied as supports in tissue engineering, carriers for drugs, and as model extracellular matrices for biological studies. These applications necessitate the presence of a number of physical properties consisting of mechanical stiffness, swelling behavior, degradation, cell attachment, and binding or release of bioactive molecules. Polysaccharide or its gel from ALG may be either chemically or physically altered to render these properties. The effectiveness of these modified ALG gels in the form of biomaterials has been confirmed in numerous *in vitro* and *in vivo* studies (Augst et al., 2006).

The polymer cross-linked by chemical or physical ways may lead to the formation of an ALG hydrogel. The behaviors of the ALG gels are reliant on numerous factors such as the molecular weight, kind of cross-linking, cross-linking density, and composition of the ALG (Lee and Mooney, 2012). Complexing agents such as phosphate or citrate have a crucial role in cross-linking of ALG composite systems (Williams and Phillips, 2009). Ionic cross-linking with multivalent cations is the usual process employed for the making of ALG gels. ALG solutions can be gelled by three methods, that is, external gelation, internal gelation, and gelation on cooling. Externally gelated ALG is usually added dropwise into calcium chloride solution and a gelled ALG matrix is produced by diffusion from the continuous phase into the inner part of the ALG drops. Cations diffuse outside moving to the center of the ALG droplet which is also referred as "diffusion method" (Klostranec and Chan, 2006; Liu et al., 2002). Internal gelation method which is also denoted as "internal setting" or *in situ* gelation involves water-insoluble calcium salts like $CaCO_3$; immixed with the ALG solution. Diminishing the pH of the system and/or enhancing the solubility of the calcium may result in the release of the calcium ions from the ALG eventually forming the ALG gel (Sun and Tan, 2013). The molecular weight of the ALG poses a greater impact on strength of the gel when compared with external gelation. ALG gels formulated by internal gelation are more inclined to syneresis as compared with externally generated gels. Few properties such as matrix strength, mechanical stiffness, pore size and permeability of ALG gels formulated by internal and external gelation are quite different (Liu et al., 2002; Ozaki et al., 2015).

An extensive study has been done on the relation between the chemical structure and its gel-forming abilities. For example, polysaccharides separated from brown algae such as *Laminaria hyperborea* and *lessonia* occur in coastal waters across the world (Lanktree et al., 2011; Md et al., 2011). Fractional precipitation with manganese and calcium salts depicted that the ratio of guluronic to mannuronic acid deviates between sources and that ALGs are block polymers (Huber et al., 2006; Khotimchenko et al., 2001). The linear unbranched copolymers which consist of homopolymeric blocks of (1, 4)-linked b-D-mannuronic acid (M) and its C-5 epimer, a-L-guluronic acid (G) residues, respectively, are attached with each other by covalent bond linkage in different sequences or blocks. D-Mannuronic acid is $^4C_1$ with diequatorial links while L-guluronic acid is $^1C_4$ with diaxial links. These blocks are either alike or solely alternating (MMMMM, GGGGGG, or GMGMGM), and the proportional amount depends on the origin of the ALG because of the diaxial links, G blocks are firmer than alternating blocks, which fit more soluble at low pH (Lee and Mooney, 2012). ALGs can be formed with a varying range of molecular weights (MWs, 50–100,0000 kDa), and aqueous solutions of ALGs possess non-Newtonian characteristics, that is, the viscosity reduces with rising shear rate (shear thinning) (Wee and Combotz, 1998). The concentration of the polymer and the MW distribution influence the viscosity of an ALG solution (Yi et al., 1999). The cross-linking of two G blocks of adjacent polymer chains with multivalent cations (e.g., Ca^{2+} or Ba^{2+}) can be done by exchange with the carboxylic groups in the sugars heading to the generation of a gel network.

15.2.3 ALG MICROPARTICLES COMPOSITE SYSTEM

ALG is the polymer being widely utilized for the formulation of microparticles (de Vos et al., 2006). Abundant formation methods have been recognized to formulate ALG microparticles of numerous sizes. Most popular and easily employed technique used is based on an external gelation method. In such a method, the ALG solution is allowed to fall dropwise into the cationic calcium chloride solution. The material which has to be incorporated is usually mixed with the solution of ALG earlier to the formation of particle and gelation (Ribeiro et al., 2014). Normally, the solution of ALG is extruded by a needle to prepare ALG droplets having a diameter of size ranges 500–5000 µm (Koch et al., 2003). More innovative droplet generation techniques, which have particles of small size and narrow size distribution, are taken into the consideration (Brun-Graeppi et al., 2011; Zimmermann et al., 2007). Systems in which a coaxial laminar airflow is applied at the outlet, shears off the droplet and harvests droplets with size ranges with a diameter of 300–1000 µm. The application of electrostatic fields jerks the droplet from the outlet to the gelation bath, making particles of diameter 50–1000 µm (Paques et al., 2014; Seifert and Phillips, 1997). In the vibrating nozzle system, the laminar flowing liquid jet nozzle helps to break up the droplets into identical size by a superimposed vibration, yielding particles of diameter 150–2000 µm (Poncelet et al., 1999). Another method that cuts the nonstop fluid jet into the segments of similar sizes is by the laminar jet break-up and generates beads having size range with diameter 120–3000 µm (Paques et al., 2014; Schwinger et al., 2002). All the methods which have been discussed above are generally syringe-based systems and show troubles in large-scale manufacturing owing to the employment of a multitude of needles/nozzles, and operational problems such as blockage of needles, sanitation, cleaning, and so forth. Moreover, these ALG microparticles are achieved by drenching the solution of ALG in a gelation bath which may be deformed by dragging forces and it creates a teardrop shape (Reis et al., 2006). Besides the nozzle-based methods, air atomization techniques also help to develop ALG particles with the combination of external gelation system and prepare particles with a diameter of 5–200 µm (Cui et al., 2000). In addition to this technique, another external gelation method could be used which has a spinning disk that forms droplets and as a consequence, ALG particles having a diameter of size 300–3000 µm are produced (Senuma et al., 2000). Emulsification methods such as mechanical emulsification and membrane emulsification can be applied for making ALG microparticles (You et al., 2001). In these methods, the solution of ALG is emulsified in an oil phase resulting in a w/o emulsion and gelation of the droplets of ALGs occurs by the technique of external gelation or internal gelation methods. By regulating the circumstances under which the water-in-oil dispersion is formed, the particle size ranges from a few microns to millimeters in diameter.

15.2.4 ALG NANOPARTICLES COMPOSITE SYSTEMS

NP composite systems generally comprise of nanocapsules, nanospheres, and nanoaggregates, having diameters from 10–1000 nm (Hamidi et al., 2008; Sahoo and Labhasetwar, 2003). These systems have the capability to incorporate enzymes, drugs and other compounds to the particle's matrix (Soppimath et al., 2001). Nanoaggregates are smaller sized colloidal systems depicting different morphologies and the drug is dispersed physically in them. ALG nanoaggregates have efficiently been loaded with insulin (Sarmento et al., 2006), antisense oligonucleotide (Aynie et al., 1999) and anticancer drugs, such as methotrexate (Santhi et al., 2005) and 5-Fluorouracil (5-FU)(Yu et al., 2008). Recently, supermagnetic ALG nanoaggregates were established for immobilization of lipase, and were then functionalized with polyethylene glycol (Liu et al., 2012). Nanocapsules are vesicular systems having polymeric membranes which contain the drug in an oily or aqueous liquid core (Hamidi et al., 2008; Mora-Huertas et al., 2010). The simplest technique employed for developing nanocapsules is the deposition of polymers on the interface of a template droplet, with consecutive solvent removal (Fessi et al., 1989; Lertsutthiwong et al., 2008; Mora-Huertas et al., 2010). Then, the polymer is deposited on the droplet interface and stabilized by intermolecular cross-linking. ALG nanocapsules of different sizes were used to encapsulate acyl derivatives (having antitumor activity) (Grebinişan et al., 2011), essential oil (turmeric oil) (Lertsutthiwong et al., 2009) and the extract of *Phyllanthus amarus* (Deepa et al., 2012). Nanospheres are spherical particles having gelled interior where the entrapped constituent is dispersed by a physical method (Lambert et al., 2001; Sarmento et al., 2006). Nanocapsules with a structured core have also been developed and are frequently prepared by first developing a nanosphere and later making a shell on the interface of the nanosphere.

15.2.4.1 METHODS OF FORMATION OF ALG NPS

15.2.4.1.1 Complexation method

In this method, formation of the complex can occur with the help of an aqueous solution producing ALG nanoaggregates (Fessi et al., 1989; Raja-onarivony et al., 1993) or on the surface of an oil droplet, creating ALG nanocapsules (Mora-Huertas et al., 2010), calcium can be taken from calcium chloride solution and is utilized as a cross-linker for the formation of ALG complex. Complexation can also occur by mixing ALG with an oppositely charged polymer-like chitosan (CS) (Sæther et al., 2008).

15.2.4.1.2 ALG-in-oil emulsification method

ALG-in-oil emulsification method, coupled with gelation of the ALG emulsion droplet, produces an ALG nanospheres composite system. Table 15.1 enlists the various ALG composite systems which have been exploited in drug delivery along with their preparation methods and applications in drug delivery.

15.3 STIMULI-RESPONSIVE ALG-BASED COMPOSITE SYSTEMS

ALG shows mild gelation on the admission of divalent cations like Ca^{2+} and so forth. Various free carboxyl groups existing in the backbone of ALG bestow it with good pH sensitivity. Therefore, it has been commonly employed in pharmaceuticals for the development of pH-based delivery systems. Microspheres of calcium ALG were prepared in an aqueous solution of poly-[(3-acrylamidopropyl)-trimethylammonium chloride-b-N-isopropylacrylamide] which depicted an enhanced drug carrying capability and efficiently delivered both hydrophobic and hydrophilic drugs at human body temperature when compared with unmodified CaAlg microspheres (Oddo et al., 2010). Various ALG-based composites have been explored for evaluating the release from the ALG networks like micelles prepared from block copolymer of poly(ε-caprolactone)-block-(dimethlyamino)

TABLE 15.1 An Overview of Some Alginate (ALG) Composite Systems, Methods of Preparation/Cross-Linking Agents with Active Ingredients and their Applications.

Alginate (ALG) composite systems	Method of preparation/ crosslinking agents	Active ingredients/drugs/ biomolecules	Uses	Reference
ALG microspheres	ALG suspension method	Doxorubicin, Irinotecan	Intratumoral drug delivery and anticancer drug delivery system	(Glage et al., 2012)
ALG microspheres	Emulsion/external gelation with layer-by-layer nanofilm coatings method	Transforming growth factor β₃, human MSCs	Cartilage tissue engineering	(Bian et al., 2011)
ALG microspheres	Water-in-oil emulsion method	Chemokines; CCL21, CCL19, CXCL12, CXCL10	Chemoattractant delivery and chemotaxis studies	(Wang and Irvine, 2011)
ALG microspheres	Antigen encapsulation ultrasonic nozzle spray method	Live porcine rotavirus, recom-binant VP6 rotavirus protein	Oral vaccine delivery system	(Nograles et al., 2012)
ALG microspheres	Water-in-oil emulsion method	Plasmid DNA	Oral DNA vaccine delivery	(Kim et al., 2002)
Calcium-ALG beads	Emulsion dehydration method	Diloxanide furoate	Colon-targeting delivery for the treatment of amebic dysentery	(Shukla et al., 2010)
Mucoadhesive ALG microspheres	Emulsification phase separation method	Acyclovir	Gastro retentive targeting system	(Md et al., 2011)
Coralline hydroxyapatite (HA)-ALG composite microspheres	Dispersion polymerization method	Gentamicin	Bone-targeting drug delivery system	(Poojari and Srivastava, 2013)
Silicate-ALG composite microspheres	Combining calcium-silicate shell with an ALG core	Bovine serum albumin (BSA)	Bone-targeting drug delivery system	(Wu et al., 2011)
ALG-chitosan (CS) microspheres	Membrane emulsification in combination with calcium and CS solidification method	Insulin	Oral drug delivery for the treatment of diabetes	(Zhang et al. 2011a)

TABLE 15.1 *(Continued)*

Alginate (ALG) composite systems	Method of preparation/ crosslinking agents	Active ingredients/drugs/ biomolecules	Uses	Reference
Calcium-ALG beads	Octadecanol, berberine in sodium-ALG suspension dipped in calcium chloride	Berberine	Stomach-specific targeting system	(Zhang et al., 2011b)
Magnetic-ALG microspheres	ALG-Fe$_3$O$_4$ cross-linked by Ca^{2+}	Sylibin	Controlled delivery, Magnetic targeting, and imaging	(Xu et al., 2010)
Thermoresponsive/ pH-sensitive ALG microspheres	Calcium-ALG microspheres soaked in poly [(3-acrylamidopropyl)-trimethylammonium chloride-b-N-isopropylacrylamide] using electrostatic microbead generator	Pyroxicam,Horseradish peroxidase	Temperature/pH-sensitive Drug delivery system	(Oddo et al., 2010)
ALG poly-l-lysine nanoaggregates	Cross-linking between calcium chloride and poly-l-lysine	Doxorubicin	Anticancer drug delivery system	(Rajaonarivony et al., 1993)
ALG poly-l-lysine or ALG CS nanoaggregates	CaCl$_2$ and CS or CaCl$_2$ and poly-l-lysine	Methylene blue	Controlled drug delivery system	(De and Robinson, 2003)
ALG/poly-l-lysine with SiO$_2$ nanoaggregates composites	CaCl$_2$ and CoCl$_2$	Magnetic cobalt silicates	Incorporating magnetic NPs for biomedical applications	(Boissière et al., 2006)
ALG-Cisplatin/CS nanoaggregates	CaCl$_2$ and CS	Cisplatin	Anticancer drug delivery system	(Cafaggi et al., 2007)
ALG/CS nanoaggregates	CaCl$_2$ and CS	Insulin	Oral drug delivery system of insulin	(Sarmento et al., 2007)
ALG/EugragitE100 nanoaggregates	CaCl$_2$ and Eudragit E100	Gliclazide	Antidiabetic drug delivery system	(Sonavane and Devarajan, 2007)

TABLE 15.1 (Continued)

Alginate (ALG) composite systems	Method of preparation/ crosslinking agents	Active ingredients/drugs/ biomolecules	Uses	Reference
ALG/CS nanoaggregates	CS	DNA	Vaccine preparation	(Douglas et al., 2006)
ALG/CS nanoaggregates	CS	Gatifloxacin	Oral drug delivery system of antibiotic	(Motwani et al., 2008)
Thiolated sodium ALG nanoaggregates composite	Disulfide linkage	5-aminosalicylic acid (5-ASA)	Oral drug delivery system of 5-ASA for the treatment of inflammatory bowel disease	(Chang et al., 2012)
ALG nanocapsule composites	CaCl$_2$ and CS	Turmeric oil	Preparation of turmeric oil-loaded CS ALG biopolymeric system.	(Lertsutthiwong et al. 2009)
ALG/CS nanocapsule composites	CaCl$_2$ and CS	Formyl or acyl derivatives	Antitumor drug delivery system	(Grebinişan et al., 2011)
ALG nanocapsule composites	CaCl$_2$	Extract of *Phyllanthus amarus*	For analgesic preparations	(Deepa et al., 2012)
ALG nanosphere composites	CaCl$_2$	Cytochrome-C	Protein drug delivery system	(Monshipouri and Rudolph, 1995)
ALG-BSA nanosphere composites		5-FU	Anticancer drug delivery system	(Yi et al., 1999)
ALG/dextran nanosphere composites	CaCO$_3$	Insulin	Oral drug delivery system of insulin for the treatment of diabetes	(Reis et al., 2007)
ALG/CS	CaCl$_2$ and CS	Plasmid DNA	Preparation of vaccine drug delivery system	(You et al., 2006)

TABLE 15.1 *(Continued)*

Alginate (ALG) composite systems	Method of preparation/ crosslinking agents	Active ingredients/drugs/ biomolecules	Uses	Reference
ALG/CS nanosphere composites	CaCl₂ and CS	5-ASA	Oral drug delivery system	(Mladenovska et al., 2007)
ALG dextran with CS/ albumin nanosphere composites	CaCO₃	Insulin	Oral antidiabetic drug delivery system	(Reis et al., 2008)
ALG nanospheres	CaCl₂	Doxorubicin	Anticancer drug delivery system	(Liu et al., 2010)
ALG/oligoCS nanospheres	OligoCS	BSA	Vaccine preparation	(Wang and He, 2010)
ALG nanospheres	CaCl₂	Doxorubicin	Antitumour targeting system	(Chen et al., 2012)
ALG nanospheres	CaCl₂	Capsasin	Antitumour targeting system	(Tachaprutinun et al., 2013)
Superparamagnetic carboxymethyl CS/sodium ALG nanospheres	Hydrothermal method, molecular self-assembly technology, electrostatic interaction and an amide linkage	Enzyme	Ideal carrier for immobilizing enzyme.	(Jiang et al., 2016)
Poly(methyl methacrylate)-grafted ALG/Fe3O4 nanocomposites	Oxidative-free radical-graft copolymerization reaction	Heavy metals	Adsorption of Pb (II) and Cu (II)/removal of heavy metal ions.	(Mittal et al., 2016)
Zein and Propylene Glycol ALG (PGA) composites	Anti-solvent coprecipitation method	Quercetagetin	A synergistic effect was remarked between zein and PGA on ameliorating the entrapment efficiency and loading capacity of quercetagetin.	(Sun et al., 2016)

TABLE 15.1 *(Continued)*

Alginate (ALG) composite systems	Method of preparation/ crosslinking agents	Active ingredients/drugs/ biomolecules	Uses	Reference
ALG-ceramic composites/Calcium phosphate composite	ALG and HA		Tissue-engineered scaffolds for bone and cartilage targeting system.	(Venkatesan et al., 2015)
Iron-ALG thin films	Iron-ion-cross-linked ALG with embedded protein molecules	Protein (BSA)	For the maximal encapsulation and release of the Protein BSA from the film.	(Jin et al., 2012)
Composite CS/ALG hydrogel	Hydrogel alone or co-formulated with poly(D, L-lactide-co-glycolide) microspheres were prepared.	Deferoxamine	For the treatment of iron dysregulation diseases	(Rassu et al., 2016)
ALG-terephthalic acid composites matrices	Cross-linking metal ions (zinc, calcium, and aluminum)		Potential controlled release drug delivery system.	(Al-Otoum et al., 2014)
ALG/Gelatin/hyaluronic acid composite film	Prepared by the combination of bone ash (0–10 v.%) into gelatin/sodium ALG/hyaluronic acid	5-FU	For controlled drug delivery systems of colon-specific drug targeting system.	(Alemdar, 2016)
ALG/CS/multilayer film	By using self-assembled polyelectrolyte multilayer method (using CS/ALG)	Indomethacin	Release duration of indomethacin rises with the increment in the thickness of the indomethacin containing CS/ALG multilayer film.	(Tian et al., 2013)
ALG glucono-delta-lactone (GDL) hydrogel composite	ALG, glass and GDL		For the treatment of aneurysms/Intracranial drug delivery system.	(Brady et al., 2017)

TABLE 15.1 *(Continued)*

Alginate (ALG) composite systems	Method of preparation/ crosslinking agents	Active ingredients/drugs/ biomolecules	Uses	Reference
ALG-brushite hydrogel beads	Cross-linking process of ALG matrix	Ibuprofen	Fabricated to optimize the release profile of ibuprofen.	(Dabiri et al., 2017)
ALG/Gelatin Hydrogels composite	Cross-linked ALG/gelatin matrix	MDA-MB-231 triple negative breast cancer cells and IMR-90 fibroblast cells.	Anticancer drug delivery for breast cancer	(Jiang et al., 2017)
Composite of microporous tri calcium phosphate filled with ALG	Cross-linking the ALG with calcium ions	Antibiotic/Vancomycin	Used for the treatment of bone infections/Prolong the release behavior of the antibiotic up to nearly one month.	(Seidenstuecker et al., 2017)
ALG, CS, and pluronic NP composite	ALG, CS, and pluronic by ionotropic pre-gelation followed by the polycationic cross-linking method.	Curcumin	Anticancer drug delivery system	(Das et al., 2010)
ALG-keratin composite nanogels	Simple cross-linking of ALG-keratin	Doxorubicin hydrochloride	Anticancer/antitumor drug delivery system	(Sun et al., 2017)
ALG/ halloysite nanotubes (composite hydrogels)	Ca^{2+} cross-linking method	-	Improve the mechanical properties of ALG hydrogel and used in bone tissue engineering.	(Huang et al., 2017)
ALG and HA composite	Calcium phosphate—HA	Ascorbic acid.	Used in biological testing: bioactivity, biocompatibility, and osteoconductivity.	(Ilie et al., 2016)
ALG/Poly(γ-glutamic acid) Composite microparticles	Emulsification/internal gelation method, ion chelation interaction between Ca^{2+} and the carboxylate groups of ALG and PGA.	-	Applied in the field of wound dressing for hemostasis or rapid removal of exudates techniques.	(Tong et al., 2017)

TABLE 15.1 *(Continued)*

Alginate (ALG) composite systems	Method of preparation/ crosslinking agents	Active ingredients/drugs/ biomolecules	Uses	Reference
ALG thin-film composite nanofiltration membranes (NFMs)	Ultrathin cross-linked ALG coatings.	-	For NFMs with high performance and maximizes the reactant usage rate, minimizes the waste discharge.	(Du et al., 2017)
ALG hydrogel/CS micelle composites	Cross-linked between CaCl$_2$ and CS	Emodin	Sustained-release or site-specific drug delivery system for unstable or hydrophobic drugs	(Cong et al., 2017)
Diethanolamine-modified high-methoxyl pectin ALG-based core shell composites	Ionotropic gelation technique employing zinc acetate as cross-linker	Metformin HCl (MFM)	Controlled intragastric drug delivery of MFM for type 2 diabetes management.	(Bera and Kumar, 2017)

ethyl methacrylate containing indomethacin entrapped in calcium ALG beads depicting a rapid drug release at pH 1.2, 6.8, and 7.4 (Alvarez-Lorenzo et al., 2013). pH-sensitive ALG-g-poly(N-vinyl-2-pyrrolidone)/gelatin (SA-g-PVP/Gel) blend beads entrapped with nifedipine were also developed as controlled release delivery system. The pH-sensitive drug release was displayed by SA-g-PVP/Gel beads at pH 1.2 and 7.4 (İnal et al., 2017).

15.4 TARGET-SPECIFIC ALG-BASED COMPOSITE SYSTEMS

ALG-based composites have been very remarkably used in the formulation of targeted drug delivery systems. Various ligands may be anchored on the surface of nanocarriers for achieving targeted delivery of drugs to specific organs (Jain and Jain, 2016; Jain and Jain, 2015a). NPs bearing cisplatin, possessing an anionic or cationic surface charge, were developed by electrostatic interaction of a cisplatin–ALG complex (anionic in nature) with a positively charged polyelectrolyte, CS or N-trimethyl CS which exhibit better anticancer activity than plain cisplatin on A549 tumor cells. They have also revealed a similar potential in stimulating apoptosis in A2780 human cells. The outcomes reported that cisplatin complexes with polycarboxylate polymers could be successfully converted into a carrier system with high potential (Cafaggi et al., 2007). The composite NPs had been also formulated with the help of biocompatible polymers like ALG, CS, and pluronic through ionotropic pre-gelation accompanied by polycationic cross-linking. Pluronic F127 was employed to raise the solubility of curcumin in NPs. A cytotoxicity assay demonstrated that composite NPs depicted nontoxicity to HeLa cells at 500 µg/mL (Das et al., 2010). pH-sensitive composite films were formulated by employing bone ash in different concentrations ranging from 0–10 w/v% into gelatin/sodium ALG/hyaluronic acid (Gel/SA/HyA) polymeric structure for colon-specific delivery. The developed system revealed increased mechanical characteristics. Berberine floating beads employing calcium ALG were also developed for targeting the GIT mucosal membrane and extending their residence time in gastric mucosa which revealed a noteworthy enhancement in gastric residence time of beads (Zhang et al., 2011b). The targeted delivery in colonic disease like inflammatory bowel disease has similarly been achieved by reducible sodium ALG nanospheres which were cross-linked by the help of disulfide linkages (Chang et al., 2012). The drug targeting colorectal cancer can also be attained by using folic acid-conjugated liposomes loaded in ALG beads coated with

Eudragit. These target-specific systems delivered 21.52 ± 2.76 μg oxaliplatin at the tumor site after 12 h (Bansal et al., 2016).

15.5   APPLICATIONS

Selectively modifying and developing a novel generation of ALG composites with amended processing systems has brought a revolution in ALG-based drug delivery systems. The idea can be applied to the controlled release systems with improved bioavailability of poorly soluble drug entities, preventing enzymatic degradation of proteins, site-specific targeted delivery, enhancing the gene transfection efficiency, and the therapeutic efficacy. Therefore, these composite ALG-based carrier systems would discover their significance in the delivery of chemotherapeutics, immune vaccines, tissue engineering, and diagnostic, imaging and so forth. Various ALGs-based composite systems, such as microspheres, beads, hydrogels, matrices, films, microparticles, etc. have been prepared for use in drug delivery (Jain et al., 2013; Jain and Jain, 2015b; Jain and Bar-Shalom, 2014; Petchsomrit et al., 2017). Das et al. (2010) encapsulated curcumin in composite NPs made from ALG, CS, and pluronic for cancer cells delivery. A cytotoxicity assay depicted that at 500 μg/mL concentration, composite NPs were discovered to be nontoxic to HeLa cells. The half-maximal inhibitory concentrations obtained for free curcumin and encapsulated curcumin were 13.28 and 14.34 μM, respectively (Das et al., 2010). Cellulose nanocrystals (CNs) and CNs-based ALG composite coatings were developed by Chen et al. (2014) which could show potential application in drug delivery. Al-Otoum et al. (2014) prepared ALG-terephthalic acid composite matrices for controlled drug delivery and employed methylene blue as the model drug. It was observed that all the beads depicted higher dye loadings and controlled release profiles in comparison to their corresponding terephthalate-free ALG counterparts (Al-Otoum et al., 2014). Iliescu et al. (2014) developed and characterized montmorillonite-based irinotecan nanocomposite beads and sodium ALG as drug carriers. The results disclosed that the beads depicted a sustained release and may show a promising applicability in drug delivery, especially in chemotherapy (Iliescu et al., 2014). Díaz-Rodríguez and Landin (2015) prepared indomethacin-loaded ALG-poloxamer-silicon carbide composites-based hydrogels which depicted potent anti-inflammatory effects in osteo-arthritic conditions. Cheng et al. (2015) developed bovine serum albumin (BSA)-encapsulated ALG CS-Carrageenan composite NPs (Cheng et al., 2015). The drug release study depicted an initial burst in the early hours of the trial, accompanied by a slower steady release and was found to follow Fickian diffusion. Hasnain et al. (2016) prepared ALG-based bipolymeric-nanobioceramic composite matrices for sustained drug release (Hasnain et al., 2016). Various nano-hydroxyapatite-ALG- poly(vinyl pyrrolidone) beads loaded with diclofenac sodium showed prolonged sustained drug release profile and complied with the Korsmeyer-Peppas model of release pattern by Fickian mechanism. Khanal et al. (2016) prepared ALG-encapsulated magnesium sulfate microbeads using the electrospraying technique for Mg^{2+} delivery. The outcomes depicted that this strategy could be potentially utilized for enhancing the therapeutic efficacy of magnesium for the targeted local delivery in case of tissue injury (Khanal et al., 2016). Petchsomrit et al. (2017) developed ALG-Based Composite Sponges containing self-micro-emulsifying curcumin (SME-Cur) with the help of freeze drying method employing various grades of HPMC. The outcomes revealed that the HPMC-based sponges containing SME-Cur can be effectively employed for enhancing the oral bioavailability and might be applicable as they could be delivered at a comparatively lower dose as that of curcumin (Petchsomrit et al., 2017). Cong et al. (2017) developed pH-sensitive hydrogel/micelle composites. The outcomes of the research proved that they could be used as a sustained-release delivery system for hydrophobic drugs (Cong et al., 2018). Zhang et al. (2017) prepared a colon-specific drug delivery based on graphene oxide functionalized with sodium ALG system, employing 5-FU as the drug. The results depicted that tumor proliferation and liver metastasis were suppressed remarkably and the survival time of mice was prolonged (Zhang et al., 2017).

15.6 CONCLUSION

Among natural biopolymers, ALGs are extensively explored for drug delivery potential owing to a number of advantageous unique properties that have brought forth fabrication of various composites for a vista of applications using nanotechnology-based techniques. ALG composites have been very promising for controlled delivery of diversified therapeutic agents. These composites can be formulated on a large scale with ease and cost-effectiveness. Recent advancements in regard of improved safety and efficacy include stimuli-responsive systems and modifications endowing multiple characteristics. This chapter encompasses the principal fabrication techniques and characterization of various ALG-based composites emphasizing their application potential in the arena of drug delivery. Moreover, there is an urge to take care of the regulatory aspects and clinical concern for achieving the fullest potential of all such investigated composites.

SUMMARY

ALGs are natural biopolymers which have been widely employed in drug delivery owing to bioadhesivity, biocompatibility, biodegradability, non-toxicity and the ease of availability. They possess numerous distinct properties for developing different composites with polymers such as polycaprolactone, CS, poly(lactic-co-glycolic) acid, pectin, poloxamer, etc. for a broad arena of applications like drug delivery and so forth. Using fabricated ALG composites, various systems can be developed such as microspheres, gels, microparticles, matrices, nanospheres, membranes, and so forth. ALG-based composite systems are the exclusive carriers for applications in controlled drug delivery owing to their potency to entrap numerous therapeutic agents, for example, anticancer, antimicrobial, anti-inflammatory, antitubercular, and so forth. Besides the simpler processing techniques, mechanical strength, good bioavailability, well-ordered release rates, stability, targeted delivery of various agents and large-scale manufacturing with cost-effectiveness are other advantages of these systems. Moreover, stimuli-responsive systems such as pH/ion-sensitive and electrical field sensitive carrier systems have been formulated for oral delivery of therapeutic agents. This chapter presents a detailed account of the fabrication techniques and characterization of various ALG-based composites and their applications in drug delivery.

KEYWORDS

- alginate
- composite
- drug delivery
- microspheres
- microparticles

REFERENCES

Al-Otoum, R.; Abulateefeh, S.; Taha, M. Preparation of Novel Ionotropically Crosslinked Beads Based on Alginate-Terephthalic Acid Composites as Potential Controlled Release Matrices. *Pharmazie* **2014,** *69*(1), 10–18.

Alemdar, N. Fabrication of a Novel Bone Ash-Reinforced Gelatin/Alginate/Hyaluronic Acid Composite Film for Controlled Drug Delivery. *Carbohydr. Polym.* **2016,** *151,* 1019–1026.

Alvarez-Lorenzo, C., Blanco-Fernandez, B.; Puga, A. M.; Concheiro, A. Crosslinked Ionic Polysaccharides for Stimuli-Sensitive Drug Delivery. *Adv. Drug Delivery Rev.* **2013,** *65*(9), 1148–1171.

Augst, A. D.; Kong, H. J.; Mooney, D. J. Alginate Hydrogels as Biomaterials. *Macromol. Biosci.* **2006,** *6*(8), 623–633.

Aynie, I.; Vauthier, C.; Chacun, H.; Fattal, E.; Couvreur, P. Spongelike Alginate Nanoparticles as a New Potential System for the Delivery of Antisense Oligonucleotides. *Antisense Nucleic Acid Drug Dev.* **1999,** *9*(3), 301–312.

Bansal, D.; Gulbake, A.; Tiwari, J.; Jain, S. K. Development of Liposomes Entrapped in Alginate Beads for the Treatment of Colorectal Cancer. *Int. J. Biol. Macromol.* **2016,** *82,* 687–695.

Bera, H.; Kumar, S. Diethanolamine-Modified Pectin Based Core-Shell Composites as Dual Working Gastroretentive Drug-Cargo. *Int. J. Biol. Macromol.* **2017,** *108,* 1053–1062.

Bian, L.; Zhai, D. Y.; Tous, E.; Rai, R.; Mauck, R. L.; Burdick, J. A. Enhanced MSC Chondrogenesis Following Delivery of TGF-B3 from Alginate Microspheres within Hyaluronic Acid Hydrogels in Vitro and in Vivo. *Biomaterials* **2011,** *32*(27), 6425–6434.

Boissière, M.; Meadows, P. J.; Brayner, R.; Hélary, C.; Livage, J.; Coradin, T. Turning Biopolymer Particles Into Hybrid Capsules: the Example of Silica/Alginate Nanocomposites. *J. Mater. Chem.* **2006,** *16*(12), 1178–1182.

Brady, S.; Fox, E.; Lally, C.; Clarkin, O. Optimisation of a Novel Glass-Alginate Hydrogel for the Treatment of Intracranial Aneurysms. *Carbohydr. Polym.* **2017,** *176,* 227–235.

Brun-Graeppi, A. K. A. S.; Richard, C.; Bessodes, M.; Scherman, D.; Merten, O.-W. Cell Microcarriers and Microcapsules of Stimuli-Responsive Polymers. *J. Controlled Release* **2011,** *149*(3), 209–224.

Cafaggi, S.; Russo, E.; Stefani, R.; Leardi, R.; Caviglioli, G.; Parodi, B.; Viale, M. Preparation and Evaluation of Nanoparticles Made of Chitosan or N-Trimethyl Chitosan and a Cisplatin–Alginate Complex. *J. Controlled Release* **2007,** *121*(1), 110–123.

Chang, D.; Lei, J.; Cui, H.; Lu, N.; Sun, Y.; Zhang, X.; Yin, Y. Disulfide Cross-Linked Nanospheres from Sodium Alginate Derivative for Inflammatory Bowel Disease: Preparation, Characterization, and in Vitro Drug Release Behavior. *Carbohydr. Polym.* **2012,** *88*(2), 663–669.

Chen, T.; Yan, Q. P.; Li, F. R.; Tang, S. Q. Nanospheres Conjugated with Hab18 as Targeting Carriers for Antitumor Drug. *Adv. Mater. Res.* **2012,** *535–537,* 2381–2384.

Cheng, L.; Bulmer, C.; Margaritis, A. Characterization of Novel Composite Alginate Chitosan-Carrageenan Nanoparticles for Encapsulation of BSA as a Model Drug Delivery System. *Curr. Drug Delivery* **2015,** *12*(3), 351–357.

Cong, Z.; Shi, Y.; Wang, Y.; Wang, Y.; Chen, N.; Xue, H. A Novel Controlled Drug Delivery System Based on Alginate Hydrogel/Chitosan Micelle Composites. *Int. J. Biol. Macromol.* **2018,** *107,* 855–864.

Cui, J.-H.; Goh, J.-S.; Kim, P.-H.; Choi, S.-H.; Lee, B.-J. Survival and Stability of Bifidobacteria Loaded in Alginate Poly-l-Lysine Microparticles. *Int. J. Pharm.* **2000,** *210*(1), 51–59.

Dabiri, S. M. H.; Lagazzo, A.; Barberis, F.; Shayganpour, A.; Finocchio, E.; Pastorino, L. New in-Situ Synthetized Hydrogel Composite Based on Alginate and Brushite as a Potential pH Sensitive Drug Delivery System. *Carbohydr. Polym.* **2017,** *177,* 324–333.

Das, R. K.; Kasoju, N.; Bora, U. Encapsulation of Curcumin in Alginate-Chitosan-Pluronic Composite Nanoparticles for Delivery to Cancer Cells. *Nanomed. Nanotechnol. Biol. Med.* **2010,** *6*(1), 153–160.

De, S.; Robinson, D. Polymer Relationships During Preparation of Chitosan–Alginate and Poly-l-Lysine–Alginate Nanospheres. *J. Controlled Release* **2003,** *89*(1), 101–112.

de Vos, P.; Faas, M. M.; Strand, B.; Calafiore, R. Alginate-Based Microcapsules for Immunoisolation of Pancreatic Islets. *Biomaterials* **2006,** *27*(32), 5603–5617.

Deepa, V.; Sridhar, R.; Goparaju, A.; Reddy, P. N.; Murthy, P. B. Nanoemulsified Ethanolic Extract of Pyllanthus Amarus Schum and Thonn Ameliorates CCl4 Induced Hepatotoxicity in Wistar Rats. *Indian J. Exp. Biol.* **2012,** *50,* 785–794.

Díaz-Rodríguez, P.; Landin, M. Controlled Release of Indomethacin from Alginate–Poloxamer–Silicon Carbide Composites Decrease in-Vitro Inflammation. *Int. J. Pharm.* **2015,** *480*(1), 92–100.

Domb, A. J.; Kumar, N. *Biodegradable Polymers in Clinical Use and Clinical Development;* John Wiley & Sons: Hoboken, New Jersey, 2011.

Douglas, K. L.; Piccirillo, C. A.; Tabrizian, M. Effects of Alginate Inclusion on the Vector Properties of Chitosan-Based Nanoparticles. *J. Controlled Release* **2006,** *115*(3), 354–361.

Du, Y.; Zhang, C.; Zhong, Q.-Z.; Yang, X.; Wu, J.; Xu, Z.-K. Ultrathin Alginate Coatings as Selective Layers for Nanofiltration Membranes with High Performance. *ChemSusChem* **2017,** *10*(13), 2788–2795.

Fessi, H.; Puisieux, F.; Devissaguet, J. P.; Ammoury, N.; Benita, S. Nanocapsule Formation by Interfacial Polymer Deposition Following Solvent Displacement. *Int. J. Pharm.* **1989,** *55*(1), R1–R4.

Glage, S.; Lewis, A. L.; Mertens, P.; Baltes, S.; Geigle, P.; Brinker, T. Evaluation of Biocompatibility and Anti-Glioma Efficacy of Doxorubicin and Irinotecan Drug-Eluting Bead Suspensions in Alginate. *Clin. Transl. Oncol.* **2012,** *14*(1), 50–59.

Grebinişan, D.; Holban, M.; Şunel, V.; Popa, M.; Desbrieres, J.; Lionte, C. Novel Acyl Derivatives of N-(p-Aminobenzoyl)-L-Glutamine Encapsulated in Polymeric Nanocapsules with Potential Antitumoral Activity. *Cellul. Chem. Technol.* **2011,** *45*(9), 571.

Hamidi, M.; Azadi, A.; Rafiei, P. Hydrogel Nanoparticles in Drug Delivery. *Adv. Drug Delivery Rev.* **2008,** *60*(15), 1638–1649.

Hasnain, M. S.; Nayak, A. K.; Singh, M.; Tabish, M.; Ansari, M. T.; Ara, T. J. Alginate-Based Bipolymeric-Nanobioceramic Composite Matrices for Sustained Drug Release. *Int. J. Biol. Macromol.* **2016,** *83,* 71–77.

Huang, B.; Liu, M.; Long, Z.; Shen, Y.; Zhou, C. Effects of Halloysite Nanotubes on Physical Properties and Cytocompatibility of Alginate Composite Hydrogels. *Mater. Sci. Eng. C* **2017,** *70,* 303–310.

Huber, G. W.; Iborra, S.; Corma, A. Synthesis of Transportation Fuels from Biomass: Chemistry, Catalysts, and Engineering. *Chem. Rev.* **2006,** *106*(9), 4044–4098.

Ilie, A.; Ghiţulică, C.; Andronescu, E.; Cucuruz, A.; Ficai, A. New Composite Materials Based on Alginate and Hydroxyapatite as Potential Carriers for Ascorbic Acid. *Int. J. Pharm.* **2016,** *510*(2), 501–507.

Iliescu, R. I.; Andronescu, E.; Ghitulica, C. D.; Voicu, G.; Ficai, A.; Hoteteu, M. Montmorillonite–Alginate Nanocomposite as a Drug Delivery System–Incorporation and in Vitro Release of Irinotecan. *Int. J. Pharm.* **2014,** *463*(2), 184–192.

İnal, M.; Işıklan, N.; Yiğitoğlu, M. Preparation and Characterization of pH-Sensitive Alginate-g-Poly (*N*-Vinyl-2-Pyrrolidone)/Gelatin Blend Beads. *J. Ind. Eng. Chem.* **2017,** *52,* 128–137.

Jain, D.; Bar-Shalom, D. Alginate Drug Delivery Systems: Application in Context of Pharmaceutical and Biomedical Research. *Drug Dev. Ind. Pharm.* **2014,** *40*(12), 1576–1584.

Jain, A.; Jain, S. K. Environmentally Responsive Chitosan-Based Nanocarriers (CBNs). In *Handbook of Polymers for Pharmaceutical Technologies: Biodegradable Polymers;* Thakur, V. K. and Thakur, M. K., Eds., John Wiley & Sons Inc.: Hoboken, NJ, 2015a; Vol. 3, pp 105–126.

Jain, A.; Jain, S. K. Ligand-Appended BBB-Targeted Nanocarriers (LABTNs). *Crit. Rev. Ther. Drug Carrier Syst.* **2015b,** *32*(2), 149–180. DOI: 10.1615/CritRevTherDrugCarrier Syst.2015010903.

Jain, A.; Jain, S. Ligand-Mediated Drug-Targeted Liposomes. In *Liposomal Delivery Systems: Advances and Challenges;* 2016; pp 144–158. DOI: 10.4155/FSEB2013.14.251.

Jain, A.; Gulbake, A.; Shilpi, S.; Jain, A.; Hurkat, P.; Jain, S. K. A New Horizon in Modifica-tions of Chitosan: Syntheses and Applications. *Crit. Rev. Ther. Drug Carrier Syst.* **2013,** *30*(2), 91–181.

Jiang, J.; Chen, Y.; Wang, W.; Cui, B.; Wan, N. Synthesis of Superparamagnetic Carboxymethyl Chitosan/Sodium Alginate Nanosphere and Its Application for Immobilizing α-Amylase. *Carbohydr. Polym.* **2016,** *151,* 600–605.

Jiang, T.; Munguia-Lopez, J. G.; Flores-Torres, S.; Grant, J.; Vijayakumar, S.; De Leon-Rodriguez, A.; Kinsella, J. M. Directing the Self-Assembly of Tumour Spheroids by Bioprinting Cellular Heterogeneous Models Within Alginate/Gelatin Hydrogels. *Sci. Rep.* **2017,** *7*(1), 4575.

Jin, Z.; Güven, G.; Bocharova, V.; Halámek, J.; Tokarev, I.; Minko, S.; Katz, E. Electrochemically Controlled Drug-Mimicking Protein Release from Iron-Alginate Thin-Films Associated with an Electrode. *ACS Appl. Mater. Interfaces* **2012,** *4*(1), 466–475.

Khanal, S.; Adhikari, U.; Rijal, N. P.; Pai, D.; Sankar, J.; Bhattarai, N. In *Synthesis and Characterization of Alginate-Based Hydrogel Microbeads for Magnesium Release,* Paper Presented at the ASME 2016 International Mechanical Engineering Congress and Exposition, 2016, pp. V014T11A022–V014T11A022.

Khotimchenko, Y. S.; Kovalev, V.; Savchenko, O.; Ziganshina, O. Physical–Chemical Properties, Physiological Activity, and Usage of Alginates, the Polysaccharides of Brown Algae. *Russ. J. Mar. Biol.* **2001,** *27*(1), S53–S64.

Kim, B.; Bowersock, T.; Griebel, P.; Kidane, A.; Babiuk, L.; Sanchez, M.; Mutwiri, G. Mucosal Immune Responses Following Oral Immunization with Rotavirus Antigens Encapsulated in Alginate Microspheres. *J. Controlled Release* **2002,** *85*(1), 191–202.

Klostranec, J. M.; Chan, W. C. Quantum Dots in Biological and Biomedical Research: Recent Progress and Present Challenges. *Adv. Mater.* **2006,** *18*(15), 1953–1964.

Koch, S.; Schwinger, C.; Kressler, J.; Heinzen, C.; Rainov, N. Alginate Encapsulation of Genetically Engineered Mammalian Cells: Comparison of Production Devices, Methods and Microcapsule Characteristics. *J. Microencapsulation* **2003**, *20*(3), 303–316.

Lambert, G.; Fattal, E.; Couvreur, P. Nanoparticulate Systems for the Delivery of Antisense Oligonucleotides. *Adv. Drug Delivery Rev.* **2001**, *47*(1), 99–112.

Lanktree, M. B.; Guo, Y.; Murtaza, M.; Glessner, J. T.; Bailey, S. D.; Onland-Moret, N. C.; Johnson, T.; et al. Meta-Analysis of Dense Genecentric Association Studies Reveals Common and Uncommon Variants Associated with Height. *Am. J. Hum. Genet.* **2011**, *88*(1), 6–18.

Lee, K. Y.; Mooney, D. J. Alginate: Properties and Biomedical Applications. *Prog. Polym. Sci.* **2012**, *37*(1), 106–126.

Lertsutthiwong, P.; Noomun, K.; Jongaroonngamsang, N.; Rojsitthisak, P.; Nimmannit, U. Preparation of Alginate Nanocapsules Containing Turmeric Oil. *Carbohydr. Polym.* **2008**, *74*(2), 209–214.

Lertsutthiwong, P.; Rojsitthisak, P.; Nimmannit, U. Preparation of Turmeric Oil-Loaded Chitosan-Alginate Biopolymeric Nanocapsules. *Mater. Sci. Eng. C* **2009**, *29*(3), 856–860.

Liu, X.; Yu, W.; Zhang, Y.; Xue, W.; Yu, W.; Xiong, Y.; Yuan, Q. Characterization of Structure and Diffusion Behaviour of Ca-Alginate Beads Prepared with External or Internal Calcium Sources. *J. Microencapsulation* **2002**, *19*(6), 775–782.

Liu, J.; Zhang, Y.; Wang, C.; Xu, R.; Chen, Z.; Gu, N. Magnetically Sensitive Alginate-Templated Polyelectrolyte Multilayer Microcapsules for Controlled Release of Doxorubicin. *J. Phys. Chem. C* **2010**, *114*(17), 7673–7679.

Liu, D.; Xu, H.; Tian, B.; Yuan, K.; Pan, H.; Ma, S.; Pan, W. Fabrication of Carvedilol Nanosuspensions Through the Anti-Solvent Precipitation-Ultrasonication Method for the Improvement of Dissolution Rate and Oral Bioavailability. *AAPS PharmSciTech* **2012**, *13*(1), 295–304.

Lopes, M.; Abrahim, B.; Veiga, F.; Seiça, R.; Cabral, L. M.; Arnaud, P.; Ribeiro, A. J. Preparation Methods and Applications Behind Alginate-Based Particles. *Expert Opin. Drug Delivery* **2017**, *14*(6), 769–782.

Md, S.; Ahuja, A.; Khar, R. K.; Baboota, S.; Chuttani, K.; Mishra, A.; Ali, J. Gastroretentive Drug Delivery System of Acyclovir-Loaded Alginate Mucoadhesive Microspheres: Formulation and Evaluation. *Drug Delivery* **2011**, *18*(4), 255–264.

Mittal, A.; Ahmad, R.; Hasan, I. Poly (Methyl Methacrylate)-Grafted Alginate/Fe_3O_4 Nanocomposite: Synthesis and its Application for the Removal of Heavy Metal Ions. *Desalin. Water Treat.* **2016**, *57*(42), 19820–19833.

Mladenovska, K.; Raicki, R.; Janevik, E.; Ristoski, T.; Pavlova, M.; Kavrakovski, Z.; Goracinova, K. Colon-Specific Delivery of 5-Aminosalicylic Acid from Chitosan-Ca-Alginate Microparticles. *Int. J. Pharm.* **2007**, *342*(1), 124–136.

Monshipouri, M.; Rudolph, A. Liposome-Encapsulated Alginate: Controlled Hydrogel Particle Formation and Release. *J. Microencapsulation* **1995**, *12*(2), 117–127.

Mora-Huertas, C.; Fessi, H.; Elaissari, A. Polymer-Based Nanocapsules for Drug Delivery. *Int. J. Pharm.* **2010**, *385*(1), 113–142.

Motwani, S. K.; Chopra, S.; Talegaonkar, S.; Kohli, K.; Ahmad, F. J.; Khar, R. K. Chitosan–Sodium Alginate Nanoparticles as Submicroscopic Reservoirs for Ocular Delivery: Formulation, Optimisation and in Vitro Characterisation. *Eur. J. Pharm. Biopharm.* **2008**, *68*(3), 513–525.

Nograles, N.; Abdullah, S.; Shamsudin, M. N.; Billa, N.; Rosli, R. Formation and Characterization of pDNA-Loaded Alginate Microspheres for Oral Administration in Mice. *J. Biosci. Bioeng.* **2012,** *113*(2), 133–140.

Oddo, L.; Masci, G.; Di Meo, C.; Capitani, D.; Mannina, L.; Lamanna, R.; Matricardi, P. Novel Thermosensitive Calcium Alginate Microspheres: Physico-Chemical Characterization and Delivery Properties. *Acta Biomater.* **2010,** *6*(9), 3657–3664.

Ozaki, C. K.; Hamdan, A. D.; Barshes, N. R.; Wyers, M.; Hevelone, N. D.; Belkin, M.; Nguyen, L. L. Prospective, Randomized, Multi-Institutional Clinical Trial of a Silver Alginate Dressing to Reduce Lower Extremity Vascular Surgery Wound Complications. *J. Vasc. Surg.* **2015,** *61*(2), 419–427.e411.

Paques, J. P.; van der Linden, E.; van Rijn, C. J.; Sagis, L. M. Preparation Methods of Alginate Nanoparticles. *Adv. Colloid Interface Sci.* **2014,** *209,* 163–171.

Petchsomrit, A.; Sermkaew, N.; Wiwattanapatapee, R. Alginate-Based Composite Sponges as Gastroretentive Carriers for Curcumin-Loaded Self-Microemulsifying Drug Delivery Systems. *Sci. Pharm.* **2017,** *85*(1), 11.

Poncelet, D.; Neufeld, R.; Goosen, M.; Burgarski, B.; Babak, V. Formation of Microgel Beads by Electric Dispersion of Polymer Solutions. *AIChE J.* **1999,** *45*(9), 2018–2023.

Poojari, R.; Srivastava, R. Composite Alginate Microspheres as the Next-Generation Egg-Box Carriers for Biomacromolecules Delivery. *Expert Opin. Drug Delivery* **2013,** *10*(8), 1061–1076.

Rajaonarivony, M.; Vauthier, C.; Couarraze, G.; Puisieux, F.; Couvreur, P. Development of a New Drug Carrier Made from Alginate. *J. Pharm. Sci.* **1993,** *82*(9), 912–917.

Rassu, G.; Salis, A.; Porcu, E. P.; Giunchedi, P.; Roldo, M.; Gavini, E. Composite Chitosan/Alginate Hydrogel for Controlled Release of Deferoxamine: A System to Potentially Treat Iron Dysregulation Diseases. *Carbohydr. Polym.* **2016,** *136,* 1338–1347.

Reis, C. P.; Neufeld, R. J.; Ribeiro, A. J.; Veiga, F. Nanoencapsulation I. Methods for Preparation of Drug-Loaded Polymeric Nanoparticles. *Nanomedicine* **2006,** *2*(1), 8–21. DOI: 10.1016/j.nano.2005.12.003.

Reis, C. P.; Ribeiro, A. J.; Houng, S.; Veiga, F.; Neufeld, R. J. Nanoparticulate Delivery System for Insulin: Design, Characterization and in Vitro/in Vivo *Bioactivity. Eur. J. Pharm. Sci.* **2007,** *30*(5), 392–397.

Reis, C. P.; Veiga, F. J.; Ribeiro, A. J.; Neufeld, R. J.; Damgé, C. Nanoparticulate Biopolymers Deliver Insulin Orally Eliciting Pharmacological Response. *J. Pharm. Sci.* **2008,** *97*(12), 5290–5305.

Ribeiro, L. N.; Alcantara, A. C.; Darder, M.; Aranda, P.; Araujo-Moreira, F. M.; Ruiz-Hitzky, E. Pectin-Coated Chitosan-LDH Bionanocomposite Beads as Potential Systems for Colon-Targeted Drug Delivery. *Int. J. Pharm.* **2014,** *463*(1), 1–9. DOI: 10.1016/j.ijpharm.2013.12.035.

Sæther, H. V.; Holme, H. K.; Maurstad, G.; Smidsrød, O.; Stokke, B. T. Polyelectrolyte Complex Formation Using Alginate and Chitosan. *Carbohydr. Polym.* **2008,** *74*(4), 813–821.

Sahoo, S. K.; Labhasetwar, V. Nanotech Approaches to Drug Delivery and Imaging. *Drug Discovery Today* **2003,** *8*(24), 1112–1120.

Santhi, K.; Dhanraj, S.; Nagasamyvenkatesh, D.; Sangeetha, S.; Suresh, B. Preparation and Optimization of Sodium Alginate Nanospheres of Methotrexate. *Indian J. Pharm. Sci.* **2005,** *67*(6), 691.

Sarmento, B.; Ferreira, D.; Veiga, F.; Ribeiro, A. Characterization of Insulin-Loaded Alginate Nanoparticles Produced by Ionotropic Pre-Gelation Through DSC and FTIR Studies. *Carbohydr. Polym.* **2006,** *66*(1), 1–7.

Sarmento, B.; Ribeiro, A.; Veiga, F.; Ferreira, D.; Neufeld, R. Oral Bioavailability of Insulin Contained in Polysaccharide Nanoparticles. *Biomacromolecules* **2007,** *8*(10), 3054–3060.

Schwinger, C.; Koch, S.; Jahnz, U.; Wittlich, P.; Rainov, N.; Kressler, J. High Throughput Encapsulation of Murine Fibroblasts in Alginate Using the Jetcutter Technology. *J. Microencapsulation* **2002,** *19*(3), 273–280.

Seidenstuecker, M.; Ruehe, J.; Suedkamp, N. P.; Serr, A.; Wittmer, A.; Bohner, M.; Mayr, H. O. Composite Material Consisting of Microporous β-TCP Ceramic and Alginate for Delayed Release of Antibiotics. *Acta Biomater.* **2017,** *51,* 433–446.

Seifert, D. B.; Phillips, J. A. Production of Small, Monodispersed Alginate Beads for Cell Immobilization. *Biotechnol. Prog.* **1997,** *13*(5), 562–568.

Senuma, Y.; Lowe, C.; Zweifel, Y.; Hilborn, J.; Marison, I. Alginate Hydrogel Microspheres and Microcapsules Prepared by Spinning Disk Atomization. *Biotechnol. Bioeng.* **2000,** *67*(5), 616–622.

Shukla, S.; Jain, D.; Verma, K.; Verma, S. Formulation and in Vitro Characterization of Alginate Microspheres Loaded with Diloxanide Furoate for Colon-Specific Drug Delivery. *Asian J. Pharm.* **2010,** *4*(4), 199.

Sonavane, G. S.; Devarajan, P. V. Preparation of Alginate Nanoparticles Using Eudragit E100 as a New Complexing Agent: Development, in-Vitro, and in-Vivo Evaluation. *J. Biomed. Nanotechnol.* **2007,** *3*(2), 160–169.

Soppimath, K. S.; Aminabhavi, T. M.; Kulkarni, A. R.; Rudzinski, W. E. Biodegradable Polymeric Nanoparticles as Drug Delivery Devices. *J. Controlled Release* **2001,** *70*(1), 1–20.

Sun, J.; Tan, H. Alginate-Based Biomaterials for Regenerative Medicine Applications. *Materials* **2013,** *6*(4), 1285–1309.

Sun, C.; Dai, L.; Gao, Y. Binary Complex Based on Zein and Propylene Glycol Alginate for Delivery of Quercetagetin. *Biomacromolecules* **2016,** *17*(12), 3973–3985.

Sun, Z.; Yi, Z.; Zhang, H.; Ma, X.; Su, W.; Sun, X.; Li, X. Bio-Responsive Alginate-Keratin Composite Nanogels with Enhanced Drug Loading Efficiency for Cancer Therapy. *Carbohydr. Polym.* **2017,** *175,* 159–169.

Tachaprutinun, A.; Pan-In, P.; Wanichwecharungruang, S. Mucosa-Plate for Direct Evaluation of Mucoadhesion of Drug Carriers. *Int. J. Pharm.* **2013,** *441*(1), 801–808.

Tian, K.; Xie, C.; Xia, X. Chitosan/Alginate Multilayer Film for Controlled Release of IDM on Cu/LDPE Composite Intrauterine Devices. *Colloids Surf B* **2013,** *109,* 82–89.

Tong, Z.; Chen, Y.; Liu, Y.; Tong, L.; Chu, J.; Xiao, K.; Chu, X. Preparation, Characterization and Properties of Alginate/Poly (γ-Glutamic Acid) Composite Microparticles. *Mar. Drugs* **2017,** *15*(4), 91.

Venkatesan, J.; Bhatnagar, I.; Manivasagan, P.; Kang, K.-H.; Kim, S.-K. Alginate Composites for Bone Tissue Engineering: A Review. *Int. J. Biol. Macromol.* **2015,** *72,* 269–281.

Wang, T.; He, N. Preparation, Characterization and Applications of Low-Molecular-Weight Alginate–Oligochitosan Nanocapsules. *Nanoscale* **2010,** *2*(2), 230–239.

Wang, Y.; Irvine, D. J. Engineering Chemoattractant Gradients Using Chemokine-Releasing Polysaccharide Microspheres. *Biomaterials* **2011,** *32*(21), 4903–4913.

Wee, S.; Combotz, W. Protein Release from Alginate Matrics. Adv. *Drug Delivery Rev.* **1998,** *31,* 267–285.

Williams, P. A.; Phillips, G. Gum Arabic. In *Handbook of Hydrocolloids;* 2nd ed.; Woodhead Publishing Ltd.: Cambridge, UK, 2009; pp 252–273.

Wu, C.; Fan, W.; Gelinsky, M.; Xiao, Y.; Chang, J.; Friis, T.; Cuniberti, G. In Situ Preparation and Protein Delivery of Silicate–Alginate Composite Microspheres with Core-Shell Structure. *J. R. Soc. Interface* **2011,** *8*(65), 1804–1814.

Xu, P.; Guo, F.; Huang, J.; Zhou, S.; Wang, D.; Yu, J.; Chen, J. Alginate-Based Ferrofluid and Magnetic Microsphere Thereof. *Int. J. Biol. Macromol.* **2010,** *47*(5), 654–660.

Yi, Y.-M.; Yang, T.-Y.; Pan, W.-M. Preparation and Distribution of 5-Fluorouracil [125]I Sodium Alginate-Bovine Serum Albumin Nanoparticles. *World J. Gastroenterol.* **1999,** *5*(1), 57.

You, J.-O.; Park, S.-B.; Park, H.-Y.; Haam, S.; Chung, C.-H.; Kim, W.-S. Preparation of Regular Sized Ca-Alginate Microspheres Using Membrane Emulsification Method. *J. Microencapsulation* **2001,** *18*(4), 521–532.

You, J.-O.; Liu, Y.-C.; Peng, C.-A. Efficient Gene Transfection Using Chitosan–Alginate Core-Shell Nanoparticles. *Int. J. Nanomed.* **2006,** *1*(2), 173.

Yu, D. G.; Zhu, L. M.; Branford-White, C. J.; Yang, X. L. Three-Dimensional Printing in Pharmaceutics: Promises and Problems. *J. Pharm. Sci.* **2008,** *97*(9), 3666–3690. DOI: 10.1002/jps.21284.

Zhang, Y.; Wei, W.; Lv, P.; Wang, L.; Ma, G. Preparation and Evaluation of Alginate–Chitosan Microspheres for Oral Delivery of Insulin. *Eur. J. Pharm. Biopharm.* **2011a,** *77*(1), 11–19.

Zhang, Z.-H.; Sun, Y.-S.; Pang, H.; Munyendo, W. L.; Lv, H.-X.; Zhu, S.-L. Preparation and Evaluation of Berberine Alginate Beads for Stomach-Specific Delivery. *Molecules* **2011b,** *16*(12), 10347–10356.

Zhang, B.; Yan, Y.; Shen, Q.; Ma, D.; Huang, L.; Cai, X.; Tan, S. A Colon Targeted Drug Delivery System Based on Alginate Modified Graphene Oxide for Colorectal Liver Metastasis. *Mater. Sci. Eng. C* **2017,** *79*, 185–190.

Zimmermann, H.; Shirley, S. G.; Zimmermann, U. Alginate-Based Encapsulation of Cells: Past, Present, and Future. *Curr. Diabetes Rep.* **2007,** *7*(4), 314–320.

CHAPTER 16

HYDROXYAPATITE-ALGINATE COMPOSITES IN DRUG DELIVERY

SITANSU SEKHAR NANDA[1,*], DONG KEE YI[1],
MD SAQUIB HASNAIN[2], and AMIT KUMAR NAYAK[3,*]

[1]*Department of Chemistry, Myongji University, Yongin, South Korea*

[2]*Department of Pharmacy, Shri Venkateshwara University, Rajabpur, Gajraula, Amroha, Uttar Pradesh 244236, India*

[3]*Department of Pharmaceutics, Seemanta Institute of Pharmaceutical Sciences, Mayurbhanj, Odisha 757086, India*

Corresponding author. E-mail: nandasitansusekhar@gmail.com; amitkrnayak@yahoo.co.in

16.1 INTRODUCTION

During last few decades, a variety of biopolymers have been exploited as raw materials for the drug delivery and contrive of formulations due to their fantabulous properties, such as biocompatibility, environmental sensitivity non-toxicity, biodegradability, and so forth (Wu et al., 2007; Hasnain et al., 2010; Maji et al., 2012; Das et al., 2013; Nayak et al., 2013a, 2013b; Malakar et al., 2014; Pal and Nayak, 2015a, 2015b; Nayak et al., 2018a). Biopolymers like alginates (Malakar and Nayak, 2012a; Malakar et al., 2012a), chitosan (Jana et al., 2013a; Nayak and Pal, 2015; Verma et al., 2017), pectin (Nayak et al., 2013c, 2014a, 2014b; Guru et al., 2018), locust bean gum (Prajapati et al., 2014), tamarind gum (Nayak, 2016; Nayak and Pal, 2018), guar gum (Chourasia et al., 2006), sterculia gum (Nayak and Pal, 2016a), okra gum (Sinha et al., 2015a, 2015b), gellan gum (Nayak et al., 2014c, 2014d, 2014e), fenugreek gum (Nayak et al., 2012a, 2013c), hydroxypropyl methylcellulose (Bodmeier and Paeratakul, 1991), polycaprolactone (Nithya et al., 2015), Carbopol (Das et al., 2013), poly(vinyl alchohol) (Hua et al., 2010), poly(vinyl pyrrolidone) (Nayak et al., 2013c), and so forth, have been utilized in the designing of controlled releasing drug delivery systems. Nevertheless, the drawbacks like admitting the burst release of drugs and washy mechanical properties are tough when these biopolymers are utilized to formulate various effective drug delivery systems (Pal and Nayak, 2015a). These drawbacks are caused primarily due to properties of the biopolymers, the poor interactions in-between the drugs and biopolymers, faster disintegration of the biopolymers during drug releasing, and so forth (Nayak and Pal, 2016b; Nayak et al., 2018a). In addition, various methodologies to fabricate drug delivery systems such as grafting with the monomers (Sen and Pal, 2009; Nayak et al., 2018b), formation of interpenetrating polymer networks (Jana et al., 2013b; Bera et al., 2015a), formation of polyelectrolyte complexes (Kumar and Ahuja, 2013; Jana et al., 2013a), chemical cross-linkings (Chourasia et al., 2006), physical blending with other biopolymers (Pal and Nayak, 2011; Malakar et al., 2012b), and so forth, have been enforced to ameliorate the characteristics of the biopolymer-based drug releasing systems. Beside these, biopolymers are also being fabricated to develop numerous composite systems for controlling the drug releasing property (Angadi et al., 2012; Hezaveh and Muhamad, 2012). In the recent years, a variety of inorganic materials such as silica (Kim et al., 2006), clays (Khlibsuwan et al., 2017), hydroxyapatite (HAp) (Nithya et al., 2015; Hasnain et al., 2016), calcium phosphate (Fullana et al., 2010), and so forth, have been reinforced within the biopolymers in the formulations of composites to control the drug releasing over a longer period. The synergistic effect of these inorganic materials–biopolymers combinations as well as the substantial interfacial interactions in-between these through the hydrogen bonding and the electro-statically interactions could ameliorate the swelling behavior, mechanical properties, and controlled releasing behavior of the pristine biopolymers. In accumulation, these characteristics could be tuned by modifying the content and the type of inorganic materials reinforced in the composite formula. The current chapter deals with a comprehensive discussion on the reported researches on the HAp–alginate composites for the use in drug-releasing applications.

16.2 ALGINATES

Alginates are regarded as the instinctive natural polysaccharide groups obtained from brown sea algae, which consist of C-5 epimer α-L-guluronate (G) residues and (1 → 4) linked β-D-mannuronate (M) residues (Lee and

Mooney, 2012; Pawar and Edgar, 2012). Alginates are anionic linear poly-saccharides. Because of the desirable rheological characteristics, alginates have been extensively utilized as thickener, gelling agent, colloidal stabi-lizing agent and also, as blood expander material (Smidsrod and Draget, 1996; Goh et al., 2012). Alginates utilized in various biomedical applications including drug delivery, cell and enzyme encapsulations, wound dressings, tissue engineering, dentistry, and so forth, owing to its excellent biocompat-ibility and biodegradability (Lin and Yeh, 2004; Sun and Tan, 2013; Priddy et al., 2014). Sodium alginate is capable of producing ionotropically gelled physical hydrogels by the influence of various divalent metal cations, such as Ba^{2+}, Ca^{2+}, Zn^{2+}, and so forth, (except Mg^{2+}) and trivalent cations, such as Al^{3+} (Nayak and Pal, 2015; Pal and Nayak, 2015). This is because of the interaction between G-block monomers and divalent/trivalent cations in the polymer chains contributing to ionic bridge formation in-between adjacent polymer chains. The ionotropically cross-linking gelation process consti-tutes alginate an attractive material for drugs as well as cell encapsulations (Goh et al., 2012). However, the significant limitation of these ionotropi-cally cross-linked alginate hydrogels is the lower degradability, *in vivo*. Such alginate-based hydrogels degrade slowly in an irregular manner through the dissociation of the ionotropic cross-linking traced by the loosing of low and high molecular weight alginate strands. The only comparatively low molecular weight alginate strands (bearing the molecular weight lower than 50 kDa) can be eliminated from the body through the kidney. On the other side, alginates having high molecular weight are difficult to eliminate from the body because mammals lack alginate degrading enzymes (Kim et al., 2012). Therefore, the alginate-based systems demonstrate the poor cell infil-tration and adhesion because of its deficiency of specific molecular interac-tion capacity with mammalian cells (Bai et al., 2013; Balakrishnan et al., 2014). It is now well-understood that the oxidation of alginate can intensify its biodegradability (Liang et al., 2011) and the number of probes focusing on the oxidized alginate for various biomedical applications is rapidly increasing (Balakrishnan et al., 2014). In addition, alginates are also being cross-linked covalently using glutaraldehyde to prepare nanoparticles, microspheres, beads, and so forth, for the modified releasing of different drugs (Babu et al., 2007; Kulkarni et al., 2012). Various drugs are also being encapsulated in different cross-linked alginate gel microsphere/bead matrices and the already developed cross-linked alginate gel systems were found to be demonstrated different patterns of drug encapsulations and release profiles reliant on their method of preparations as well as their physicochemical properties (Pal and Nayak, 2015b). However, the drug releasing properties of these cross-linked alginate hydrogels were found to experience some severe problems (Hua et al., 2010). Principally, the encapsulated drugs may leak owing to the long immersion time during the gel formation, which may cause diminutions of the drug encapsulation efficiency. Furthermore, the burst releasing of drugs from the pure cross-linked alginate microspheres/beads may be caused due to the quick degradation of the matrices in the release procedure. Recent years, much attention has been paid for bettering the operation of cross-linked (chemical as well as physical) alginates and non-cross-linked alginate composite systems by reinforcing the second biopolymer(s) or bioinorganic material(s) for drug delivery applications (Hua et al., 2010; Pal and Nayak, 2015a, 2015b; Hasnain et al., 2016; Jain and Datta, 2016). Some examples of already reported alginate-based composite systems, which are developed for the use in drug delivery applications, are presented in Table 16.1.

TABLE 16.1 Some Examples of Alginate-Based Composite Systems for Drug Delivery Applications.

Alginate-based composite systems for drug delivery	References
Calcium alginate-methyl cellulose mucoadhesive microcapsules of gliclazide	Pal and Nayak 2011
Hydroxypropyl methylcellulose-alginate systems for sustained release of indomethacin	Bodmeier and Paeratakul 1991
Alginate-poly(vinyl alcohol) hydrogel beads of diclofenac sodium	Hua et al., 2010
Fenugreek seed mucilage-calcium alginate mucoadhesive beads of metformin HCl	Nayak et al., 2013d
Calcium alginate-gum Arabic beads of glibenclamide	Nayak et al., 2012b
Okra gum-zinc alginate beads for sustained releasing of diclofenac sodium	Sinha et al., 2015a
Okra gum-calcium alginate mucoadhesive beads of glibenclamide	Sinha et al., 2015b
Tamarind seed polysaccharide-alginate mucoadhesive microspheres of gliclazide	Pal and Nayak 2012
Tamarind seed polysaccharide-alginate beads of diclofenac sodium	Nayak and Pal 2011
Tamarind seed polysaccharide-alginate mucoadhesive beads of metformin HCl	Nayak and Pal 2013; Nayak et al., 2016
Locust bean gum-alginate systems containing aceclofenac	Prajapati et al., 2014
Jackfruit seed starch–calcium alginate mucoadhesive beads of pioglitazone	Nayak et al., 2013a
Jackfruit seed starch–calcium alginate mucoadhesive beads of metformin HCl	

TABLE 16.1 *(Continued)*

Alginate-based composite systems for drug delivery	References
Calcium alginate-ispaghula mucilage mucoadhesive beads for controlled glibenclamide release	Nayak et al., 2013b
Calcium alginate-ispaghula mucilage mucoadhesive beads of gliclazide	Nayak et al., 2010a
Cationized starch-alginate beads containing aceclofenac	Malakar et al., 2013a
Soluble starch-Ca^{2+}-Zn^{2+}-alginate microparticles of aceclofenac	Nayak et al., 2018c
Potato starch-calcium alginate beads of tolbutamide	Malakar et al., 2013b
Zinc alginate-carboxymethyl cashew gum microbeads of isoxuprine hydrochloride	Das et al., 2014
Unsaturated esterified alginate-gellan gum microspheres of aceclofenac	Jana et al., 2013c
Composite microbeads of sodium alginate coated with chitosan for controlled release of amoxicillin	Angadi et al., 2012
Calcium alginate-poly(vinyl pyrrolidone) microbeads of diclofenac sodium	Nayak et al., 2011a
Calcium alginate-poly(vinyl pyrrolidone)-nanoHAp beads containing diclofenac sodium	Hasnain et al., 2016
Montmorillonite-alginate composite microspheres of venlafaxine hydrochloride	Jain and Datta 2016
Montmorillonite-alginate nanocomposite of irinotecan	Illiescu et al., 2014
Montmorillonite-alginate nanocomposites of vitamin B1 and vitamin B6	Kevadiya et al., 2010
Alginate-magnesium stearate oil-entrapped buoyant beads of ibuprofen	Malakar and Nayak 2012b
Alginate-sterculia gum gel-coated oil-entrapped alginate beads of risperidone	Bera et al., 2015b
Alginate gel-coated oil-entrapped alginate–tamarind gum–magnesium stearate buoyant beads of risperidone	Bera et al., 2015c
Calcium phosphate-alginate microspheres	Ribeiro et al., 2004
Alginate-HAp nanocomposite beads containing diclofenac sodium	Zhang et al., 2010
Alginate-HAp nanocomposite beads of ofloxacin	Roul et al., 2013
Alginate-calcium carbonate hybrid nanoparticles	Wu et al., 2014
Chitosan-sodium alginate nanocomposites blended with cloisite 30b	Nayak and Sahoo 2011

16.3   HYDROXYAPATITE (HAP)

HAp is a bioceramic material, having chemical formula of $[Ca_{10}(PO_4)_6(OH)_2]$ (Nayak, 2010). In the pure HAp molecules, calcium to phosphorus ratio is maintained at 1.67. HAp can be synthetically produced by a variety of methods such as wet precipitation method (Santos et al., 2004), hydrothermal method (Manafi and Joughehdoust, 2009), solgel method (Chai and Ben-Nissan, 1999), biomimetic deposition method (Tas, 2000), and so forth. It is the inorganic constituents of the bone mineral composition and it can be promptly reabsorbed into the bone tissue (Oonishi, 1991). HAp displays outstanding properties such as high osteoconductivity and osteoinduction when implanted in the human body (Uskoković and Uskoković, 2011; Zhou and Lee, 2011). Because of the osteoconductive and osteoinduction characteristics, HAp can perform better in bone regeneration applications (Komlev et al., 2002; Uskoković and Uskoković, 2011). HAp has been employed in the enzyme and drug delivery systems because of its fantabulous characteristics, such as the capability to adsorb a wide range of chemical species and good biocompatibility (Pharm et al., 2002; Ribeiro et al., 2004; Mizushima et al., 2006). Nevertheless, the drug releases from HAp-based scaffolds has established to be primarily very quick, owing to the fragile interaction between HAp particles and the drugs (Ribeiro et al., 2010). HAp loaded with therapeutic concentrations of antibiotics such as norfloxacin, cephalexin, ciprofloxacin, gentamycin, amoxicillin, gatifloxacin, and so forth has been verified for the treatment of osteomyelitis and hence, HAp can be a suitable drug delivery system (Baro et al., 2002; Nayak and Sen, 2009; Nayak et al., 2010b, 2011b, 2011c, 2013e). Recently, HAp has been exposed to accelerate the healing of bone fractures with help of electrical stimulation (Quilitz et al., 2010). This response to electrical stimulation has been credited to the microstructure and porosity of HAp. Such approaches have been recognized in the treatment of osteonecrosis and osteoarthritis (Hoepfner and Case, 2002; Gittings et al., 2009).

Recently, various natural polymers such as collagen, gelatin, chitosan, alginate, cellulose, and so forth are widely employed to fabricate composites for drug delivery and tissue engineering applications referable to the biodegradation and biocompatibility of HAp (Narbat et al., 2006; Grande et al., 2009). Thus, the combinations of HAp and biopolymers in the form of composite structures appear to be an attractive direction to sustain the release of drugs toward long-term controlled release systems. A few HAp–biopolymer composites for drug releasing applications have successfully derived by several methods (Xu and Czernuszka, 2008; Uskoković and Uskoković, 2011). Burst releasing of drug from poly(lactic-co-glycolic acid) was noticed due to the interaction between micron-sized HAp and poly(lactic-co-glycolic acid) particles, and the release order can be controlled by tuning the concentration of HAp (Xu and Czernuszka, 2008). Surface coating of HAp with poly(lactic-co-glycolic acid) microspheres through a two-fold constant composition method help upturn the entrapment efficiency of drug and sustain its release. Thus, the probability continues of contriving HAp-biopolymer composites at a molecular level and then further ameliorating their characteristics. Since past few years, numerous HAp-based composites are being fabricated for the use as drug-releasing matrices by various research teams. Some examples of already reported HAp-based composite systems, which are developed for the use in drug delivery applications, are presented in Table 16.2.

TABLE 16.2 Some Examples of Hydroxyapatite-Based Composite Systems Employed in Drug Delivery Applications.

Hydroxyapatite (HAp)-based composite systems in drug delivery applications	References
HAp–ciprofloxacin composites	Nayak and Sen 2009; Nayak et al., 2010b, 2011b, 2011c
HAp–ofloxacin composites	Nayak et al., 2013e
Alginate-HAp microspheres	Ribeiro et al. 2004
Alginate-HAp nanocomposite beads containing diclofenac sodium	Zhang et al., 2010
Alginate-HAp nanocomposite beads of ofloxacin	Roul et al., 2013
Calcium alginate-poly(vinyl pyrrolidone)-nanoHAp beads containing diclofenac sodium	Hasnain et al., 2016
HAp-coated poly(lactic-co-glycolic acid) microspheres	Xu and Czernuszka 2008
HAp-polycaprolactone nanocomposite film of ciprofloxacin	Nithya and Meenakshi Sundaram 2015
HAp–anionic collagen composites for controlled antibiotic release	Martin et al., 1998
HAp-collagen–alginate composite as carrier of bone morphogenetic protein	Sotome et al., 2004
HAp/poly(ethyl methacrylate)/poly(methyl methacrylate) composites for gentamicin release	Real et al., 2000

TABLE 16.2 *(Continued)*

Hydroxyapatite (HAp)-based composite systems in drug delivery applications	References
Agarose encapsulated mesoporous carbonated HAp nanocomposites powder for drug delivery	Kolanthai et al., 2017
Glass-reinforced HAp composites of sodium ampicillin	Queiroz et al., 2001
Nanocrystalline HAp-calcium sulfate composite for local antibiotic delivery	Rauschmann et al., 2005
HAp-magnetite-MWCNT nanocomposite for multifunctional drug delivery	Pistone et al., 2014
Mesoporous nanocomposite of MCM-48/HAp for ibuprofen release	Aghaei et al., 2014

16.4 VARIOUS ALGINATE–HAP COMPOSITE-BASED DRUG RELEASING SYSTEMS

In recent decades, alginate-HAp composites have attracted much attention for their applications as the matrices for drug releasing and repairing/regenerating diverse tissues/organs (Docherty-Skogh et al., 2010). Alginate–HAp composites are based on the water-soluble polymer network; the hydrophilic part combines with water particles and holds water inside the net. These bipolymeric-bioceramic composite materials are being synthesized or fabricated to meet the specific chemical and mechanical attributes. Various alginate–HAp composites can influence the geometry, adhesion and proliferation of the cellular level when they serve as the mimics for the extracellular matrix (Suárez-González et al., 2010; Chae et al., 2013). The migration, growth and differentiation of the cells are sensitive to the elastic modulus of alginate–HAp composites (Lin and Yeh, 2004). In some reported works, alginate-HAp composite based scaffolds with improved mechanical properties were prepared by direct mixing of sodium alginate with HAp powders (Lin and Yeh, 2004; Turco et al., 2009). However, the straight mixing is an abandoned method and consequences of a lack of homogeneity of particle distribution in the polymer matrix with limited bioactivity. Soaking the scaffolds in simulated body fluid and/or modified simulated body fluid is another useful second-hand method to formulate alginate–HAp composites (Zhang and Ma, 2004) For example, Suárez-González et al. (2010) fabricated alginate–HAp composite scaffolds by incubating the alginate scaffolds in modified simulated body fluid. After 28 days of incubation, a layer of HAp was noticed to locate along the surface of alginate scaffolds. However, these methods usually include a longtime of incubation, which consequences in a decrease of stability because of the conversation of the cross-linking ions (Ca^{2+}) and the partial degradation. Furthermore, a longtime of incubation also changes the release features of any encapsulated biological factors or therapeutic agents during storing in simulated body fluid over such a longtime. In situ mineralization is another effective and simple method for making alginate–HAp composites (Xie et al., 2012). This method was also used for constructing alginate–HAp microspheres for growth factor delivery, drug delivery, such as alginate–HAp composite microspheres (Zhang et al., 2010). Alginate solution was equipped by dissolving alginate powder in a solution containing phosphate ions, and then this solution was released into a calcium chloride solution. The alginate was cross-associated with calcium ions and molded stable microspheres, and simultaneously, calcium ions responded with phosphate ions to form HAp. Although the alginate-HAp composite microspheres presented a sustained drug delivery, they bore no apparent core/shell structure. Fibrous alginate-HAp nanocomposite scaffolds are also being prepared through in situ mineralization by the electrospinning method (Chae et al., 2013). In the literature, several alginate–HAp composite-based systems for controlling drug release are already reported by various research groups.

16.4.1 IN SITU GENERATED ALGINATE–HAP NANOCOMPOSITE BEADS

Zhang et al. (2010) synthesized and evaluated alginate–HAp nanocomposite beads as controlled drug releasing carriers. Within these alginate–HAp nanocomposites, a nonsteroidal anti-inflammatory drug, namely diclofenac sodium was loaded as model drug to resolve the issue of the burst release of drugs from the synthesized calcium alginate beads. These alginate–HAp nanocomposite beads were synthesized through the in situ generation of HAp particles during the solgel transition procedure of sodium alginate with the influence of calcium ions. The solgel transition procedure of sodium alginate occurred when the solution of sodium alginate reacted with the solution of $Ca(NO_3)_2$ and the formation of HAp was found to be started as the calcium ions present in the surrounding environment penetrated into the alginate beads and met the phosphate ions. Calcium ions in the reaction system reacted with $(NH_4)_2HPO_4$, carboxyl groups of sodium alginate to form calcium alginate–HAp nanocomposite beads. The HAp particles grew slowly within the calcium ion cross-linked ionotropically gelled alginate chains and the interactions between sodium alginate, HAp and the encapsulated drug (i.e., diclofenac sodium), occurred at the molecular level because of the uniform dispersing of the phosphate ions in these calcium alginate–HAp nanocomposite beads. The reaction of the *in situ* synthesis of HAp is shown below:

$$10Ca\,(NO_3)_2 + 6(NH_4)_2\,HPO_4 + 8NH_3 \cdot H_2O \rightarrow Ca_{10}\,(PO_4)_6$$
$$(OH)_2 \downarrow +6H_2O + 20NH_4NO_3$$

The *in situ* synthesized alginate–HAp nanocomposite beads loaded with diclofenac sodium displayed a coarse bead-surface with the occurrences of several typical wrinkles. The occurrence of the *in situ* synthesized HAp crystals within the calcium alginate matrices would contract by restricting the movability of the ionotropically gelled alginate chains. The *in vitro* drug releasing from these alginate–HAp nanocomposite was found dependent on the reaction temperature as well as reaction time of the synthesis procedure. The *in situ* formed HAp crystals displayed the influence on the drug releasing pattern (*in vitro*) of the nanocomposite beads the synthesized HAp enhanced the drug loadings. A pH-sensitive *in vitro* drug releasing pattern was noticed by these nanocomposite beads. This occurrence can be attributed by the fact that the *in situ*-formed HAp crystals could hindrance the encapsulated drug releasing and also, overcome the burst effects of drug releasing from the pure calcium alginate gel beads.

16.4.2   CALCIUM ALGINATE-HAP NANOCOMPOSITE BEADS OF OFLOXACIN

Roul et al. (2013) have prepared and evaluated ofloxacin (a fluroquinolone) loaded calcium alginate–HAp nanocomposite beads. The particle size of calcium alginate–HAp nanocomposite beads of ofloxacin was measured and it was found to have the diameter of 5 mm (approximately). These beads also were of spherical in shape with a smoother surface morphological feature. The drug (ofloxacin) encapsulation efficiencies (%) of the nanocomposite bead systems were within 55.90 ± 4.25–$93.52\pm2.21\%$. The drug encapsulation of these calcium alginate–HAp nanocomposite-based beads was improved with the rise in HAp and sodium alginate amounts to these bead formulas. This result could be explained by the incorporation of HAp powders within the alginate matrices might construct a thicker coating around the encapsulated drug particles, which may possibly control the drug leakage during the nanocomposite bead preparation. The *in vitro* ofloxacin releasing from these HAp-based nanocomposite beads demonstrated a prolonged release pattern at pH 7.4 as compared to that of the pure calcium alginate beads. Additionally, in the *in vitro* release study, it was observed that the reinforcement of HAp powders slower the release of encapsulated ofloxacin.

16.4.3   CALCIUM ALGINATE-POLY (VINYL PYRROLIDONE)/ NANO-HAP COMPOSITE BEADS

In a research, diclofenac sodium-loaded composite beads made of calcium alginate, poly(vinyl pyrrolidone), and nano-HAp was developed and evaluated by Hasnain et al. (2016) for the usage as sustained releasing carrier matrices. These biopolymeric–bioceramic composite-based calcium alginate-poly(vinyl pyrrolidone)/nano-HAp beads were synthesized by the reinforcement of synthetic nano-HAp within ionotropically gelled calcium alginate–poly(vinyl pyrrolidone) polymeric systems. 65.82 ± 1.88–$94.45 \pm 3.72\%$ of diclofenac encapsulation efficiency was measured for these composite beads. The mean sizes of these calcium alginate–poly(vinyl pyrrolidone)/nano-HAp composite beads were within the range, 0.98 ± 0.07–1.23 ± 0.15 mm. The diclofenac encapsulation within these composite beads was found to be enhanced with the reduction of sodium alginate to poly(vinyl pyrrolidone) ratio in the polymeric raw material formula. Possibly, the intermolecular hydrogen bonding between–OH groups of the alginate structure and –C=O groups of poly(vinyl pyrrolidone) structure in these biopolymeric-bioceramic composite-based calcium alginate–poly(vinyl pyrrolidone)/nano-HAp beads, which might lessen the leaching of encapsulated drug during bead synthesis. This occurrence could make possible to encapsulate drug increasingly. The schematic presentation of the proposed interactions to form the calcium alginate–poly(vinyl pyrrolidone)/nano-HAp composite beads of diclofenac sodium are presented (Figure 16.1). These calcium alginate–poly(vinyl pyrrolidone)/nano-HAp composite beads of diclofenac sodium demonstrated a spherically shaped morphological view (Figure 16.2). The surface topographical morphology of these biopolymeric–bioceramic composite beads revealed a rough surface with some cracks and wrinkles. In addition, porous structure with numerous micropores was noticed by examining the surface topographic morphological view of these composite beads by scanning electron microscopy. Various calcium alginate–poly(vinyl pyrrolidone)/nano-HAp composite beads of diclofenac sodium exhibited prolonged release over 8 h of *in vitro* drug releasing study, when tested in 0.1 N HCl (pH 1.2) for first 2 h and then, in phosphate buffer (pH 7.4) for the remaining period (Figure 16.3). These composite beads also revealed to follow the Koresmeyer-Peppas model with non-Fickian release (anomalous transport) mechanism during the course of drug release.

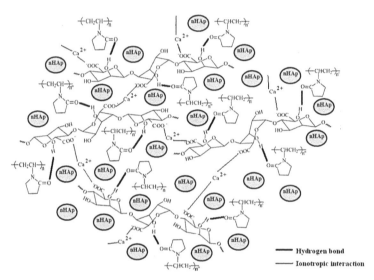

FIGURE 16.1 Schematic presentation of the proposed interactions to form calcium alginate–poly(vinyl pyrrolidone)/nano-hydroxyapatite (HAp) composite beads of diclofenac sodium.

Source: Adapted with permission from Hasnain et al. (2016) (Copyright © 2014 Elsevier B. V.).

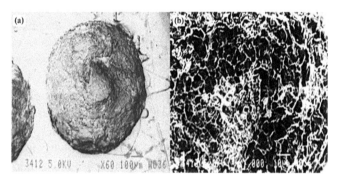

FIGURE 16.2 (See color insert.) Scanning electron microscopy photographs of the calcium alginate–poly(vinyl pyrrolidone)/nano-HAp composite beads of diclofenac sodium at lower magnification (60x) and bead surface topography at higher magnification (1000x).

Source: Adapted with permission from Hasnain et al. (2016) (Copyright © 2014 Elsevier B. V.).

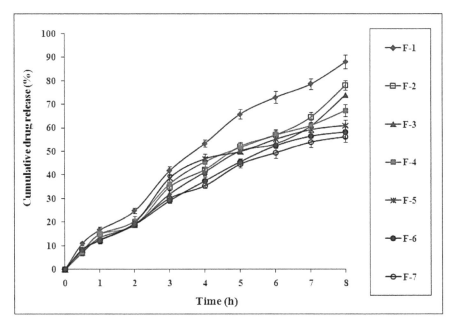

FIGURE 16.3 *In vitro* drug release from various calcium alginate-poly(vinyl pyrrolidone)/ nano-HAp composite beads of diclofenac sodium in 0.1 N HCl (pH 1.2) for first 2 h and then, in phosphate buffer (pH 7.4) for next 6 h.

Source: Adapted with permission from Hasnain et al. (2016) (Copyright © 2014 Elsevier B. V.).

16.5 CONCLUSION

The drug-releasing applications of various alginate–HAp composite systems has also been discussed in this chapter. All the reported alginate–HAp composites exhibited sustained drug release behavior with new functionalities. Finally, the use of alginate–HAp composites for delivering therapeutic cells is another interesting aspect to consider in regenerative medication. In this case, the objective is to use alginate–HAp composites as platforms where cells can reorganize into more sophisticated tissues. This strategy together with the use of drug could be applied, for example, to neuronal growth. Drugs have already shown to have a remarkable affinity for alginate–HAp, and their integration could contribute to the developing of drug delivery systems. The combination of new approaches using microengineering will be a potent tool in the design and development of drug delivery systems in the near future.

SUMMARY

This chapter is focusing on the synergies resulting from the combination of HAp–alginate materials through the fabrication of composites. HAp is a bioceramic material having a broad range of biomedical applications, especially in orthopedics and dentistry. HAp can be synthesized through many chemical methods such as wet precipitation, solgel transformation, hydrothermal, and so forth. To intensify the usage of HAp as composite material, it is being processed with other inorganic materials as well as organic materials (mainly polymers). During past few years, various HAp–alginate composites have been modulated in a versatile way with the incorporation of different drugs for the use in drug delivery. Within these HAp–alginate composites, HAp crystallites were well inviolate with the alginate molecules. Almost all reported HAp–alginate composites were found to release the incorporated/encapsulated drugs over prolonged periods.

KEYWORDS

- alginate
- hydroxyapatite
- composites
- drug delivery

REFERENCES

Aghaei, H.; Nourbakhsh, A. A.; Karbasi, S.; Kalbasid, R.; Rafienia, M.; Nourbakhsh, N.; Bonakdar, S.; Mackenzie, K. J. D. Investigation on Bioactivity and Cytotoxicity of Mesoporous Nano-Composite MCM-48/Hydroxyapatite for Ibuprofen Drug Delivery. *Ceram. Int.* **2014,** *40,* 7355–7362

Angadi, S. C.; Manjeshwar, L. S.; Aminabhavi, T. M. Novel Composite Blend Microbeads of Sodium Alginate Coated with Chitosan for Controlled Release of Amoxicillin. *Int. J. Biol. Macromol.* **2012,** *51,* 45–55.

Babu, V. R.;Sairam, M. Hosamani, K. M.; Aminabhavi, T. M. Preparation of Sodium Alginate-Methyl Cellulose Blend Microspheres for Controlled Release of Nifedipine. *Carbohydr. Polym.* **2007,** *69,* 241–250.

Bai, X.; Fang, R.; Zhang, S.; Shi, X.; Wang, Z.; Chen, X.; Yang, J.; Hou, X.; Nie, Y.; Li, Y.; Tian, W. Self-Cross-Linkable Hydrogels Composed of Partially Oxidized Alginate and Gelatin for Myocardial Infarction Repair. *J. Bioact. Compat. Polym.* **2013,** *28*(2), 126–140.

Balakrishnan, B.; Joshi, N.; Jayakrishnan, A.; Banerjee, R. Self-Crosslinked Oxidized Alginate/Gelatin Hydrogel as Injectable, Adhesive Biomimetic Scaffolds for Cartilage Regeneration. *Acta Biomater.* **2014,** *10,* 3650–3663.

Baro, M.; Sánchez, E.; Delgado, A.; Perera, A.; Évora, C. In Vitro-in Vivo Characterization of Gentamicin Bone Implants. *J. Controlled Release* 2002, *83,* 353–364.

Bera, H.; Boddupalli, S.; Nayak, A. K. Mucoadhesive-Floating Zinc-Pectinate-Sterculia Gum Interpenetrating Polymer Network Beads Encapsulating Ziprasidone HCl. *Carbohydr. Polym.* **2015a,** *131,* 108–118.

Bera, H.; Kandukuri, S. G.; Nayak, A. K.; Boddupalli,S. Alginate-Sterculia Gum Gel-Coated Oil-Entrapped Alginate Beads for Gastroretentive Risperidone Delivery. *Carbohydr. Polym.* **2015b,** *120,* 74–84.

Bera, H.; Boddupalli,S.; Nandikonda, S.; Kumar, S.; Nayak. A. K. Alginate Gel-Coated Oil-Entrapped Alginate–Tamarind Gum–Magnesium Stearate Buoyant Beads of Risperidone. *Int. J. Biol. Macromol.* **2015c,** *78,* 102–111.

Bodmeier, R.; Paeratakul, O. A Novel Multiple-Unit Sustained Release Indomethacin-Hydroxypropyl Methylcellulose Delivery System Prepared by Ionotropic Gelation of Sodium Alginate at Elevated Temperatures. *Carbohydr. Polym.* **1991,** *16,* 399–408.

Chae, T.; Yang, H.; Leung, V.; Ko, F.; Troczynski, T. Novel Biomimetic Hydroxyapatite/Alginate Nanocomposite Fibrous Scaffolds for Bone Tissue Regeneration. *J. Mater. Sci. Mater. Med.* **2013,** *24,* 1885–1894.

Chai, C. S.; Ben-Nissan, B. Bioactive Nanocrystalline Sol-Gel Hydroxyapatite Coatings. *J. Mater. Sci. Mater. Med.* **1999,** *10,* 465–469.

Chourasia, M.; Chourasia, M. K.; Jain, N. K.; Jain, A.; et al. Cross-Linked Guar Gum Microspheres: A Viable Approach for Improved Delivery of Anticancer Drugs for the Treatment of Colorectal Cancer. *AAPS PharmSciTech* **2006,** *7,* E1–E9.

Das, B.; Nayak, A. K.; Nanda, U. Topical Gels of Lidocaine HCl Using Cashew Gum and Carbopol 940: Preparation and in Vitro Skin Permeation. *Int. J. Biol. Macromol.* **2013,** *62,* 514–517.

Das, B.; Dutta, S.; Nayak, A. K.; Nanda, U. Zinc Alginate-Carboxymethyl Cashew Gum Microbeads for Prolonged Drug Release: Development and Optimization. *Int. J. Biol. Macromol.* **2014,** *70,* 505–515.

Docherty-Skogh, A. C.; Bergman, K.; Waern, M. J.; Ekman, S.; Hultenby, K.; Ossipov, D.; Hilborn, J.; Bowden, T. Engstrand, T. Bone Morphogenetic Protein-2 Delivered by Hyaluronan-Based Hydrogel Induces Massive Bone Formation and Healing of Cranial Defects in Minipigs. *Plast. Reconstr. Surg.* **2010,** *125,* 1383–1392.

Fullana, S. G.; Ternet, H.; Freche, M.; Lacout, J. L.; Rodriguez, F. Controlled Release Properties and Final Macroporosity of a Pectin Microspheres-Calcium Phosphate Composite Bone Cement. *Acta Biomater.* **2010,** *6,* 2294–2300.

Gittings, J. P.; Bowen, C. R.; Turner, I. G.; Dent, A. C. E.; Baxter, F. R.; Chaudhuri, J. B. Electrical Characterization of Hydroxyapatite-Based Bioceramics. *Acta Biomater.* **2009,** *5,* 743–754.

Goh, C. H.; Heng, P. W. S.; Chan, L. W. Alginates as a Useful Natural Polymer for Microencapsulation and Therapeutic Applications. *Carbohydr. Polym.* **2012,** *88,* 1–12.

Grande, C. J.; Torres, F. G.; Gomez, C. M.; Bañó, M. C. Nanocomposites of Bacterial Cellulose/Hydroxyapatite for Biomedical Applications. *Acta Biomater.* **2009,** *5,* 1605–1615.

Guru, P. R.; Bera, H.; Das, M.; Hasnain, M. S.; Nayak, A. K. Aceclofenac-Loaded *Plantago ovata* F. Husk Mucilage-Zn^{+2}-Pectinate Controlled-Release Matrices. *Starch Stärke* **2018,** *70,* 1700136.

Hasnain, M. S.; Nayak, A. K.; Singh, R.; Ahmad, F. Emerging Trends of Natural-Based Polymeric Systems for Drug Delivery in Tissue Engineering Applications. *Sci. J. UBU* **2010,** *1*(2), 1–13.

Hasnain, M. S.; Nayak, A. K.; Singh, M.; Tabish, M.; Ansari, M. T.; Ara, T. J. Alginate-Based Bipolymeric-Nanobioceramic Composite Matrices for Sustained Drug Release. *Int. J. Biol. Macromol.* **2016,** *83,* 71–77.

Hezaveh, H.; Muhamad, I. I. The Effect of Nanoparticles on Gastrointestinal Release from Modified K-Carrageenan Nanocomposite Hydrogels. *Carbohydr. Polym.* **2012,** *89,* 138–145.

Hoepfner, T. P.; Case, E. D. The Porosity Dependence of the Dielectric Constant for Sintered Hydroxyapatite. *J. Biomed. Mater. Res.* **2002,** *60,* 643–650.

Hua, S.; Ma, H.; Li, X.; et al. pH-Sensitive Sodium Alginate/Poly(Vinyl Alchohol) Hydrogel Beads Prepared by Combined Ca^{2+} Cross-Linking and Freeze-Thawing Cycles for Controlled Release of Diclofenac Sodium. *Int. J. Biol. Macromol.* **2010,** *46,* 517–523.

Illiescu, R. I.; Andronescu, E.; Ghitulica, C. D.; Voicu, G.; Ficai, A.; Hotetu, M. Montmorillonite-Alginate Nanocomposite as a Drug Delivery System-Incorporation and in Vitro Release of Irinotecan. *Int. J. Pharm.* **2014,** *463,* 184–192.

Jain, S.; Datta, M. Montmorillonite-Alginate Microspheres as a Delivery Vehicle for Oral Extended Release of Venlafaxine Hydrochloride. *J. Drug Delivery. Sci. Technol.* **2016,** *33,* 149–156.

Jana, S.; Saha, A.; Nayak, A. K.; Sen, K. K.; Basu, S. K. Aceclofenac-Loaded Chitosan-Tamarind Seed Polysaccharide Interpenetrating Polymeric Network Microparticles. *Colloids. Surf. B. Biointerf.* **2013a,** *105,* 303–309.

Jana, S.; Das, A.; Nayak, A. K.; Sen, K. K.; Basu, S. K. Aceclofenac-Loaded Unsaturated Esterified Alginate/Gellan Gum Microspheres: In Vitro and in Vivo Assessment. *Int. J. Biol. Macromol.* **2013b,** *57,* 129–137.

Jana, S.; Maji, N.; Nayak, A. K.; Sen, K. K.; Basu, S. K. Development of Chitosan-Based Nanoparticles Through Inter-Polymeric Complexation for Oral Drug Delivery. *Carbohydr. Polym.* **2013c,** *98,* 870–876.

Kevadiya, B. D.; Joshi, G. V.; Patel, H. A.; Ingole, P. G.; Mody, H. M.; Bajaj, H. C. Montmorillonite-Alginate Nanocomposites as a Drug Delivery System: Intercalation and in Vitro Release of Vitamin B1 and Vitamin B6. *J. Biomater. Appl.* **2010,** *25*(2), 161–177.

Khlibsuwan, R.; Siepmann, F.; Siepmann, J.; Pongjanyakul, T. Chitosan-Clay Nanocomposite Microparticles for Controlled Drug Delivery: Effects of the MAS Content and TPP Crosslinking. *J. Drug Delivery Sci. Technol.* **2017,** *40,* 1–10.

Kim, H. J., Matsuda, H.; Zhou, H. S.; Honma, I. Ultrasound-Triggered Smart Drug Release from a Poly(Dimethylsiloxane)-Mesoporous Silica Composite. *Adv. Mater.* **2006,** *18,* 3083–3088.

Kim, W. S.; Mooney, D. J.; Arany, P. R.; Lee, K.; Huebsch, N.; Kim, J. Adipose Tissue Engineering Using Injectable, Oxidized Alginate Hydrogels. *Tissue Eng. Part A* **2012,** *18*(7–8), 737–743.

Kolanthai, E.; Sindu, P. A.; Arul, K. T.; Chandra, V. S.; Manikandan, E.; Kalkura, S. N. Agarose Encapsulated Mesoporous Carbonated Hydroxyapatite Nanocomposites Powder for Drug Delivery. *J. Photochem. Photobiol. B Biol.* **2017,** *166,* 220–231.

Komlev, V. S.; Barinov, S. M.; Koplik, E. V. A Method to Fabricate. Porous Spherical Hydroxyapatite Granules Intended for Time-Controlled Drug Release. Biomaterials **2002,** *23,* 3449–3454.

Kulkarni, R. V.; Mutalik, S.; Mangond, B. S.; et al. Novel Interpenetrated Polymer Network Microbeads of Natural Polysaccharides for Modified Release of Water Soluble Drug: In Vitro and in Vivo Evaluation. *J. Pharm. Pharmacol.* **2012**, *64,* 530–540.

Kumar, A.; Ahuja, M. Carboxymethyl Gum Kondagogu-Chitosan Polyelectrolyte Complex Nanoparticles: Preparation and Characterization. *Int. J. Biol. Macromol.* **2013**, *62,* 80–84.

Lee, K. Y.; Mooney, D. J. Alginate: Properties and Biomedical Applications. *Prog. Ploym. Sci.* **2012**, *37,* 106–126.

Liang, Y.; Liu, W.; Han, B.; Yang, C.; Ma, Q.; Song, F.; Bi, Q. An in Situ Formed Biodegradable Hydrogel for Reconstruction of the Corneal Endothelium. *Colloids Surf. B* **2011**, *82,* 1–7.

Lin, H. R.; Yeh, Y. J. Porous Alginate/Hydroxyapatite Composite Scaffolds for Bone Tissue Engineering: Preparation, Characterization, and in Vitro Studies. *J. Biomed. Mater. Res. Part B* **2004**, *71,* 52–65.

Maji, R.; Das, B.; Nayak, A. K.; Ray, S. Ethyl Cellulose Microparticles Containing Metformin HCl by Emulsification-Solvent Evaporation Technique: Effect of Formulation Variables. *ISRN Polym. Sci.* **2012**, *2014,* Article ID 801827.

Malakar, J.; Nayak, A. K. Formulation and Statistical Optimization of Multiple-Unit Ibuprofen-Loaded Buoyant System Using 2^3-Factorial Design. *Chem. Eng. Res. Des.* **2012a**, *9,* 1834–1846.

Malakar, J.; Nayak, A. K. Theophylline Release Behavior for Hard Gelatin Capsules Containing Various Hydrophilic Polymers. *J. Pharm. Educ. Res.* **2012b**, *3,* 10–16.

Malakar, J.; Nayak, A. K.; Goswami, S. Use of Response Surface Methodology in the Formulation and Optimization of Bisoprolol Fumarate Matrix Tablets for Sustained Drug Release. *ISRN Pharm.* **2012a**, *2014,* Article ID 730628.

Malakar, J.; Nayak, A. K.; Pal, D. Development of Cloxacillin Loaded Multiple-Unit Alginate-Based Floating System by Emulsion–Gelation Method. *Int. J. Biol. Macromol.* **2012b**, *50*(1), 138–147.

Malakar, J.; Nayak, A. K.; Jana, P.; Pal, D. Potato Starch-Blended Alginate Beads for Prolonged Release of Tolbutamide: Development by Statistical Optimization and in Vitro Characterization. *Asian J. Pharm.* **2013a**, *7,* 43–51.

Malakar, J.; Nayak, A. K.; Das, A. Modified Starch (Cationized)-Alginate Beads Containing Aceclofenac: Formulation Optimization Using Central Composite Design. *Starch Stärke* **2013b**, *65,* 603–612.Malakar, J.; Das, K.; Nayak, A. K. In Situ Cross-Linked Matrix Tablets for Sustained Salbutamol Sulfate Release – Formulation Development by Statistical Optimization. *Polym. Med.* **2014**, *44,* 221–230.

Manafi, S. A.; Joughehdoust, S. Synthesis of Hydroxyapatite Nanostructure by Hydrothermal Condition for Biomedical Application. *Iran. J. Pharm. Sci.* **2009**, *5,* 89–94.

Martin, V. C.; Goissis, G.; Rebeiro, A. C.; Marcantinio, E., Jr.; Bet, M. R. The Controlled Release of Antibiotic by Hydroxyapatite: Anionic Collagen Composites. *Artif. Org.* **1998**, *22,* 215–221.

Mizushima, Y.; Ikoma, T.; Tanaka, J.; Hoshi, K.; Ishihara, T.; Ogawa, Y.; et al. Injectable porous Hydroxyapatite Microparticles as a New Carrier for Protein and Lipophilic Drugs. *J. Controlled Release* **2006**, *110,* 260–265.

Narbat, M. K.; Orang, F.; Hashtjin, M. S.; Goudarzi, A. Fabrication of Porous Hydroxyapatite-Gelatin Composite Scaffolds for Bone Tissue Engineering. *Iran. Biomed. J.* **2006**, *10,* 215–223.

Nayak, A. K. Hydroxyapatite Synthesis Methodologies: An Overview. *Int. J. ChemTech Res.* **2010**, *2,* 903–907.

Nayak, A. K. Tamarind Seed Polysaccharide-Based Multiple-Unit Systems for Sustained Drug Release. In *Biodegradable and Bio-based Polymers: Environmental and Biomedical Applications;* Kalia, S., Averous, L., Eds.; WILEY-Scrivener: USA, 2016; pp 471–494.

Nayak, A. K.; Pal, D. Development of pH-Sensitive Tamarind Seed Polysaccharide-Alginate Composite Beads for Controlled Diclofenac Sodium Delivery Using Response Surface Methodology. *Int. J. Biol. Macromol.* **2011,** *49,* 784–793.

Nayak, A. K.; Pal, D. Ionotropically-Gelled Mucoadhesive Beads for Oral Metformin HCl Delivery: Formulation, Optimization and Antidiabetic Evaluation. *J. Sci. Ind. Res.* **2013,** *72,* 15–22.

Nayak, A. K.; Pal, D. Chitosan-Based Interpenetrating Polymeric Network Systems for Sustained Drug Release. In *Advanced Theranostics Materials;* Tiwari, A., Patra, H. K., Choi, J.-W., Eds.; Wiley-Scrivener: USA, 2015; pp 183–208.

Nayak, A. K.; Pal, D. Sterculia Gum-Based Hydrogels for Drug Delivery Applications. In *Polymeric Hydrogels as Smart Biomaterials;* Kalia, S., Ed.; Springer Series on Polymer and Composite Materials; Springer International Publishing: Switzerland, 2016a; pp 105–151.

Nayak, A. K.; Pal, D. Plant-Derived Polymers: Ionically Gelled Sustained Drug Release Systems. In *Encyclopedia of Biomedical Polymers and Polymeric Biomaterials;* Mishra, M., Ed.; Taylor & Francis Group: New York, NY 10017, U.S.A., 2016b; Vol. VIII, pp 6002–6017.

Nayak, A. K.; Pal, D. Functionalization of Tamarind Gum for Drug Delivery. In *Functional Biopolymers;* Thakur, V. K., Thakur, M. K., Eds.; Springer International Publishing: Switzerland, 2018; pp 35–56.

Nayak, P. L.; Sahoo, D. Chitosan-Sodium Alginate Nanocomposites Blended with Cloisite 30b as a Novel Drug Delivery System for Anticancer Drug Curcumin. *Int. J. Appl. Biol. Pharm. Technol.* **2011,** *2,* 402–411.

Nayak, A. K.; Sen, K. K. Hydroxyapatite-Ciprofloxacin Implantable Minipellets for Bone Delivery: Preparation, Characterization, in Vitro Drug Adsorption and Dissolution Studies. *Int. J. Drug Dev. Res.* **2009,** *1*(1), 47–59.

Nayak, A. K.; Hasnain, M. S.; Beg, S.; Alam, M. I. Mucoadhesive Beads of Gliclazide: Design, Development and Evaluation. *ScienceAsia* **2010a,** *36*(4), 319–325.

Nayak, A. K.; Bhattacharya, A.; Sen, K. K. Hydroxyapatite-Antibiotic Implantable Minipellets for Bacterial Bone Infections Using Precipitation Technique: Preparation, Characterization and in-Vitro Antibiotic Release Studies. *J. Pharm. Res.* **2010b,** *3*(1), 53–59.

Nayak, A. K.; Khatua, S.; Hasnain, M. S.; Sen, K. K. Development of Alginate-PVP K 30 Microbeads for Controlled Diclofenac Sodium Delivery Using Central Composite Design. *DARU J. Pharm. Sci.* **2011a,** *19*(5), 356–366.

Nayak, A. K.; Laha, B.; Sen, K. K. Development of Hydroxyapatite-Ciprofloxacin Bone-Implants Using "Quality by Design". *Acta Pharm.* **2011b,** *61*(1), 25–36.

Nayak, A. K.; Bhattacharyya, A.; Sen, K. K. In Vivo Ciprofloxacin Release from Hydroxyapatite-Ciprofloxacin Bone-Implants in Rabbit Tibia. *ISRN Orthop.* **2011c,** Article ID 420549.

Nayak, A. K.; Pal, D.; Pradhan, J.; Ghorai, T. The Potential of *Trigonella foenum-graecum* L. Seed Mucilage as Suspending Agent. *Indian J. Pharm. Educ. Res.* **2012a,** *46,* 312–317.

Nayak, A. K.; Das, B.; Maji, R. Calcium Alginate/Gum Arabic Beads Containing Glibenclamide: Development and in vitro Characterization. *Int. J. Biol. Macromol.* **2012b,** *51,* 1070–1078.

Nayak, A. K.; Hasnain, M. S.; Malakar, J. Development and Optimization of Hydroxyapatite-Ofloxacin Implants for Possible Bone-Implantable Delivery in Osteomyelitis Treatment. *Curr. Drug Deliv.* **2013a,** *10,* 241–250.

Nayak, A. K.; Pal, D.; Das, S. Calcium Pectinate-Fenugreek Seed Mucilage Mucoadhesive Beads for Controlled Delivery of Metformin HCl. *Carbohydr. Polym.* **2013b,** *96,* 349–357.

Nayak, A. K.; Pal, D.; Hasnain, M. S. Development, Optimization and in Vitro-in Vivo Evaluation of Pioglitazone-Loaded Jackfruit Seed Starch-Alginate Beads. *Curr. Drug Delivery* **2013c,** *10,* 608–619.

Nayak, A. K.; Pal, D.; Santra, K. *Plantago ovata* F. Mucilage-Alginate Mucoadhesive Beads for Controlled Release of Glibenclamide: Development, Optimization, and in vitro-in Vivo Evaluation. *J. Pharm.* **2013d,** *2013,* Article ID 151035.

Nayak, A. K.; Kalia, S.; Hasnain, M. S. Optimization of Aceclofenac-Loaded Pectinate-Poly(Vinyl Pyrrolidone) Beads by Response Surface Methodology. *Int. J. Biol. Macromol.* **2013e,** *62,* 194–202.

Nayak, A. K.; Pal, D.; Santra, K. Ispaghula Mucilage-Gellan Mucoadhesive Beads of Metformin HCl: Development by Response Surface Methodology. *Carbohydr. Polym.* **2014a,** *107,* 41–40.

Nayak, A. K.; Pal, D.; Santra, K. Tamarind Seed Polysaccharide-Gellan Mucoadhesive Beads for Controlled Release of Metformin HCl. *Carbohydr. Polym.* **2014b,** *103,* 154–163.

Nayak, A. K.; Pal, D.; Santra, K. Development of Calcium Pectinate-Tamarind Seed Polysaccharide Mucoadhesive Beads Containing Metformin HCl. *Carbohydr. Polym.* **2014c,** *101,* 220–230.

Nayak, A. K.; Pal, D.; Santra, K. *Artocarpus heterophyllus* L. Seed Starch-Blended Gellan Gum Mucoadhesive Beads of Metformin HCl. *Int. J. Biol. Macromol.* **2014d,** *65,* 329–339.

Nayak, A. K.; Pal, D.; Santra, K. Development of Pectinate-Ispagula Mucilage Mucoadhesive Beads of Metformin HCl by Central Composite Design. *Int. J. Biol. Macromol.* **2014e,** *66,* 203–221.

Nayak, A. K.; Pal, D.; Santra, K. Swelling and Drug Release Behavior of Metformin HCl-Loaded Tamarind Seed Polysaccharide-Alginate Beads. *Int. J. Biol. Macromol.* **2016,** *82,* 1023–1027.

Nayak, A. K.; Hasnain, M. S.; Pal, D. Gelled Microparticles/Beads of Sterculia Gum and Tamarind Gum for Sustained Drug Release In *Handbook of Springer on Polymeric Gel;* Thakur, V. K., Thakur, M. K., Eds.; Springer International Publishing: Switzerland, 2018a, pp 361–414.

Nayak, A. K.; Bera, H.; Hasnain, M. S.; Pal, D. Graft-Copolymerization of Plant Polysaccharides. In *Biopolymer Grafting;* Thakur, V. K., Ed.; Elsevier: Netherlands, 2018b; pp 1–62.

Nayak, A. K.; Beg, S.; Hasnain, M. S.; Malakar, J.; Pal, D. Soluble Starch-Blended Ca^{2+}-Zn^{2+}-Alginate Composites-Based Microparticles of Aceclofenac: Formulation Development and in Vitro Characterization. *Future J. Pharm. Sci.* 2018c, *4*(1), 63–70. Accepted; In Press.

Nithya, R.; Meenakshi Sundaram, N. Biodegradation and Cytotoxicity of Ciprofloxacin-Loaded Hydroxyapatite-Polycaprolactone Nanocomposite Film for Sustainable Bone Implants. *Int. J. Nanomed.* **2015,** *10,* 119–127.

Oonishi, H. Orthopaedic Applications of Hydroxyapatite. *Biomaterials* **1991,** *12,* 171–178.

Pal, D.; Nayak, A. K. Development, Optimization and Anti-Diabetic Activity of Gliclazide-Loaded Alginate-Methyl Cellulose Mucoadhesive Microcapsules. *AAPS PharmSciTech* **2011,** *12*(4), 1431–1441.

Pal, D.; Nayak, A. K. Novel tamarind Seed Polysaccharide-Alginate Mucoadhesive Microspheres for Oral Gliclazide Delivery. *Drug Delivery* **2012,** *19,* 123–131.

Pawar, S. N.; Edgar, K.J. Alginate Derivatization: A Review of Chemistry, Properties and Applications. *Biomaterials* **2012, 33,** 3279–3305.

Pal, D.; Nayak, A. K. Interpenetrating Polymer Networks (IPNs): Natural Polymeric Blends for Drug Delivery. In *Encyclopaedia of Biomedical Polymers and Polymeric Biomaterials;* Mishra, M., Ed.; Taylor & Francis Group: New York, NY 10017, U.S.A., 2015a; Vol. VI, pp 4120–4130.

Pal, D.; Nayak, A. K. Alginates, Blends and Microspheres: Controlled Drug Delivery. In *Encyclopedia of Biomedical Polymers and Polymeric Biomaterials;* Mishra, M., Ed.; Taylor & Francis Group: New York, NY 10017, U.S.A., 2015b; Vol. I, pp 89–98.

Pharm, H. H.; Luo, P.; Genin, F.; Dash, A. K. Synthesis and Characterization of Hydroxyapatite-Ciprofloxacin Delivery Systems by Precipitation and Spray Drying Technique. *AAPS PharmSciTech.* **2002,** *3,* E1.

Pistone, A.; Iannazzo, D.; Panseri, S.; Montesi, M.; Tampieri, A.; Galvagno, S. Hydroxyapatite-Magnetite-MWCNT Nanocomposite as a Biocompatible Multifunctional Drug Delivery System for Bone Tissue Engineering. *Nanotechnology* **2014,** *25,* 425701.

Prajapati, V. D.; Jani, G. K.; Moradiya, N. G.; Randeria, N. P.; Maheriya, P. M.; Nagar, B. J. Locust Bean Gum in the Development of Sustained Release Mucoadhesive Macromolecules of Aceclofenac. *Carbohydr. Polym.* **2014,** *113,* 138.

Priddy, L. B.; Chaudhuri, O.; Stevens, H. Y.; Krishnan, L.; Uhrig, B. A.; Willett, N. J.; Guldberg, R. E. Oxidized Alginate Hydrogels for Bone Morphogenetic Protein-2 Delivery in Long Bone Defects. *Acta Biomater.* **2014,** *10,* 4390–4399.

Queiroz, A. C.; Santos, J. D.; Monteiro, F. J.; Gibson, I. R.; Knowles, J. C. Adsorption and Release Studies of Sodium Ampicillin from Hydroxyapatite and Glass-Reinforced Hydroxyapatite Composites. *Biomater.* **2001,** *22,* 1393–1400.

Quilitz, M.; Steingröver, K.; Veith, M. Effect of the Ca/P Ratio on the Dielectric Properties of Nanoscaled Substoichiometric Hydroxyapatite. *J. Mater. Sci. Mater. Med.* **2010,** *21,* 399–405.

Rauschmann, M. A.; Wichelhaus, T. A.; Stirnal, V.; Dingeldein, E.; Zichner, L.; Schnettler, R.; et al. Nanocrystalline Hydroxyapatite and Calcium Sulphate as Biodegradable Composite Carrier Material for Local Delivery of Antibiotics in Bone Infections. *Biomaterials* **2005,** *26,* 2677–2684.

Real, R. P.; Padilla, S.; Vallet-Regi, M. Gentamicin Release from Hydroxyapatite/Poly(Ethyl Methacrylate)/Poly(Methyl Methacrylate) Composites. *J. Biomed. Mater. Res.* **2000,** *52,* 1–7.

Ribeiro, C. C.; Barrias, C. C.; Barbosa, M. A. Calcium Phosphate-Alginate Microspheres as Enzyme Delivery Matrices. *Biomaterials* **2004,** *25,* 4363–4373.

Ribeiro, N.; Sousa, S. R.; Monteiro, F. J. Influence of Crystallite Size of Nanophased Hydroxyapatite on Fibronectin and Osteonectin Adsorption and on MC3T3-E1 Osteoblast Adhesion and Morphology. *J. Colloid Interface Sci.* **2010,** *351,* 398–406.

Roul, J.; Mohapatra, R.; Sahoo, S. K. Preparation, Characterization and Drug Delivery Behavior of Novel Biopolymer/Hydroxyapatite Nanocomposite Beads. *Asian J. Biomed. Pharm. Sci.* **2013,** *3,* 33–38.

Santos, M. H.; Oliveira, M. D.; Souza, L. P. D. F.; Mansur, H. S.; Vasconcelos, W. L. Synthesis Control and Characterization of Hydroxyapatite Prepared by Wet Precipitation Process. *Mater. Res.* **2004,** *7*(4), 625–630.

Sen, G.; Pal, S. Microwave Initiated Synthesis of Polyacrylamide Grafted Carboxymethyl Starch (CMS-g-PAM): Application as a Novel Matrix for Sustained Drug Release. *Int. J. Biol. Macromol.* **2009,** *45,* 48–55.

Sinha, P.; Ubaidulla, U.; Hasnain, M. S.; Nayak, A. K.; Rama, B. Alginate-Okra Gum Blend Beads of Diclofenac Sodium from Aqueous Template Using $ZnSO_4$ as a Cross-Linker. *Int. J. Biol. Macromol.* **2015a,** *79,* 555.

Sinha, P.; Ubaidulla, U.; Nayak, A. K. Okra (*Hibiscus esculentus*) Gum-Alginate Blend Mucoadhesive Beads for Controlled Glibenclamide Release. *Int. J. Biol. Macromol.* **2015b,** *72,* 1069.

Smidsrod, O.; Draget, K. I. Chemistry and Physical Properties of Alginates. *Carbohydr. Eur.* **1996,** *14,* 6–13.

Sotome, S.; Uemura, T.; Kikuchi, M.; Chen, J.; Itoh, S.; Tanaka, J.; Tateishi, T.; Shinomiya, K. Synthesis and in Vivo Evaluation of a Novel Hydroxyapatite/Collagen–Alginate as a Bone Filler and a Drug Delivery Carrier of Bone Morphogenetic Protein. *Mater. Sci. Eng. C* **2004,** *24,* 341–347.

Suárez-González, D.; Barnhart, K.; Saito, E.; Vanderby, R.; Hollister, S. J.; Murphy, W. L. Controlled Nucleation of Hydroxyapatite on Alginate Scaffolds for Stem Cell-Based Bone Tissue Engineering. *J. Biomed. Mater. Res. Part A* **2010,** *95,* 222–234.

Sun, J.; Tan, H. Alginate-Based Biomaterials for Regenerative Medicine Applications. *Materials* **2013,** *6,* 1285–1309.

Tas, A. C. Synthesis of Biomimetic Ca-Hydroxyapatite Powders at 37°C in Synthetic Body Fluids. Biomaterials **2000,** *21,* 1429–1438.

Turco, G.; Marsich, E.; Bellomo, F.; Semeraro, S.; Donati, I.; Brun, F.; Grandolfo, M.; Accardo, A.; Paoletti, S. Alginate/Hydroxyapatite Biocomposite for Bone Ingrowth: A Trabecular Structure with High and Iisotropic Connectivity. *Biomacromolecules* **2009,** *10,* 1575–1583.

Uskoković, V.; Uskoković, D. P. Nanosized Hydroxyapatite and other Calcium Phosphates: Chemistry of Formation and Applicationas Drug and Gene Delivery Agents. *J. Biomed. Mater. Res. Part B* **2011,** *96,* 152–191.

Verma, A.; Dubey, J.; Verma, N.; Nayak, A. K. Chitosan-Hydroxypropyl Methylcellulose Matricesas Carriers for Hydrodynamically Balanced Capsules of Moxifloxacin HCl. *Curr. Drug Delivery* **2017,** *14,* 83–90.

Wu, J.; Wei, W.; Wang, L. Y.; Su, Z. G.; Ma, G. H. A Thermosensitive Hydrogel Based on Quaternized Chitosan and Poly(Ethylene Glycol) for Nasal Drug Delivery System. *Biomaterials* **2007,** *28,* 2220–2232.

Wu, J. L.; Wang, C. Q.; Zhou, R. X.; Cheng, S. X. Multi-Drug Delivery Systems Based on Alginate/Calcium Carbonate Hybrid Nanoparticles for Combination Chemotherapy. *Colloids Suf. B* **2014,** *123,* 498–505.

Xie, M.; Olderøy, M. Ø.; Zhang, Z.; Andreassen, J. P.; Strand, B. L.; Sikorshi, P. Biocomposites Prepared by Alkaline Phosphatase Mediated Mineralization of Alginate Microbeads. *RSC Adv.* **2012,** *2,* 1457–1465.

Xu, Q.; Czernuszka, J. T. Controlled Release of Amoxicillin from Hydroxyapatite-Coated Poly(Lactic-Co-Glycolic Acid) Microspheres. *J. Controlled Release* **2008,** *127,* 146–153.

Zhang, R.; Ma, P. X. Biomimetic Polymer/Apatite Composite Scaffolds for Mineralized Tissue Engineering. *Macromol. Biosci.* **2004,** *4,* 100–111.

Zhang, J.; Wang, Q.; Wang, A. In Situ Generation of Sodium Alginate/Hydroxyapatite Nano-composite Beads as Drug-Controlled Release Matrices. *Acta Biomater.* 2010, 6, 445–454.

Zhou, H.; Lee, J. Nanoscale Hydroxyapatite Particles for Bone Tissue Engineering. *Acta Biomater.* **2011,** *7,* 2769–2781.

CHAPTER 17

ALGINATE-BASED GASTROINTESTINAL TRACT DRUG DELIVERY SYSTEMS

SOUGATA JANA[1,2,*], KALYAN KUMAR SEN[1], and
SABYASACHI MAITI[3]

[1]*Department of Pharmaceutics, Gupta College of Technological
Sciences, Ashram More, G.T. Road, Asansol, West Bengal 713301,
India*

[2]*Department of Health and Family Welfare, Directorate of Health
Services, Government of West Bengal, Salt Lake, Kolkata,
West Bengal, 700091, India*

[3]*Department of Pharmacy, Indira Gandhi National Tribal University,
Amarkantak, Madhya Pradesh, India*

Corresponding author. E-mail: janapharmacy@rediffmail.com

17.1 INTRODUCTION

Oral drug delivery systems are important due to drug release from the formulation in the gastrointestinal tract (GIT), solubilization in the GI mediums, drug transport across the gastric/intestinal membrane, and absorption into systemic circulation in its active form after hepatic metabolism (Banerjee and Mitragotri, 2017; Ku, 2008). Some drug/bioactive molecules have disadvantages to deliver by oral route such as highly water-soluble, low bioavailability, labile in acidic environment, and short half-life. In these circumstances, different design strategies can be adopted to deliver the bioactive molecules effectively (Jana et al., 2016a; Jana et al., 2015c; Banerjee and Onyuksel, 2012)

Designing a drug delivery system based on natural polymers showed prolonged release with biodegradability, biocompatibility, and reduced toxicity, which are the major challenges faced by researchers/scientist all over the world. Biopolymeric nanoparticles (BNPs) are one of the promising delivery systems for the delivery of therapeutics. BNPs showed good therapeutic efficiency and decrease in the side effects and site-specific prolonged release of drug (Łukasiewicz et al., 2015; Jana et al., 2016b; Jana et al., 2013b; Jana et al. 2014). Biopolymeric microparticles (BMPs) are another system with a particle size range 1–1000 μm. BMPs showed excellent drug–plasma profile within a therapeutic range, minimized dosing frequency, decreased side effects, and increased patient compliance (Jana et al., 2015c).

Among natural biopolymers, alginate (ALG) is a widely used polymer for the fabrication of drug carriers systems. Sodium ALG (Na-ALG), an anionic linear polymer, is obtained from brown algae, biocompatible, nontoxic, and biodegradable. Chemically, ALG is made up of 1,4-α-l-guluronic acid and β-d-mannuronic acid residues. It is utilized in the different pharmaceuticals, food, and biomedical fields. In this chapter, we focused on the ALG-based composites in drug delivery through GIT. Different approaches are given below (Jana et al., 2016b; Yin et al., 2018).

17.2 ALGINATE-BASED SYSTEMS FOR GASTROINTESTINAL TRACT DELIVERY

17.2.1 INSULIN DELIVERY

Diabetes mellitus (DM) is a worldwide epidemic disease, currently affecting more than 415 million people globally. DM is occurred by either the lack of or a resistance to the insulin (INS), which is a glucose-regulating hormone, in a patient (Lim et al. 2017). Therefore, INS is the most important drug of choice to control blood glucose levels. INS is mainly used in the form of injection via subcutaneous route, which leads to painful and possible infections, that causes higher patient compliance. Oral INS administration is a more convenient form of drug administration because it is less invasive. Oral INS delivery to the GIT is one of the most challenging tasks to overcome the different barriers of therapeutic INS delivery. There are two main approaches for an effective and therapeutic oral route of INS delivery: (i) barrier of encapsulated INS from the GI acidic pH in the stomach and (ii) sustained release of INS at the targeted GI site of absorption. INS-loaded ALG/chitosan (CS) blend gel beads were prepared by Tahtat et al. 2013 for oral delivery of INS. The beads were formulated by dual cross-linking such as calcium chloride ($CaCl_2$) (2%) and glutaraldehyde (GA) (2%) solution. ALG/CS ratio (6:4) showed 72% of INS in simulated intestinal fluid (SIF, pH 6.5) at 6 h. Further, Mukhopadhyay et al. 2015 developed ALG/CS polyelectrolyte complex for INS delivery

Particle size range of the ALG/CS NPs was 100–200 nm and ~85% encapsulation efficiency. ALG/CS core–shell NPs were characterized by Fourier transform infrared (FTIR), dynamic light scattering (DLS), and scanning electron microscopy (SEM) techniques. In vitro INS release study is performed in GI pH (i.e., 1.2, 6.8, and 7.4). In vitro result showed ~26% INS released in pH 1.2 after 2 h and sustained release observed 79–84% in SIF up to 24 h. Oral toxicity studies of ALG/CS NPs were performed in Swiss albino mice. In vivo relative bioavailability of ~8% was observed in diabetic mice model. Lim et al. (2017) fabricated ALG–κ-carrageenan hydrogel beads by Ca^{2+} cross-linking, for oral delivery of INS. They characterized the beads by FTIR, field emission scanning electron microscopy (FESEM), swelling studies, and so forth. In vitro release study of INS in simulated gastric fluid (SGF) (pH 1.2), the ALG hydrogel beads released INS about 50% of the encapsulated INS as part within 2 h of incubation, when the concentration of κ-carrageenan (>0.05%·w/v) used in the hydrogel bead showed full retention of all the entrapped INS as part in the composite. After incubation of ALG–κ-carrageenan (1% w/v κ-carrageenan) beads in SGF, there was approximately 65% of INS as part remained biologically active in the composites. INS bioactivity assay was performed in the SGF. The beads were first incubated in an enzyme-free SGF solution for 2 h, before the released insulin as part in SIF at pH 7.4. FESEM were used for the evaluation of surface morphology and internal structure of the lyophilized ALG/κ-carrageenan beads and ALG beads. FESEM result revealed that κ-carrageenan concentration (0.1% w/v) beads had a macroporous structure similar to the ALG beads, but κ-carrageenan concentration (1%·w/v) beads, the internal structure, had dense matrix that, due to the Ca-κ-carrageenan network matrices, is formed alongside with the ALG matrices. Bhattacharyya et al. (2017) fabricated polyurethane (PU)–ALG/CS core–shell NPs for oral INS delivery. Average particle size range of PU–ALG/CS NPs was 90–110 nm examined by of SEM and transmission electron microscope (TEM) analyses. In vitro release study of INS from PU–ALG/CS was performed in different GI pH mediums such as pH 1.2, pH 6.8, and pH 7.4. PU–ALG/CS NPs were released ~50% at 10 h in pH 6.8 medium, whereas sustained release of INS, that is, 98% at 20 h was observed in pH 7.4 buffer.

17.2.2   PROTEIN DELIVERY

Omera et al. (2016) synthesized ALG and aminated CS-coated microbeads (ALG-AmCS) for the oral delivery of protein bovine serum albumin (BSA). BSA release from ALG-AmCS microbeads was evaluated in SGF (pH 1.2), SIF (pH 6.8), and simulated colonic fluids (SCF) (pH 7.4). The stability of ALG-AmCS microbeads in SCF was improved with increasing AmCS concentration. This is due to the hydroxyl groups (–OH) and/or the additional amine groups (NH_3^+) of AmCS could hydrophobically interact with protein (BSA) under mild conditions (>pH 5) leading to strong ionic interactions that showed a little amount of cumulative BSA release. In vitro result of microbeads containing 0.25% AmCS showed that BSA reached ~63% in SIF and ~86% in SCF. Yang et al. (2013) developed ALG–methoxypolyethylene glycol-grafted carboxymethyl CS (mPEG-g-CMCS), interpenetrating polymer network (IPN) beads for the oral GI delivery of BSA. The SEM result showed that mPEG was grafted into CMCS; the structure of the ALG/mPEG-g-CMCS IPN beads became more rigid cross-linking with Ca^{2+}. The prepared beads (mPEG-g-CMC: ALG ratio 1:1, wt.%) showed good pH sensitivity and the loading capacity (~62%). The in vitro result showed that burst release of the BSA was decreased slightly at SGF (pH 1.2) and the release at pH 7.4 (SCF) was 90% in 9 h. Kim et al. (2012) fabricated ALG–carboxymethyl cellulose (CMC) beads by ionically cross-linked with Fe^{3+} for the delivery of BSA. FTIR analysis stated that the formation of a three-dimensional bonding structure between the anionic polymeric chains of ALG–CMC and the trivalent cation Fe^{3+}. The size range of the ALG–CMC beads was 1.3–1.7 mm and the surface roughness of the microbeads increased with increase in CMC concentration that is evaluated by the FESEM. In vitro result revealed ~69.85% at 24 h in pH 7.4 medium. Wen et al. (2017) synthesized ALG–CS core–shell nanofilm for the delivery of BSA to the colon. Coaxial electrospinning technique was used for the fabrication of nanofilm, where BSA-loaded CS NP is core part and ALG is shell part. SEM analysis revealed that the film formed was a smooth surface. TEM result showed that the average size of single NP was ~20 nm and spherical in shape. DLS analysis showed mean diameter of ~270.5 nm and polydispersity index (PDI) of 0.265. In vitro release of BSA in SCF was ~75% at 16 h. Rahmani et al. (2018) prepared protein–ALG complexes for the delivery of protein. In this experiment, they have used different types of model protein such as lysozyme, cytochrome C, chymotrypsin, myoglobin, and BSA. In vitro data of protein release kinetics from the complexes depend on the ionic strength and changes in pH.

17.2.3 ANTICANCER DRUG DELIVERY

Cancer is a main health problem worldwide; this is due to uncontrolled growth and survival of mutated or transformed cells. Jayapal et al. (2017) developed exemestane (EXE)-loaded ALG NPs for the treatment of breast cancer. EXE is an irreversible steroidal aromatase inactivator and inhibits the synthesis of estrogen. EXE–ALG NPs are prepared by simple cross-linked (2% $CaCl_2$) method. In vitro dissolution study was performed in pH 6.8. The average particle sizes of 197 nm and zeta potential of -18.3 mV for EXE–ALG NPs were observed by using DLS. Iliescu et al. (2014) developed irinotecan-loaded montmorillonite (MT)–ALG nanocomposites. The surface morphology of the nanocomposites was evaluated by the FTIR, X-ray diffraction (XRD), and SEM analysis. The in vitro release profiles of irinotecan were evaluated in pH 7.4 up to 10 h. Agarwal et al. (2015) prepared AL–CMC beads containing 5-fluorouracil (5-FU) for oral colon drug delivery. In vitro release study of ALG–CMC beads showed drug release ($>90\%$) in the colonic enzymes medium. 5-FU–ALG–CMC formulations were evaluated in colon adenocarcinoma cells (HT-29) by flow cytometry and result showed the therapeutic potential of the 5-FU–ALG–CMC formulations. Azhar and Olad (2014) formulated 5-FU-loaded ALG–MT nanocomposites (ALG–CS/5-FU/MT) by an intercalation technique. In vitro 5-FU release study was performed in pH 7.4, and result showed controlled burst release and formulated nanocomposites system containing MT (30 wt.%) 50% release of FU (i.e. $T_{50\%}$ is about 8 h); this phenomenon is called sigmoidal drug release pattern due to the intercalation of 5-FU in silicate layers of MT. Release kinetic data stated Korsmeyer–Peppas kinetic model, suggesting diffusion controlled drug release pattern. SEM image of ALG–CS/5-FU/MT nanocomposites showed dense morphology due to the formation of CS–ALG composites on the surface of the 5-FU/MT nanocomposite. Dodov et al. (2009) synthesized lectin-conjugated CS–Ca–ALG microparticles loaded with 5-FU for the colon cancer treatment. Prepared microparticles are developed by one-step spray-drying technique. Microparticles were spherical in shape, with 6.73 g/mg of wheat germ agglutinin (WGA) conjugated onto their surface. Size, zeta potential, and entrapment efficiency (EE%) of the microparticles (WGA-5FU) were 14 μm, 15.3 mV, and 72%, respectively. Bansal et al. (2016) developed oxaliplatin (L-OHP)-loaded folic acid (FA)-conjugated liposomes in ALG beads coated with Eudragit-S-100 for the treatment of colon specific tumor. In vitro releases of L-OHP were analyzed by the dialysis bag method in pH 7.4. L-OHP-loaded FA-LP formulation showed ~49% of L-OHP release after 24 h. Particle size, zeta potential, PDI, and EE% of the beads were 190 nm, 0.19, −4.52 mV, and 28%, respectively. γ-scintigraphic study revealed that Eudragit-coated ALG beads entered into the colon in mice. In vivo data revealed that L-OHP-loaded FA-LP formulation beads delivered 21 µg L-OHP/g of tissues in the tumor after 12 h. Mucoadhesive property can be increased by the modification of polymers for the drug delivery. Shtenberg et al. (2017) synthesized novel ALG–polyethylene glycol (PEG)–maleimide (ALG-PEGM) containing Ibuprofen (IBU) for GI delivery. In vitro result revealed 97% of IBU was released from ALG-PEGM tablets in the first 2.5 h in pH 6.8. Wang et al. (2015) developed folate-phytosterol-ALG (FP-ALG) core/shell NPs for anticancer drug delivery. Folate is a cancer-cell-specific ligand and phytosterols are steroid compounds with hydrophobic moieties to prevent colon, breast, ovarian, prostate, lung, and stomach cancer. Doxorubicin (DOX) was used as anticancer drug. In vitro release of DOX from DOX-FP-ALG NPs was studied in dialysis membrane method in phosphate-buffered saline solutions of different pH, that is, pH 5.5, pH 6.5, and pH 7.4. In vitro data showed DOX release of 15% in pH 7.4, 27% in pH 6.5, and 60% in pH 5.5 at 72 h. Result stated significantly rapid DOX release characteristics in acidic pH and prolonged release of drugs (hydrophobic) in the acidic condition of cancerous tissues. The cellular uptake and internalization of DOX from DOX-FP-ALG NPs were confirmed by confocal laser scanning microscopy image.

7.2.4 ANTIVIRAL DRUG DELIVERY

Joshy et al. (2017) fabricated lipid-based drug delivery system containing zidovudine (AZT). Hybrid NPs were prepared by the using ALG and stearic acid–polyethylene glycol (SA-PEG). These NPs showed dendritic morphology, where SA-PEG acts as external shell and AZT as core part. The optimized hybrid NPs showed ~407 nm size, −42.53 mV surface potential, 83% drug encapsulation, and had significant stability for 6 months. In vitro cytotoxicity and cellular uptake of the formulated NPs in glioma, neuro, and HeLa cells showed nontoxic nature. Hemolysis and aggregation sated no lysis and aggregation in RBC, WBC, and platelets. Further, Joshy et al. (2018) formulated AZT-loaded glutamic acid–ALG conjugate by emulsion solvent evaporation method for the GI delivery. Pluronic F68 (PF-68) was incorporated in the matrix as a stabilizer. The in vitro release of AZT from NPs was 54% at 24 h in pH 7.4. Particle size and EE% were 432 nm and 29%, respectively. Jana et al. (2016c) synthesized O-carboxymethyl tamarind gum (CTG) and ALG IPN hydrogel by Ca^{+2} ionic gelation techniques. Acyclovir was used as a model drug. They characterized the formulated IPN hydrogel by FESEM, energy dispersive X-ray (EDX), FTIR, and DSC analysis. The surface characteristics of acyclovir-loaded hydrogels were evaluated by FESEM (Figure 17.1). The ALG-Ca^{2+}-CTG particles showed spherical with rough surface. EDX analysis stated the elemental composition of the formulation. It was found that 20.34% chloride and 2.46% calcium were present on the sample. The elemental data confirmed that the particle surface was deposited by unreacted CaCl$_2$. Hence, the final hydrogel particles were further washed with distilled water to remove surface adsorbed Ca ions. A 12.14 wt.% of Na was also found from EDX analysis.

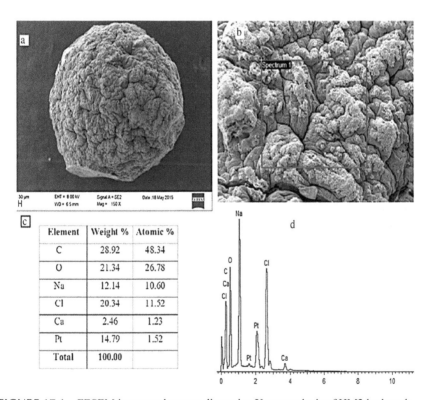

Element	Weight %	Atomic %
C	28.92	48.34
O	21.34	26.78
Na	12.14	10.60
Cl	20.34	11.52
Ca	2.46	1.23
Pt	14.79	1.52
Total	100.00	

FIGURE 17.1 FESEM image and energy dispersive X-ray analysis of HM2 hydrogels.

Source: Reprinted with permission from Jana et al., 2016c. © 2016 Elsevier. https://doi.org/10.1016/j.ijbiomac.2016.08.017

In vitro acyclovir release data of the prepared formulations were depicted in Figure 17.2. Ca-ALG particles (HM3) released~97% drug in pH 6.8 in 4 h. But at ratio 75:25 (Na-ALG:CTG), the hydrogels showed sustained release of drug of ~82% at 7 h. At equal weight-to-percentage ratio of polymers (Na-ALG: CTG=50:50), the drug release rate became faster than that observed for HM2. The drug release rate, however, was still slower for interpenetrating hydrogels (HM1) than ALG alone (HM3). The in vitro drug release from IPN hydrogels was 18–23% in pH 1.2 in 2 h. The acyclovir release became faster at pH 6.8 as the ratio of CTG was increased from 25 to 50%.

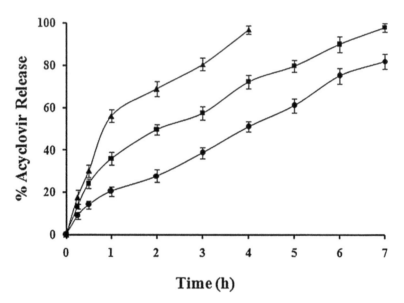

FIGURE 17.2 The release profiles of acyclovir-loaded hydrogel microparticles in phosphate buffer solution (pH 6.8). Key: (■) HM1 (sodium alginates [Na-ALG]:O-carboxymethyl tamarind gum [CTG]=50:50), (●) HM2 (Na-ALG: CTG=75:25), and (▲) HM3 (Na-ALG: CTG=100:0).

Source: Reprinted with permission from Jana et al., 2016c. © 2016 Elsevier. https://doi. org/10.1016/j.ijbiomac.2016.08.017

17.2.5 ANTIBIOTIC DELIVERY

Sarkar et al. (2017) synthesized carbon quantum dot (CQD) tailored ALG hydrogel films for the delivery of vancomycin (V). Vancomycin is a tricyclic glycopeptides, amphoteric antibiotic, used for the treatment of infections, osteomyelities, which occurs by gram-positive bacteria such *as Staphylococcus aureus*. The drug loading capacity was 96% in beta-cyclodextrin (βCD) associate dvancomycin loaded CQD-Ca^{2+}-ALG (V-βCD-CQD-ALG) nanohybrid. In vitro result showed that 56% of vancomycin in pH 1.5 at 120 h, that stated controlled release of vancomycin into the acidic environment in

GIT. Ciprofloxacin is a broad-spectrum antibiotic observed GI side effect after long oral administration. So, sustained release of ciprofloxacin by oral delivery systems was developed by the Blandón et al. (2016). Kefiran (KEF)-ALG gel microspheres were developed by ionotropic gelation. KEF is a microbial biopolymer produced by *Lactobacillus kefiranofaciens,* water-soluble glucogalactan, and has capacity to form gels. In vitro release of ciprofloxacin from Kef-ALG microspheres was ~5.0% at pH 1.2, and 5.0% and ~25.0% at pH 7.4 at 21 h.

17.2.6 ANTIDIABETIC DRUG DELIVERY

Metformin is a choice of oral hypoglycemic drug for the treatment of type 2 DM, but it has poor bioavailability (40–60%), short half-life ($t_{1/2}$) (1.5–1.6 h) chronic administration may cause hyper-lactatemia, so it is essential for the development of sustained release formulations. Maestrelli et al. (2017) developed metformin loaded ALG-based microspheres. In vitro result showed that less amount of drug release in gastric environment and sustained release of metformin hydrochloride (MTF) in SIF medium. Martínez-Gómez et al. (2017) prepared ALG-PVA hydrogels containing MTF by freeze-thaw cycle process. The formulated hydrogel released a very low amount of MTF in pH 1.2 and the ~55% in pH 8 at 6 h. Nayak and Pal (2013a) obtained a series of jackfruit seed starch-ALG hydrogels by ionotropic gelation method. The optimized formulation showed in vitro release of MTF was ~10% in pH 1.2 and ~60–90% in pH 7.4. Similarly, Nayak and Pal (2013b) developed tamarind seed polysaccharide–ALG hydrogels for the oral delivery of MTF by ionic gelation using $CaCl_2$. The loaded formulation showed that MTF released ~15% in pH 1.2 at 2 h.

17.2.7 ANTIDEPRESSANT DRUG DELIVERY

Sustained release of drugs is important for patients and is essential for the medicinal treatment in round the time. Depressed patients are one of such category patients who suffer from recurrent and chronic disorder requiring long treatment. The treatments of such types of disease are done by antidepressants drug. Jain and Datta (2016) prepared venlafaxine (VF) hydrochloride-loaded MT–ALG composite microbeads for the antidepressants drug delivery. VF is water-soluble, has $t_{1/2}$ 4–5 h, and is third generation drug, which inhibits the reuptake of serotonin, dopamine, and norepinephrine. The microbeads were synthesized by in situ ion exchange followed by ionotropic gelation method. In vitro VF release from VF–MT–ALG beads is shown as 20% at 26 h in SGF and 22% at 29 h in SIF.

17.2.8   ANTI-INFLAMMATORY DRUG

Yin et al. (2018) developed agar–ALG hydrogel beads containing indomethacin (IDMC). In vitro release of IDMC from optimized formulation showed ~63% at 720 min in SIF at pH 7.4. Rivera et al. (2015) fabricated CS–ALG nanocapsules for the delivery of bioactive compounds such as 5-aminosalicylic acid (5-ASA) and glycomacropeptide. 5-ASA is an anti-inflammatory drug that is utilized for the treatment of inflammatory bowel disease. Nanocapsules were developed through layer-by-layer deposition of CS and ALG layers on polystyrene NPs. The optimized formulation showed 70% of 5-ASA encapsulation efficiency. Duan et al. (2017) studied Zn^{2+} cross-linked ALG/N-succinyl-CS blend microspheres for the delivery of 5-ASA. Various analytical techniques were used for the characterization of fabricated microsphere such as SEM, FTIR, and EDX spectrometer. In vitro result showed that ~60% and ~71% of entrapped 5-ASA was released from prepared microspheres in pH 6.8 and 7.4 over 8 h. In vitro release studies stated that fabricated microsphere has a pH-dependent drug release characteristic. Seeli et al. (2016) developed barium ions cross-linked guar gum succinate–ALG (GGS-ALG) beads as pH-sensitive colon-targeting drug delivery systems. IBU was used as a model drug. The in vitro sequential IBU release from the GGS-ALG beads is revealed as 20% in pH 1.2 (SGF) within 3 h and ~90% of initial drug content within 2 h in pH 7.4 (SIF) after changing the dissolution buffer. In vitro result concluded that ALG beads successfully carried out colon delivery without premature drug release in the acidic medium. 3-(4,5-dimethylthiazol-2-yl)-2,5-diphenyl tetrazolium bromide assay confirmed that GGS-ALG beads (concentration range of 0–30 μg/ml) had no cytotoxic effect on the cultured mouse mesenchymal stem cells (mMSC). Treenate and Monvisade (2017) developed hydroxyl ethylacryl CS (HCS) and ALG hydrogel for the delivery of paracetamol. Hydrogel was fabricated by using ionic cross-linkers such as Zn^{2+}, Ca^{2+}, and Cu^{2+} and FTIR analysis confirmed the cross-linking reaction. Ca^{2+} cross-linking hydrogel system observed higher stability than that of Zn^{2+} or Cu^{2+} cross-linking system. In vitro result showed the paracetamol release in 2 h in SGF followed by 6 h in SIF and <20%

paracetamol release in SGF. Jana et al. (2013a) developed ALG–gellan gum microspheres for sustained aceclofenac (AC) delivery. Microspheres were developed by the maleic anhydride-induced unsaturated esterification method. The prepared microspheres were analyzed by the P-XRD, FTIR, DSC, and SEM analysis. Drug entrapment efficiency (DEE) and particle size range of the microsphere were 39–98% and 270–490 nm, respectively. The in vitro dissolution revealed prolonged release of AC up to 6 h. The in vivo results showed absorption of AC in rabbits, sustained period at 7 h (Fig 17.3), and good anti-inflammatory pharmacodynamics performed in carrageenan-induced rat model.

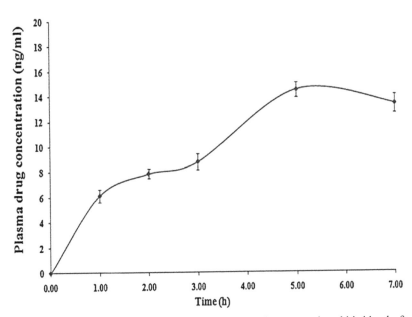

FIGURE 17.3 The plasma drug concentration versus time curve in rabbit blood after a single oral dose of microspheres.

Source: Reprinted with permission from Jana et al., 2013a. © 2013 Elsevier. https://doi. org/10.1016/j.ijbiomac.2013.03.015

In another study, Jana et al. (2015a) fabricated ALG hydrogel core–shell systems for dual drug delivery (AC and ranitidine HCl). AC-loaded Eudragit L-100-coated ALG microspheres were used as core part. The DEE and particle size range of Eudragit L-100-coated ALG microspheres were 56–68% and 551–677 μm, respectively. Particle surface morphology was evaluated by the SEM analysis (Figure 17.4)

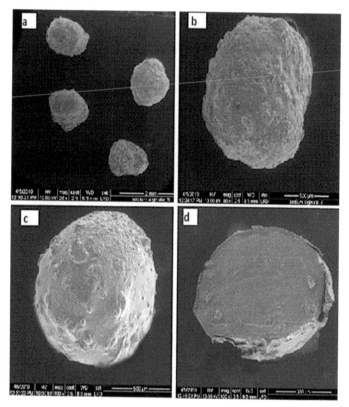

FIGURE 17.4 SEM photograph of uncoated aceclofenac (AC)-loaded ALG microspheres (a and b), AC-loaded ALG microspheres coated with Eudragit L-100 (c), and cross-sectional view of AC-loaded ALG microspheres coated with Eudragit L-100 (d).

Source: Reprinted with permission from Jana et al., 2015a. © 2015 Elsevier. https://doi.org/10.1016/j.ijbiomac.2014.11.027

Further, Jana et al. (2015b) investigated ALG–locust bean gum (LBG) containing AC with Ca^{2+} cross-linking method. DEE and size range of the microsphere was 59–93% and 406–684 μm respectively. The prepared microspheres showed sustained release of AC in pH 6.8 for a time of 8 h.

17.3 CONCLUSION

ALG is an anionic linear biopolymer which is biocompatible, biodegradable, and nontoxic in nature. Chemically, it contains 1,4-α-l-guluronic acid and β-d-mannuronic acid residues. ALG-based delivery systems are recently important to the delivery of drug to the target site. This chapter focused on the ALG-based systems delivery of therapeutics such as anti-inflammatory, antidepressant, antidiabetic, antibiotic, antiviral, anticancer, and insulin, and so forth through GIT. We also discuss the different drug release pattern in SGF, SIF, and SCF and characterization part of the different matrix systems. Finally, we can conclude that ALG-based systems are successfully delivering the bioactive molecule to the target sites to get the desired therapeutic effect.

SUMMARY

Recent trends to polymeric blends/modified chemical structures are utilized for the development of polymeric carriers systems. This physical/chemical modification leads to increase the mechanical strength and tailors the drug release to the target site. Single polymer does note to control the drug release, due to premature/burst release in the acidic environment before reaching the target site. Natural polymers have biodegradable, biocompatible, and nontoxic nature. Among natural polymers, ALG is one of the important polymers that has a versatile application in the biomedical fields. Due to its versatility, we have especially emphasized on the ALG-based systems for drug delivery through the GIT.

KEYWORDS

- alginate
- gastrointestinal delivery
- drug delivery

REFERENCES

Agarwal, T.; Narayana, S. N. G. H.; Pal, K.; Pramanik, K.; Giri, S.; Banerjee, I. Calcium Alginate-Carboxymethyl Cellulose Beads for Colon-Targeted Drug Delivery. *Int. J. Biol. Macromol.* **2015,** *75,* 409–417.

Azhar, F. F. Olad, A. A Study on Sustained Release Formulations for Oral Delivery of 5-Fluorouracil Based on Alginate–Chitosan/Montmorillonite Nanocomposite Systems. *Appl. Clay Sci.* **2014,** *101,* 288–296.

Banerjee, A.; Onyuksel, H. Peptide Delivery Using Phospholipid Micelles. *Wiley Interdiscip. Rev. Nanomed. Nanobiotechnol.* **2012,** *4,* 562–574.

Banerjee, A.; Mitragotri, S. Intestinal Patch Systems for Oral Drug Delivery. *Curr. Opin. Pharmacol.* **2017,** *36,* 58–65.

Bansal, D.; Gulbake, A.; Tiwari, J.; Jain, S. K. Development of Liposomes Entrapped in Alginate Beads for the Treatment of Colorectal Cancer. *Int. J. Biol. Macromol.* **2016,** *82,* 687–695.

Bhattacharyya, A.; Mukherjee, D.; Mishra, R.; Kundu, P. P. Preparation of Polyurethane–Alginate/Chitosan Core Shell Nanoparticles for the Purpose of Oral Insulin Delivery. *Eur. Polym. J.* **2017,** *92,* 294–313.

Blandón, L. M. B; Islan, G. A.; Castro, G. R.; Noseda, M. D.; Thomaz-Soccol, V.; Soccol, C. R. Kefiran-Alginate Gel Microspheres for Oral Delivery of Ciprofloxacin. *Colloids Surf. B* **2016,** *145,* 706–715.

Dodov, M. G.; Calis, S.; Crcarevska, M. S.; Geskovski, N.; Petrovska, V.; Goracinova, K. Wheat Germ Agglutinin-Conjugated Chitosan–Ca–Alginate Microparticles for Local Colon Delivery of 5-Fu: Development and in Vitro Characterization. *Int. J. Pharm.* **2009,** *381,* 166–175.

Duan, H.; Lü, S.; Qin, H.; Gao, C.; Bai, X.; Wei, Y.; Wu, X.; Liu, M.; Zhang, X.; Liu, Z. Co-Delivery of Zinc and 5-Aminosalicylic Acid from Alginate/N-Succinyl-Chitosan Blend Microspheres for Synergistic Therapy of Colitis. Int J Pharm **2017,** *516,* 214–224.

Iliescu, R. I.; Andronescu, E.; Ghitulica, C. D.; Voicu, G.; Ficai, A.; Hoteteu, M. Montmorillonite-Alginate Nanocomposite as a Drug Delivery System—Incorporation and in Vitro Release of Irinotecan. *Int. J. Pharm.* **2014,** *463,* 184–192.

Jain, S.; Datta, M. Montmorillonite-Alginate Microspheres as a Delivery Vehicle for Oral Extended Release of Venlafaxine Hydrochloride. *J. Drug Delivery Sci. Technol.* **2016,** *33,* 149–156.

Jana, S.; Das, A.; Nayak, A. K.; Sen, K. K.; Basu, S. K. Aceclofenac-Loaded Unsaturated Esterified Alginate/Gellan Gum Microspheres: In Vitro and in Vivo Assessment. *Int. J. Biol. Macromol.* **2013a,** *57,* 129–137.

Jana, S.; Maji, N.; Nayak, A. K.; Sen, K. K.; Basu, S. K. Development of Chitosan-Based Nanoparticles through Inter-Polymeric Complexation for Oral Drug Delivery. *Carbohydr. Polym.* **2013b,** *98,* 870–876.

Jana, S.; Manna, S.; Nayak, A. K.; Sen, K. K.; Basu, S. K. Carbopol Gel Containing Chitosan-Egg Albumin Nanoparticles For Transdermal aceclofenac Delivery. *Colloids Surf. B* **2014,** *114,* 36–44.

Jana, S.; Samanta, A.; Nayak, A. K.; Sen, K. K.; Jana, S. Novel Alginate Hydrogel Core–Shell Systems for Combination Delivery of Ranitidine HCl and Aceclofenac. *Int. J. Biol. Macromol.* **2015a,** *74,* 85–92.

Jana, S.; Gandhi, A.; Sheet, S.; Sen, K. K. Metal Ion-Induced Alginate–Locust Bean Gum IPN Microspheres for Sustained Oral Delivery of Aceclofenac. *Int. J. Biol. Macromol.* **2015b,** *72,* 47–53.

Jana, S.; Laha, L.; Maiti, S. Boswellia Gum Resin/Chitosan Polymer Composites: Controlled Delivery Vehicles for Aceclofenac. *Int. J. Biol. Macromol.* **2015c,** *77,* 303–306.

Jana, S.; Banerjee, A.; Sen, K. K.; Maiti, S.; Gelatin-Carboxymethyl Tamarind Gum Biocomposites: In Vitro Characterization and Anti-Inflammatory Pharmacodynamics. *Mater. Sci. Eng. C* **2016a,** *69,* 478–485.

Jana, S.; Sen, K. K.; Gandhi, A. Alginate Based Nanocarriers for Drug Delivery Applications. *Curr. Pharm. Des.* **2016b,** *22,* 3399–3410.

Jana, S.; Sharma, R.; Maiti, S.; Sen, K. K, Interpenetrating Hydrogels of O-Carboxymethyl Tamarind Gum and Alginate for Monitoring Delivery of Acyclovir. *Int. J. Biol. Macromol.* **2016c,** *92,* 1034–1039.

Jayapal, J. J.; Dhanaraj, S.; Exemestane Loaded Alginate Nanoparticles for Cancer Treatment: Formulation and in Vitro Evaluation. *Int. J. Biol. Macromol.* **2017,** *105,* 416–421.

Joshy, K. S.; George, A.; Jose, J.; Kalarikkal, N.; Pothen, L. A.; Thomas, S. Novel Dendritic Structure of Alginate Hybrid Nanoparticles for Effective Anti-Viral Drug Delivery. *Int. J. Biol. Macromol.* **2017,** *103,* 1265–1275.

Joshy, K. S.; Alex, S. M.; Snigdha, S.; Kalarikkal, N.; Pothen, L. A.; Thomas, S. Encapsulation of Zidovudine in PF-68 Coated Alginate Conjugate Nanoparticles for Anti-HIV Drug Delivery. *Int. J. Biol. Macromol.* **2018,** *107,* 929–937.

Kim, M. S.; Park, S. J.; Gu, B. K.; Kim, C.-H. Ionically Crosslinked Alginate–Carboxymethyl Cellulose Beads for the Delivery of Protein Therapeutics. *Appl. Surf. Sci.* **2012,** *262,* 28–33.

Ku, M. S. Use of the Biopharmaceutical Classification System in Early Drug Development. *AAPS J.* **2008,** *10,* 208–212.

Lim, H.-P.; Ooi, C.-W.; Tey, B.-T.; Chan, E.-S. Controlled Delivery of Oral Insulin Aspart Using pH-Responsive Alginate/K-Carrageenan Composite Hydrogel Beads. *React. Funct. Polym.* **2017,** *120,* 20–29.

Łukasiewicz, S.; Szczepanowicz, K.; Błasiak, E.; Dziedzicka-Wasylewska, M. Biocompatible Polymeric Nanoparticles as Promising Candidates for Drug Delivery. *Langmuir* **2015,** *31,* 6415–6425.

Maestrelli, F.; Mura, P.; González-Rodríguez, M. L.; Cózar-Bernal, M. J.; Rabasco, A. M.; Mannelli, L. D. C.; Ghelardini C.; Calcium Alginate Microspheres Containing Metformin Hydrochloride Niosomes and Chitosomes Aimed for Oral Therapy of Type 2 Diabetes Mellitus. *Int. J. Pharm.* **2017,** *530,* 430–439.

Martínez-Gómez, F.; Guerrero, J.; Matsuhiro, B.; Pavez, J. In Vitro Release of Metformin Hydrochloride from Sodium Alginate/Polyvinyl Alcohol Hydrogels. *Carbohydr. Polym.* **2017,** *155,* 182–191.

Mukhopadhyay, P.; Chakraborty, S.; Bhattacharya, S.; Mishra, R.; Kundu, P. P. pH-Sensitive Chitosan/Alginate Core-Shell Nanoparticles for Efficient and Safe Oral Insulin Delivery. *Int. J. Biol. Macromol.* **2015,** *72,* 640–648.

Nayak, A.; Pal, D.; Formulation Optimization and Evaluation of Jackfruit seed Starch-Alginate Mucoadhesive Beads of Metformin HCl. *Int. J. Biol. Macromol.* **2013a,** *59,* 264–272.

Nayak, A.; Pal, D.; Ionotropically-Gelled Mucoadhesive Beads for Oral Metformin HCl Delivery: Formulation, Optimization and Antidiabetic Evaluation. *J. Sci. Ind. Res.* **2013b,** *72,* 15–22.

Omer, A. M.; Tamer, T. M.; Hassan, M. A.; Rychter, P.; Mohy Eldin, M. S.; Koseva, N. Development of Amphoteric Alginate/Aminated Chitosan Coated Microbeads for Oral Protein Delivery. *Int. J. Biol. Macromol.* **2016,** *92,* 362–370.

Rahmani, V.; Sheardown, H. Protein-Alginate Complexes as pH-/Ion-Sensitive Carriers of Proteins. *Int. J. Pharm.* **2018,** *535,* 452–461.

Rivera, M. C.; Pinheiro, A. C.; Bourbon, A. I.; Cerqueira, M. A.; Vicente, A. A. Hollow Chitosan/Alginate Nanocapsules for Bioactive Compound Delivery. *Int. J. Biol. Macromol.* **2015,** *79,* 95–102.

Sarkar, N.; Sahoo, G.; Das, R.; Prusty, G.; Swain, S. K. Carbon Quantum Dot Tailored Calcium Alginate Hydrogel for pH Responsive Controlled Delivery of Vancomycin. *Eur. J. Pharm. Sci.* **2017,** *109,* 359–371.

Seeli, D. S.; Dhivya, S.; Selvamurugan, N.; Prabaharan, M. Guar Gum Succinate-Sodium Alginate Beads as a pH-Sensitive Carrier for Colon-Specific Drug Delivery. *Int. J. Biol. Macromol.* **2016,** *91,* 45–50.

Shtenberg, Y.; Goldfeder, M.; Schroeder, A.; Bianco-Peled, H. Alginate Modified with Maleimide-Terminated PEG as Drug Carriers with Enhanced Mucoadhesion. *Carbohydr. Polym.* **2017,** *175,* 337–346.

Tahtat, D.; Mahlous, M.; Benamer, S.; Khodja, A. N.; Oussedik-Oumehdi, H.; Laraba-Djebari, F. Oral Delivery of Insulin from Alginate/Chitosan Crosslinked by Glutaraldehyde. *Int. J. Biol. Macromol.* **2013,** *58,* 160–168.

Treenate, P.; Monvisade, P. In Vitro Drug Release Profiles of pH-Sensitive Hydroxyethylacryl Chitosan/Sodium Alginate Hydrogels Using Paracetamol as a Soluble Model Drug. *Int. J. Biol. Macromol.* **2017,** *99,* 71–78.

Wang, J.; Wang, M.; Zheng, M.; Guo, Q.; Wang, Y.; Wang, H.; Xie, X.; Huang, F.; Gong, R. Folate Mediated Self-Assembled Phytosterol-Alginate Nanoparticles for Targeted Intracellular Anticancer Drug Delivery. *Colloids Surf. B* **2015,** *129,* 63–70.

Wen, P.; Feng, K.; Yang, H.; Huang, X.; Zong, M.-H.; Lou, W.-Y.; Li, N.; Wu, H. Electrospun Core-Shell Structured Nanofilm as a Novel Colon-Specific Delivery System for Protein. *Carbohydr. Polym.* **2017,** *169,* 157–166.

Yang, J.; Chen, J.; Pan, D.; Wan, Y.; Wang, Z. pH-Sensitive Interpenetrating Network Hydrogels Based on Chitosan Derivatives and Alginate for Oral Drug Delivery. *Carbohydr. Polym.* **2013,** *92,* 719–725.

Yin, Z.-C.; Wang, Y.-L.; Wang, K. A pH-Responsive Composite Hydrogel Beads Based on Agar and Alginate for Oral Drug Delivery. *J. Drug Delivery Sci. Technol.* **2018,** *43,* 12–18.

CHAPTER 18

ALGINATE HYDROGELS AS A COLON-TARGETED DRUG DELIVERY SYSTEM

PRAMENDRA KUMAR[1,*] and DEEPAK KUMAR[1, 2]

[1]Department of Applied Chemistry, M. J. P. Rohilkhand University, Bareilly, Uttar Pradesh 243006, India

[2]Department of Applied Chemistry, Babasaheb Bhimrao Ambedkar University (Central University), Lucknow, Uttar Pradesh 266025, India

*Corresponding author. E-mail: pramendra2002@gmail.com

18.1 INTRODUCTION

The colon-targeted oral drug delivery is necessary in order to treat a variability of colon diseases such as ulcerative, Crohn's disease, colonic cancer, amebiosis, colitis, and so forth (Philip and Philip, 2010). In current years, there have been several numbers of advances for the development of target specificity of colon-targeted delivery systems (Dolmans et al., 2003). The primary approaches pertaining to the colon-specific delivery contain: (i) covalent bonded of a drug with polymers as a prodrug, (ii) drug-coated polymer, drug delivery system (Agarwal et al., 2015) with the pH-sensitive drug carrier (polymer) bioadhesive natural polymers or biodegradable natural polymers, and (iii) microbially triggered release of the drug (Aguilar et al., 2007). In addition, some of the new drug delivery methods have also been presented such as: (i) pressure-controlled drug delivery, (ii) CODESTM (combined approach of pH-dependent and microbial triggered drug delivery), (iii) osmotic pressure-controlled drug delivery through a semipermeable membrane, and (iv) multiparticulate systems like microspheres and nanoparticles (Agnihotri et al., 2004). However, several researchers highlighted that though the unique drug delivery systems have shown good potential, yet further developments are necessary before their full conversion into medical use (Talaei et al., 2013).

The colon-specific drug delivery system should be protective drug method to the colon. The drug release and absorption should not arise in the stomach and in the small intestine, and neither the bioactive agent should be degraded in either of the dissolution sites but only released and absorbed once the system reaches the colon (Bhalersao and Mahaparale, 2013). The colon is believed to be an appropriate absorption location for protein and peptides drugs for the following causes: (i) low diversity and strength of peptic enzymes, (ii) relative proteolytic action of colon mucosa is much low than that detected in the small intestine, thus colon-specific drug delivery system (CDDS) protects peptide drugs from hydrolysis and enzymatic poverty in duodenum and jejunum drug release into ileum or colon which clues to better systemic bioavailability (Philip and Philip, 2010; Qureshi et al., 2013) and finally, because the colon has a long residence time which is more than 5 days and is greatly approachable to absorption garnishes (Saha et al., 2013).

Colon-targeted drug delivery has been the effort of several studies in current years due to its potential to develop treatment of many diseases which affected the colon and decrease the systemic side effects (Amidon et al., 2015). The delivery of these drugs exactly to the colon without being absorbed first in the upper gastrointestinal (GI) zone allows for a greater concentration of the drug to reach the colon with negligible systemic preoccupation (Amidon et al., 2015; Das et al., 2010). The colonic insides have a long retention period (more than 5 days), and the colonic mucosa is known to simplify the absorption of numerous drugs and creation of this organ as an idyllic site for drug delivery. A drug can be transported to the colon through the oral or the rectal path (Figure 18.1) (Leuva et al., 2012).

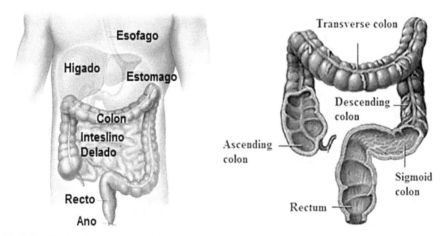

FIGURE 18.1   Anatomy of colon.

Oral dosage forms are the most favored delivery path for colon-specific delivery because of their convenience (Philip and Philip, 2010). Oral dosage forms also permit for a better degree of elasticity in their development, strategy, relatively harmless administration, and enhanced patient adherence and they do not need sterile preparation (Kumar et al., 2010). Direct rectal delivery of drugs is stimulating with respect to affecting a drug to exact sites inside the colon (Malayandi et al., 2014). Additionally, the amount of drug distribution diverges for various rectal dosage forms depending on their diffusion capacity and retention period (Kumar and Mishra, 2008).

The achievement of a CDDS depends on the drug's physicochemical characteristics (Jain et al., 2007), the type of delivery system, all other influences which may affect the GI transportation time, and the degree of interaction between the drug and the GI tract (GIT) (Amidon et al., 2015). It is necessary for oral CDDS to protect the drug from being released in the small intestine and stomach. Target sites, colonic disease conditions, and drugs used for treatment are shown in Table 18.1.

TABLE 18.1   Colon Targeting Diseases and its Sites.

S. N.	Target sites	Drug and active agents	Disease conditions
1	Systemic action	Nonsteroidal anti-inflammatory drugs Steroids Insulin Typhoid	To prevent gastric irritation To prevent first-pass metabolism of orally ingested drug oral delivery of peptides oral delivery of vaccines
2	Topical action	Hydrocortisone, budenoside, prednisolone, mesalazine, balsalazide	Inflammatory bowel diseases, irritable bowel diseases and Crohn's diseases, chronic pancreatitis
3	Local action	Digestive enzyme supplements 5-fluorouracil	Pancreatectomy and cystic fibrosis, colorectal cancer

Source: Adapted from Sreelatha and Brahma (2013)

18.2   NEED OF COLON-TARGETED DRUG DELIVERY

1. Colon-targeted dosage form lowers dosing and its frequency and reduces systemic adverse effects and dose dumping.
2. By prolonging drug release, the peptide and protein kind of drugs can be targeted to colon through oral route.
3. Both local and systemic drug release could be possible at colonic site.

4. Colon targeting could provide better and reliable treatment for colorectal cancer.

5. Drugs which are polar in nature and/or prone to acidic or enzymatic decomposition could be specifically and effectively released in the colon.

18.3 FACTORS AFFECTING COLON-TARGETED DRUG DELIVERY

18.3.1 PHYSIOLOGICAL FACTORS

18.3.1.1 GASTRIC EMPTYING

Drug delivery to the colon upon oral administration depends mainly on gastric emptying and bowel transit time. Upon reaching the colon, the transit time of dosage form depends on the size of the particles. Smaller particles have more transit time compared to larger particles. Diarrhea patients have a shorter transit time, whereas constipation patients have longer transit times.

18.3.1.2 pH IN COLON

The pH of varies between different individuals. The food intake, diseased state, and so forth influence the pH of the GIT. This change in the pH in different parts of GIT is the basis for the development of colon-targeted drug delivery systems. Coating with different polymers is done to target the drug to the site shown in Table 18. 2 (rights are reserved by Nalanda and Rangari, 2015).

TABLE 18.2   pH in Different Parts of Colon.

S. N.	Colon	pH
1.	Ascending colon	6.4
2.	Transverse colon	6.6
3.	Descending colon	7.0

Source: Adapted from Sreelantha and Brahma (2013).

18.3.1.3 COLONIC MICROFLORA AND ENZYMES

The GIT contains a variety of microorganisms that produce many enzymes needed for metabolism (Orlu et al., 2006). The growth of this microflora is controlled by the GIT contents and peristaltic movements. The enzymes released by different microorganisms *Escherichia coli*, *Clostridia*, *Lactobacilli*, *Eubacteria*, and *Streptococci* are responsible for the various metabolic reactions that take place in the GIT (Ghugarkar et al., 2015).

18.3.2 PHARMACEUTICAL FACTORS

18.3.2.1 DRUG CANDIDATES

A drug candidate appropriate for medical testing is predictable to bind to the proper receptor site on the target, to elicit the favorite functional response of the selected target molecule, and to have satisfactory bioavailability and biodistribution to elicit the favorite responses in humans and animals; it must also pass recognized venomousness evaluation in human and animals. A drug candidate proper for colon-targeted drug delivery system is expected to satisfy specific and demand conditions (Hefti, 2008). Due to great retention time of colon, colon causes an enhancement in the absorption of weakly absorbed agents such as peptides, natural polysaccharide, and so forth; drugs used for the treatment of inflammatory bowel diseases and so forth are appropriate for colon-targeted drug delivery system.

18.3.2.2 DRUG CARRIERS

The selection of a suitable drug carrier for colon-specific drug delivery system depends on the characteristics and nature of the drug targeted and disease for which the drug is used. The numerous physicochemical influences of drug that influence the carrier selection contain chemical nature, partition coefficient, permanence, functional groups of drug compound, and so forth (Sreelatha and Brahma, 2013).

18.4 POLYMERS IN COLON TARGETING

Natural polymers are the great candidates for the improvement of solid dosage forms due to their numerous properties (Sandler and Preis, 2016). They are stable, nonhazardous, and hydrophilic in nature. These polysaccharides are degraded by bacteria as well as enzymes present in the colon, which remain intact during their passage through the upper GIT. This unique property of polysaccharides can be utilized for targeting the drug to the colon (Bastiancich et al., 2016). Until last few years, it was measured that polymers are the components of system or the excipients of dosage forms which do not pass much effect on the drug release and newer drugs (Mansuri et al., 2016). The drug delivery systems, developed by using natural polymers and their derivatives, found to be active in the treatment of several diseases and can protect to deliver the gene instead of using the viruses as vectors. Though the wide range of natural polymers and their compounds with variable properties is available, but sometime natural polymers fail to fulfill the demand due to the some conditions (Debele et al., 2016). To fulfill the demands of drug delivery, development in the natural polymer properties is vital as it is very hard to get novel polymer with explicit enhanced properties, namely, enhanced thermal stability, biocompatibility, multiphase response, rigidity, and flexibility. Regular replacement of natural polysaccharides with modified natural polymers/synthetic polymers to meet favorite properties can be active for drug targeting. Natural polymers are many methods to modify the properties of polymers, including grafting, cross-linking (Kumar et al., 2017), blending, and curing (Kumar et al., 2018). Blending compounds are mixture of two or more natural polymers with essential properties. Grafting is a method in which monomers are covalently joined on the backbone of main polymer and curing is the polymerization of an oligomer mixture that forms a coating which adheres to the substrate. Among these, grafting is widely used technique for polymer modification (Kumar et al., 2016; Kumar and Kumar, 2014).

Numerous natural polymers such as sodium alginate (ALG) (Joshy et al., 2018), chitosan (CS) (Fonseca et al., 2017), guar gum (Fonseca-Santos and Chorilli, 2017), xanthan gum (Laffleur and Michalek, 2017), pectin (Marras-Marquez et al., 2015), and gellan gum (Dewan et al., 2017) have been employed either alone or in combination with their native or modified forms to control the drug release from different types of delivery system, but these just had a limited degree of success. In recent years, graft copolymers designed primarily for medical applications have entered the arena of controlled release.

18.5 ALGINATES (ALGS)

ALGs have become a very significant family of polysaccharides (Agüero et al., 2017) because of their effectiveness in preparing hydrogels at various pH and different temperature conditions, appropriate for sensitive biomolecules such as nucleic acids and proteins, and even for alive cells like islets of Langerhans (Simó et al., 2017; Venkatesan et al., 2015). In addition, the complex small monosaccharide units in sequences of ALGs, and our increasing capability to form controlled sequences through the act of isolated epimerases upon the ALG predecessor poly(mannuronic acid) (Zia et al., 2015) produce remarkable chances for understanding the relationship of possessions to sequence in natural ALGs, that is, control of monosaccharide sequence being perhaps the highest synthetic test in polysaccharide chemistry (Pawar and Edgar, 2012).

ALG is both biopolymer as well as polyelectrolyte that are measured to be biocompatible, nonhazardous, biodegradable, and nonimmunogenic. ALG is anionic and linear polysaccharide obtained from brown seaweed like *Laminaria hyperborea, Macrocystis pyrifera, and Ascophyllum nodosum* (Klöck et al., 1997) and also characterized as an anionic copolymer included of mannuronic acid (M-block) and guluronic acid (G-block) units arranged in an irregular block-wise pattern. This natural polymer possesses the alternating blocks of $\beta(1\rightarrow4)$ linkages, guluronic acid (G), and $\alpha(1\rightarrow4)$ mannuronic acid (M) units (Figure 18.2) and is obtainable as several grades depending on the cleanliness required for a given applications (Orive et al., 2002; Yang et al., 2011).

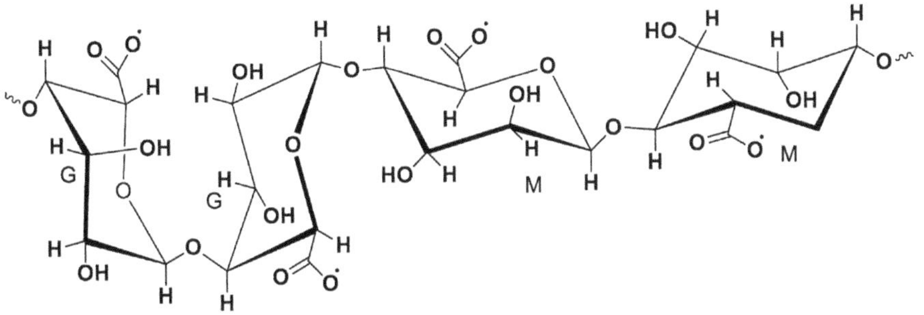

FIGURE 18.2   Structure of alginate.

While it is conceivable to form ALGs from both algal as well as bacterial sources, commercially obtainable ALGs presently come only from algae. The natural polymer composition, sequence, and molecular weights vary with the source and species that produce the natural polymer. Due to the profusion of algae in water sources, there is a great quantity of ALG material current in nature (Florentin, 2015; Pawar and Edgar, 2012). Therefore, there is important additional possible to design maintainable biomaterials based on ALGs. The combination of biochemical as well as chemical techniques offers considerable potential for generating improved alginic acid derivatives with control over monomer units sequence and nature, location, and extent of substituent. This in opportunity allows the tailoring of ALG derivative properties such as hydrophobicity, affinity for specific proteins, solubility, and many others. Such improvements are difficult through key alginic acid properties with pH sensitivity, solubility, and complexity. The consequence of ALGs as natural polymer in biomedicine can barely be excessive. ALGs are presently used as spiral dressing materials for the treatment of acute or chronic wounds (Boateng et al., 2008). They also play a crucial part in the development of cystic fibrosis, wherein bacterial biofilms designed from ALG gels are concealed by *Pseudomonas aeruginosa* (Ramsey and Wozniak, 2005). More significantly, the utility of ALG cross-linking to create hydrogels for cell encapsulation has demonstrated to be most beneficial for biomedical applications (Lee and Mooney, 2012; Soon-Shiong et al., 1993; Zimmermann et al., 2007).

18.6 ALGS USED IN DRUG DELIVERY

Zhang et al. (2017) investigated that the colon-targeted drug delivery system is one way to address this problem after the resection of colorectal cancer. Therefore, they developed the graphene oxide (GO)-based sodium ALG functionalized colon-targeting drug delivery system that is loaded with 5-fluorouracil (5-FU) as the anticancer drug (denoted as GO-ALG/5-FU). Their results exhibit that the as-prepared drug delivery system has a much minor toxicity and better colon-targeting controlled-release behaviors.

Wang et al. (2016) investigated the protective mechanism of CS–ALG microspheres loaded with icariin with trinitrobenzene sulfonic acid/ethanol-induced colonic mucosal injury in rats. The results of drug released showed that the icariin loaded into microspheres released only 10% in simulated gastric fluid and a high amount of 65.6% in the stimulated colonic fluid. The fluorescence tracer indicated high retention of targeted microspheres of more than 12 h in colon. A novel pH-sensitive drug delivery system (hydrogel/micelle):ALG-Ca^{2+} hydrogel-contained drug carriers (CS-based micelles) for controlling drug release was reported by Cong et al., 2017.

Agarwal et al. (2015) synthesized and characterized calcium ALG (CA)-carboxymethyl cellulose (CMC) beads for colon-specific oral drug delivery. They exploited pH-responsive swelling, mucoadhesivity, and colonic microflora catered biodegradability of the formulations for colon-specific drug delivery. The CA-CMC beads were prepared by ionic gelation method and its physicochemical characterization was done by SEM, XRD, EDAX, DSC, and texture analyzer. They also observed that degradation rate increased drastically in the presence of colonic microflora. In vitro release study of anticancer drug 5-FU showed a release (>90%) in the presence of colonic enzymes.

Sookkasem et al. (2015) synthesized the CA beads containing self-emulsifying curcumin (SE-Cur) for colon targeting. Encapsulation efficiency was in the range of 85–98%. The formulations containing a mixture of SE-Cur, 2–4% ALG and 0.1 or 0.3 M calcium chloride, could prevent early curcumin release in simulated gastric fluid (pH 1.2) and simulated intestinal fluid (pH 6.8) and >60% of the drug was released in simulated colonic fluid (pH 7.4) within 12 h, while the total drug release from the beads containing curcumin powder in all media was only 10–20%. The emulsion droplet sizes in simulated colonic fluid were in the range of 120–202 nm. SE-Cur released from the beads showed cytotoxic ability against the human colon adenocarcinoma cell lines (HT-29) with an IC50 of 10 µg/mL. In addition, the reducing power assay (antioxidant activity) was linearly proportional to the concentration of the SE-Cur released. Our results demonstrate the potential use of SE-Cur-loaded ALG beads for the delivery of poorly soluble drugs to the colon. Momin et al. (2013) synthesized the hydrogel-based biodegradable enteric-coated ALG beads for colon-targeted drug delivery of embelin. All investigated factors have significant effect on percentage of drug entrapment, the size of beads, and the release of embelin from ECA beads. The mechanism of drug release from ECA beads followed the diffusion-controlled model for an inert porous matrix. The natural polymer like ALG-based multiparticulate dosage form provided an intermediate erosion pattern for the colonic delivery of embelin beads. Hence, it can be concluded that the drugs like embelin can be delivered to colon without releasing in stomach and upper intestine for the better treatment of helminthiasis using natural polysaccharides as a polymer.

CA beads can be prepared by dropwise addition of the solution of sodium ALG into the solution of calcium chloride. The ALG beads have the advantage of being nontoxic, and dried ALG beads reswell in presence of dissolution media and can act as controlled-release systems. CA beads were prepared as cores and 5-ASA was spray-coated on them (Lin and Ayres, 1992). Different enteric as well as sustained release polymers were applied as a coat on CA beads. A system was prepared by coating CA beads with aqua coat that is a pH-independent polymer followed by 2% w/w coating of Eudragit L-30D. Being enteric polymer, Eudragit resisted the release of drug in acidic media and drug release was triggered at alkaline pH and controlled by the thickness of aqua coat. When drug-loaded CA beads swell sufficiently (osmotic gradient) to exceed the strength of outer sustained released coat, the film bursts to release the drug. Such a system delivers drug to the distal intestine with the minimal initial leak and provides sustained release in the colon (Chourasia and Jain, 2004). Prepared ALG beads are coated with dextran acetate. In the absence of dextranase, minimal drug release occurred, whereas it was significantly improved in the presence of dextranase (Kiyoung et al., 1999).

Wang, et al. (2014) synthesized the composite materials for the controlled release of drugs, a series of novel pH-sensitive konjac glucomannan/sodium ALG and GO hydrogels, using GO as a drug-binding effector for anticancer drug loading and release. They studied the effects of component ratio and pH on the swelling properties of hydrogels. The release amount of 5-FU incorporated into hydrogels was about 38.02% at pH 1.2 and 84.19% at pH 6.8 after 6 and 12 h, respectively.

18.7   CONCLUSION

The improvement in formulation with ALG for colon-targeted oral drug delivery system has increased an interest among the scientists because of its drug release and compatibility. Colon-specific drug delivery systems based on ALG offer important therapeutic assistances to the patients in terms of protection, efficiency, and patient acquiescence. Factors with the physicochemical nature of the drug, ALGs formulation and route variables, and the GI physiological factors impact may present a way to the successful formulation of a colon-specific drug delivery system. Hydrogel of ALG is widely used as a drug binder and it was also found that ALG-based hydro-gels have the excellent capacity to drug release at the approximately neutral pH, a long transit time, reduced enzymatic activity, and increased respon-siveness to absorption enhancers and show the good drug-binding effector for controlling the release rate of drugs. ALG-based hydrogels could be a suitable polymer carrier for the colon-targeted oral drug delivery systems.

SUMMARY

Colon-specific drug delivery system is developed to deliver the drug directly into the colon with reduced dose amount, dosage frequency, as well as systemic side effects and is widely used for the treatment of several diseases associated with colon like Crohn's disease, inflammatory bowel disease, colon cancer, and so forth. The main benefit of colon-specific drug delivery system is that to provide the near-neutral pH, an extensive transit period, decrease the enzymatic activity, and improve absorptive capacity. Hydrogels of ALG are widely used in drug delivery system, especially colon-specific drug delivery system, because of its biocompatibility, biodegradability, high absorption capacity, nontoxicity, and various peculiar physicochemical properties which make it more attractive material for drug delivery system. In this chapter, we discuss about the colon-specific drug delivery system and the various types of hydrogels of ALG which are used in colon-specific drug delivery system.

KEYWORDS

- colon cancer
- alginate
- drug delivery
- hydrogels

REFERENCES

Agarwal, T.; Narayana, S. G. H.; Pal, K.; Pramanik, K.; Giri, S.; Banerjee, I. Calcium Alginate-Carboxymethyl Cellulose Beads for Colon-Targeted Drug Delivery. *Int. J. Biol. Macromol.* **2015,** *75,* 409–417.

Agnihotri, S. A.; Mallikarjuna, N. N.; Aminabhavi, T. M. Recent Advances on Chitosan-Based Micro- and Nanoparticles in Drug Delivery. *J. Controlled Release* **2004,** *100*(1), 5–28.

Agüero, L.; Zaldivar-Silva, D.; Peña, L.; Dias, M. L. Alginate Microparticles as Oral Colon Drug Delivery Device: a Review. *Carbohydr. Polym.* **2017,** *168,* 32–43.

Aguilar, M. R.; Elvira, C.; Gallardo, A.; Vázquez, B.; Román, J. Smart Polymers and Their Applications as Biomaterials. In *Topics in Tissue Engineering;* Ashammakhi, N., Reis, R., Chiellini, E., Eds.; CiteSeer: Pennsylvania, 2007; Vol. 3, pp 1–27.

Amidon, S.; Brown, J. E.; Dave, V. S. Colon-Targeted Oral Drug Delivery Systems: Design Trends and Approaches. *Pharm. Sci. Tech.* **2015,** *16*(4), 731–741.

Bastiancich, C.; Danhier, P.; Préat, V.; Danhier, F. Anticancer Drug-Loaded Hydrogels as Drug Delivery Systems for the Local Treatment of Glioblastoma. *J. Controlled Release* **2016,** *243,* 29–42.

Bhalersao, S. D.; Mahaparale, P. R. Different approaches for colon drug delivery systems: a Review. *Int. J. Res. Rev. Pharm. Appl. Sci.* **2014,** *2*(3), 529–549..

Boateng, J. S.; Matthews, K. H.; Stevens, H. N.; Eccleston, G. M. Wound Healing Dressings and Drug Delivery Systems: a Review. *J. Pharm. Sci.* **2008,** *97*(8), 2892–2923.

Chourasia, M.; Jain, S. Polysaccharides for Colon Targeted Drug Delivery. *Drug Delivery* **2004,** *11*(2), 129–148.

Cong, Z.; Shi, Y.; Wang, Y.; Wang, Y.; Chen, N.; Xue, H. A Novel Controlled Drug Delivery System Based on Alginate Hydrogel/Chitosan Micelle Composites. *Int. J. Biol. Macromol.* **2017,** *107,* 855–864.

Das, S.; Deshmukh, R.; Jha, A. Role of Natural Polymers in the Development of Multiparticulate Systems for Colon Drug Targeting. *Syst. Rev. Pharm.* **2010,** *1*(1), 79–84.

Debele, T. A.; Mekuria, S. L.; Tsai, H. C. Polysaccharide Based Nanogels in the Drug Delivery System: Application as the Carrier of Pharmaceutical Agents. *Mater. Sci. Eng. C* **2016,** *68,* 964–981.

Dewan, M.; Sarkar, G.; Bhowmik, M.; Das, B.; Chattoapadhyay, A. K.; Rana, D.; Chattopadhyay, D. Effect of Gellan Gum on the Thermogelation Property and Drug Release Profile of Poloxamer 407 Based Ophthalmic Formulation. *Int. J. Biol. Macromol.* **2017,** *102,* 258–265.

Dolmans, D. E.; Fukumura, D.; Jain, R. K. Photodynamic Therapy for Cancer. *Nat. Rev. Cancer* **2003,** *3*(5), 380–387.

Florentin, K. D. Q. Caracterizacao estrutural e atividades farmacológicas do alginato obtido da alga Dictyopteris delicatula (JV Lamouroux., 1809) e seu derivado sulfatado. Universidade Federal do Rio Grande do Norte, 2015.

Fonseca-Santos, B.; Chorilli, M. An Overview of Carboxymethyl Derivatives of Chitosan: Their Use as Biomaterials and Drug Delivery Systems. *Mater. Sci. Eng. C* **2017,** *77,* 1349–1362.

Ghugarkar, P.; Kulat, P.; Swain, K.; Suggala, V.; Shaik, D. Colon Targeted Drug Delivery System: a Review on Primary and Novel Approaches. *Int. J. Pharm. Sci. Res.* **2015,** *6*(7), 2681–2687.

Hefti, F. F. Requirements for a Lead Compound to Become a Clinical Candidate. *BMC Neurosci.* **2008,** *9*(3), 7.

Jain, A.; Gupta, Y.; Jain, S. K. Perspectives of Biodegradable Natural Polysaccharides for Site-Specific Drug Delivery to the Colon. *J. Pharm. Pharm. Sci.* **2007,** *10*(1), 86–128.

Joshy, K.; Susan, M. A.; Snigdha, S.; Nandakumar, K.; Laly, A. P.; Sabu, T. Encapsulation of Zidovudine in PF-68 Coated Alginate Conjugate Nanoparticles for Anti-HIV Drug Delivery. *Int. J. Biol. Macromol.* **2018,** *107,* 929–937.

Kiyoung, L.; Kun, N.; Yueim, K. Polysaccharides as a Drug Coating Polymer. *Polym. Prep.* **1999,** *40,* 359–360.

Klöck, G.; Pfeffermann, A.; Ryser, C.; Gröhn, P.; Kuttler, B.; Hahn, H.-J.; Zimmermann, U. Biocompatibility of Mannuronic Acid-Rich Alginates. *Biomaterials* **1997,** *18*(10), 707–713.

Kumar, D.; Kumar, S. Grafting of Acrylic Acid on to Plantago Psyllium Mucilage. *IOSR J. Appl. Chem.* **2014,** *7,* 76–82.

Kumar, P.; Mishra, B. Colon Targeted Drug Delivery Systems—an Overview. *Curr. Drug Delivery* **2008,** *5*(3), 186–198.

Kumar, M.; Ali, A.; Kaldhone, P.; Shirode, A.; Kadam, V. J. Report on Pharmaceutical Approaches to Colon Targeted Drug Delivery Systems. *J. Pharm. Res.* **2010,** *3,* 470–473.

Kumar, D.; Khan, N.; Kumar, P. Improve the Native Characteristics of Polysaccharides by Grafting Through the Gamma Radiation: a Review. *Green Chem. Technol. Lett.* **2016,** *2*(3), 151–159.

Kumar, D.; Chandra, R.; Dubey, R. Synthesis and Characterisation of Cross-Linked Polymers of Acrylic Acid and Psyllium Mucilage (Psy-Cl-Aa). *J. Technol. Adv. Sci. Res.* **2017,** *2*(4), 185–189.

Kumar, D.; Pandey, J.; Kumar, P. Microwave Assisted Synthesis of Binary Grafted Psyllium and Its Utility in Anticancer Formulation. *Carbohydr. Polym.* **2018**, *179,* 408–414.

Laffleur, F.; Michalek, M. Modified Xanthan Gum for Buccal Delivery—a Promising Approach in Treating Sialorrhea. *Int. J. Biol. Macromol.* **2017**, *102,* 1250–1256.

Lee, K. Y.; Mooney, D. J. Alginate: Properties and Biomedical Applications. *Prog. Polym. Sci.* **2012**, *37*(1), 106–126.

Leuva, V.; Patel, B.; Chaudhary, D.; Patel, J.; Modasiya, M. Oral Colon-Specific Drug Delivery System. *J. Pharm. Res.* **2012**, *5*(4), 2293–2297.

Lin, S. Y.; Ayres, J. W. Calcium Alginate Beads as Core Carriers of 5-Aminosalicylic Acid. *Pharm. Res.* **1992**, *9*(9), 1128–1131.

Malayandi, R.; Kondamudi, P. K.; Ruby, P.; Aggarwal, D. Biopharmaceutical Considerations and Characterizations in Development of Colon Targeted Dosage Forms for Inflammatory Bowel Disease. *Drug Delivery Transl. Res.* **2014**, *4*(2), 187–202.

Mansuri, S.; Kesharwani, P.; Jain, K.; Tekade, R. K.; Jain, N. Mucoadhesion: a Promising Approach in Drug Delivery System. *React. Funct. Polym.* **2016**, *100,* 151–172.

Marras-Marquez, T.; Peña, J.; Veiga-Ochoa, M. Robust and Versatile Pectin-Based Drug Delivery Systems. *Int. J. Pharm.* **2015**, *479*(2), 265–276.

Momin, M.; Mehta, T.; Abhang, P. Hydrogel Based Biodegradable Enteric Coated Alginate Beads for Colon Targeted Drug Delivery of Embelin. *BioMedRx* **2013**, *1,* 288–292.

Nalanda, A.; Rangari, T. Review on Recent and Novel Approaches to Colon Targeted Drug Delivery Systems. *IJPPR Human J.* **2015**, *3*(1), 167–186.

Orive, G.; Ponce, S.; Hernandez, R.; Gascon, A.; Igartua, M.; Pedraz, J. Biocompatibility of Microcapsules for Cell Immobilization Elaborated with Different Type of Alginates. *Biomaterials* **2002**, *23*(18), 3825–3831.

Orlu, M.; Cevher, E.; Araman, A. Design and Evaluation of Colon Specific Drug Delivery System Containing Flurbiprofen Microsponges. *Int. J. Pharm.* **2006**, *318*(1), 103–117.

Pawar, S. N.; Edgar, K. J. Alginate Derivatization: a Review of Chemistry, Properties and Applications. *Biomaterials* **2012**, *33*(11), 3279–3305.

Philip, A.K.; Philip, B. Colon Targeted Drug Delivery Systems: a Review On Primary And Novel Approaches. *Oman Med. J.* **2010**, *25*(2), 79.

Qureshi, A. M.; Momin, M.; Rathod, S.; Dev, A.; Kute, C. Colon Targeted Drug Delivery System: a Review on Current Approaches. *Indian J. Pharm. Biol. Res.* **2013**, *1*(4), 130–147.

Ramsey, D. M.; Wozniak, D. J. Understanding the Control of *Pseudomonas aeruginosa* Alginate Synthesis and the Prospects for Management of Chronic Infections in Cystic Fibrosis. *Mol. Microbiol.* **2005**, *56*(2), 309–322.

Saha, D. N.; Sharma, R.; Rajawat, G. S.; Dev, J. A. An Investigation on Colon Drug Delivery System for Satranidazole Tablet. *Int. J. Res. Pharm. Sci.* **2013**, *3*(2), —161–182.

Sandler, N.; Preis, M. Printed Drug-Delivery Systems for Improved Patient Treatment. *Trends Pharmacol. Sci.* **2016**, *37*(12), 1070–1080.

Simó, G.; Fernández-Fernández, E.; Vila-Crespo, J.; Ruipérez, V.; Rodríguez-Nogales, J. M. Research Progress in Coating Techniques of Alginate Gel Polymer for Cell Encapsulation. *Carbohydr. Polym.* **2017**, *170,* 1–14.

Sookkasem, A.; Chatpun, S.; Yuenyongsawad, S.; Wiwattanapatapee, R. Alginate Beads for Colon Specific Delivery of Self-Emulsifying Curcumin. *J. Drug Delivery Sci. Technol.* **2015**, *29,* 159–166.

Soon-Shiong, P.; Feldman, E.; Nelson, R.; Heintz, R.; Yao, Q.; Yao, Z.; Zheng, T.; Merideth, N.; Skjak-Braek, G.; Espevik, T. Long-Term Reversal of Diabetes by the Injection of Immunoprotected Islets. *Proc. Natl. Acad. Sci.* **1993**, *90*(12), 5843–5847.

Sreelatha, D.; Brahma, C. K. Colon Targeted Drug Delivery – a Review on Primary and Novel Approaches. *J. Global Trend Pharm. Sci.* **2013,** *4*(3), 1174–1183.

Talaei, F.; Atyabi, F.; Azhdarzadeh, M.; Dinarvand, R.; Saadatzadeh, A. Overcoming Therapeutic Obstacles in Inflammatory Bowel Diseases: a Comprehensive Review on Novel Drug Delivery Strategies. *Eur. J. Pharm. Sci.* **2013,** *49*(4), 712–722.

Venkatesan, J.; Bhatnagar, I.; Manivasagan, P.; Kang, K. H.; Kim, S. K. Alginate Composites for Bone Tissue Engineering: a Review. *Int. J. Biol. Macromol.* **2015,** *72,* 269–281.

Wang, Q. S.; Wang, G. F.; Zhouc, J.; Gao, L. N.; Cui, Y. L. Colon Targeted Oral Drug Delivery System Based on Chitosan/Alginate Microspheres Loaded with Icariin in the Treatment of Ulcerative Colitis. *Int. J. Pharm.* **2016,** *515,* 176–185.

Yang, J. S.; Xie, Y. J.; He, W. Research Progress on Chemical Modification of Alginate: a Review. *Carbohydr. Polym.* **2011,** *84*(1), 33–39.

Zhang, B.; Yan, Y.; Shen, Q.; Ma, D.; Huang, L.; Cai, X.; Tan, S. A Colon Targeted Drug Delivery System Based on Alginate Modified Graphene Oxide for Colorectal Liver Metastasis. *Mater. Sci. Eng. C* **2017,** *79,* 185–190.

Zia, K. M.; Zia, F.; Zuber, M.; Rehman, S.; Ahmad, M. N. Alginate Based Polyurethanes: a Review of Recent Advances and Perspective. *Int. J. Biol. Macromol.* **2015,** *79,* 377–387.

Zimmermann, H.; Shirley, S. G.; Zimmermann, U. Alginate-Based Encapsulation of Cells: Past, Present, and Future. *Curr. Diabetes Rep.* **2007,** *7*(4), 314–320.

CHAPTER 19

ALGINATE CARRIERS FOR THE TREATMENT OF OCULAR DISEASES

RAVI SHESHALA[1] and TIN WUI WONG[1,2,*]

[1]*Particle Design Research Group, Faculty of Pharmacy, Universiti Teknologi MARA Selangor, Puncak Alam Campus, 42300 Puncak Alam, Malaysia*

[2]*Non-Destructive Biomedical and Pharmaceutical Research Centre, iPROMISE, Universiti Teknologi MARA Selangor, Puncak Alam Campus, 42300 Puncak Alam, Malaysia*

Corresponding author. E-mail: wongtinwui@salam.uitm.edu.my; wongtinwui@yahoo.com

19.1 INTRODUCTION

Alginates are random, linear, and naturally occurring water-soluble anionic polysaccharide polymers consisting of linear monomer residues, α-L-guluronic acid (G) and β-D-mannuronic acid (M) that are arranged in homogenous, that is, poly-G (GGGG), poly-M (MMM), and heterogeneous (MGMG) blocklike patterns. The homogeneous blocks (composed of either acid residue alone) are separated by blocks made of random or alternating units of mannuronic acids and guluronic acids (Szekalska et al., 2016; Lee and Mooney, 2012). The chemical structure of alginates is shown in Figure 19.1.

Alginates are isolated from brown seaweeds such as marine brown algae (Phaeophyceae) that grow rich and plentiful in consistently cold and clear water. A dilute alkaline solution is used to extract the alginic acid present in the seaweed. Free alginic acid is obtained by treating the resultant thick and viscous mass with mineral acids. The alginic acid can be converted into a water-soluble sodium salt in the presence of calcium carbonate to produce sodium alginate, which is the major form currently available commercially (Tonnesen and Karlsen, 2002). The alginate, apart from being isolated from the brown algae cell walls (Repka and Singh, 2009; Sachan et al., 2009), can be derived from several bacteria strains (*Azotobacter, Pseudomonas*) (Remminghorst and Rehm, 2006). The chemical composition and sequence of alginates may vary widely between algae species and even between different parts of the algae and the time of year when they are harvested. Although the production of alginates is technically feasible by means of microbial fermentation, the commercial alginates are exclusively extracted from algal sources as the latter meets the requirement of economic feasibility. To date, all commercially available alginates have been extracted from brown algae, mainly from *Laminaria hyperborea, Macrocystis pyrifera, Laminaria digitata, Ascophyllum nodosum, Laminaria japonica, Ecklonia maxima, Lessonia nigrescens,* and *Durvillaea antarctica* (Donati and Paoletti, 2009).

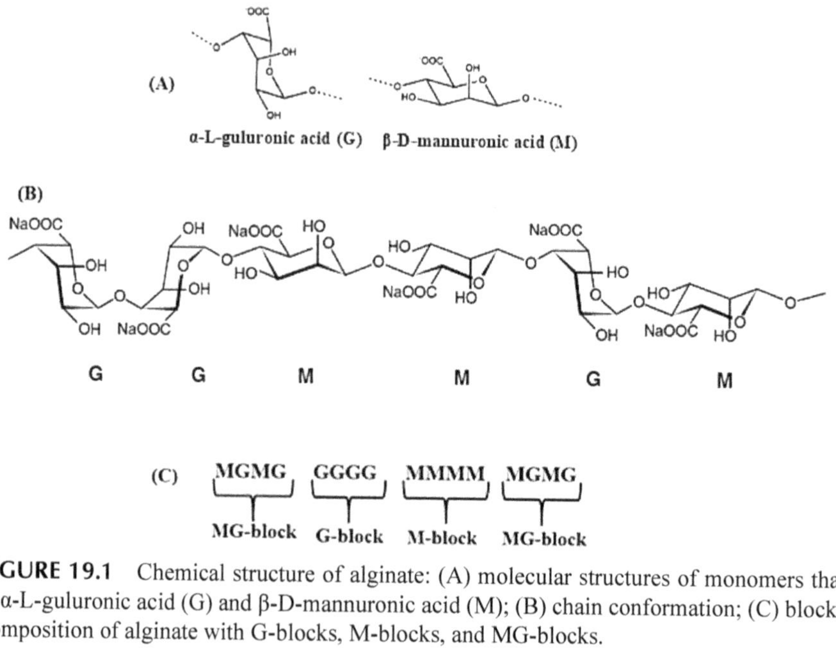

FIGURE 19.1   Chemical structure of alginate: (A) molecular structures of monomers that is α-L-guluronic acid (G) and β-D-mannuronic acid (M); (B) chain conformation; (C) blocks composition of alginate with G-blocks, M-blocks, and MG-blocks.

Source: A: Adapted with permission from Spadari et al. (2017); B: Reprinted with permission from Donati and Paoletti (2009). © 2009 Springer; C: from Szekalska et al. (2016) Creative Commons Attribution License.

Alginates are classified based on their grades, namely, low, medium, and high and those grades are defined based on the source, location, and species (Table 19.1). Low-grade alginates are used for industrial applications such as textile, paper, and pulp, whereas high-grade alginates are used in the food and pharmaceutical industries (MarketsandMarkets, 2015; CBI Product Factsheet, 2015; Imeson, 2009).

TABLE 19.1 Classification of Alginate.

Grade	Source	Prominent harvest location
High	*Laminaria hyperborea*	France, Ireland, UK, Norway
Medium – High	*Lessonia negrescens*	Chile, Peru
Medium	*Laminaria japonica*	China, Japan
Low	*Macrocystis pyrifera*	USA, Mexico, Chile
Low	*Durvillaea antarctica*	Australia, Chile
High	*Flavicans*	Chile, Peru
Medium	*Ecklonia maxima*	South Africa
Low	*Ascophyllum nodosum*	France, Iceland, Ireland, Norway, UK
-	*Laminaria digitata*	France, Norway, Ireland, Iceland
-	*Lessonia trabeculata*	Chile
High	*Sargassum*	Indonesia, India

Source: Adapted from MarketsandMarkets (2015), CBI Product Factsheet (2015), Imeson (2009).

19.2 GENERAL PROPERTIES AND APPLICATIONS OF ALGINATE

The proportion, distribution, and length of M-, G-, and MG-blocks determine the physical and chemical properties of the alginates (FMC BioPolymers). Alginates are white to yellowish fibrous or granular powder, odorless and tasteless. They are soluble in water, forming viscous, colloidal solutions and insoluble in alcohols, chloroform, ether, and aqueous acidic solution below pH 3 (Alginic acid, 2017). They are chemically very stable at pH values of 5–10 (Ramya et al., 2013).

Alginates are excellent and the most versatile biopolymers. They have a long usage history in a wide range of applications in several industries such as food and beverage, pharmaceuticals, personal care, cosmetics, castings, water treatment, and ceramics. Commercially, these natural polymers are mainly available in the forms of sodium, calcium, and magnesium salts. The main industrial applications of alginate as a natural polymeric material are linked to its stabilizing, viscosifying, and gelling properties and its ability to retain water. The alginates form gel through mild gelation by reacting with divalent cations such as calcium ions (Ca^{2+}). They are nontoxic, mucoadhesive, biodegradable, biocompatible, hemocompatible, and readily available at low cost. The summative properties render alginates being widely used in the development of drug delivery systems (Figure 19.2). Alginates have been largely used in wound dressings, dental impression, and formulations for preventing gastric reflux and as encapsulation agents in the biotechnology sector (Ramya et al., 2013). The alginate gel can be produced through ionotropic gelation under mild conditions. It takes a simple step to entrap drugs and living cells in alginate gels, which in turn allows a widespread application of alginate as scaffolds or matrices for tissue engineering, drug delivery systems, and cell encapsulation and transplantation (Mishra and Gilhotra, 2008). Table 19.2 summarizes the pharmaceutical and biomedical applications of alginates.

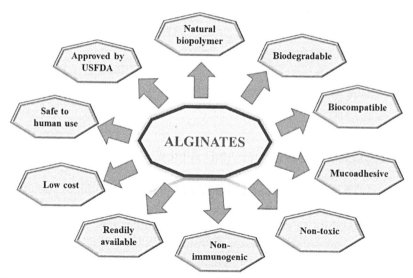

FIGURE 19.2   Advantages of alginate for industrial applications.

19.3   ANATOMICAL AND PHYSIOLOGICAL BARRIERS OF EYE IN TREATMENT OF OCULAR DISEASES

The eyes are an important organ of vision and also a delicate organ of the body. It takes the form of a sphere with a diameter of about 2.5 cm. The anatomy of eyes can be divided into the accessory structure of eye and structure of eyeball (Sheshala et al., 2015). The schematic representation of the eye with anterior (conjunctiva, cornea, lens, anterior chamber, and pupil)

TABLE 19.2 Pharmaceutical and Biomedical Applications of Alginates.

Alginate type	Brand name*	Pharmaceutical/biomedical application
Alginic acid	Protacid	Anti-reflux tablets, natural tablet binder, and disintegrant, sustained-release and release-modifying agent, taste-masking agent, thickener, suspending and viscosifying agent, stabilizer
Sodium alginate	Protanal	Anti-reflux suspensions, controlled-release tablets, wound dressings, dental impression material, denture fixatives, films, foams, suspending and viscosifying agent, tablet and capsule disintegrant, tablet binder, stabilizer, diluent in capsule formulation, thickener
Magnesium alginate	Protanal	Anti-reflux suspensions for infants
Potassium alginate	Protanal	Dental impression material
Propylene glycol alginate	Protanal ester	Suspending agent, stabilizer, plasticizer, binder, emulsifier, viscosifying agent
Ammonium alginate	-	Color diluent, emulsifier, film former, humectant
Calcium alginate	-	Tablet disintegrant

*Products of FMC BioPolymers.

Source: Adapted from Szekalska et al. (2016), FMC BioPolymers.

and posterior (retina and vitreous chamber) segments is shown in Figure 19.3 (adopted and modified from Virtual Medical Centre). Understanding both structures enables us to design an effective ocular product to treat various eye diseases such as glaucoma, dry eye syndrome, trachoma, keratitis, and conjunctivitis.

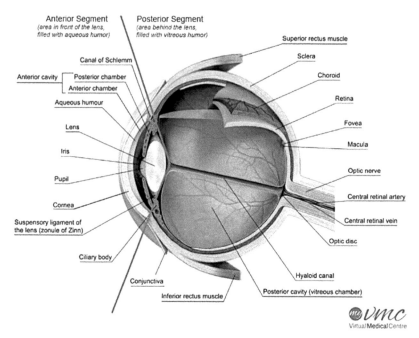

FIGURE 19.3   Schematic representation of eye with anterior and posterior segments. *Source:* Adapted and modified with permission from Virtual Medical Centre, www.myvmc.com

Cornea and conjunctiva are primary anatomical permeation barriers to drug applied topically. Cornea, the front part of the eye globe, consists of three major layers, namely, outer epithelium, middle stroma, and inner endothelium. It is clear, colorless, and does not contain blood vessels but rich in nerve endings. The lipophilic nature of epithelium and endothelium of cornea (rich in lipid content) makes them barriers to the permeation of polar, water-soluble compounds, whereas hydrophilic nature of stroma (consisting of 70–80% water) makes it a barrier to the permeation of nonpolar, lipid-soluble compounds (Gibson, 2009). Sclera, another boundary layer to eye front, also acts as a significant permeation barrier to most of the drugs. It is white in color, opaque, has rich a supply of blood vessels and nerves, and provides attachment for the external muscles of the eye. The outer surface of sclera is loosely covered by the conjunctival membrane. The drugs are absorbed into the general circulation through permeating both sclera and conjunctiva.

Tear production and blinking reflex of eyes are the major physiological barriers to drug absorption into the eye. As these two processes occur simultaneously, the drug can be removed rapidly from the eye (16%/min of the total volume) upon topical administration of eye drops (25–56 μL). The pre-corneal volume is about 7 μL but the cornea can hold up to 20–30 μL before spillage occurs. Instillation of an excess volume of liquid translates to spillage onto the cheek or loss with tears through draining into the nasolachrymal duct. The latter is aided by the blink reflex where each blink pumps approximately 2 μL of tear fluid into the nasolachrymal fluid (Sheshala et al., 2015; Virtual Medical Centre; Gibson, 2009). Overall, less than 10% (typically 1% or less) of topically administered dose actually permeates the cornea and absorbs into the eye due to the combined effect of short pre-corneal contact time and poor corneal permeability. Hence, frequent instillation of solutions with higher drug concentrations is imperative in order to achieve desired therapeutic benefits (Laddha and Mahajan, 2017).

Protein binding and enzymatic metabolism of drugs are also considered as physiological factors which result in poor drug absorption by ocular route. The increased size of protein–drug complex makes the bounded drug unavailable for the absorption and has it rapidly removed from the eye through nasolachrymal drainage. The enzymes present in tear fluids, such as esterases, monoamine oxidases, and aminopeptidases, are responsible for drug degradation during or after drug absorption into the eye and render them inactive (Gibson, 2009).

In short, cornea, conjunctiva, and sclera act as anatomical barriers and rapid pre-corneal elimination of drugs is due to dilution with tear fluids and blinking reflux as well as nasolachrymal drainage of drug into systemic circulation, binding of drug to lachrymal protein and metabolism by ocular enzymes as physiological barriers are responsible for poor ocular drug bioavailability and therapeutic response.

19.4 OCULAR ALGINATE CARRIERS

19.4.1 IN SITU GELLING SYSTEM

Alginic acid/sodium alginate is a natural hydrophilic, mucoadhesive, biodegradable, and nontoxic polymer that has been approved by the US Food and Drug Administration for human use. It is widely used as anion-triggered in situ gelling polymeric system for ocular drug delivery. Alginates are ion-sensitive polymers and polymeric chains presenting negative charges can self-organize around the cations (monovalent and divalent) present in the lacrimal fluid to form a gel on the ocular surface. The gelling property of alginates enhances the retention time of drug in the eye by overcoming the rapid pre-corneal elimination and therefore leads to increased drug bioavailability. Typically, G units of alginates can cross-link with Ca^{2+} present in the ocular fluid and form an inhomogeneous 3-dimensional ionotropic gel. Alginates with G-rich content form a low viscosity, stable but free-flowing liquid at concentrations suitable for gel formation in the lacrimal fluid upon exposure to divalent cations, and such liquid gel is not easily eroded by the tear fluid (Jain et al., 2016; Destruel et al., 2017). The mechanism of alginate gel formation in the form of egg-box model is shown in Figure 19.4.

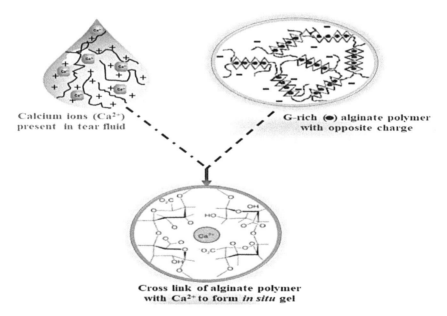

Calcium ions (Ca^{2+})
present in tear fluid

G-rich (●) alginate polymer
with opposite charge

Cross link of alginate polymer
with Ca^{2+} to form *in situ* gel

FIGURE 19.4 Mechanism of ion-activated in situ gel formation of alginates through cross-linking with Ca^{2+} in tear fluid.

Source: Adapted and modified from Destruel et al. (2017), FMC BioPolymers d/b/a NovaMatrix.

The alginates have been used alone and in combination with other polymers for an effective ocular delivery of various therapeutic uses (Table 19.3). Cohen et al. (1997) demonstrate that alginates with guluronic acid contents

TABLE 19.3 Examples of Alginate-Based Drug Delivery Systems for Ocular Application.

Material	Drug	Carrier	Therapeutic goal	Reference
Sodium alginate and NaCMC	Gatifloxacin	In situ gel	To enhance drug bioavailability through longer pre-corneal residence time and ability to sustain release of drug	Kesavan et al. (2010)
Sodium alginate and gellan gum	Ketotifen fumarate	In situ gel	To enhance drug bioavailability by using in situ gelling and mucoadhesive vehicle	Kumar and Muralidharan (2012)
Sodium alginate and HPMC K4M	Levofloxacin hemihydrates	In situ gel	To prolong the release of an active substance by crosslinking with cations present in tear fluid	Swapnil et al. (2014)
Sodium alginate and HPMC K4M	Neomycin sulfate	In situ gel	To sustain the drug release for a longer duration to have an effective antimicrobial action for the treatment of various bacterial eye infections caused by microorganisms such as *Pseudomonas aeruginosa*	Singh et al. (2017)
Sodium alginate, PF127, and PF68	Lomefloxacin	In situ gel	To increase the residence time and sustain the drug release for reducing the dosing frequency of lomefloxacin	Gadad et al. (2016)
Sodium alginate and hydroxypropyl cellulose	Dorzolamide hydrochloride	In situ gel	For the effective treatment of glaucoma by sustaining the drug release for a prolonged period	Bhalerao and Singh (2011)
Sodium alginate and HPMC K15M	Voriconazole	In situ gel	To increase ocular residence time, to reduce the dose, and sustain the release profile of the antifungal agent, voriconazole	Puranik and Tagalpallewar (2015)
Alginic acid	Carteolol	In situ gel	To reduce the frequency of carteolol dosing from twice to only once a day	Séchoy et al. (2000)
Sodium alginate	Pilocarpine nitrate	In situ gel	To overcome the poor bioavailability of drugs caused by dilution and drainage of the eye drop solutions from the eye	Cohen et al. (1997)

TABLE 19.3 *(Continued)*

Material	Drug	Carrier	Therapeutic goal	Reference
Sodium alginate and HPMC	Gatifloxacin	In situ gel	To improve patient compliance through sustaining drug release with excellent ocular tolerance	Liu et al. (2006)
Sodium alginate and PF127	Cromolyn sodium	In situ gel	To reduce the ocular irritation caused by high concentrations of pluronics and to increase the patient compliance by reducing the side effects without comprising the gelling capacity and rheology of the system	Shastri et al. (2010)
Sodium alginate and methylcellulose	Sparfloxacin	In situ gel	To avoid the side effects caused by pulsed dosing of sparfloxacin by sustaining the drug release for a longer period of time	Khan et al. (2015)
Sodium alginate and chitosan	Gatifloxacin sesquihydrate	Films	To enhance ocular drug bioavailability and patient compliance by surface treated alginate–chitosan films	Gilhotra and Mishra (2008)
Sodium alginate and HPMC K14M	Azithromycin	Ocular inserts	To enhance the antibiotic's usefulness for topical treatment of ocular surface bacterial infections and Lid Margin diseases	Gilhotra et al. (2011)
Sodium alginate and chitosan	Gatifloxacin sesquihydrate	Ocular inserts	To improve the retention of drug in pre-corneal region and release the drug for a longer period of time in a sustained manner	Mishra and Gilhotra (2008)
Sodium alginate and lipid	Flurbiprofen	Nanostructured lipid carrier-based ocular inserts	To decrease systemic side effects and increase effective drug concentration in the eye for the treatment of ocular inflammation	Gokce and Okur (2016)
Chitosan-coated sodium alginate	Daptomycin	Nanoparticles	To develop a potential delivery system for daptomycin permeation across ocular epithelia for an effective treatment of bacterial endophthalmitis	Costa et al. (2015)

TABLE 19.3 *(Continued)*

Material	Drug	Carrier	Therapeutic goal	Reference
Chitosan and sodium alginate	Ketorolac tromethamine	Nanodispersions	To sustain the release of drug and to enhance its trans-corneal permeation in comparison to the conventional drug carrier without corneal damage	Morsi et al. (2015)
Chitosan/thiolated chitosan and sodium alginate	Fluorescein isothiocyanate	Nanoparticles	To synthesize mucoadhesive polymer, thiolated chitosan from chitosan and to prepare nanoparticles for ocular drug delivery with potential applications	Zhu et al. (2012)
Chitosan-coated sodium alginate–chitosan	5-Fluorouracil	Nanoparticles	To enhance mucoadhesiveness of polymeric system and improve drug bioavailability against that of uncoated system with the aim to reduce drug dose and dosing frequency	Nagarwal et al. (2012)
Chitosan and sodium alginate	Azelastine hydrochloride	Microspheres	To develop mucoadhesive microspheres and overcome the limitations of ocular drug delivery with prolonged drug presence in cul-de-sac and improved therapeutic efficacy	Shinde et al. (2014)
Alginate–anthracene cross-link by polyethylene glycol chains	Protein	Photoreversible gels	To develop controllable drug delivery systems that are suited for the treatment of macular degeneration and diabetic retinopathy in the posterior segment of the eye	Wells and Sheardown (2007)

>65% gel instantaneously instead of slowly and forming weak gels. The high G alginate gel of pilocarpine nitrate provides intraocular pressure reduction in rabbit eyes for a longer duration (10 h) than the neat drug solution (3 h) and low G alginate gel carrier. The high G alginate gel improves ocular drug bioavailability by overcoming drug dilution and drainage. A combination of one or more polymers with different gelling mechanisms has been investigated for the purpose of reducing the polymer fraction required for gelation to avoid ocular tissue irritation and designing gels with improved gelling and drug delivery properties (Jain et al., 2016; Gratieri et al., 2010). Commonly, the alginates have been formulated with pluronics, hydroxylpropyl methylcellulose (HPMC), and sodium carboxymethylcellulose (NaCMC) to produce in situ gelling systems.

Liu et al. (2006) develop an ion-activated in situ gelation system of sodium alginate (Kelton®) with HPMC (Methocel E50LV) as the viscosifying agent to introduce sustained drug delivery characteristics, reduce drug administration frequency, and improve patient compliance. The combination retains drug in a capacity superior to those of alginate or HPMC alone. The combination sustains gatifloxacin release for 10 h and demonstrates excellent ocular tolerance without any sign of irritation.

Singh et al. (2017) formulated neomycin sulfate in situ gels using a combination of sodium alginate (0.2–0.7%) and HPMC K4M. Optimized formulations consisting of 0.5% sodium alginate/1.5% HPMC K4M, 0.3% sodium alginate/1.7% HPMC K4M, and 0.4% sodium alginate/2% HPMC K4M are liquid before instillation and undergo rapid gelation upon instillation into the eye. This alginate-based polymeric network sustains the drug release for 6 h and the developed formulations are found to be stable for 6 months with no changes in clarity, pH, and drug content.

Shastri et al. (2010) developed a combination in situ gelling system of pluronic F127 (PF127) (thermoreversible gelling polymer) with HPMC, Carbopol®, xanthan gum, and high G sodium alginate to avoid the ocular irritation caused by high concentrations of PF127. Formulations with a combination of PF127 (15%)/Carbopol® (0.4%), PF127 (15%)/xanthan gum (0.5%), and PF127 (15%)/sodium alginate (0.9%) demonstrate clear gels with low viscosity and higher gelling abilities. The combinations other than xanthan gum exhibit fast gelling without any initial burst release of the drug. The combinations can sustain drug release for 10 h compared to individual polymers. The combination in situ gelling system shows an excellent ocular tolerance.

Lin et al. (2004) formulated a series of combination systems of sodium alginate and pluronic F127 in situ gelling vehicles for ocular delivery of pilocarpine. The optimum polymer concentrations for in situ gel formation are 2% for alginate and 14% for pluronic. However, the mixture of 0.1% alginate and 14% pluronic exhibits a free-flowing nature at pH 4.0 and 25°C with a significant increase in its gel strength under the physiological condition. Both in vitro drug release and in vivo pharmacological studies indicate that the alginate/pluronic solution retains pilocarpine better than the alginate or pluronic alone and aids in enhancing ocular drug bioavailability.

Sparfloxacin loaded in situ gelling system consisting of sodium alginate as ion-sensitive polymer and methylcellulose as viscosifying agent has been formulated by Khan et al. (2015) to avoid the side effects associated with pulsed dosing. Optimized formulation presents as a liquid at pH 4.7 and converts into a gel at pH 7.4 of tear fluid. The drug releases from this in situ gelling system can sustain over a period of 24 h. The formulation is found to be nonirritant, exhibits significant antimicrobial effect and good ocular tolerance with enhanced corneal drug permeation. It is physicochemically stable for a long period of time with a shelf life of 2.28 years.

Kesavan et al. (2010) formulated sodium-alginate-based ophthalmic mucoadhesive system of gatifloxacin. An increase in the concentration of sodium alginate and NaCMC from 0.4 to 2% and 0.1 to 0.5%, respectively, enhances the mucoadhesive force significantly with the formulation containing 2% sodium alginate showing maximum bioadhesive strength. The mucoadhesion behavior of alginate is brought about by its good spreading property as its surface tension (31.5 mN/m) is lower than the critical surface tension of the mucin-coated cornea (38 mN/m) (Séchoy et al., 2000). The drug release is significantly sustained over a period of 12 h when the sodium alginate concentration increases from 0.4 to 2%. Alginate forms 3-dimensional ionotropic hydrogel matrices through interacting with Ca^{2+} in the tear fluid via G moieties. It is able to retain the drug in the matrix and prevent premature drug release.

Swapnil et al. (2014) formulated ocular in situ gels of levofloxacin hemihydrate based on the concept of ion-activated gelation using sodium alginate as a gelling agent in combination with HPMC as a viscosifying agent. This ion-activated polymer undergoes gelation on the ocular surface by cross-linking with the divalent/polyvalent cations, that is, Ca^{2+} present in tear fluids due to the interaction with the guluronic acid block. The formulation is prepared in deionized water as the gelling agent forms a stiff gel when interacts with the ions of a buffer system. The combination use of sodium alginate and HPMC sustains the levofloxacin release for a period of 8 h and induces no irritation upon administration into the eye.

Gadad et al. (2016) formulated thermoreversible solution–gel (solgel) of lomefloxacin hydrochloride using a combination of PF127 (18%), PF68 (1–3%), and sodium alginate (0.5–1.5%). A gradual increase in the gel strength of formulations is observed with an increase in the concentration of PF68 due to enhancement in the ethylene oxide/propylene oxide ratio of PF127 when combined with it. Formulations composed of 1.5% sodium alginate show higher gel strength than that of 0.5% in concentration. This may be due to a larger propensity of interaction between sodium alginate with pluronic. The gelation temperature of the formulation ranges between 31.1 and 39.3°C. The formulation containing 2% PF68 and 1% sodium alginate is characterized by gelation at 37°C (physiological temperature of the eye). With an increase in the concentration of sodium alginate from 0.5 to 1.5%, the gelation temperature decreases. At higher alginate fractions, more alginate molecules will bind to the polyoxyethylene chains present in the pluronic molecules. This induces dehydration of pluronic, causing an increase in the entanglement of the adjacent chains extensively, thereby increasing intermolecular hydrogen bonding which leads to gelation occurring at lower temperatures (Kolsure and Rajkapoor, 2012). In vitro drug release studies indicate that the drug release rate decreases with an increase in the concentration of PF68 and sodium alginate due to increased ease of polymer entanglement, giving rise to denser chain arrangement in the gel which in turn functions as a drug release barrier.

Séchoy et al. (2000) compared in situ gelling performances of alginic acid and hydroxyethyl cellulose for prolonged delivery of carteolol. The viscosity of the solutions prepared by both polymers is almost similar but alginic acid gels show better adhesive properties with mucin-coated corneal surface and slower drug diffusion compared to that of hydroxyethyl cellulose. The ionic interaction between carteolol and alginic acid may be the cause for slow in vitro drug diffusion. Carteolol–alginic acid formulations show excellent ocular tolerance without any irritation and histopathological changes. The use of alginic acid overall increases the area under the curve from 0–8 h (AUC_{0-8h}) of the drug in the aqueous humor by 50%. The alginic-acid-based in situ gelling system reduces the frequency of dosing administration from twice to once daily with improved patient compliance and convenience.

19.4.2 OCULAR FILM/INSERT

The polymeric ocular film and ocular inserts are sterile preparations with a solid or semisolid consistency usually composed of a polymeric vehicle containing the drug whose size and shape are especially designed to be placed in cul-de-sac or conjunctival sac for therapeutic application (Kumari et al., 2010). These polymeric ocular devices should be nontoxic, biodegradable, and biocompatible. They represent a significant advancement in the ocular treatment and currently being developed to overcome the ocular barriers and prevent loss of drug through the nasolacrimal drainage system. The ocular film is usually applied to treat anterior segment ocular diseases such as conjunctivitis, glaucoma, and dry eye syndrome. The film is mucoadhesive and hydrophilic. It undergoes swelling and forms a chain interaction with mucin and such interaction will be stronger with anionic and cationic polymers compared to nonionic polymers (Maiti and Jana, 2017).

Gilhotra and Mishra (2008) compared the characteristics of alginate–chitosan films with the same composition of ionically surface-cross-linked films consisting of gatifloxacin sesquihydrate intended for ocular drug delivery. Surface-cross-linked films consisting of 2% sodium alginate and 1% chitosan show the most prolonged drug release within 24 h of the test. The drug release mechanism changes from erosion to diffusion upon surface-cross-linking of the film. The surface-treated alginate–chitosan film can be a potential vehicle to enhance ocular drug bioavailability and patient compliance.

Gilhotra et al. (2011) formulated a sustained-release bioadhesive ocular insert of azithromycin using alginate, Carbopol®, and HPMC as the matrix former as well as bioadhesive polymer. Film casting method is used to prepare these ocular inserts. The alginate films exhibit greater bioadhesion and show higher tensile strength and elasticity than the Carbopol® films. These films are characterized by higher swelling or water uptake degree than Carbopol® films at their initial contact with biological fluids. The introduction and an increase in the content of HPMC in alginate films (0.6–1.4%) enhance the swelling degree of the films, attributing to the water-retaining capacity of HPMC. The combination use of HPMC and alginate in film preparation aids to sustain drug release.

Mishra and Gilhotra (2008) developed polymeric ocular inserts of gatifloxacin sesquihydrate using sodium alginate and chitosan with glycerin as the plasticizer by a solvent casting method. The tensile strength of this ocular insert increases with the total amount of polymer employed. It is primarily governed by the sodium alginate content as inserts with higher sodium alginate content show greater tensile strengths. As sodium alginate forms hydrogels and swells considerably in an aqueous medium, an increase in the amount of alginate content increases the swelling capacity of ocular inserts. The combination of 2% sodium alginate and 1% chitosan sustains the drug release for the longest period of time (12 h) and has its kinetics following zero-order release mechanism. The sustained drug release property is brought about by alginate conferring tensile strength and swellability, and egg-box structure of the cross-linked matrix in the presence of Ca^{2+}, as well as, chitosan imparting coacervate formation with alginate and increased bioadhesiveness which improves drug retention in the pre-corneal area.

19.4.3 MICRO- AND NANOPARTICULATE SYSTEMS

The prospective of alginate-based novel drug delivery systems, that is, micro- and nanoparticulate systems has been explored as a novel vehicle to address the drug permeation issues. Specifically, these systems are used to extend topical ophthalmic delivery with the aim to delay the elimination of drug from eye upon administration by remaining at the site of application (cul-de-sac) for a prolonged period of time, to provide sustained drug release and to improve the corneal penetration of drug molecules (Jain et al., 2016). Polymeric microparticles and nanoparticles can be the best drug delivery tools to treat ocular diseases. They exhibit a relatively large specific surface area for drug encapsulation and ocular mucosa contact. They facilitate dissolution of poorly water-soluble drugs by reducing their particle size in a formulation (Maiti and Jana, 2017).

Gokce and Okur (2016) developed a nanostructured lipid carrier of flurbiprofen-loaded within the sodium alginate insert for the treatment of ocular inflammation. The flurbiprofen-loaded nanostructured lipid carrier is prepared by high shear homogenization with sodium alginate added into the formed nanocarrier thereafter as insert carrier. The combination of nanostructured lipid carrier and alginate insert sustains drug release almost two times than insert without sodium alginate. The nanostructured lipid-carrier-based ocular insert is stable physicochemically and microbiologically. It may be useful in clinical practice for maintaining mydriasis during cataract or other eye surgical treatments.

Costa et al. (2015) developed mucoadhesive chitosan-coated alginate nanoparticles containing daptomycin through ionotropic pre-gelation of an alginate core followed by chitosan polyelectrolyte complexation for effective drug permeation across ocular epithelia to treat bacterial endophthalmitis. Daptomycin-loaded chitosan–alginate nanoparticles are negatively charged and have a size range of 380–420 nm. They are suitable for ocular application. The daptomycin permeability is up to 16% for chitosan nanoparticles and 9% for chitosan–alginate nanoparticles through corneal cell monolayer, and

18% for chitosan nanoparticles and 12% for chitosan–alginate nanoparticles through retinal cell monolayer after 4 h of incubation. The use of nanoparticulate systems entails epithelial retention of the drug compared to free drug.

Morsi et al. (2015) developed ketorolac tromethamine-loaded alginate–chitosan nanodispersions for ocular sustained drug delivery and improved trans-corneal drug permeation using modified coacervation and ionotropic pre-gelation techniques. Both size and zeta potential attributes of nanodispersions, which may govern the extent of drug permeation, are affected by alginate content. The nanodispersions show an initial burst drug release followed by a more gradual and sustained-release phase. The nanodispersions significantly retard the release of ketorolac tromethamine and provide a higher extent of trans-corneal drug permeation when compared to the commercial eye drops (Acular®).

Zhu et al. (2012) synthesized thiolated chitosan from chitosan with improved permeation enhancement and mucoadhesive properties. They then prepared chitosan/thiolated chitosan–sodium alginate nanoparticles using a modified ionic gelation method for ocular drug delivery. Fluorescein isothiocyanate is employed as the model drug. The nanoparticles are formed through electrostatic interaction between the negatively charged alginate and the positively charged chitosan or thiolated chitosan. The thiolated chitosan–alginate nanoparticles are smaller in size than chitosan–alginate nanoparticles and deliver greater amounts of drugs into human corneal epithelium in vitro as well as in vivo with rats.

Nagarwal et al. (2012) formulated chitosan-coated sodium alginate–chitosan nanoparticles loaded with 5-fluorouracil for ophthalmic delivery. The drug-loaded nanoparticles are produced by coacervation technique and the formed nanoparticles are coated with chitosan thereafter. In the latter, the alginate shell is solidified by reacting with chitosan, which occurs spontaneously through electrostatic interactions between the negatively charged carboxylate groups on alginate and the protonated amino groups on chitosan. The particle size significantly increases from 329–412 to 412–505 nm with changed morphology after coating of chitosan onto sodium alginate–chitosan nanoparticles. The chitosan-coated sodium alginate–chitosan nanoparticles show higher burst drug release (43.47%) than the uncoated counterparts (30.46%). A release of 74.15 and 81.20% of the drug is noted from uncoated and coated nanoparticles, respectively, over a period of 8 h of dissolution, where 99.82% drug is released in 4 h with a high burst effect (51.74% in 1 h) when the free drug solution is concerned. The complex formation between sodium alginate and chitosan enhances drug encapsulation and limits drug release more effectively than either polymer alone. Albeit faster in drug release, the chitosan coat increases the mucoadhesiveness of the dosage form. The coated nanoparticles are characterized by a higher drug bioavailability than the uncoated nanoparticles. The coated layer of chitosan not only endows positive surface charge but also prolongs the interaction of nanoparticles with oppositely charged mucin (negative charge). It increases the viscosity of mucin which translates to the mucoadhesive nature of the formulation. Further, the positive charge of nanoparticles enhances ocular drug absorption through paracellular transport by opening the tight junctions of corneal epithelia (Sarmento et al., 2007).

Shinde et al. (2014) fabricated azelastine-hydrochloride-loaded chitosan–sodium alginate microspheres for ocular delivery with improved therapeutic efficacy using modified ionotropic gelation technique. The microspheres have an average particle size in the range of 3.55–6.70 µm and zeta potential ranging from $+24.55$ to $+49.56$ mV. The resultant microspheres demonstrate maximum drug entrapment of 73.05% with 65% mucin binding efficiency. The drug is released in a controlled manner over a period 8 h, following a non-Fickian diffusion release mechanism. In vivo study using rats concludes that the microspheres are effective in prolonging the drug's presence in cul-de-sac with improved therapeutic efficacy.

Motwani et al. (2008) investigated mucoadhesive chitosan–alginate nanoparticles as a novel vehicle for extended topical ocular delivery of gatifloxacin. In vitro drug release results demonstrated that nanoparticles provide a quick drug release throughout the first hour, and followed by a steady drug release for a period of 24 h through a non-Fickian diffusion process, which is favorable in ocular drug delivery.

19.4.4   PHOTOREVERSIBLE ALGINATE GEL

Wells and Sheardown (2007) synthesized photoreversible alginate gels by covalent cross-linking of alginate (intravitreally inert polymer) by photo-sensitive molecule, anthracene via polyethylene glycol chains for tunable controlled-release systems which may be particularly suited for disease treatment in the posterior segment of the eye. Photoreversible anthracene provides chains the ability to photodimerize. The developed gels respond to ultraviolet-induced cross-linking and are expected to reversibly cross-link alginate. The release of protein from physically cross-linked alginate microspheres can be modulated for over 8 months. The proposed system responding to light stimuli is under development to control the rate of drug delivery intravitreally in accordance to disease progression or regression, resulting in a tunable treatment profile ideal for macular degeneration and diabetic retinopathy therapies.

Alginates have been extensively studied for a wide range of applications. These include in situ gel formation, controlled drug release, targeted drug delivery, and medical purposes. Various products are available commercially for oral, dermal, rectal, periodontal, and arthroscopic applications. However, to the best of our knowledge, only one product is available in the market for ocular application, that is, an in situ forming gel Carteol® LP containing carteolol hydrochlorate in alginic acid for the treatment of chronic open-angle glaucoma by once a day administration in the morning (Destruel et al. 2017).

19.6 CONCLUSIONS AND FUTURE PERSPECTIVES

Owing to unique properties of natural and multifunctional alginate polymeric carriers such as mucoadhesiveness, swelling capacity, solgel transition ability, tailoring of drug release, biodegradability, and biocompatibility, they have gained a preferential place in the development of advanced drug delivery systems. To date, considerable efforts have been devoted to design and develop alginate-based dosage forms such as in situ forming gels, ocular films, and nanoparticulate systems for the effective treatment of ocular diseases. The late formulations overcome drawbacks associated with the existing conventional ocular dosage forms. Principally, they enhance corneal drug penetration and drug bioavailability with good tolerance and safety. They provide accurate dosing administration with easy administration method, are retained at the site of application with prolonged pre-corneal contact time due to increased mucoadhesive property, release drug from the dosage form in a sustained manner, and reduce the frequency of dosing administration. The nanoparticulate drug delivery systems have gained a widespread attention in ocular applications. Nonetheless, their drug permeation enhancement action and toxicity have yet to be fully understood. Future studies are required in order to develop such technology for commercial application.

SUMMARY

Alginate is a water-soluble polysaccharide made of homopolymeric regions of β-D-mannuronic acid (M)-blocks and α-L-guluronic acid (G)-blocks, interdispersed with regions of alternating structure of α-L-guluronic acid and β-D-mannuronic acid blocks. It is commonly isolated from brown algae such as *Laminaria hyperborea, Ascophyllum nodosum,* and *Macrocystis pyrifera.* Alginate is nontoxic, biodegradable, and biocompatible. It inherently possesses biological effects such as anticholesterolemic, antihypertensive, antidiabetic, antiobesity, antimicrobial, anticancer, antihepatotoxicity, wound healing, anticoagulation, and coagulation activities. Alginate has been used as emulsion thickener, stabilizer, emulsifier, carrier polymer for antigen, enzyme, microbe, animal cell and recombinant gene product, bone and cartilage tissue engineering scaffold, peripheral nerve regeneration implant, wound dressing, dental impression material, anti-heartburn, and gastric reflux raft-forming formulation, radioactive and heavy metal absorption agent and plasma expander. Pharmaceutically, alginate has been used as a drug carrier in the form of microspheres, microcapsules, nanoparticles, gel beads, hydrogel, film, and tablets. With reference to ocular diseases, alginate-based carrier systems, that is, sodium alginate alone and/or in combination with in situ gel polymers (poloxamers, sodium carboxymethylcellulose, hydroxypropyl methylcellulose), alginate-based inserts/films, alginate/chitosan nanodispersions, chitosan–alginate nanoparticles, and microparticles have been investigated as a potential drug delivery vehicle. This chapter intends to highlight alginate formulations and mechanisms of action of ocular dosage forms for use in the treatment of eye disorders.

KEYWORDS

- alginate
- film
- gel
- insert
- microparticle
- nanoparticle
- ocular

REFERENCES

Alginic Acid. National Center for Biotechnology Information. PubChem Compound Database; CID=6850754. https://pubchem.ncbi.nlm.nih.gov/compound/6850754 (accessed Nov 13, 2017).

Bhalerao, A. V.; Singh, S. S. In Situ Gelling Ophthalmic Drug Delivery System for Glaucoma. *Int. J. Pharma Bio. Sci.* **2011,** *2,* P-7–P-14.

CBI Product Factsheet: Alginates in Europe. CBI Market Intelligence, Hague, The Netherlands, 2015, pp 1–13.

Cohen, S.; Lobel, E.; Trevgoda, A.; Peled, Y. A Novel in Situ-Forming Ophthalmic Delivery System from Alginates Undergoing Gelation in the Eye. *J. Controlled Release* **1997,** *44,* 201–208.

Costa, J. R.; Silva, N. C.; Sarmento, B.; Pintado, M. Potential Chitosan-Coated Alginate Nanoparticles for Ocular Delivery of Daptomycin. *Eur. J. Clin. Microbiol. Infect. Dis.* **2015,** *34,* 1255–1262.

Destruel, P.-L.; Zeng, N.; Maury, M.; Mignet, N.; Boudy, V. In Vitro and in Vivo Evaluation of in Situ Gelling Systems for Sustained Topical Ophthalmic Delivery: State of the Art and Beyond. *Drug Discovery Today* **2017,** *22,* 638–651.

Donati, I., Paoletti, S. *Material properties of alginates.* In *Alginates: Biology and applications;* Rehm, B. H. A., Ed.; Springer: New York, 2009; pp 1–53.

FMC BioPolymers. Alginates. www.fmcbiopolymer.com (accessed Jun 10, 2017).

FMC BioPolymers d/b/a NovaMatrix, DuPont Nutrition and Health (Formerly FMC Health and Nutrition). Alginate Applications. PRONOVA UP Sodium Alginate Gelation. www.novamatrix.biz (accessed Jun 10, 2017).

Gadad, A. P.; Wadklar, P. D.; Dandghi, P.; Patil, A. Thermosensitive in Situ Gel for Ocular Delivery of Lomefloxacin. *Indian J. Pharm. Educ. Res.* **2016,** *50,* S96-S105.

Gibson, M. *Ophthalmic Dosage forms.* In *Pharmaceutical Preformulation and Formulation: A Practical Guide from Candidate Drug Selection to Commercial Dosage form;* Gibson, M., Ed.; CRC Press: Florida, 2009; Vol. 199; pp 431.

Gilhotra, R. M.; Mishra, D. N. Alginate-Chitosan Film for Ocular Drug Delivery: Effect of Surface Cross-Linking on Film Properties and Characterization. *Pharmazie* **2008,** *63,* 576–579.

Gilhotra, R. M.; Nagpal, K.; Mishra, D. N. Azithromycin Novel Drug Delivery System for Ocular Application. *Int. J. Pharma. Invest.* **2011,** *1,* 22–28.

Gokce, E. H.; Okur, N. U. Novel Nanostructured Lipid Carrier Based Flurbiprofen Loaded Sodium Alginate Inserts for Ocular Drug Delivery. *Lat. Am. J. Pharm.* **2016,** *35,* 972–979.

Gratieri, T.; Gelfuso, G. M.; Rocha, E. M.; Sarmento, V. H.; de Freitas, O., Lopez, R. F. A Poloxamer/Chitosan in Situ Forming Gel with Prolonged Retention Time for Ocular Delivery. *Eur. J. Pharm. Biopharm.* **2010,** *75,* 186–193.

Imeson, A. *Food stabilisers, Thickeners and Gelling Agents,* 1st ed.; Wiley-Blackwell: New Jersey, 2009.

Jain, D.; Kumar, V.; Singh, S.; Mullertz, A.; Bar-Shalom, D. Newer trends in in Situ Gelling Systems for Controlled Ocular Drug Delivery. *J. Anal. Pharm. Res.* **2016,** *2,* 1–16.

Kesavan, K.; Nath, G.; Pandit, J. K. Sodium Alginate Based Mucoadhesive System for Gatifloxacin and Its in Vitro Antibacterial Activity. *Sci. Pharm.* **2010,** *78,* 941–957.

Khan, N.; Aqil, M.; Imam, S. S.; Ali, A. Development and Evaluation of a Novel in Situ Gel of Sparfloxacin for Sustained Ocular Drug Delivery: In vitro and ex vivo Characterization. *Pharm. Dev. Technol.* **2015,** *20,* 662–669.

Kolsure, P. K.; Rajkapoor, B. Development of Zolmitriptan Gel for Nasal Administration. *Asian J. Pharm. Clin. Res.* **2012,** *5,* 88–94.

Kumar, J. R.; Muralidharan, S. Formulation and in Vitro Evalution of Gellan Gum/Carbopol and Sodium Alginate Based Solution to Gel Depot of Ketotifen Fumarate System. *J. Pharm. Sci. Res.* **2012,** *4,* 1973–1977.

Kumari, A.; Sharma, P. K.; Garg, V. K.; Garg, G. Ocular Inserts—Advancement in Therapy of Eye Diseases. *J. Adv. Pharm. Technol. Res.* **2010,** *1,* 291–296.

Laddha, U. D.; Mahajan, H. S. An Insight to Ocular in Situ Gelling Systems. *Int. J. Adv. Pharm.* **2017,** *6,* 31–40.

Lee, K. Y.; Mooney, D. J. Alginates: Properties and Biomedical Applications. *Prog. Polym. Sci.* **2012,** *37,* 106–126.

Lin, H. R.; Sung, K. C.; Vong, W. J. In situ gelling of Alginate/Pluronic Solutions for Ophthalmic Delivery of Pilocarpine. *Biomacromolecules* **2004,** *5,* 2358–2365.

Liu, Z.; Li, J.; Nie, S.; Liu, H.; Ding, P.; Pan, W. Study of an Alginate/HPMC-Based in Situ Gelling Ophthalmic Delivery System for Gatifloxacin. *Int. J. Pharm.* **2006,** *315,* 12–17.

Maiti, S.; Jana, S. Biocomposites in Ocular Drug Delivery. In *Biopolymer-Based Composites: Drug Delivery and Biomedical Applications;* Maiti, S.; Jana, S., Eds.; Woodhead Publishing: United Kingdom, 2017; pp 139.

MarketsandMarkets. Alginates and Derivatives Market-Global Trends and Forecast to 2019: By type (Sodium Alginate, Calcium Alginate, Potassium Alginate, PGA, others), Application (Food and beverage, Industrial, Pharmaceuticals, others), and by Region. 2015. http://www.marketresearch.com/MarketsandMarkets-v3719/; https://www.marketresearch.com/product/sample-8778477.pdf

Mishra, D. N.; Gilhotra, R. M. Design and Characterization of Bioadhesive in-Situ Gelling Ocular Inserts of Gatifloxacin Sesquihydrate. *DARU* **2008,** *16,* 1–8.

Morsi, N.; Ghorab, D.; Refai, H.; Teba, H. Preparation and Evaluation of Alginate/Chitosan Nanodispersions for Ocular Delivery. *Int. J. Pharm. Pharm. Sci.* **2015,** *7,* 234–240.

Motwani, S. K.; Chopra, S.; Talegaonkar, S.; Kohli, K.; Ahmad, F. J.; Khar, R. K. Chitosan-Sodium Alginate Nanoparticles as Submicroscopic Reservoirs for Ocular Delivery: Formulation, Optimisation and in Vitro Characterisation. *Eur. J. Pharm. Biopharm.* **2008,** *68,* 513–525.

Nagarwal, R. C.; Kumar, R.; Pandit, J. K. Chitosan Coated Sodium Alginate-Chitosan Nanoparticles Loaded with 5-FU for Ocular Delivery: in Vitro Characterization and in Vivo Study in Rabbit Eye. *Eur. J. Pharm. Sci.* **2012,** *47,* 678–685.

Puranik, K. M.; Tagalpallewar, A. A. Voriconazole In situ Gel for Ocular Drug Delivery. *SOJ Pharm. Pharm. Sci.* **2015,** *2,* 1–10.

Ramya, R.; Ali, Z. A.; Sudha, P. N. Chitosan Composites for Biomedical Applications: An Overview. In *Natural Polymers, Biopolymers, Biomaterials and their Composites, Blends and IPNs;* Thomas. S., Ninan, N., Mohan, S., Francis, E., Ed.; CRC Press: New Jersey, 2013; Vol. 2, p 20.

Remminghorst, U.; Rehm, H. A. Bacterial alginates: From Biosynthesis to Applications. *Biotechnol. Lett.* **2006,** *28,* 1701–1712.

Repka, M. A.; Singh, A. Alginic Acid. *Handbook of Pharmaceutical Excipients,* 6th ed.; Rowe, R. C., et al., Pharmaceutical Press: London, 2009; pp 20–22.

Sachan, K. N.; Pushkar, S.; Jha, A.; Bhattcharya, A. Sodium Alginate: the Wonder Polymer for Controlled Drug Delivery. *J. Pharm. Res.* **2009,** *2,* 1191–1199.

Sarmento, B.; Ribeiro, A.; Veiga, F.; Sampaio, P.; Neufeld, R.; Ferreira, D. Alginate/Chitosan Nanoparticles are Effective for Oral Insulin Delivery. *Pharm. Res.* **2007,** *24,* 2198–2206.

Séchoy, O.; Tissié, G.; Sébastian, C.; Maurin, F.; Driot, J. Y.; Trinquand, C. A new Long Acting Ophthalmic Formulation of Carteolol Containing Alginic Acid. *Int. J. Pharm.* **2000,** *207,* 109–116.

Shastri, D. H.; Patel, L. D.; Parikh, R. K. Studies on in Situ Hydrogel: A Smart Way for Safe and Sustained Ocular Drug Delivery. *J. Young Pharm.* **2010,** *2,* 116–120.

Sheshala, R.; Kok, Y. Y.; Ng, J. M.; Thakur, R. R. S.; Dua, K. In Situ Gelling Ophthalmic Drug Delivery System: An Overview and Its Applications. *Recent Pat. Drug Delivery Formulation* **2015,** *9,* 242–253.

Shinde, U. A.; Shete, J. N.; Nair, H. A.; Singh, K. H. Design and Characterization of Chitosan-Alginate Microspheres for Ocular Delivery of Azelastine. *Pharm. Dev. Technol.* **2014,** *19,* 813–823.

Singh, N.; Mazumder, R.; Paul, S. D. Preparation and in Vitro Evaluation of an Anti-Bacterial in Situ Ophthalmic Gel. *Curr. Nanomed.* **2017,** *7,* 67–72.

Spadari, C. C.; Lopes, L. B.; Ishida, K. Potential Use of Alginate-Based Carriers as Antifungal Delivery System. *Front. Microbiol.* **2017,** *8,* 1–11.

Swapnil, D.; Sonawane, Lahoti, S. Design and Evaluation of Ion Induced in situ Gel Formulation for Levofloxacin Hemihydrateocular Delivery. *Int. J. Pharm. Sci. Invent.* **2014,** *3,* 38–43.

Szekalska, M.; Pucilowska, A.; Szymańska, E.; Ciosek, P.; Winnicka, K. Alginate: Current Use and Future Perspectives in Pharmaceutical and Biomedical Applications. *Int. J. Polym. Sci.* **2016,** *2016,* 1–17.

Tonnesen, H. H.; Karlsen, J. Alginate in Drug Delivery Systems. *Drug Dev. Ind. Pharm.* **2002,** *28,* 621–630.

Virtual Medical Centre. The Eye and Vision. www.myvmc.com; https://www.myvmc.com/anatomy/the-eye-and-vision/28/ (accessed Nov 8, 2017).

Wells, L. A.; Sheardown, H. Photoreversible Alginate for Drug Delivery. *ARVO Annual Meeting Abstract, May 2007, Invest. Ophthalmol. Vis. Sci.* **2007,** *48,* 5817.

Zhu, X.; Su, M.; Tang, S.; Wang, L.; Liang, X.; Meng, F.; Hong, Y.; Xu, Z. Synthesis of Thiolated Chitosan and Preparation Nanoparticles with Sodium Alginate for Ocular Drug Delivery. *Mol. Vision* **2012,** *18,* 1973–1982.

CHAPTER 20

ALGINATE CARRIERS FOR BIOACTIVE SUBSTANCES: HERBAL NATURAL COMPOUNDS AND NUCLEIC ACID MATERIALS

MARIA ROSARIA LAURO[1,*], GIOVANNI AMATO[2],
FRANCESCA SANSONE[1], CLAUDIA CARBONE[2], and
GIOVANNI PUGLISI[2]

[1]*Department of Pharmacy, University of Salerno, Via Giovanni Paolo II, 84084 Fisciano, Italy*

[2]*Department of Drug Sciences, University of Catania, Viale A. Doria, 95100 Catania, Italy*

Corresponding author. E-mail: lauro@unisa.it

20.1 INTRODUCTION

In 1994, US food and drug law specifically called out "an herb or other botanical" as ingredients that can be used to constitute dietary supplements. Since 1991, the WHO considers phytotherapy in its health programs and suggests basic procedures for the validation of drugs from plant origin in developing countries. In recent years, natural products derived from plants have been growing interest as alternative therapeutic compounds. In fact, the US government has considered botanicals (herbal or traditional medicines) a category of "complementary or alternative medicine" (Hoffman et al, 2015). The renaissance of plants derivatives is due to several reasons such as the higher side effects of the conventional medicine. However, they have a series of factors that limit their use in therapy such as poor solubility, limited dissolution rate, and instability in extreme pH, rapid degradation/oxidation resulting in less nutritional value of plant derivatives or no therapeutic effect, with high doses required for an effect (Lauro et al., 2007; Sansone et al., 2011a; Puglia et al., 2017). The peculiar properties of alginate (ALG)-based biomaterials (biocompatibility, biodegradability, gelling ability in presence of multivalent ions) make them attractive polymers for the development of different delivery systems such as beads, sponges, micro- and nanoparticles, fibers and sponges for nutraceutical, or biomedical applications (De Cicco et al., 2014; Del Gaudio et al., 2015). These polymers also protect, themselves or together with other polymers, the natural biocompounds from high temperature, oxidation, improving their shelf life, prolonging their antioxidant efficacy and sometimes acting synergistically with them in biological activity.

Moreover, ALG derivatives are able gene delivery carriers allowing the development of efficient non-viral methods, such as the formulation of nanosystems, to encapsulate deoxyribonucleic acid (DNA), polycations, and vesicular materials. On these bases, in this chapter, we analyze recent literature (last five years) about the application of pure ALG derivatives, or in mixture with other polymers, as carriers for nutraceutical or drug natural compounds or for nucleic acid materials.

20.2 REGULATORY ASPECTS OF ALGINATES (ALGS): FOOD/NUTRACEUTICAL AND PHARMACEUTICAL ASPECTS

The use of natural polymers has increased in recent times; also due to the advocacy of "green" materials from "green" chemistry and technologies.

The food and beverage industry accounts for 20–30% of ALGs demand. Industrial (e.g., textile printing), pharmaceutical, and cosmetic applications account for the remaining market. In nutraceuticals, ALGs are used as carriers of active or functional food ingredients or edible coating or films. In pharmaceutical, naturapolyceutics is a word coined from natural polymers and pharmaceutics. It is the art, science, and technology of utilizing natural polymers for the design and development of drug delivery systems. Since the mid-1970s, different forms of ALGs such as ALG salt, alginic acids (AAs), and propylene glycol ALGs have been used successfully in pharmaceutical applications. In cosmetics, wherein it is used for its functionality as a moisture retainer and thickener.

Alginate is a linear copolymer of β-D-Mannuronic acid and α±-L-Guluronic acid. Low G/M ratios are mostly destined for industrial applications (CBI Foreign Ministry, 2015).

The FDA has outlined the specific uses and levels of concentration that are allowed for the different types of ALGs (ammonium, calcium, potassium, sodium, and propylene glycol) in food products (USDA, 2015) and recognizes ALG as a "generally referred as safe" material, by experts (Sosnik, 2014). These products are also included in FDA Inactive Ingredient Guide for use in oral preparation and in non-parenteral medicines licensed in the UK (Rowe et al., 2012).

In April 1995, the American National Organic Standards Board, a Federal Advisory Board established by the Organic Foods Production Act and governed by the Federal Advisory Committee Act, allowed ALGs as synthetic materials for use in organic food processing and, in December 2000, included them in the National Organic Program Rule, a regulatory program responsible for developing national standards for organically produced agricultural products. AA, sodium ALG, and potassium ALG are classified as food additives in Canada. In Codex Alimentarius only potassium and sodium ALGs are listed as the food additives of non-agricultural origin. Moreover in Europe, ALG is classified as non-agricultural and are permitted because they are included in the list of allowed food additives for use as thickeners and stabilizers. In particular, sodium ALG is listed as an approved food additive for use in certain unprocessed fruit and vegetables (Sosnik, 2014).

Also for pharmaceutical and biomedical application, safety of ALGs is a big issue and, regulatory approval by national and international authority is fundamental. Before a natural polymer can obtain approval, three main areas in the regulatory issue must be documented: characterization and functionality, based on product specification, analysis using a validation method, and product stability; product reproducibility of the manufactured compound by GMP guidelines and documentation of manufacture, specifications, and safety described in Drug Master File; documented toxicology and safety by basic and application-specific studies (USDA, 2015).

The conventional role of ALGs in pharmaceutics includes serving as thickening, gel forming, and stabilizing agents, as ALG can play a significant role in controlled release drug products. Multiple drugs can be loaded into ALG-based gels for simultaneous or sequential delivery (Szekalska et al., 2016).

Because the functionality of ALG is related to its chemical and structural composition, key parameters relevant for the development of new commercial applications of ALGs for the biomedical and pharmaceutical industries, are referenced in ASTM standards (ASTM International, 2006).

20.3 ALGS CARRIERS FOR NATURAL COMPOUNDS: USE IN FOOD/NUTRACEUTICAL FIELD

ALGs offer various applications also to deliver the natural biomolecules such as in modulating gastrointestinal (GI) release. ALGs form a biodegradable, nontoxic, and edible film that not degraded within the upper GI tract (GIT), so it is possible to design a hydrogel that remains intact in certain regions of the upper GIT, but then disintegrates and delivers the nutraceuticals in the colon (McClements, 2017), protecting the active from pH degradation and applying to it a controlled delivery. It also protects natural actives from high temperature, oxidation, improving their shelf life, prolonging their anti-oxidant efficacy and acting synergistically in biological activity with some compounds (Table 20.1).

TABLE 20.1 A List of Research Articles on Alginates (ALGs), Natural Compounds in Nutraceutical/Food Field Published During the Last 5 Years (2013–2017).

Compound	Type of ALG	Preparation methods	Carrier	Authors	Year
Anthocyanins	Sodium ALG calcium ALG	In situ gelling system	Beads	Celli et al.	2016
Hesperidin	Sodium ALG calcium ALG	Ionotropic gelation	Beads	Tsirigotis-Maniecka et al.	2017
Blood orange extract	Sodium ALG	Spray drying	Microsystems	Lauro et al.	2017
Quercetin	Chitosan ALG	Electrostatic gelation	Nanoparticles	Aluani et al.	2017
Gallic acid	Sodium ALG calcium ALG	Electrospray technique	"Egg-box" structure	Li et al.	2016
Resveratrol	Sodium ALG	Emulsification followed by external gelation	Reservoir submicron particles	Isteniĉ et al.	2015
Resveratrol	Ca ALG, ALG sucrose, ALG chitosan	Extrusion	Microbeads-containing liposomes	Balanc et al.	2016
Betalains	Calcium ALG bovine serum albumin	Ionic gelation	Beads	Otálora et al.	2016
White tea extract	ALG-poly (ε-caprolactone)	Nanoprecipitation method	Nanoparticles	Sanna et al.	2015

Celli et al. (2016) developed an innovative ALG-based in situ gastroretentive gelling system as a platform to modulate the release and increase the retention time of anthocyanins (ACNs)-rich freeze-dried extract from Haskap berries (var. Indigo Gem) in sites where their absorption and stability are favored. ACNs are absorbed in the upper digestive tract (stomach and initial sections of the small intestine) (Felgines et al., 2007). An insufficient residence time of ACNs and their metabolism in these organs could result in limited absorption and contribute to degradation at high pHs found in the intestines. For these purposes, Thirteen base formulations with varying concentrations of sodium ALG (1.5, 2.5, and 3.5%), sodium bicarbonate (1.5, 2.0, and 2.5%), and calcium carbonate (0.5, 1.25, and 2.0%) were evaluated. All the formulations investigated in this study exhibited a high gelling capacity at 0.1 N HCl maintained at 37°C. They is gelled instantaneously when in contact with the acidic medium and retained the gel structure for more than 24 h undisturbed. For all formulations, the release profile was characterized by a biphasic pattern, with a burst effect of ACNs release into the acid solution, followed by a reduction in release rate. The release rate from these systems is controlled by diffusion through channels formed into hydrogel structure due to its swelling properties. The viscosity of the ALG solution does not seems to play a role in the gelling process (Celli et al., 2016).

Unlike ANCs, flavones such as hesperidin (Hd) are unstable in acidic medium (Sansone et al., 2009; Sansone et al., 2011b), so, sodium ALG hydrogel microbeads by means of the extrusion/external gelation technique, are developed by Tsirigotis-Maniecka (2016) to protect Hd, isolated from orange peels, in harsh gastric conditions and to improve its bioavailability. In order to enhance its protection and decrease its leakage from the porous matrix, polyelectrolyte films (chitosan; gelatin; polyallylamine hydrochloride/poly-sodium 4-styrenesulfonate) were deposited on the ALG matrices. Microbeads FTIR spectra confirmed that Hd was well incorporated in the ALG core. The best balance between Hd protection against aggressive gastric conditions, and its further controlled release were obtained combining ALG with chitosan (ACP) and ALG with gelatin (AGP) yielded. A swelling index (SI) was introduced and the microbeads behavior within the liquid media of different pHs were investigated to evaluate their swelling properties and stability, respectively. The swelling properties of the particles were determined by the composition of the core and the coating material, as expression affinity of the polymers for the selected environment and may significantly influence their release properties. In an acidic medium (pH 2.0), ALG core material was probably crucial in maintaining the stability of the food grade microparticles and preventing their excessive swelling. The swelling profiles of ACP (Figure 20.1) indicate a longer reabsorption process (90 min), probably due to longer diffusion into the entire volume of the shrunken core, whereas for AGP the rehydration process was accomplished within the first 30 min of the experiment (Figure 20.1), and then the microcapsules were in a steady state for further 90 min. Then their mass started to decrease, probably as a result of denaturation of gelatin induced by the low pH of the medium. Therefore, in the acidic medium (pH 2.0; 10 mM of HCl) SI (SI2) of ACP and AGP were elevated, because under low pH conditions the protonation of amine groups leads a strong charge density of gelatin and chitosan. This produces chain repulsions, protons diffusion, phenomena that along with entrapped water inside the gel, results in noticeable swelling of the particle. In this case, ALG core material was probably crucial in maintaining the stability of the MPs and preventing their excessive swelling in an acidic medium. In fact, considering that the process was conducted in an acid medium, this effect could even be exacerbated with in situ shrinkage of the matrix facilitated by the protonation of the carboxyl groups of the uronic residues of ALG. In neutral pH (pH 7.0; distilled water), ACP showed a slight variation of SI (SI7) probably due to pH-promoted changes upon the ALG core microenvironment disrupted by the chitosan membrane. Instead, AGP SI7 is the lower, indicating a compact gelatin coat structure as a result of low electrostatic repulsion between their chains in media of pH close to its isoelectric point. In alkaline medium (pH 10; 0.1 mM NaOH), the SI10 values and swelling profiles (Figure 20.1) of all types of particles exhibited intensive swelling as a result of the physical expansion of the hydrogel core. This behavior was caused by electrostatic repulsive forces between the ALG chains caused by deprotonation of the carboxyl groups of uronic acids residues. Experimental data revealed that the application of chitosan and gelatin films onto the ALG microspheres effectively reduced the uncontrolled leaching of Hd from the microparticles. Considering the results obtained, it may be concluded that chitosan membrane seems to be the most efficient release-limiting factor in acidic and neutral environments. However, gelatin is also very promising as a coating factor (Tsirigotis-Maniecka et al., 2017)

ACNs and Hd are polyphenols present in different plants, in particular in citrus species (Picerno et al., 2011; Lauro et al., 2015; Lauro et al., 2017). Lauro et al. (2017) reported that sodium ALG/beta-cyclodextrin (ALG/CD) matrix as edible film enhances the dissolution/release of a blood orange extract, rich in polyphenols from spray-dried microparticles, due to ALG characteristic of swellable hydrophilic polymer, and CD hydroxyl group. ALG also improves extract shelf life, and wettability. Instead, CD improves mitochondrial membrane potential (MMPs) inhibitory activity of the extract presumably because of the presence of free hydroxyl groups that support the hydrogen bond with the enzyme active site and preserved the extract antioxidant efficiency and stability. Both polymers also acted synergistically improving the in vitro advanced glycation end products direct inhibition and protecting the extract and its components from degradation phenomena.

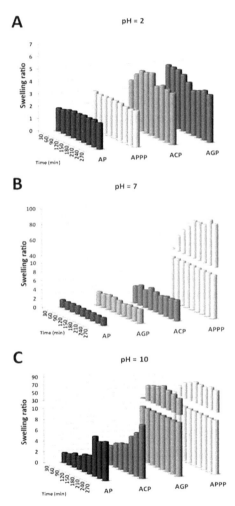

FIGURE 20.1 Swelling characteristics of the hesperidin-loaded microparticles: uncoated ALG microparticles (AP), chitosan-coated ALG microcapsules (ACP), gelatin-coated ALG microcapsules (AGP), PAH/PSS-coated ALG microcapsules (APPP), compared in three different pH media types: pH=2 (10 mMHCl) (a), pH=7 (distilled water) (b), and pH=10 (0.1 mMNaOH) (c), (t=30–270 min).

Source: Reprinted with permission from Tsirigotis-Maniecka et al., 2017. © 2017 Elsevier.

Other polyphenols and herbal extracts rich in polyphenols are formulated with pure ALGs or in combination with other polymers to improve
their technological and biological characteristics. Quercetin is a flavonol
with numerous health benefits particularly due to its antioxidant properties. However, its low solubility, bioavailability, and stability limit its use
as components for functional foods, nutraceuticals, and pharmaceutical
agents (Sansone et al., 2011b). Aluani et al. (2017), evaluated chitosan/ALG
nanoparticles as a platform for quercetin delivery providing preservation of
its antioxidant activity without elevating any systemic toxicity. Two types
of chitosan/ALG (1:10 and 10:1 w/w ratio) nanoparticles, differing in their
size and charge due to the different ratio between both biopolymers, were
prepared. Respect to the empty nanoparticles with higher concentration of
chitosan (NP2), the empty nanoparticles prepared with the higher concentration of sodium ALG (NP1) was characterized by smaller size and negative
values for zeta potential. Particles size and charge are some factors correlate
with formulation toxicity responses after the contact with the cells and tissues
in the biological system. Two different liver cells were chosen for in vitro
cytotoxicity assays – cultivated human hepatoma cells HepG2 and isolated
primary rat hepatocytes. For NP1 and NP2 nanoparticles, no apparent cytotoxicity was observed on HepG2 cells in the concentration range between
50 and 1000 g/ml. The results from MTT-assay (marker for mitochondrial
function) showed lack of toxicity of both the empty and quercetin – loaded
nanoparticles in human HepG2 cells after 24 h exposure. On marker of cell
membrane integrity (lactate dehydrogenase; LDH-leakage) only NP1 slight
increase (17%) LDH-leakage, but no signs of significant cytotoxicity were
observed in HepG2 cells when the exposure period was extended to 48 and
72 h. In vivo toxicity study showed that no mortality of male Wistar rats
was observed after 14 days of treatment, confirming the safety profile of
the chitosan/ALG nanoformulations. To study the immune responses after
stimulation, two types of murine cells, isolated spleen lymphocytes and
peritoneal macrophages, were used as cell models. The both empty and
loaded nanoparticles, stimulated significantly the proliferation of these
cells with superior effects of QR-NP1 formulated with higher concentration of ALG, respect to QR-NP2. Because free quercetin did not stimulate
the proliferation of isolated lymphocytes, a possible explanation for such
stimulation might be the finding that polysaccharide easily taken by the
macrophages (Gupta et al., 2015). In fact, the mechanisms of sodium ALG's
stimulation include induction in cytokine release and activation of the innate
immune system through activation of macrophage such as cells. Interesting
finding was that the empty chitosan/ALG nanoparticles possessed protective

activity themselves. In the end, experimental data about antioxidant activity of quercetin-loaded chitosan/ALG nanoparticles on in vitro oxidative stress models (iron/ascorbic acid; Fe2+/AA)-induced lipid peroxidation in microsomes and tert-butyl hydroperoxide (t-BuOOH) oxidative stress in isolated rat hepatocytes were performed. The empty chitosan/ALG nanoparticles showed to possess protective activity themselves. Moreover, the encapsulation of quercetin into the nanoparticles with higher concentration of chitosan (QR-NP2) provided better protection on cell viability and glutatione (GSH) content compared to free quercetin and QR-NP1, and comparable effects on malondialdehyde (MDA) levels and LDH release in a model of t-BuOOH-induced oxidative stress in isolated hepatocytes. (Aluani et al., 2017).

Sodium ALG beads were prepared by Li et al. (2016) to encapsulated water-soluble phenolic compounds such as gallic acid (GA) (water solubility of about 12 g/L at room temperature) through the electrospray technique with different voltage value (0, 5, 7.5, or 10 kV). During the gelling process, sodium ALG is cross-linked by the Ca^{2+} forming the "egg-box" structure. The impacts of beads size and loading amount of GA on the release profile in simulated digestion fluid were investigated. About 50 or 33% of GA was incorporated into 1:1 or 1:2 (w/w) sodium ALG beads, respectively. Higher voltage values of 7.5 or 10 kV reduce the ALG blank beads size significantly (from 1359 to 400 or 200, respectively). This is probably due to the ALG solution change flow from drip to jet reducing size at high voltage. Moreover, the voltage at 10 kV produced smaller GA-loaded ALG beads than that of blank ones. Meanwhile, the GA may have impact on the water absorption ability of the ALG beads. ALG can absorb large amount of water due to its hydroscopic nature which may be affected by the interaction with GA. GA interact with the calcium ALG matrix, reducing the water bonds and, consequently, the ALG beads water content. After freeze drying, the size tended to decrease but was there the presence of residues water (30 g/100 g) not removed because strongly bound to the ALG calcium complex. The loading ability and efficiency were much lower than theoretical values. In fact, the loading ability for 50% varied from 7.58/100 to 12.76/100 g. For 33% beads, the loading ability was around 7/100 g. These results were probably due to true concentration of GA inside ALG beads higher than that of collection solution which induced GA migrating into the collection solution. In this way, GA was squeezed out of the beads into the surrounding solution which led to the lower encapsulation ability than expected. Considering the loading ability results reported in the literature (50 mg/kg body weight would effectively suppress high fat diet-induced dyslipidemia, hepatosteatosis, and oxidative stress), the authors reported that about 30 g of dried beads are required for daily consumption to exert its nutraceutical properties. In the in vitro release test in simulated GI fluid without enzymes, GA was quickly released from ALG beads which are influenced by both the loading amount of active and the bead size. About 70–80% of GA was released from ALG beads when incubated in SGF within 30 min. Beads 33% at 0 kV had large size as well as low level of GA loading which correlated with its slow release speed. Beads with small size possess high surface area which provides large transfer interface for GA. The release level of GA in the simulated intestinal fluid was higher than that in the simulated gastric fluid because ALG is stable at acid pH but swells and degrades under higher pH value. In fact, more than 90% of GA was released in all the beads samples within 60 min of incubation (Figure 20.2) (Li et al., 2016).

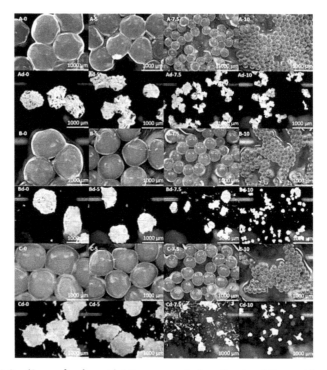

FIGURE 20.2   (See color insert.) Microscope photos of wet and freeze-dries ALG beads prepared under various voltages. A-0, A-5, A-7.5, and A-10 are the blank wet ALG beads prepared with voltage of 0, 5, 7.5, and 10 kV, respectively, while Ad-0, Ad-5, Ad-7.5, and Ad-10 are the blank freeze dried ALG beads prepared with the same conditions, respectively; photos numbered with B stands for 50% ALG beads and C is 33% ALG beads loaded with of gallic acid (numbers are voltages applied and d means freeze-dried form, scale bar is 1000 μm).

Source: Reprinted with permission from Li et al., 2016. © 2016 Elsevier.

Resveratrol-loaded ALG submicron particles were prepared by emulsification followed by external gelation. The release studies showed an initial "burst" effect in both acid (pH 1.2) and buffer medium (pH 7.0). The maximum of 17.3% (±0.3%) of the resveratrol was released at both pH values. After 10 min, the diffusion rate decrease, indicating that the ALG submicron particles were able to reproduce a reservoir system. This could be considered suitable for oral administration, confirming good protection to incorporated resveratrol and allowing prolonged release after uptake. The intermolecular interactions between ALG and resveratrol (via hydroxyl groups of resveratrol) confirmed by FTIR and differential scanning calorimetry (DSC) analysis is the possible reason for such a low release percentage. The ALG submicron particles present a pH-dependent release pattern. In order to evaluate the mechanism of resveratrol release at both pH values, the experimental results are fitted by two models: Fick's second law and linear superimposition model (Figure 20.3). Nevertheless, the transport mechanism does not strictly follow Fick's diffusion behavior; it is the main release mechanism. In fact, the Fickian diffusion rate constant is higher for pH 1.2 due to the conversion of the carrier material to insoluble alginic acid (AA). In particle size analyses, the presence of resveratrol seems to reduce the dimensions. In fact, empty ALG size varied from 110 to 630 nm with average particle size of 360 nm, while the size of the ALG–resveratrol submicron particles varied from 30–630 nm with average particle size of 250 nm. It is because resveratrol is an amphiphilic molecule, characterized

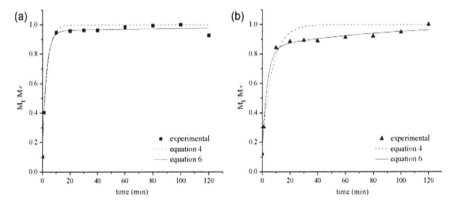

FIGURE 20.3 Fick's and Linear Superimposition Model description of resveratrol release from ALG–resveratrol submicron particles at 37°C in 0.1 M HCl (pH 1.2) (a) and in phosphate-buffered saline (pH 7.2) (b).

Source: Reprinted with permission from Istenič et al., 2015. © 2015 Elsevier.

by a hydrophobic aromatic ring and a hydrophilic phenolic hydroxyl group, and acts as a surface active compound along with the surfactant PGPR (polyglycerol polyricinoleate) used to prepare the ALG-in-oil formulation. The authors reported that due to their submicron particles size, the encapsulation of resveratrol offers wide range of application and represents a potential delivery system in food products (Istenič et al., 2015).

Hybrid delivery systems based on Ca-ALG, ALG-sucrose (ALG/SUC), and ALG-chitosan (ALG/CH) particles with entrapped resveratrol-bearing liposomes (multilamellar lipid vesicles, MLV) were also prepared by Balanč et al. (2016) to encapsulated bioactive poorly soluble compounds into functional food products. DSC analysis revealed the interactions between resveratrol and phospholipids and between liposomes and ALG. In fact, the nanostructure of ALG hydrogel has been changed after the liposome inclusion (Figure 20.4). At temperatures between 220 and 250°C, blank Ca-ALG beads exhibited an exothermic peak resulted from degradation of ALG due to dehydration and depolymerization of the protonated carboxylic groups and oxidation reactions of the macromolecule. This thermal event was not recorded in the case of samples containing liposomes, probably due to the interactions between ALG and phospholipids, albeit the repulsive forces between liposomes and ALGs minimize possible interactions between them. The sample containing sucrose (ALG/SUC-LIP/RES) displayed a distinct sharp endothermic peak at 181°C, while a second double endothermic peak at 230°C typical for sucrose, did not appear in the DSC thermogram of ALG/SUC-LIP/RES formulation. This behaviour suggests that sucrose interferes with the thermal behaviour of ALG beads containing resveratrol-loaded liposomes. Moreover, ALG/SUC microbeads showed better rehydration properties than pure ALG beads. Sucrose reduces aggregation of ALG eggboxes and interferes with the formation of dimers grown into larger structures during drying (Vreeker et al., 2008). The same effect on rehydration seems to have liposomes incorporated within junction zones of ALG but at far less extent. Chitosan coating did not show significant impact on d50 upon rehydration. Instead, resveratrol incorporated within the lipid bilayer had a destabilizing effect due to hydrophobic interactions between resveratrol and phospholipids with some contribution of hydrogen bonding. The efficiency of encapsulation of resveratrol into liposomes loaded microbeads was high (85–91%). ALG/CH-LIP/RES microbeads exhibited the lowest encapsulation efficiency (EE%) due to their smallest dimensions. This involved a shorter path for the resveratrol diffusion from the inside of the microbeads and a more pronounced leakage of resveratrol to the collecting solution during preparation method. It is interesting that the presence of chitosan prolongs the sustained release time of a bioactive compounds from the ALG matrix by making the denser structure due to interactions between two polymers (polyanionic ALG and cationic chitosan), while sucrose crystals probably act as a physical barrier to mass transfer, reducing the resveratrol diffusion (Balanč et al., 2016).

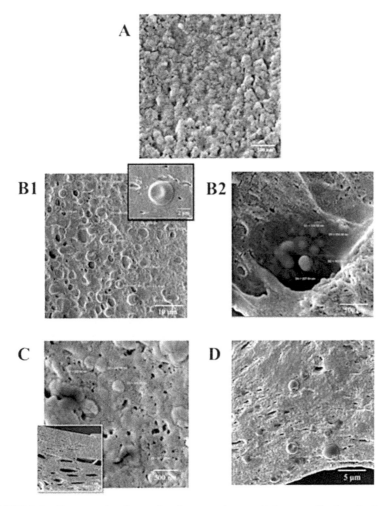

FIGURE 20.4   Cross-sectional scanning electron microscopic images of hydrogel microbead samples: ALG (A) (×231.000), ALG-LIP/RES (B1) low magnification (×14.000), with the insert showing flattening of a single liposome; ALG-LIP/RES (B2) high magnification (×276.000), ALG/CH-LIP/RES (×231.000) with the insert showing the surface membrane (C), ALG/SUC-LIP/RES (D) (×26.700).

Source: Reprinted with permission from Balanč et al., 2016. © 2016 Elsevier.

Betalains from *Opuntia ficus Indica* fruits were encapsulated in calcium-ALG (CA) and in combination of calcium ALG and bovine serum albumin (CAB), by ionic gelation, to stabilize this pigment during storage conditions. Stability is an important aspect for natural colorant and antioxidant compounds in foods. Betalain stability is strongly affected by pH, water activity, temperature, oxygen, light exposure, among others. In particular, hydrolysis was the main mechanism of betalain degradation leading to the betalamic acid formation during storage under non-favorable conditions, such as either high temperature or high %RH (34.6, 57.6, 74.8, and 84.3% at 25°C for 25 days). The encapsulation can be used for stabilization, protection, and extending the shelf life of sensitive compounds as well as for many applications in the food industry, including controlled release, delivery and masking of flavors, colors, and odors. Both, CA and CAB encapsulated betalains showed higher storage stability at low %RH (34.6%RH at 25°C) with the best storage conditions for CA beads with retentions of betalain content of 48.8% and antiradical activity of 88.5% Otálora et al. (2016).

White tea extract was nanoencapsulated into polymeric nanoparticles (NPs) based on poly(ε-caprolactone) (PCL) and ALG by a nanoprecipitation method to control the release in GI fluids of tea polyphenols and to preserve their antioxidant activity and stability. The major polyphenolic constituents, the flavan-3-ols, also known as catechins, include (+)-epigallocatechin-3-gallate (EGCG), (+)-epigallocatechin (EGC), (+)-epicatechin-3-gallate (ECG), and (+)-epicatechin (EC). Considering that the composition of NPs strongly influenced their size and distribution, to optimize the NPs formulation conditions, different amounts of ALG (0.1, 0.5, and 1.0%·w/v) were initially employed. In particular, NPs obtained with ALG at lower concentration (0.1% w/v) are characterized by a mean particle size (300 nm) with a wide distribution (PDI 0.397 ± 0.27). By increasing the ALG concentration, a rise in particle size distribution was observed. These results were probably due to the high viscosity of ALG solution that promoted a larger particle precipitation with a tendency to separation. The optimal ALG concentration was found to be 0.5% w/v that produced NPs with spherical shape, a mean diameter of 380.80 ± 37.97 nm, and a unimodal distribution (PDI 0.15 ± 0.06). NPs (0, 5% of ALG) showing a good capacity to control the polyphenols delivery. In simulated gastric medium (pH 1.2) after 5 h, 20% of polyphenols were released with a classical Fickian diffusion-controlled mechanism facilitated by the swelling of ALG. Instead, 80% was released at pH 7.4 at the same time, through drug diffusion in the hydrated matrix and polymer relaxation mechanisms. Furthermore, DPPH·assay confirmed that the antioxidant activity of tea extract is concentration-dependent and that white tea extract maintained a good free radical scavenging activity after encapsulation into NPs. Moreover, the stability studies conducted by authors at different temperatures (25 and 40°C) over 30 days showed that the polyphenols content was strongly influenced by the storage temperature. The total polyphenol content (TPC) was of 65% at 25°C and decrease to $43.7 \pm 3.2\%$ for the samples stored at 40°C. Interesting results were obtained from the encapsulation of white tea extract into NPs that largely prevented the extract degradation with providing a TPC loss of 12.6% and 24% of the initial content with increasing storage temperature (Sanna et al., 2015).

20.4 ALG-BASED NANOCARRIERS FOR NATURAL COMPOUNDS DELIVERY

Among different compounds, a great attention has been paid to the delivery of natural compounds by ALG-based delivery systems by topical and oral administration (Table 20.2). Deol and Kaur (2013) developed calcium ALG beads coated with Eudragit S100 for the colon cancer targeted release of ginger extract (GE). GE is a highly antioxidant compound with free radicals scavenging properties and peculiar activity in inhibiting the synthesis of prostaglandin and leukotriene, without the occurrence of the side effects typical of the activity of non-selective cyclooxygenase inhibitors (Grzanna et al., 2005). The ability of Eudragit S100 in dissolving at pH 7.4, avoiding the release of the natural compound in the upper GIT, was herein applied for the first time for the specific GE prolonged targeted release in the colon. The authors reported the beads reached the ileocecal junction after 8 h, with a release pattern of super class II controlled by swelling and relaxation of the polymer. It is important to underline that the presence of calcium ALG, under acidic conditions, led to the occurrence only of a low swelling ratio process due to the proton–calcium ion exchange forming insoluble alginic aid regions. Increasing in pH values determines an increase in swelling, due to the enhanced solubility of the polymer. GE-loaded Ca-ALG beads swelling at higher pH values are enhanced by the presence of phosphate ions that are able to capture the calcium ions of the beads. The ionotropy strongly affects the release rate at higher pH, with the coated GE beads releasing the natural compound through swelling and erosion mechanisms only after the dissolution of the Eudragit coating. The formulation was evaluated in terms of protective effect against colon cancer, post-induction, in terms of oxidative stress, mitochondrial enzyme complex activity, β-glucuronidase and ammonia concentration determination, and colon cancer-induced histopathological

TABLE 20.2 A List of Research Articles on ALGs, Natural Compounds in the Drug Delivery Field Published During the Last 5 Years (2013-2017).

Title	Type of ALG	Topic/therapeutic area	Drug carrier	Authors	Year
Ginger extract	Eudragit S100-coated calcium ALG	Oral delivery, colon cancer	Beads	Deol and Kaur	2013
Lakshadi Guggul	Chitosan–calcium phosphate ALGs	Oral delivery, osteoarthritis	ALG enclosed chitosan–calcium phosphate nanocarriers	Samarasinghe et al.	2014
Glycyrrhizin	Calcium ALG	Oral delivery, stomach	Beads	Rathore et al.	2017
Naringenin	ALG-chitosan	Oral delivery, diabetes mellitus	Core–shell nanoparticles	Maity et al.	2017
Quercetin	ALG-chitosan	Oral delivery, diabetes	Microparticles	Mukhopadhyay et al.	2016
Quercetin	ALG-chitosan	Oral delivery	Microparticles	Hazra et al.	2015
Icariin	ALG-chitosan	Oral delivery, colon, ulcerative colitis	Microspheres	Wang et al.	2016
Capsaicin	ALG	Oral delivery, colon delivery	Nanoliposomes	Giri et al.	2017
Nobiletin	ALG	Oral delivery	Nanoemulsions	Lei et al.	2017
Riboflavin	Sodium ALG	Oral delivery	Beads and Hydrogels	Abd El-Ghaffar et al.	2012
Riboflavin	ALG	Oral delivery	Liquid-core macro and microcapsules	Messaoud et al.	2016
Curcumin	ALG	Oral delivery, gastroretentive	Self-microemulsifying drug delivery systems	Petchsomrit et al.	2017
Curcumin	Galactosylated ALG	Oral delivery, hepatocarcinoma	Polymer–drug conjugate micelle	Sarika et al.	2016a
Curcumin	ALGs	Cancer	Polymer–drug conjugate micelle	Dey and Sreenivasan	2014

TABLE 20.2 (Continued)

Title	Type of ALG	Topic/therapeutic area	Drug carrier	Authors	Year
Curcumin	ALG aldehyde	Cancer	Nanogels	Sarika, et al.	2016b
Curcumin	Calcium ALG	Topical delivery	Nanoemulsions	Nguyen et al.	2015
Hydroxytyrosol	ALG	Topical chemotherapy	Hydrocolloid films	Ng and Tan	2015
Centella asiatica	Sodium ALG	Wound healing	Hydrocolloid	Jin et al.	2015
Eucalyptus oil	Sodium ALG	Topical delivery, antimicrobic	Microcapsules	Noppakundilograt et al.	2015
Lithospermum erythrorhizon	Sodium ALG	Topical delivery, wound healing, antibacterial	Microcapsules	Lou et al.	2015
Silibinin	ALG/Gelatine scaffolds	Bone tissue regeneration	Chitosan nanoparticles	Leena et al.	2017
Chlorpheniramine maleate	Sodium ALG	Different medical fields	Magnetic beads with caffeine as precursor	Amiri et al.	2017

changes. In vivo studies on male Wistar rats showed the potential effectiveness of GE beads for the treatment of colon cancer post-induction, thanks to the coating with Eudragit S100 able to ensure a majority GE delivery to the concerned target site (distal part of the colon) (Grzanna et al., 2005). Recently, ALG-enclosed chitosan–calcium phosphate nanocarriers have been developed for the oral treatment of osteoarthritis, exploiting the activity of Lakshadi Guggul (LG) (Samarasinghe et al., 2014). LG is a combination of several herbal products including *Cissus quadrangularis*, *Withania somnifera*, *Azadirachta indica*, *Sida alba*, and *Terminalia arjuna*. *C. quadrangularis,* was widely used for its antifungal, antibacterial, antioxidant, analgesic, and anti-inflammatory activities (Mishra et al., 2010). This study, performed on chondrocytes exposed to inflammation conditions, showed the ability of LG in enhancing protective activity by stimulating their growth, improving viability by decreasing apoptotic and mitochondrial depolarization, inhibiting nitric oxide and PGE_2, increasing GAG, and aggrecan synthesis. The encapsulation of the natural product significantly increased it's in vivo antiarthritic potential compared to the treatment with the pure LG. Interestingly, the authors report the ability of the nanoformulation in reversing disease severity by regenerating cartilage formation and down-regulating inflammation-activated signaling pathways by specifically entering inflamed sites through the circulation. ALGs are considered promising candidates for designing targeted oral colon delivery systems with biomimetic approach of variation of pH value through the GIT in human body, due to their many advantages: hydrophilicity, ability to form microparticles, high stability at low pH that protects the drug in the stomach, the pH-responsive behavior promoting drug release and their mucoadhesive properties. The stability of ALGs in colonic fluid still limit their application thus promoting the continuous research and development of strategies to reach and reside in the colonic region. Among different type of ALGs, calcium ALG has been widely used for targeting gastric mucosa (Zhang et al., 2011). Recently, floating calcium ALG beads of glycyrrhizin, the main constituent of *Glycyrrhiza glabra* (liquorice) root, have been developed and characterized by a physicochemical and technological point of view for targeting the gastric mucosa and prolonging their gastric residence time (Rathore et al., 2017). Different flavonoids have been studied for the encapsulation into ALGs-based delivery systems, such as naringerin, quercetin, nobiletin, and icariin. Naringenin-loaded chitosan/ALG core–shell nanoparticles were developed by Maity et al. (2017). Naringenin is a poorly water-soluble flavanone present in citrus fruits, having antioxidant and antihyperglycemic activities, able in preventing absorption of glucose from the intestine of diabetes-induced rats

(Ortiz-Andrade et al., 2008). In order to improve its absorption in the intestine preventing its rapid elimination due to enzymatic metabolism in gut and liver after oral administration, modified drug delivery systems represent a promising strategy. In this work, ALG-coated chitosan nanoparticles, having mean sizes of 150–300 nm and pH-controlled slow sustained release, have been successfully developed for the treatment of diabetes after oral administration, exploiting the presence of chitosan to achieve controlled drug delivery and ALGs for their mucoadhesive properties. Ex vivo and in vivo studies demonstrated the safety of the nanoparticles, as confirmed by the histological study of treated rats' liver and intestine, and their strong mucoadhesive properties to the rat intestinal lumen, thus allowing a slow and sustained drug release enhancing the permeability of the natural compound from the intestinal microvilli to the circulatory system. The effectiveness of naringerin-loaded core–shell nanoparticles in reducing free iron content along with arachidonic acid and deoxyribose degradation was found to be higher compared to the free compound, thus showing the high potential of the oral administration of naringerin. Another interesting flavonoid, quercetin, has been deeply investigated in different delivery systems for overcoming its instability, low water solubility, and extensive first-pass metabolism, thus exploiting its many activities (antidiabetic, antioxidant, anticarcinogenic, antiradical, antiinammatory, antimutagenic, antiangiogenic, antiviral, antibacterial, and antiaging) (Montenegro et al., 2007; Caddeo et al., 2016a; Caddeo et al., 2016b). Recently, this bioflavonoid has been studied for its antidiabetic properties using carboxypropionylated pH-responsive porous microparticles for sustained oral delivery (Mukhopadhyay et al., 2016). Quercetin-loaded ALG microparticles showed excellent EE% (94%) of the bioflavonoid with a controlled release that was retarded in the stomach and complete in alkaline intestine. The authors demonstrated the safety of this novel ALG microparticles, since any significant changes in body weight, food intake, water intake, hair loss or hair color difference and behavior were noticed in polymeric microparticle treated rats as compared to control animals. Furthermore, a significant and sustained (up to 24 h) hypoglycemic response after 2–3 h of oral delivery in diabetic rats was observed, being this data related to quercetin retarded (acid pH in the stomach) and sustained (alkaline intestine) release that helps in achieving significant glycemic control in diabetics. Quercetin was also encapsulated in chitosan-coated ALG microspheres prepared by a simple ionic cross-linking technology with sodium ALG and chitosan (Hazra et al., 2015). The technological and physicochemical characterization of these microparticles confirmed the presence of spherical microspheres with rough and nonporous surface. With high EE% (80%) of quercetin, with no significant differences depending on the amount of polymers. Interestingly, release studies showed that the amount of drug delivered depends on the chitosan concentration, since it appreciably decreased and become steady with the increase on the polymer concentration, probably related to an increase in the densities of the polymer matrix and the formation of larger microspheres. ALG-chitosan microparticles have been recently developed for the delivery of icariin, the main active flavonoid glucoside isolated from Herba epimedii (*Epimedium brevicornum Maxim.*), for the potential oral treatment of ulcerative colitis induced in rats by trinitrobenzensulfonic acid (TNBS) (Wang et al., 2016). Herein, authors evaluated whether pretreatment with icariin-loaded microspheres could protect against TNB/ethanol-induced colon injury, used as the classical model of inflammatory bowel disease, because it is the most similar animal model closed to the pathogenesis of human. In vivo results showed that the group pre-treated orally with icariin-loaded microspheres could significantly decrease the colon mucosa damage index. Furthermore, histological observations showed the presence of a slight damage in colonic mucosa of animals pre-treated with microspheres, while the model group treated with TNBS showed serious injury of colonic mucosa, related to the increase of the pro-inflammatory mediator expressions. The targeted icariin-loaded microspheres were able to decrease the production and gene expression of inflammatory mediators (TNF-a, IL-6 and IL-1b) and cytokines. Furthermore, the carriers cross-linked by glutaraldehyde were able to increase the residence of drugs in the colon, thus avoiding drug loss in the upper regions of the digestive system (Wang et al., 2016). Giri et al. (2017) recently reported a novel formulation of liposome encapsulated ALG beads coated with Eudragit S-100 as a carrier for colon targeting of capsaicin. Capsaicin is an alkaloid with a strong effectiveness on relieving pain and a chemopreventive activity in various human cancer models (Clark et al., 2016). Unfortunately, its many drawbacks such as poor bioavailability, quick first-pass metabolism, and the short half-life strongly limit capsaicin clinical use. In order to overcome these limits, liposomes coated with a specific polymer such as sodium ALG, could represent a promising solution for the oral target colonic delivery. The preliminary physicochemical and technological characterization of capsaicin-loaded liposomes confirmed their incorporation into ALG hydrogel beads and coating with Eudragit S-100, with only a minimum interaction between the natural compound and other excipients. Interestingly, Eudragit-coated ALG beads allowed a slight drug release (<30%) in stomach and intestine and released the largest amount of drug (>70%) into the colonic region. The increasing interest for pH-sensitive ALG properties is confirmed by the increasing number of recent articles in which different approaches on ALG responsiveness to pH variation along the GIT are exploited as attractive option for the development of oral colon-specific drug delivery devices. To confirm this, recently, ALG hydrogel was exploited by Lei et al. (2017) to encapsulate nobiletin-loaded nanoemulsion droplets, aiming to control drug crystallization and release rate. Nobiletin is a characteristic citrus polymethoxylated flavone with interesting bioactivities such as anticancer, anti-dementia, anti-atherosclerosis, and anti-inflammatory effects. In this work, a nanoemulsion filled ALG hydrogel matrix was developed by the in situ internal gelling method of $CaCO_3$-GDL (D-glucono-d-lactone) system, to stabilize nobiletin in nanoemulisons thus preventing nobiletin precipitation in the GIT. The morphological studies showed that nanoemulsion-filled ALG hydrogels had a flat and slight porous structure, with droplets homogenously embedded in the network of the hydrogels. The hydrogel was able to ensure a controlled release of nobiletin at low pH (1.2) and a burst effect at pH 7.4, related to the corrosion of the hydrogel (Figure 20.5). Authors showed that nobiletin had worse physical stability and higher bioaccessibility when loaded in nanoemulsions, while ALG hydrogels provided better EE%, with lower lipolysis rate/extent and bioaccessibility due to the controlled release, thus potentially supporting the sustainable absorption of functional components. Furthermore, hydrogel was able to prevent the formation of nobiletin crystals during digestion, whose separation were clearly evident in case of nanoemulsion systems, thus confirming the potential of these delivery systems for the oral delivery of nobiletin. Abd El-Ghaffar et al. (2012) described an improved and simplified emulsification method for the preparation of polyglycidyl methacrylate grafted sodium ALG (PGMA-g-SA) hydrogels for the oral delivery of the vitamin riboflavin. In particular, PGMA was used to reinforce the structure of sodium ALG and increase its strength. Scanning electron microscopic SEM images showed that PGMA-g-SA hydrogels morphology had very narrow micropores with smooth layers and cracks on their surface. Riboflavin entrapment efficiency was found to be higher in the PGMA-g-SA hydrogels. The PGMA grafting onto sodium ALG affected the release of riboflavin, since a slowest release was found with the increase of PGMA grafting degree. Furthermore, the release was found to be pH sensitive, with a much higher amount of riboflavin released at pH 7.5 in respect to acidic pH value (1.2). Riboflavin controlled release was also studied by Messaoud and co-workers by shellac-coated ALG liquid-core capsules produced by reverse spherification (Messaoud et al., 2016). In this work, different combinations of ALG and shellac (a purified resinous secretion of lac insects [*Kerria lacca*]), were evaluated to control the physicochemical properties of the final liquid-core capsules, testing three different concentrations (1, 5 and 10% wt.) of shellac and two shellac coating mechanisms (Ca^{2+} reticulation and acid precipitation). Shellac is a nontoxicity and biodegradable complex mixture of polar and non-polar components having excellent film forming and protective properties, widely used as adhesives, thermoplastics, sealants, and coating materials in food and pharmaceutical industries (Aulton et al., 1995). In this work, riboflavin retarded release was achieved by coating the ALG capsules with an additional layer of shellac, whose structure was confirmed by SEM images. Interestingly, the retention efficiency of the prepared shellac-coated capsules was affected by the procedure employed to add the external shellac layer, since Ca^{2+} shellac reticulation leads to a higher retention of riboflavin along the GIT, especially after heating above the glass transition temperature of shellac. Based on the obtained results, the authors conclude asserting that this system could represent a promising strategy for the development of macro and microcapsules with pH-sensitive release behavior for the oral delivery of low molecular weight drugs, thus ensuring the intestine targeting. The increased interest of researchers on ALG microparticles in pharmaceutical and biomedical fields confirms its potential use as an effective matrix for drug and cell delivery. Concerning oral delivery of natural compounds, increasing attention has been paid to polyphenols (curcumin, resveratrol) due to their many different activities such as antioxidant, anti-inflammatory, anti-carcinoma, antimicrobial, antiviral, and cardioprotective properties able in reducing the risk of chronic diseases (Hu et al., 2016). Unfortunately, the poor oral bioavailability, low solubility, and instability in acidic pH, strongly limit the clinical application of polyphenols. In particular, curcumin, a natural polyphenol derived from the rhizome of turmeric (*Curcuma longa Linn.*), is been widely studied and different drug delivery systems have been developed for improving its oral bioavailability. Among different strategies, Petchsomrit et al. (2017) recently reported the development of curcumin-loaded floating ALG-based sponges, constitutes by self-microemulsifying drug delivery systems (SMEDDS) within a floating sponge (microporous polymeric materials), as a novel gastroretentive delivery system for the treatment of GI diseases The preliminary physicochemical and technological characterization of this formulation highlight its potentiality as novel floating oral dosage form, thanks to the possibility to overcome the typical problems of SMEDDS, mainly related to instability and drug precipitation during storage, exploiting the peculiar low-density flotation properties of sponges. Loading curcumin-SMEDDS in composite sponges, a gradual and sustained release of curcumin was obtained after 8 h, related to sponges flotation. In particular, ALG-based sponges prepared with 4% ALG and 15% curcumin-SMEDDS were selected as the best formulation based on its physical appearance, drug loading capacity, and in vitro drug release profile. Furthermore, this formulation exhibited no oil leakage in sponges, uniform weight, high drug loading, and the highest value of entrapment efficiency (92%). In order to overcome the instability problem of curcumin, different encapsulation strategies have been developed such as liposomes, nanoparticles, inclusion complexes, and micelles. Among them, the polymer–drug conjugation represents a valid approach for the delivery of hydrophobic drugs (Zhou et al., 2010). In this field, Sarika et al. (2016a) recently reported an ALG–curcumin conjugate for the oral administration of this drug and target activity on hepatocytes by attaching a galactose moiety on ALG through Schiff's base reaction involving amino and aldehyde groups. In vitro release studies showed a faster and higher delivery of curcumin at low pH value when loaded in the galactosylated ALG–curcumin conjugate, due to the breakage of the Schiff's base. Interestingly, a significant enhanced target activity to HepG2 cells was observed in the galactosylated polymer–drug conjugate in respect to the non galactosylated ALG–drug conjugate, with a significantly higher cytotoxicity, probably due to the presence of the galactose moiety that enhanced the cell internalization capability (Sarika et al., 2016a). Another interesting aspect related to drug conjugates is their ability in promoting passive tumor targeting through enhanced permeation and retention (EPR) effect, as recently reported (Figure 20.6) (Maeda, 2010). Based on this, curcumin was covalently conjugated to the C-6 carboxylate functionality of hydrophilic, biodegradable, and biocompatible natural polymer sodium ALG through esterification reaction (Dey and Sreenivasan, 2014). ALG–curcumin conjugate was found to increase drug water solubility in respect of the free curcumin, and able in self-aggregating in nanosized micelles when dispersed in aqueous solution, thus enhancing curcumin stability in water. Interestingly, Alg–curcumin conjugate showed a greater cytotoxic effect, even at low concentration, compared to free curcumin. The authors related this data to the presence of the coating layer of the hydrophilic ALG that would improve the systemic circulation time of curcumin due to the enhanced aqueous solubility, better cellular internalization, and improved stability of curcumin, with enhanced EPR effect. Another strategy involving ALGs for curcumin delivery is represented by nanogel, nanoscale sized hydrogels formed from hydrophilic or amphiphilic polymer networks by physical/chemical interactions. Sarika et al. (2016b) reported the preparation of nanogels prepared by inverse miniemulsion technique using ALG and gelatin nanogel (Alg Ald-Gel), for improving the therapeutic efficacy of curcumin in breast cancer cells. Herein,

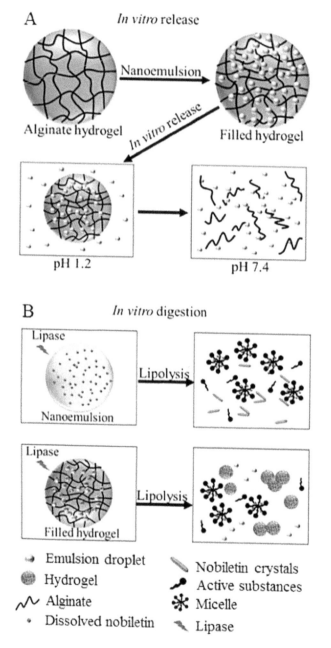

FIGURE 20.5   (See color insert.) Schematic illustrations of (A) in vitro release behavior and (B) in vitro digestion behavior for nanoemulsions and filled ALG hydrogels.

Source: Reprinted with permission from Lei et al., 2017. © 2017 Elsevier.

nanogels showed spherical morphology, higher curcumin loading capacity and fast release at acidic pH. The nanogels were found to be safe, since less than 5% of hemolysis was found, thus highlighting their high compatibility with only a minimum interaction with blood components in the blood stream. Results of in vitro anticancer activity of unloaded and curcumin-loaded Alg Ald-gel, performed on human breast carcinoma cells (MCF-7), showed that unloaded nanogels had no cytotoxic effect on MCF-7 cells at all concentrations. Interestingly, curcumin-loaded Alg Ald-gel showed lower toxicity compared to the free drug, probably due to the controlled release of the drug. Furthermore, intracellular uptake studies confirmed that curcumin is localized within the nanogel, thus it is protected from degradation and hydrolysis in physiological condition (Sarika et al., 2016b).

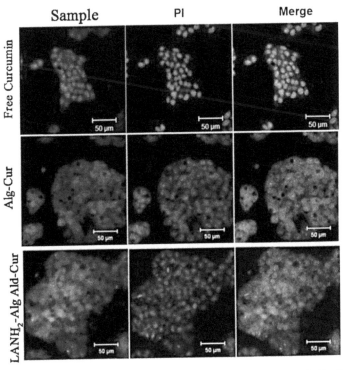

FIGURE 20.6   (See color insert.) Cellular uptake of free curcumin (row 1) Alg-Cur (row 2) and LANH$_2$-Alg Ald-Cur (row 3) by HepG2 cells observe under CLSM signal from curcumin (column 1) and PI (column 2) was separately obtained and merged (column 3). LANH$_2$-Alg Ald-Curcumin shows higher intensity as a result of increased level of particle internalization compared to Alg-Curcumin and free curcumin.

Source: Reprinted with permission from Sarika et al., 2016a. © 2016 Elsevier.

ALGs have also used for the development of drug delivery systems for topical administration. In particular, nanocarriers with an oily core (made of triglycerides) and a protective shell of calcium ALG (calcium ALG-based nanocarriers, CaANCs) were prepared by an accelerated nanoemulsification polymer cross-linking method, for the topical delivery of curcumin (Nguyen et al., 2015). CaANCs were found to form a stable dispersion in a carbomer-based hydrogel, thus representing a promising potential topical formulation. Curcumin loading allowed increasing its water solubility and antioxidant activity, thanks to the presence of the calcium ALG shell able in protecting the drug dissolved in the oil phase. Furthermore, the delivery system allowed increasing the amount of curcumin penetrated into the skin from the aqueous galenic formulation, without the addition of enhancers or occlusion systems. Results of ex vivo cutaneous penetration experiments demonstrated that curcumin-loaded CaANCs were able to improve the amount of drug into the epidermis with no risk of transdermal delivery or systemic undesired side effects, thus being a suitable delivery system for both cosmetic use and the treatment of superficial skin diseases with no damage to the dermis (Nguyen et al., 2015). Among topical application, topical chemotherapy is reaching increasing attention for its potentiality in the treatment of breast cancer directly onto the skin, in those cases in which cancer cells are limited to the superficial layer. In this field, an ALG and gelatin bilayer film containing Hidrox® was developed as a novel potential topical chemotherapeutic agent (Ng and Tan, 2015). Hidrox® is a commercial olive extract enriched in hydroxytyrosol, a phenolic compound from olives with protective effect on normal cells and selective antitumor activities on cancerous cells. In this work, Hidrox® loaded bilayer films were prepared by a smooth and homogenous morphology, confirming the compatibility between the polymer matrix and Hidrox, and probably related to the presence of gelatin in sodium ALG films able in promoting homogenous dispersion of the drug in the film. Film characterization confirmed that Hidrox was uniformly distributed and that the combination of ALG and gelatin might play a critical role in drug dispersion. Results of in vitro release experiments confirmed that hydrogels were able to release greater amount of Hidrox compared to films, in which several mechanisms are involved including the hydration of polymeric films, swelling and diffusion of the gel and drug in the polymer matrix. Herein, the authors reported that the involved patterns in drug release were mainly related to their swelling properties. At the first stage of release experiments, both hydrogel and films showed a fast release of hydroxytyrosol, due to the presence of drug molecules at their surface. Afterward, the drug release rate from the films decreased depending on the time required for the drug to diffuse from the inner polymer matrix onto the film surface. Cell proliferation assay performed on human breast cancer cells (MCF-7) showed a dose-dependent effect, with Hidrox film having a lower cytotoxic effect due to the lower drug concentration. On the base of these results, the authors conclude that bilayer film containing Hidrox could represent a valid new approach for topical chemotherapy (Ng and Tan, 2015). Interestingly, sodium ALG hydrocolloids have been proposed also for the delivery of *Centella asiatica* with antimicrobial activity in various wound models such as abrasion, excision, and infection wound models in comparison with the commercial product (Jin et al., 2015). *Centella asiatica* is constituted by different components (asiaticoside, asiatic acid, and madecassic acid) with many activities in treating systemic scleroderma and keloids, and excellent bacteriostatic and anti-inflammatory activity (Jin et al., 2015). The effectiveness of this formulation after the topical application was confirmed by in vivo results, highlighting its capability in promoting the healing effect in excision, infection, and abrasion wounds in rats. In this study, sodium ALG was used as the base of the hydrocolloid system due to its high biocompatibility and excellent hydrocolloid forming properties. In fact, previous studies confirmed the ability of ALG hydrogels to retain fluids and maintain a moist environment at the wound site thus accelerating the wound healing process (Boateng et al., 2008). Concerning hydrogels, increasing attention has been paid to their artificial conjugation with inorganic components. In this field, the combination of ALG hydrogel beads with magnetic $CoFe_2O_4$ nanoparticles (MCFO) was recently proposed by Amiri et al. (2017) through a co-precipitation method using caffeine as a green novel precursor in order to alkalinize the medium. In this work, chlorpheniramine maleate was used as model drug. Physicochemical and technological characterization showed the presence of homogeneous small MCFO nanoparticles of almost 10 nm in diameter. Furthermore, CFO/chlorpheniramine maleate ALG beads were found to be spherical, fine unique and homogenous gel structure, related to the interfacial interactions between ALG chains and magnetic nanoparticles that could possibly act as inter-molecular cross-linkers. Hydrogel properties such as swelling behavior, EE%, and release rate, varied based on the pH and composition of the beads. Swelling behavior was lower at pH 1.2 in respect to pH 7.4, and rises with time since it was fast at the beginning and then slow. Interestingly, swelling degree reduced with increasing nanoparticles and ALG content, probably because of the formation of rigid and compacted network with higher cross-linker concentration. Authors found that pH values affected both EE% (higher at pH 7.4) and drug release, with a more controlled and prolonged release due to the chlorpheniramine maleate trapping inside the carbon pores and cavities. In particular, drug diffusion is controlled by the protonation and deprotonation of carboxylic acids, since deprotonation of bead's carboxylic acid group occurring at neutral pH value, promotes higher swelling with consequent greater drug diffusion through polymeric hydrogel beads. The prepared hydrogels were biocompatible, since no cytotoxic effect was found on U87 human glioblastoma cancer cell line. Based on these results, authors conclude that the prepared stimuli-responsive beads can be exploited as novel application in different fields such as biomedical, pharmaceutical, regenerative medicine, and tissue engineering (Amiri et al., 2017).

ALG-based delivery systems for topical application of natural compounds is not only restricted to hydrocolloids but also even include microparticles. In this field, Noppakundilograt et al. 2015 developed sodium ALG microcapsules prepared by the Shirasu Porous Glass membrane emulsification and subsequent cross-linking by $CaCl_2$ for the delivery of eucalyptus oil, an essential oil with antimicrobial activity against Gram-positive bacteria (Noppakundilograt et al., 2015). Herein, the authors focused on investigating the effects of varying the concentration of sodium ALG, eucalyptus oil, and $CaCl_2$ on physicochemical and technological properties of microcapsules. In particular, microcapsules mean diameter increased with increasing encapsulating sodium ALG concentrations, but it was found that average size decreased with increasing the amount of eucalyptus oil loading and $CaCl_2$ cross-linking concentrations. Even if the cross-linking time did not significantly affect the microcapsule diameters, a significant influence on the release efficiency was found. In particular, using 0.1% w/v sodium ALG, 20%v/v eucalyptus oil and cross-linked with 1.0% w/v of $CaCl_2$ for 30 min, allowed obtaining microcapsules with 88% eucalyptus oil loading concentration. ALG microcapsules provided a controlled release following the Ritger–Peppas model, with a complete release of the encapsulated oil over 10 days, demonstrating that the rate-limiting step was affected by ionic cross-link density between the ALG and Ca^{2+} ions. At the same time, Lou et al. (2015) developed slow-release sodium ALG and pectin microcapsules for the delivery of *Lithospermum erythrorhizon* extract, recently proven to promote wound healing, accelerate epithelialization, angiogenesis, cell proliferation, induce granulation tissues proliferation, also showing anti-bacterial activity against Gram-negative and Gram-positive bacteria (Kontogiannopoulos et al., 2011; Liang et al., 2013). Animals studies confirmed that sodium ALG/pectin L. erythrorhizon microcapsules were able to significantly reduce the wound area (91.3%) after 11 days of treatment, due to the presence of the β, β-dimethylacrylshikonin that promotes cell growth and collagen growth,

growth factor synthesis, and wound healing (Lou et al., 2015). A recent medical application of ALG regards the bone tissue regeneration. It has been recently reported the preparation of chitosan nanoparticles incorporated into scaffolds containing ALG and gelatin, for the sustained and prolonged release of silibinin, a plant-derived flavonolignan (Leena et al., 2017). The idea of this work was to exploit the specific properties of selected raw materials in terms of controlled degradation and similarity to bone extracellular matrix, for tissue engineering applications, thus investigating the potential activity of silibinin in the promotion of bone formation. Silibinin-loaded chitosan nanoparticles prepared by ionic gelation technique showed a mean diameter of about 200–250 nm. Nanoparticles were incorporated into scaffolds containing ALG and gelatin, synthesized by freeze-drying technique, and then analyzed in terms of swelling, biodegradation and protein adsorption, critical design variables in fabricating scaffold materials. Swelling of scaffolds in phosphate-buffered saline at 37°C was found to increase in the first hour then decrease after 24 h, probably related to a decrease in water uptake ability. The presence of ALG and gelatin favors protein adsorption, whose amount affects the rate of cell adhesion onto scaffolds and the growth of the cells, both important for bone tissue engineering application. Furthermore, scaffolds were found to be biocompatible as they were nontoxic to mouse mesenchymal stem cells (MSCs, C3H10T1/2). Interestingly, scaffolds loaded with 50 M of silibinin–chitosan nanoparticles were able to stimulate osteoblast differentiation at cellular and molecular levels. Furthermore, the authors showed that silibinin release regulated microRNAs involved in the bone morphogenetic protein pathway, thus promoting osteoblast differentiation. Based on these evidences, authors suggested the potential activity of silibinin-loaded chitosan nanoparticles loaded in ALG–gelatin scaffolds for promoting a sustained and prolonged drug release, and their use as promising candidates for bone tissue engineering applications (Leena et al., 2017).

20.5 GENE THERAPY

Gene therapy is a potent approach to the treatment of potentially lethal diseases such as cancer and genetic disorders by insertion of genetic material (e.g., plasmid, siRNA, etc.) within the cells. This technique has been conceived as a result of the great progress of molecular biology methods developed since the 1980s. In particular, gene therapy involves transferring one or more healthy genes in a diseased cell, in order to cure disorders caused by their absence or defect. Therefore, it is first necessary to identify the single gene or the different genes responsible for the genetic disease. Second, it is possible to try replacing diseased genes, employing a suitable vector and, by which defective sequences can be replaced consenting the proteins' synthesis necessary for proper metabolic function. This technique is known as "transfection."

Gene therapy concerns large DNA molecules (plasmids, pDNAs), oligonucleotides, and RNA such as small interfering (siRNA) or messenger RNA. The clinic use limitation of this nucleic material is hindered by the lack of optimal delivery systems. In fact, administered as naked molecules, the siRNAs/pDNAs are rapidly degraded by serum nuclease and by RNAse A. Furthermore, the anionic charge of the phosphate groups present on the siRNAs/pDNAs backbone, leads to an unfavorable interaction with the anionic phospholipids of cell membranes, resulting in a negligible cellular uptake. Among the many types of carriers useful for delivery of genetic material, polymers play a fundamental role in this field as polycations for plasmids (Licciardi et al., 2012) and siRNA delivery (Cavallaro et al., 2014). The polycations characteristic is conferred by protonable amine groups at physiological or neutral pH, that allow them to interact with the numerous negative DNA charges, due to the presence of phosphate groups, and consequently preventing the electrostatic repulsion between DNA and cell surface. Furthermore, these polymers have also been efficacy used for the nanoparticles formulation to transport and deliver different genetic material (Nograles et al., 2012; Israel et al., 2015).

20.5.1 ALG APPLICATIONS FOR NUCLEIC MATERIALS

The presence of carboxyl groups in ALG molecules, render this polymer unsuitable for use in gene therapy. The use of the chemical derivatization of ALG chain to obtain polycations together with emulsion method or iono-tropic gel technologies are strategies used to apply ALGs in gene therapy (Table 20.3).

Wang et al. (2015) engineered a novel lipopolysaccharide-amine (LPSA) brush copolymer as a cytosolic delivery vector by introducing anionic polysaccharide of oxidized ALG and cholesterol to polyethyleneimine (PEI; 1.8 kDa) acting as backbone and side chains, respectively. Encouragingly, LPSA can spontaneously and quickly self-assemble into nanopolymersomes in water at a concentration higher than $1.38 \times 10-3$ mg/mL. As a gene vector, NPs obtain higher than 95% transfection efficiency in MSCs in vitro and induce significant angiogenesis in zebrafish when delivering plasmid encoding vascular endothelial growth factor DNA (pVEGF). To explore their extracellular delivery stability and storage stability, the authors have investigated the stability of empty or pDNA-loaded LPSA NPs (pNPs) under analogous physiological environments and different storage conditions, monitoring the changes in size, zeta potential, disassembly, and transfection efficiency. In particular, considering that pNPs will be exposed to a poly-anionic environment during in vivo application, their relative stability has been evaluated using heparin as polyanion model. At 15 min of incubation, increasing the heparin concentration, the amount of displaced pDNA increases and the complete displacement occurs at heparin concentration ≥ 20 mg/mL, equivalently the complete displacement concentration of ~ 10 mg heparin/µg pDNA (~ 1000 IU heparin/µg pDNA), which is much higher than the value of PEI derivatives (0.4 IU heparin/µg pDNA). In order to estimate the toxicity of pNPs, the authors also evaluated the damage of vectors to mito-chondria of MSCs after transfection. In fact, it has been reported that PNPs can induce significant damage to mitochondria and will lead to the release of cytochrome C, subsequent induction of executioner caspases and apoptosis induction (Hunter et al., 2010). The estimated parameter was the loss of MMP. pNPs do not cause severe loss of MMP; MMP of MSCs decreases with the increase of N/P ratio; the pNP groups at any N/P ratio have higher MMP compared with the PEI 25 k group, which loses about 20% of MMP. At N/P of 60, the optimal for in vitro transfection, the MMP of pNP group is close to that of the untreated group (N/P = 0) (Wang et al., 2015).

TABLE 20.3 A List of Research Articles on ALGs and Genetic Material Delivery Published During the Last Years.

Type of ALG	Preparation methods	Carrier	Authors	Year
Sodium ALG	Chemical modification	Nanopolymersomes	Wang et al.	2015
Sodium ALG	Ionotropic gelation	Nanogels	Zhao et al.	2012
Sodium ALG	Ionotropic gelation	Nanoparticles	Jain et al.	2012
Alginic acid (AA)	Electrostatic interaction	Ternary complexes	Kurosaki et al.	2009
AA	Self-assembled/ electrostatic interaction	Cationic liposomes	Chen et al.	2015
Sodium ALG	Emulsion method	Microspheres	Nograles et al.	2012

The most commonly used methods for formulation of ALG-based genetic delivery systems is the ionic interaction method. In particular, ALG molecules are used either for the formation of nanogels or for coating of DNA–polycations complexes in order to reduce their toxicity.

Zhao et al. (2012) formulated nanocarriers of ALG/CaCO$_3$/DNA mixing a solution containing Ca^{2+} ions and DNA with a solution containing CO$_3{}^{2-}$ ions and different amounts of sodium ALG (0.1–5.0 µg) by co-precipitation method. The influence of ALG on nanoparticles stability and DNA transfection activity were evaluated. Considering that, as it is well known, carriers for genetic material delivery require a high level of gene expression as well as a low level of cytotoxicity, the nanoparticles toxicology was also evaluated. Owing to the presence of ALG, the growth of CaCO$_3$-based co-precipitates was retarded and, consequently, the size of the nanoparticles could be controlled and the stability of the nanoparticles enhance. As know, ALG has a pKa around 3.5 and in the basic and neutral solutions, the ALG chains exist in the form of stretching conformation due to the repulsion between the deprotonated carboxyl groups. ALG chains have the ability to bind Ca^{2+} cations reducing the electrostatic repulsion between –COO$^-$ groups in the ALG chains and improving their affinity with water molecules. As a result, ALG/CaCO$_3$/DNA nanoparticles with the high ALG content in the surface layer were formed. The negatively charged ALG chains improve the colloidal stability of the nanoparticles in the aqueous medium. The results also showed that the transfection efficiency of ALG/CaCO$_3$/DNA nanoparticles is strongly dependent on the ALG amount. In fact, the gene expression increases with increasing ALG achieves a maximum value at the ALG of 1 µg and, then, decreases with further ALG increase. Furthermore, the authors have been studied also the effect of a second plasmid (pEGFP-C1) to verify the efficiency of ALG/CaCO$_3$/DNA nanoparticles in the transfection activities. The intensity of green fluorescence in the cells transfected by ALG/CaCO$_3$/DNA nanoparticles is much higher than that of CaCO$_3$/DNA nanoparticles. For both reported plasmids (pGL3-Luc and pEGFP-C1), ALG modification results in the significantly enhanced gene expressions (Zhao et al 2012). In the end, regarding the nanoparticles toxicity, MTT test showed that their cell viabilities are higher than 90% after being transfected by ALG/CaCO$_3$/DNA nanoparticles for 48 h, implying that these nanoparticles do not have apparent cytotoxicity.

The advantage of employing polymers such as ALG is that it facilitates the controlled release of DNA from the polymer matrix system. Moreover, physical encapsulation of DNA enables protection from the enzymes and other plasma proteins during its transit from blood to the site of action. Jain et al (2012) have developed tuftsin-modified cross-linked ALG nanoparticles with encapsulated reporter (green fluorescent protein, GFP) and murine interleukin-10 (mIL-10) expressing plasmid DNA. Tuftsin is a tertapeptide made up of L-threonine, L-lysine, L-proline, and L-arginine that is known to stimulate the immune function of various cells, including macrophages (primarily), neutrophils, and monocytes. It has been found to increase the macrophage-mediated phagocytosis, macrophage migration index, spleno-cytes proliferation, and bactericidal and tumoricidal activities. Nanopar-ticles were prepared by premixing a solution of ALG with the plasmid DNA (EGFP-N1 or mIL-10) and a calcium chloride solution dripped in the ALG solution. Then, the surface of the particles was modified using the peptide sequences with tuftsin and scrambled amino acid residues. The peptides had six positively charged L-arginine (i.e., RRRRRR) residues for anchoring to the negatively charged ALG nanoparticle surface; four L-glycine (i.e., GGGG) spacer residues; and either Thr–Lys–Pro–Arg residues of tuftsin or Pro–Thr–Lys–Arg residues of the scrambled sequence. When the concentra-tion of nanoparticles increased, the ζ potential values became increasingly negative as the peptide surface coverage decreased. Additionally, at higher nanoparticle concentrations, there was significant aggregation and precipita-tion. After surface modification, the variation of hydrodynamic diameter and the surface charge values showed a decreasing of diameter from 420 to 430 nm to around 280 – 290 nm. The relatively higher polydispersity index observed in the case of the blank (0.66 ± 0.08) and unmodified nanopar-ticles (0.67 ± 0.01) may have been due to more aggregated nanoparticles relative to more uniformly dispersed peptide-modified ALG nanoparticles (0.26 ± 0.01). The average ζ potential of DNA-encapsulated unmodified ALG nanoparticles was −45.8 mV, similar to the values observed for blank unmodified nanoparticles. These results confirm that the plasmid DNA was physically encapsulated in the ALG matrix and not adsorbed to the surface. When the ALG nanoparticle surface was modified with either scrambled peptide or tuftsin constructs, the average ζ potential values changed to 23.6 and 19.7 mV, respectively, due to the neutralization of the surface negative charge with excess of the positively charged L-arginine residues that anchored the peptides on the ALG surface. The stability study of encapsulated plasmid DNA due to processing conditions as well as upon exposure to DNase-I using agarose gel electrophoresis was also performed. This study showed that the ALG nanoparticles encapsulated DNA is highly stable and that DNA is also protected from enzymatic degradation by DNase-I. To assess the potential cytotoxicity of the control and surface-modified EGFP-N1 plasmid DNA-encapsulated ALG nanoparticles, the formulations were incubated at different amounts with J774A.1 macrophages. The cell viability showed that neither the blank, unmodified and scrambled peptide-modified nor the tufts unmodified ALG nanoparticle formulations induced any significant cytotox-icity when added to cells at 0.2 and 0.5 mg amounts per 200,000 cells. A significant decrease in cell viability to 60% with scrambled peptide-modified nanoparticles at 1 mg amount happened, indicating that higher concentration of the positive charge, imparted due to the scrambled peptide, is causing rupture of the cell membrane. However, this effect was not observed with tuftsin-modified nanoparticles even at 1 mg levels, where the cell viability was around 90%. The difference in the cytotoxicity profile of the tuftsin and scrambled peptide modified nanoparticles can be attributed to the uptake kinetics and mechanism of internalization of the two different versions of the nanoparticles. The tuftsin-modified nanoparticles are phagocytized through receptor-mediated endocytosis, whereas scrambled peptide nanoparticles may solely interact with negative charged cell membrane by electrostatic interactions and, hence, may cause some additional cytotoxicity. DNA encapsulated in unmodified nanoparticles and scrambled peptide-modified nanoparticles showed a transient expression for up to 72 h; the levels were significantly lower than those of tuftsin-modified nanoparticles. The maximum GFP concentration of 0.54 ng/mg of intracellular protein was observed after 48 h of transfection with tuftsin-modified nanoparticles. An initial transgene expression of naked plasmid and Lipofectin-complexed DNA was observed up to 24. However, the levels were significantly lower than any of the ALG formulations tested. Finally, in order to confirmation of GFP transfection with control and tuftsin-modified ALG nanoparticles, mIL-10 expressing plasmid DNA (i.e., pORF-mIL-10) was encapsulated in the same formulations and the transgene expression was evaluated at the transcriptional and translational levels. The polymerase chain reaction confirmed the presence of mIL-10 transcript from cells transfected with Lipofectin-complexed DNA and DNA-encapsulated in both scrambled peptide- and tuftsin-modified nanoparticles (Jain et al., 2012).

Another way to use ALG for genetic material delivery is the coating of nanocarriers characterized by a positive ζ potential which gives toxicity. ALG molecules coating the surface of carriers changing the ζ potential value from positive to negative showing a decreased cytotoxicity.

Kurosaki et al (2009) prepared ternary complexes composed by pDNA (pCMV-Luc)–PEI-polysaccharide in two steps. In the first step, pDNA and PEI solution (pH 7.4) were mixed and left for 15 min at room temperature, subsequently different polysaccharides (PL) such as Fucoidan, xanthan gum, AA, hyaluronic acid (HA), and chondroitin sulfate (CS) were mixed with pDNA/PEI complex at various charge ratios, ranging from 1:8:0 to 1:8:8, and left for another 15 min at room temperature. The addition of polysaccharides to the pDNA/PEI complex decreased its

ζ potential and reached a plateau at a charge ratio 1:8:6 of phosphate of pDNA: nitrogen of PEI: sulfate or carboxylate of polysaccharide; therefore, the ternary complex at a charge ratio of 1:8:6 was used throughout the study. The size and the potential changed from 72.0 ± 11.1 nm particle size and $+48.6 \pm 0.6$ mV for pDNA/PEI complex to 26.7 ± 6.1 nm and -29.0 ± 1.9 mV for pDNA/PEI/AA complex, which showed smaller dimensions between the various ternary complexes and a potential value comparable to other complexes.

Agglutination activities of complexes were evaluated (Figure 20.7) using erythrocytes from mice, and in particular a 2% (v/v) stock suspension was prepared. The pDNA/PEI complex agglutinated a lot of erythrocytes. On the other hand, in the ternary complexes pDNA/PEI/PL, any agglutination was not observed. Furthermore, cell viability of systems was determinate on B16-F10 cell line after 2 h of incubation and measured at 24 h after treatment. The pDNA/PEI complex significantly decreased cell viability, obtaining a value around 20%, whereas each ternary complex showed a value around 100% and more, as for the complex with AA which showed a value of 120%.

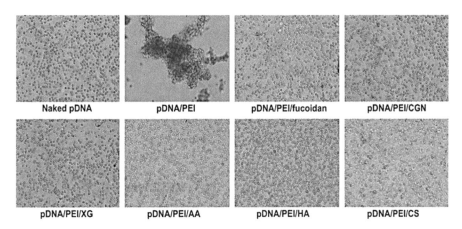

FIGURE 20.7 Agglutination with erythrocytes. Each complex was added to erythrocytes, and agglutinations were assessed. Agglutination was observed by phase microscopy (400 × magnification).

Source: Reprinted with permission from Kurosaki et al., 2009. © 2009 Elsevier.

Lastly, each complex containing pCMV-Luc was added to the B16-F10 cells to quantify uptake and gene expression. The pDNA/PEI/AA complex showed significantly lower uptakes than pDNA/PEI complex. Gene expression of each complex was evaluated by luciferase activity. The pDNA/PEI complex showed extremely high gene expression exceeded 10^{10} RLU/mg protein. On the other hand, ternary complexes were significantly lower than the pDNA/PEI complex, only the pDNA/PEI/CS complex, however, showed high gene expression exceeded 10^{10} RLU/mg protein (Kurosaki et al., 2009)

Biocompatible anionic polyelectrolytes, such as AA, HA, pectin (PC) from citrus peels, and polyglutamic acid (PG), has been widely used in gene delivery as coating for cationic liposome, due to positive charges can lead to serious cytotoxicity, which is the main reason limiting the clinical use of cationic liposome (Figure 20.8). In this field, Chen et al (2015) have evaluated the influence of polysaccharide coating on gene transfection efficiency and cytotoxicity of cationic liposome. Surface charge is an important indicator for the biocompatibility of gene carriers in bloodstream, the noncoated surface charge of liposome/pDNA is 30 mV, which is the main cause of cell toxicity. However, by adding anionic polyelectrolytes, the surface became negatively charged ranging from −10 to −30 mV in function of the amount of polyanionic chains. Despite the great reverse of surface charge to negative value, vectors have still maintained high transfection efficiency. In particular, transfection studies were performed in HeLa, MCF-7, and HepG2 cells at an initial cell density of 2×10^5 and the cells were kept under standard incubation conditions for 48 h. To further quantitatively determine the transfection efficiency, flow cytometry was measured for all coated liposomes (Figure 20.9) in all three cell lines considered. With increasing the coating of HA and PG, the fluorescence intensity observed in Hela cells showed little change, and that for AA and PC coating, the expression level just slightly decreased. The level of GFP expression with HA and PC coating was higher than liposome in MCF-7 cells, especially for PC coating, the GFP expression almost increased 10%. With increasing the coating of AA, the fluorescence intensity first increased, and then decreased with further increasing the concentration of AA. The GFP expression level observed in MCF-7 cells greatly reduced with increased coating of PG. To be noted, with PG coating, especially for PGL2, the percentage of HepG2 cells expressed GFP increased considerably, almost two-fold increase over liposome, which is a very intriguing result, because HepG2 cell is one of the notoriously difficult transfected cell lines (Munkonge et al., 2009; Miller et al., 2009). Further increasing PG coating, however, the cells produced with GFP decreased a lot. For HA coating, all the ratios (HAL1, HAL2 and HAL3) tested showed appreciably increased GFP expression of HepG2 cells. Through AA coating, the level of GFP expression reduced greatly especially at higher concentration.

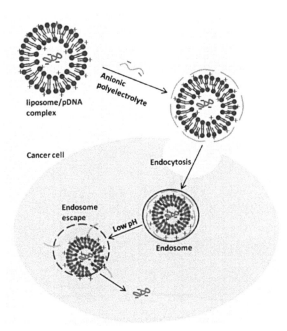

FIGURE 20.8   Schematic illustrations showing the self-assembly of various anionic poly-electrolytes (AA, HA, PC, and PG) with cationic liposome/pDNA complex and the process of cellular uptake and gene release.

Source: Reprinted with permission from Chen et al., 2015. © 2015 Elsevier.

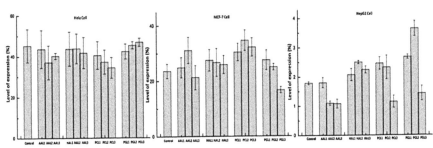

FIGURE 20.9   Transfection efficiency of liposome/pDNA complex (Control), AAL1, AAL2, AAL3, HAL1, HAL2, HAL3, PCL1, PCL2, PCL3, PGL1, PGL2, and PGL3 for Hela, MCF-7, and HepG2 cells as assessed by flow cytometry.

Source: Reprinted with permission from Chen et al., 2015. © 2015 Elsevier.

By coating with anionic polyelectrolyte, the surface positive charges could be shielded to reduce nonspecific interaction with serum components and minimize the cytotoxicity. In order to demonstrate the shielding effect of polyanionic, MTT assay was performed to determine the in vitro cytotoxicity of coated liposomes in Hela, MCF-7, and HepG2 cells. Figure 20.10 shows that coating with anionic polyelectrolyte exhibited improved cytocompatibility as compared to liposome/pDNA precursor (control) in all tested cells.

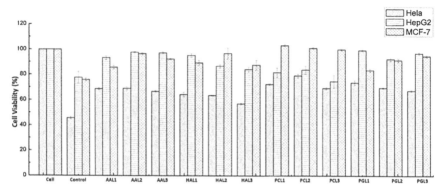

FIGURE 20.10   Cell viability of different polyanionic coated liposome/pDNA complex after incubation with Hela, MCF-7, and HepG2 cells.

Source: Reprinted with permission from Chen et al., 2015. © 2015 Elsevier.

Finally, the protective effect of coated polyanionic on pDNA from nuclease degradation was examined by DNase I, where naked pDNA shows complete degradation, in comparison, more pDNA could be recovered from coated liposome/pDNA complexes than the liposome/pDNA complex after sequential incubation with DNase I. These results indicate that polyanionic coating renders a significant protection to the plasmid against nuclease digestion (Chen et al., 2015).

In the end, another method widely used to form nanocarriers for genetic material delivery is the emulsion method. In their study, Nograles et al. (2012) have employed ALG to produce microspheres through emulsification technique for delivery of genetic material in a form of oral suspension dose delivered through the GIT of mice. In particular, the aim of work was to assess the capacity of orally administered pDNA loaded ALG microspheres to deliver pDNA carrying GFP reporter gene, into intestinal cells of mice. ALG microspheres were prepared through water-in-oil emulsion method,

1 ml of 9:1 isoamyl alcohol:3.5% (w/v) sodium ALG solution and 1% Span 80 were homogenized for about 20–30 s using homogenizer, after, a volume of 500 µl of 0.1 M CaCl$_2$ was added as a gelling agent. Plasmid DNA, which is to be encapsulated within microspheres, was added to CaCl$_2$ solution for improved "bio-beads"; and the volume of CaCl$_2$ was adjusted when prepared with appropriate amount of DNA, for instance, 20 µl of pDNA (5 µg) was added to 480 µl 0.1 M CaCl$_2$. The emulsion was vortexed vigorously at high speed for 1 min. The average diameter of microspheres was recorded at 46.88±3.07 µm. Results showed that there was no significant effect of pDNA loading on the overall size of pDNA-loaded microspheres. Significant reduction in microsphere size was noted upon incorporation of the emulsifier, Span 80, into the formulation. Therefore, subsequent experiments employed empty and pDNA-loaded microspheres that were formed in the presence of 1% Span 80 emulsifier in the formulation. A relatively higher loading capacities were observed at an initial load of 4, 5, or 6 µg of pDNA, whereby higher encapsulation efficiencies (EE%) were observed within the mean ranges of 72.9–74.4%. The EE% decreased significantly upon comparison of EE% for the initial load of 5 and 10 µg (74 vs. 56.3%, respectively). The maximum initial pDNA load, which showed both the highest EE% (72.9%) with an accompanying highest pDNA load (4.47 µg) were obtained with initial load of 6 µg pDNA as compared to other initial loads.

The in vitro pDNA release was evaluated using pDNA loaded (10 µg) microspheres in both acidic and basic environment of simulated GI conditions. The microspheres demonstrated shrinkage (Martoni et al., 2007) in acidic pH resulting to the minimal release of pDNA from the microspheres into the surrounding medium as measured from the absorbance of supernatant in pDNA release studies. Microsphere shrinkage offer protection of encapsulated material against the external environment (Vandenberg et al., 2001) while membrane swelling at alkaline pH (Martoni et al., 2007) increase the membrane pore sizes and cause the subsequent release of encapsulated material into suspending medium. Therefore, ALG microspheres may serve as efficient delivery vehicles for plasmid DNA molecules into the intestinal tissues; where alkaline pH ensues and whereby absorption and antigen presentation occur; rather than release within the acidic environment of the stomach.

pDNA delivery following oral administration of loaded ALG microspheres was evaluated among target tissues in animals. In vivo results of GFP biodistribution and dose–response assessments performed in this study suggest delivery of pVAX-GFP within the alkaline intestines environment where encapsulated pDNA are released from loaded ALG microspheres.

Within the intestinal epithelium, several mechanisms of transport and uptake of substances may occur which may involve both Peyer's patches (PP) and other non-PP tissue, such as enterocytes (Coppi et al., 2010). BALB/c mice were orally dosed with en(pVAX-GFP) ALG microspheres, and expression of GFP among cell suspensions of various organs were assessed in a 24 and 48 h timeframe. After oral delivery of en(pVAX-GFP) ALG microspheres, intestinal tissue samples showed the higher level of GFP expression with respect to blood, esophagus, and stomach. No GFP expression was observed in the liver and spleen (Nograles et al., 2012). These results indicate that ALG microspheres demonstrated efficient entrapment of plasmid DNA and showed good transfection ability after oral administration, showing a more consistent GFP expression in intestinal tissue samples.

SUMMARY

ALGs are natural polymers with biocompatible, biodegradable and nontoxic characteristics and possess well-defined physical and chemical properties. In particular, sodium ALG is an edible biocompatible coating polymer, water-soluble, approved by the US FDA as food additive and capable of forming a hydrogel polymer matrix which allows a good diffusion of the bioactive compounds. These aspects together with fine chemical modifications by combining ALGs with other natural and synthetic polymers have sustained the greater interest of the scientific community to use these natural polymers in a wide range of applications in different fields, pharmaceutical, nutraceutical, and gene delivery. The present chapter focuses on ALGs applied to herbal natural compounds and gene materials to improve their performance. In fact, they form a film able to avoid natural products from oxidation/degradation phenomena; are excellent carriers to enhance their shelf life, prolong their antioxidant efficiency, and also for adding nutritive value and functional properties to nutraceutical compounds. Moreover, in the delivery of nucleic acid materials, ALG derivatives have been widely used as polymeric backbones for the formation of systems which can be provided as valuable gene delivery carriers. Many efforts have been made to develop efficient non-viral methods, which include the creation of nanoparticles with encapsulated DNA, polycations, and vesicular systems.

KEYWORDS

- alginate derivatives
- alginate/chitosan
- alginate/sucrose
- Eudragit/alginate
- alginate/gelatin herbal products
- regulatory aspects
- nutraceutical
- pharmaceutical
- gene delivery
- nano- and microsystems

REFERENCES

Abd El-Ghaffar, M. A.; Hashem, M. S.; El-Awady, M. K.; Rabie, A. M. pH-Sensitive Sodium Alginate Hydrogels for Riboflavin Controlled Release. *Carb. Polymer.,* **2012,** *89,* 667–675.

Aluani, D.; Tzankova, V.; Kondeva-Burdina, M.; Yordanov, Y.; Nikolova, E.; Odzhakov, F.; Apostolov A.; Markova, T.; Yoncheva, K. Evaluation of Biocompatibility and Antioxidant Efficiency of Chitosan-Alginate Nanoparticles Loaded with Quercetin. *Int. J. Biol. Macromol.* **2017,** *103,* 771–782.

Amiri, M.; Salavati-Niasari, M.; Pardakhty, A.; Ahmadi, M.; Akbari, A. Caffeine: A novel Green Precursor for Synthesis of Magnetic CoFe$_2$O$_4$ Nanoparticles and pH-Sensitive Magnetic Alginate Beads for Drug Delivery. *Mater. Sci. Eng. C* **2017,** *76,* 1085–1093.

ASTM International. Standard Guide for Characterization and Testing of Alginates as Starting Materials Intended for Use in Biomedical and Tissue- Engineered Medical Products Application. 2006. ftp://185.72.26.245/Astm/2/01/Section%2013/ASTM1301/PDF/F2064.pdf (accessed Aug 31, 2017).

Aulton, M.; Cole, G.; Hogan, J. *Pharmaceutical Coating Technology;* Taylor &Francis: London, UK; 1995.

Balanč, B.; Đordevič, V.; Markovic, S.; Pjanovic, R.; Nedovic, V.; Bugarski, B. M. Novel Resveratrol Delivery Systems Based on Alginate-Sucrose and Alginate-Chitosan Microbeads Containing Liposomes. *Food Hydrocolloids* **2016,** *61,* 832–842.

Boateng, J. S.; Matthews, K. H.; Stevens, H. N.; Eccleston, G. M. Wound Healing Dressings and Drug Delivery Systems: A Review. *J. Pharm. Sci.* **2008,** *97,* 2892–2923.

Caddeo, C.; Díez-Sales, O.; Pons, R.; Carbone, C.; Ennas, G.; Puglisi, G.; Fadda, A. M.; Manconi, M. Cross-Linked Chitosan/Liposome Hybrid System for the Intestinal Delivery of Quercetin. *J. Colloid. Interface Sci.* **2016a,** *461,* 69–78.

Caddeo, C.; Nacher, A.; Vassallo, A.; Armentano, M. F.; Pons, R.; Fernàndez-Busquets, X.; Carbone, C.; Valenti, D.; Fadda, A. M.; Manconi, M. Effect of Quercetin and Resveratrol

Co-Incorporated in Liposomes Against Inflammatory/Oxidative Response Associated with Skin Cancer. *Int. J. Pharm.* **2016b,** *513,* 153–163.

Cavallaro, G.; Licciardi, M.; Amato, G.; Sardo, C.; Giammona, G.; Farra, R.; Dapas, B.; Grassi, M.; Grassi, G. Synthesis and Characterization of Polyaspartamide Copolymers Obtained by ATRP for Nucleic Acid Delivery. *Int. J. Pharm.* **2014,** *466,* 246–257.

CBI Ministry of Foreign Affairs. Product Factsheet: Alginates in Europe, 2015. https://www.cbi.eu/market-information/natural-food-additives/alginates/ (accessed Aug 28, 2017).

Celli, B. G.; Brooks, M. S.; Ghanem, A. Development and Evaluation of a Novel Alginate-Based in Situ Gelling System to Modulate the Release of Anthocyanins. *Food Hydrocolloids* **2016,** *60,* 500–508.

Chen, M.; Zeng, Z.; Qu, X.; Tang, Y.; Long, Q.; Feng, X. Biocompatible Anionic Polyelectrolyte for Improved Liposome Based Gene Transfection. *Int. J. Pharm.* **2015,** *490,* 173–179.

Clark, R.; Lee, S. H. Anticancer Properties of Capsaicin Against Human Cancer. *Anticancer Res.* **2016,** 36(3), 837–843.

Coppi, G.; Montanari; M.; Rossi, T.; Bondi, M.; Iannuccelli, V. Cellular Uptake and Toxicity of Microparticles in a Perspective of Polymyxin B Oral Administration. *Int. J. Pharm.* **2010,** *385,* 42–44.

De Cicco, F.; Porta, A.; Sansone, F.; Aquino, R. P.; Del Gaudio, P. Nanospray Technology for an in Situ Gelling Nanoparticulate Powder as a Wound Dressing. *Int. J. Pharm.* **2014,** *473,* 30–37.

Del Gaudio, P.; De Cicco, F.; Sansone, F.; Aquino, R. P.; Adami, R.; Ricci, M.; Giovagnoli, S. Alginate Beads as a Carrier for Omeprazole/SBA-15 Inclusion Compound: A Step Towards the Development of Personalized Pediatric Dosage Forms. *Carbohydr. Polym. 133,* **2015,** 464–472.

Deol, P. K.; Kaur, I. P. Improving the Therapeutic Efficiency of Ginger Extract for Treatment of Colon Cancer Using a Suitably Designed Multiparticulate System. *J. Drug Target* **2013,** *21*(9), 855–865.

Dey, S.; Sreenivasan, K. Conjugation of Curcumin onto Alginate Enhances Aqueous Solubility and Stability of Curcumin. *Carbohydr. Polym.* **2014,** *99,* 499–507.

Felgines, C.; Texier, O.; Besson, C.; Lyan, B.; Lamaison, J. L.; Scalbert, A. Strawberry Pelargonidin Glycosides are Excreted in Urine as Intact Glycosides and Glucuronidated Pelargonidin Derivatives in Rats. *Br. J. Nutr.* **2007,** *98,* 1126–1131.

Giri, T. K.; Bhowmick, S.; Maity, S. Entrapment of Capsaicin Loaded Nanoliposome in pH Responsive Hydrogel Beads for Colonic Delivery. *J. Drug Delivery. Sci. Technol.* **2017,** *39,* 417–422.

Grzanna, R.; Lindmark, L.; Frondoza, C. G. Ginger—An Herbal Medicinal Product with Broad Anti-Inflammatory Actions. *J. Med. Food.* **2005,** *8,* 125–132.

Gupta, P. K.; Jaiswal, A. K.; Asthana, S.; Verma, A.; Kumar, V.; Shukla, P.; Dwivedi, P.; Dube, A.; Mishra, P. R. Self-Assembled Ionically Sodium Alginate Cross-Linked Amphotericin B Encapsulated Glycol Chitosan Stearate Nanoparticles: Applicability in Better Chemotherapy and Non-Toxic Delivery in Visceral Leishmaniasis. *Pharm. Res.* **2015,** *32*(5), 1727–1740.

Hazra, M.; Mandal, D. D.; Mandal, T.; Bhuniya, S.; Ghosh, M. Designing Polymeric Microparticulate Drug Delivery System for Hydrophobic Drug Quercetin. *Saudi Pharm. J.* **2015,** *23,* 429–436.

Hoffman, F. A. Botanicals as "new" Drugs: US Development. *Epilepsy Behav.* **2015,** *52,* 338–343.

Hu, B.; Liu, X.; Zhang, C.; Zeng, X. Food Macromolecule Based Nanodelivery Systems for Enhancing the Bioavailability of Polyphenols. *J. Food Drug Anal.* **2016,** 1–13.

Hunter, A. C.; Moghimi, S. M. Cationic Carriers of Genetic Material and Cell Death: A Mitochondrial Tale. *Biochim. Biophys. Acta* **2010**, *1797,* 1203–1209.

Israel, L. L.; Lellouche, E.; Ostrovsky, S.; Yarmiayev, V.; Bechor, M.; Michaeli, S.; Lellouche, J. P. Acute in Vivo Toxicity Mitigation of PEI-Coated Maghemite Nanoparticles Using Controlled Oxidation and Surface Modifications toward siRNA Delivery. *ACS Appl. Mater. Interfaces* **2015**, *7,* 15240–15255.

Istenič, K.; Balanč, B. D.; Djordevjć, V. B.; Bele, M.; Nedović, V. A.; Bugarski, B. M.; Ulrih, N. P. Encapsulation of Resveratrol into Ca-Alginate Submicron Particles. *J. Food Eng.* **2015**, *167,* 196–203.

Jain, S., Amiji, M. Tuftsin-Modified Alginate Nanoparticles as a Noncondensing Macrophage-Targeted DNA Delivery System. *Biomacromolecules* **2012**, *13,* 1074–1085.

Jin, S. G.; Kim, K. S.; Yousaf, A. M.; Kim, D. W.; Jang, S. W.; Son, M. W.; Kim, Y. H.; Yong, C. S.; Kim, J. O.; Choi, H. G. Mechanical Properties and in Vivo Healing Evaluation of a Novel Centella Asiatica-Loaded Hydrocolloid Wound Dressing. *Int. J. Pharm.* **2015**, *490,* 240–247.

Kontogiannopoulos, K. N.; Assimopoulou, A. N.; Tsivintzelis, I.; Panayiotou, C.; Papageorgiou, V. P. Electrospun Fiber Mats Containing Shikonin and Derivatives with Potential Biomedical Applications. *Int. J. Pharm.* **2011**, *409,* 216–228.

Kurosaki, T.; Kitahara, T.; Kawakami, S.; Nishida, K.; Nakamura, J.; Teshima, M.; Nakagawa, H.; Kodama, Y.; To, H.; Sasaki, H. The Development of a Gene Vector Electrostatically Assembled with a Polysaccharide Capsule. *Biomaterials* **2009**, *30,* 4427–4434.

Lauro, M. R.; De Simone, F.; Iannelli, P.; Aquino, R. P. Preparations and Release Characteristics of Naringin and Naringenin Gastro-Resistant Microparticles by Spray-Drying. *J. Drug Delivery Sci. Technol.* **2007**, *17,* 119–124.

Lauro, M. R.; Crasci, L.; Carbone, C.; Aquino, R. P; Panico, A. M.; Puglisi, G. Encapsulation of a Citrus By-Product Extract: Development, Characterization And Stability Studies of a Nutraceutical with Antioxidant and Metalloproteinases Inhibitory Activity. *LWT Food Sci. Technol.* **2015**, *62,* 169–176.

Lauro, M. R.; Crasci, L.; Giannone, V.; Ballistreri, G.; Fabroni, S.; Sansone, F.; Rapisarda, P.; Panico, A. M.; Puglisi, G. An Alginate/Cyclodextrin Spray Drying Matrix to Improve Shelf Life and Antioxidant Efficiency of a Blood Orange By-Product Extract Rich in Polyphenols: MMPS Inhibition and Antiglycation Activity in Dysmetabolic Diseases. *Oxid. Med. Cell. Long.* **2017**, *2017.* https://doi.org/10.1155/2017/2867630 (accessed Nov 6, 2017).

Leena, R. S.; Vairamani, M.; Selvamurugan, N. Alginate/Gelatin Scaffolds Incorporated with Silibinin-Loaded Chitosan Nanoparticles for Bone Formation in Vitro. *Colloids Surf. B* **2017**, *158,* 308–318.

Lei, L.; Zhang, Y.; He, L.; Wu, S.; Li, B.; Li, Y. Fabrication of Nanoemulsion-Filled Alginate Hydrogel to Control the Digestion Behavior of Hydrophobic Nobiletin. *LWT Food Sci. Technol.* **2017**, *82,* 260–267.

Li, J.; Kim, S. Y.; Chen, X.; Park, H. J. Calcium-Alginate Beads Loaded with Gallic Acid: Preparation and Characterization. *Food Sci. Technol.* **2016**, *68,* 667–673.

Liang, D.; Sun, Y.; Shen, Y.; Li, F.; Song, X.; Zhou, E.; Zhao, F.; Liu, Z.; Fu, Y.; Guo, M.; Zhang, N.; Yang, Z.; Cao, Y. Shikonin Exerts Anti-Inflammatory Effects in a Murine Model of Lipopolysaccharide-Induced Acute Lung Injury by Inhibiting the Nuclear Factor-kappaB Signaling Pathway. *Int. Immunopharmacol.* **2013**, *16,* 475–480.

Licciardi, M.; Cavallaro, G.; Amato, G.; Fiorica, C.; Giammona, G. New Copolymers Graft of α,β-poly(N-2-hydroxyethyl)-D,L-Aspartamide Obtained from Atom Transfer Radical Polymerization as Vector for Gene Delivery. *React. Funct. Polym.* **2012**, *72,* 268–278.

Lou, C. W.; Chang, C. Y.; Wu, Z. H.; Lin, J. H. The Optimal Extracting Process, Manufacturing Technique and Biological Evaluation of Lithospermum Erythrorhizon Microcapsules. *Mater. Sci. Eng. C* **2015,** *48,* 165–171.

Maeda, H. Tumor-Selective Delivery of Macromolecular Drugs via the EPR Effect: Background and Future Prospects. *Bioconjugate Chem.* **2010,** *21,* 797–802.

Maity, S.; Mukhopadhyay, P.; Kundu, P. P.; Chakraborti, A. S. Alginate Coated Chitosan Core-Shell Nanoparticles for Efficient Oral Delivery of Naringenin in Diabetic Animals—An in Vitro and in Vivo Approach. *Carbohydr. Polym.* **2017,** *170,* 124–132.

Martoni, C.; Bhathena, J.; Jones, M. L.; Urbanska, A. M.; Chen, H.; Prakash, S. Investigation of Microencapsulated BSH Active Lactobacillus in the Simulated Human GI Tract. *J. Biomed. Biotechnol.* **2007,** *2007,* 13684.

McClements, D. J. Recent Progress in Hydrogel Delivery Systems for Improving Nutraceutical Bioavailability. *Food Hydrocolloids* **2017,** *68,* 238–245.

Messaoud, G. B.; Sánchez-González, L.; Probst, L.; Jeandel, C.; Arab-Tehrany, E.; Desobry, S. Physico-Chemical Properties of Alginate/Shellac Aqueous-Corecapsules: Influence of Membrane Architecture on Riboflavin Release. *Carbohydr. Polym.* **2016,** *144,* 428–437.

Miller, A. M.; Dean, D. A. Tissue-Specific and Transcription Factor-Mediated Nuclear Entry of DNA. *Adv. Drug Delivery Rev.* **2009,** *61,* 603–613.

Mishra, G.; Srivastava, S.; Nagori, B. P. Pharmacological and Therapeutic Activity of Cissus Quadrangularis: An Overview. *Int. J. Pharm. Tech. Res.* **2010,** 2(2), 1298–1310.

Montenegro, L.; Carbone, C.; Maniscalco, C.; Lambusta, D.; Nicolosi, G.; Ventura, C. A.; Puglisi, G. In Vitro Evaluation of Quercetin-3-O-Acyl Esters as Topical Prodrugs. *Int. J. Pharm.* **2007,** 336(2), 257–262.

Mukhopadhyay, P.; Maity, S.; Chakraborty, S.; Rudra, R.; Ghodadara, H.; Solanki, M.; Chakraborti, A. S.; Prajapati, A. K.; Kundu, P. P. Oral Delivery of Quercetin to Diabetic Animals using Novel pH Responsive Carboxypropionylated Chitosan/Alginate Microparticles. *RSC Adv.* **2016,** *6,* 73210–73221.

Munkonge, F. M.; Amin, V.; Hyde, S. C.; Green, A. M.; Pringle, I. A.; Gill, D. R.; Smith, J. W.; Hooley, R. P.; Xenariou, S.; Ward, M. A.; Leeds, N.; Leung, K. Y.; Chan, M.; Hillery, E.; Geddes, D. M.; Griesenbach, U.; Postel, E. H.; Dean, D. A.; Dunn, M. J.; Alton, E. W. Identification and Functional Characterization of Cytoplasmic Determinants of Plasmid DNA Nuclear Import. *J. Biol. Chem.* **2009,** *284,* 26978–26987.

Ng, S. F.; Tan, S. L. Development and in Vitro Assessment of Alginate Bilayer Films Containing the Olive Compound Hydroxytyrosol as an Alternative for Topical Chemotherapy. *Int. J. Pharm.* **2015,** *495,* 798–806.

Nguyen, H. T. P.; Munnier, E.; Souce, M.; Perse, X.; David, S.; Bonnier, F.; Vial, F.; Yvergnaux, F.; Perrier, T.; Cohen-Jonathan, S.; Chourpa, I. Novel Alginate-Based Nanocarriers as a Strategy to Include High Concentrations of Hydrophobic Compounds in Hydrogels for Topical Application. *Nanotechnology* **2015,** *26*(25), 1–14.

Nograles, N.; Abdullah, S.; Shamsudin, M. N.; Billa, N.; Rosli, R. Formation and Characterization of pDNA-Loaded Alginate Microspheres for Oral Administration in Mice. *J. Biosci. Bioeng.* **2012,** *113,* 133–140.

Noppakundilograt, S.; Piboon, P.; Graisuwan, W.; Nuisin, R.; Kiatkamjornwong, S. Encapsulated Eucalyptus Oil in Ionically Cross-Linked Alginate Microcapsules and its Controlled Release. *Carbohydr. Polym.* **2015,** *131,* 23–33.

Ortiz-Andrade, R. R.; Sánchez-Salgado, J. C.; Navarrete-Vázquez, G.; Webster, S. P.; Binnie, M.; García-Jiménez, S.; León-Rivera, I.; Cigarroa-Vazquez, P.; Villalobos-Molina,

R.; Estrada-Soto, S. Antidiabetic and Toxicological Evaluations of Naringenin in Normoglycaemic and NIDDM Rat Models and its Implications on Extra-Pancreatic Glucose Regulation. *Diabetes Obes. Metab.* **2008,** *10,* 1097–1104.

Otálora, M. C.; Carriazo, J. G; Iturriaga, L.; Osorio, C.; Nazareno, M. A. Encapsulating Betalains from Opuntia Ficus-Indica Fruits by Ionic Gelation: Pigment Chemical Stability During Storage of Beads. *Food Chem.* **2016,** *202,* 373–382.

Petchsomrit, A.; Sermkaew, N.; Wiwattanapatapee, R. Alginate-Based Composite Sponges as Gastroretentive Carriers for Curcumin-Loaded Self-Microemulsifying Drug Delivery Systems. *Sci. Pharm.* **2017,** *85,* 11.

Picerno, P.; Sansone, F.; Mencherini, T.; Prota, L.; Aquino, R. P; Rastrelli, L.; Lauro, M. R. Citrus Bergamia Juice: Phytochemical and Technological Studies. *Nat. Prod. Commun.* **2011,** *6,* 951–955.

Puglia, C.; Lauro, M. R.; Tirendi, G. G.; Fassari, G. E.; Carbone, C.; Bonina, F.; Puglisi, G. Modern Drug Delivery Strategies Applied to Natural Active Compounds. *Expert Opin. Drug Delivery* **2017,** *14*(6), 755–768.

Rathore, M.; Shriwas, S.; Dwivedi S.; Dubey, R. Formulation and Evaluation of Glycyrrhizin Alginate Beads for Stomach-Specific Delivery. *Asian J. Med. Pharm. Res.* **2017,** *7*(1), 06–08.

Rowe, R.; Sheskey, P.; Fenton, M. *Handbook of Pharmaceutical Excipients,* 7th ed.; Pharmaceutical Press: North Yorkshire, UK, 2012.

Samarasinghe, R. M.; Kanwar, R. K.; Kumar, K.; Kanwar, J. R. Antiarthritic and Chondroprotective Activity of Lakshadi Guggul in Novel Alginate-Enclosed Chitosan Calcium Phosphate Nanocarriers. *Nanomedicine* **2014,** *9*(6), 819–837.

Sanna, V.; Lubinu, G.; Madau, P.; Pala, N.; Nurra, S.; Mariani, A.; Sechi, M. Polymeric Nanoparticles Encapsulating White Tea Extract for Nutraceutical Application. *J. Agric. Food Chem.* **2015,** *63,* 2026–2032.

Sansone, F.; Rossi, A.; Del Gaudio, P.; De Simone, F.; Aquino, R. P.; Lauro M. R. Hesperidin Gastroresistant Microparticles by Spray-Drying: Preparation, Characterization, and Dissolution Profiles. *AAPS PharmSciTech.* **2009,** *10*(2), 391–401.

Sansone, F.; Mencherini, T.; Picerno, P.; D'Amore, M.; Aquino, R. P; Lauro, M. R. Maltodextrin/Pectin Microparticles by Spray Drying as Carrier for Nutraceutical Extracts. *J. Food Eng.* **2011a,** *105,* 468–476.

Sansone, F.; Picerno, P.; Mencherini, T.; Villecco, F.; D'Ursi, A. M.; Aquino, R. P.; Lauro, M. R. Flavonoid Microparticles by Spray-Drying: Influence of Enhancers of the Dissolution Rate on Properties and Stability. *J. Food Eng.* **2011b,** *103,* 188–196.

Sarika, P. R.; James, N. R.; Kumar, P. R. N.; Raj, D. K. Galactosylated Alginate-Curcumin Micelles for Enhanced Delivery of Curcumin to Hepatocytes. *Int. J. Biol. Macromol.* **2016a,** *86,* 1–9.

Sarika, P. R.; James, N. R.; Anil Kumar, P. R.; Raj, D. K. Preparation, Characterization and Biological Evaluation of Curcumin Loaded Alginate Aldehyde–Gelatin Nanogels. *Mater. Sci. Eng. C* **2016b,** *68,* 251–257.

Sosnik, A. Alginate Particles as Platform for Drug Delivery by the Oral Route: State-of-the-Art. *ISRN Pharm.* **2014.** https://www.hindawi.com/journals/isrn/2014/926157/ (accessed Jul 24, 2017).

Szekalska, M.; Puciłowska, A.; Szymańska, E.; Ciosek, P.; Winnicka, K. Alginate: Current Use and Future Perspectives in Pharmaceutical and Biomedical Applications. *Int. J. Pol. Sci.* **2016.** http://dx.doi.org/10.1155/2016/7697031 (accessed Jul 30, 2017).

Tsirigotis-Maniecka, M.; Gancarz, R.; Wilk, K. A. Preparation and Characterization of Sodium Alginate/Chitosan Microparticles Containing Esculin. *Colloids Surf. A* **2016,** *510,* 22–23.

Tsirigotis-Maniecka, M.; Lamch, L.; Chojnacka, I.; Gancarz, R.; Wilk, K. A. Microencapsulation of Hesperidin in Polyelectrolyte Complex Microbeads: Physico-Chemical Evaluation and Release Behavior. *J. Food Eng.* **2017,** *214,* 104–116.

USDA, United States Department of Agriculture. Alginates: Handling/Processing, 2015. https://www.ams.usda.gov/sites/default/files/media/Alginates%20TR%202015.pdf (accessed Aug 31, 2017).

Vandenberg, G.; Drolet, C.; Scott, S.; De la Noüe, J. Factors Affecting Protein Release from Alginate-Chitosan Coacervate Microcapsules During Production and Gastric/Intestinal Simulation, *J. Controlled Release* **2001,** *77,* 297–307.

Vreeker, R.; Li, L.; Fang, Y.; Appelqvist, I.; Mendes, E. Drying and Rehydration of Calcium Alginate Gels. *Food Biophys.* **2008,** *3,* 361–369.

Wang, Q. M.; Chen, Y.; Wang, L. C.; Zhang, X. C.; Huang, H. Z.; Teng, W. Stability and Toxicity of Empty or Gene-Loaded Lipopolysaccharide-Amine Nanopolymersomes. *Int. J. Nanomed.* **2015,** *10,* 597–608.

Wang, Q. S.; Wang, G. F.; Zhou, J.; Gao, L. N.; Cui, Y. L. Colon Targeted Oral Drug Delivery System Based on Alginate-Chitosan Microspheres Loaded with Icariin in the Treatment of Ulcerative Colitis. *Int. J. Pharm.* **2016,** *515,* 176–185.

Zhang, Z. H.; Sun, Y.-S.; Pang, H.; Munyendo, W. L. L.; Hui-Xia, L.; Zhu, S. L. Preparation and Evaluation of Berberine Alginate Beads for Stomach-Specific Delivery. *Molecules* **2011,** *16,* 10347–10356.

Zhao, D.; Zhuo, R. X.; Cheng, S. X. Alginate Modified Nanostructured Calcium Carbonate with Enhanced Delivery Efficiency for Gene and Drug Delivery. *Mol. Biosyst.* **2012,** *8,* 753–759.

Zhou, P.; Li, Z.; Chau, Y. Synthesis, Characterization and in Vivo Evaluation of poly (ethyleneoxide-co-glycidol)-platinate Conjugate. *Eur. J. Pharm. Sci.* **2010,** *41,* 464–472.

INDEX

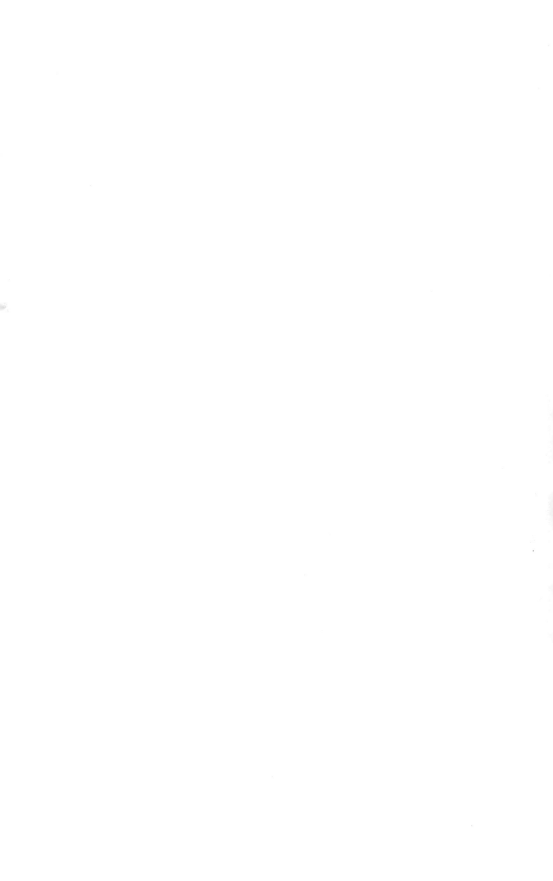

Milton Keynes UK
Ingram Content Group UK Ltd.
UKHW030901141024
449569UK00025B/1285